D1485983

NUTRITIONAL AND THERAPEUTIC INTERVENTIONS FOR DIABETES AND METABOLIC SYNDROME

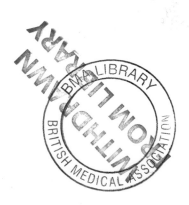

NUTRITIONAL AND THERAPEUTIC INTERVENTIONS FOR DIABETES AND METABOLIC SYNDROME

Edited by

DEBASIS BAGCHI
*University of Houston College of
Pharmacy, Houston, TX, USA*

NAIR SREEJAYAN
*University of Wyoming
School of Pharmacy
Laramie, WY, USA*

AMSTERDAM • BOSTON • HEIDELBERG • LONDON
NEW YORK • OXFORD • PARIS • SAN DIEGO
SAN FRANCISCO • SINGAPORE • SYDNEY • TOKYO
Academic Press is an imprint of Elsevier

Academic Press is an imprint of Elsevier
32 Jamestown Road, London NW1 7BY, UK
225 Wyman Street, Waltham, MA 02451, USA
525 B Street, Suite 1800, San Diego, CA 92101-4495, USA

First edition 2012

Notice
No responsibility is assumed by the publisher for any injury and/or damage to persons or property as a matter of products liability, negligence or otherwise, or from any use or operation of any methods, products, instructions or ideas contained in the material herein. Because of rapid advances in the medical sciences, in particular, independent verification of diagnoses and drug dosages should be made

British Library Cataloguing-in-Publication Data
A catalogue record for this book is available from the British Library

Library of Congress Cataloging-in-Publication Data
A catalog record for this book is available from the Library of Congress

ISBN: 978-0-12-385083-6

For information on all Academic Press publications
visit our website at elsevierdirect.com

Typeset by TNQ Books and Journals Pvt Ltd.

www.tnq.co.in

Printed and bound in United States of America

12 13 14 15 16   10 9 8 7 6 5 4 3 2 1

Working together to grow
libraries in developing countries

www.elsevier.com | www.bookaid.org | www.sabre.org

ELSEVIER   BOOK AID
International   Sabre Foundation

Dedicated to My Beloved and Respected Teacher: Professor Amalendu Banerjee

Debasis Bagchi

Contents

III
MOLECULAR INSIGHTS OF DIABETES AND METABOLIC SYNDROME

IV
PATHOPHYSIOLOGY

V
PREVENTION AND TREATMENT 1: DIET, EXERCISE, SUPPLEMENTS AND ALTERNATIVE MEDICINES

VI
PREVENTION AND TREATMENT 2: DRUGS AND PHARMACEUTICALS

VII
DIABETES IN ANIMALS AND TREATMENT

Preface

Diabetes is a metabolic disease wherein the body does not produce or adequately use the hormone insulin leading to a dysregulation of glucose. The disease is growing at epidemic proportions, affecting over 220 million people worldwide, and is expected to double by 2030.[1] The number of people suffering from type 1 and type 2 diabetes has doubled over the past three decades.[2] In the US, diabetes affects 25.8 million people of all ages, which is approximately 8.3% of the population.[3,4] In 2010, approximately 10.9 million people over 65 years of age had diabetes, approximately 215,000 people below the age of 20 years had either type 1 or type 2 diabetes, and 1.9 million people over the age of 20 years were newly diagnosed with diabetes.[3–5]

What is more worrying is that about 7 million of those 25.8 million diabetics remain undiagnosed until they develop a major complication such as stroke, neuropathy, amputation or blindness, which further adds to the economic burden of diabetes on society. Understanding the nature of the disease and its complications will help in designing effective therapeutic strategies to curb the epidemic. This book is aimed at providing a comprehensive approach to understanding diabetes, its complications, and the various strategies for its prevention and treatment. The wide range of topics covered here will be of interest to patient caregivers, basic research scientists, graduate students and anybody interested in knowing more about this disease.

Section I discusses the epidemiology and gives a general overview of type 1 and type 2 diabetes. Type 1 diabetes is a condition wherein the pancreas produces little or no insulin and is more common during adolescence; whereas type 2 diabetes, the more prevalent form, results when the body becomes resistant to the effects of insulin or does not produce sufficient insulin. In addition, this section also deals with "prediabetes", a condition associated with higher than normal blood sugar that precedes classification as frank diabetes, which affects about 79 million people worldwide. It is believed that some of the vascular complications attributed to diabetes begin during the prediabetic stage; therefore, addressing prediabetes may help preempt the development to full-blown diabetes. This section also has a chapter on childhood diabetes which had previously been assumed to be type 1 diabetes. The alarming increase in childhood obesity and sedentary lifestyle has resulted in an increasing prevalence of type 2 diabetes among children. Together with a broad overview of diabetes, this section also offers perspectives from physicians, nurses, epidemiologists, and dietitians.

Poorly controlled diabetes can lead to a variety of macrovascular and microvascular complications (retinopathy, nephropathy, and neuropathy). Atherosclerosis is the major macrovascular complication of diabetes, as well as the leading cause of morbidity and mortality in the advanced world, resulting in heart disease, stroke, and peripheral circulatory disorders. Diabetic retinopathy is the most frequent cause of new cases of blindness among adults aged 20–74 and about 28.5% of diabetic individuals > 40 years of age are afflicted with diabetic retinopathy. Diabetes is the leading cause of nephropathy, and end-stage renal disease which accounts for 44% of new cases of kidney failure. Diabetes is also the major cause of neuropathy, and vasculopathy which accounts for more than 60% of non-traumatic lower-limb amputations. Section II discusses these devastating complications associated with diabetes and various measures of prevention and management.[3]

Diabetes is a polygenic disorder, and the pathogenesis of diabetes involves multitudes of both genetic and environmental factors that adversely affect insulin secretion and tissue response to insulin. Genome-wide association studies have attempted to identify genetic variants that contribute to the development of diabetes.[6] Recent evidence suggests that epigenetic phenomenon plays a major role in the development of diabetes.[7] These newer developments are addressed in Section III, which deals with molecular insights on diabetes and metabolic syndrome. In recognition of the role of inflammation in the pathogenesis of diabetes and its complication, two chapters that deal with targeting inflammatory response in diabetes have also been included in this section.

Continuing with this theme, Section IV moves into the pathophysiology of various complications associated with diabetes and metabolic syndrome with reference to the different organ systems. Several aspects, including sleep, hypertension, and liver and pancreatic cell functions are discussed in this section.

A number of authors contributed twelve chapters in Section V demonstrating the prevention and treatment of diabetes using appropriate diet, physical exercise, proper dietary supplements, including antioxidants, and alternative medicines. Authors highlight the beneficial effects of structurally diverse antioxidants, healthy diet, nutraceuticals, and dietary supplements, including dietary fiber, fucoxanthin, chromium, vanadium, selenium, resveratrol, omega-3, and omega-6 polyunsaturated fatty acids. Because caloric input and diabetic diet play key roles in the management of diabetes, a chapter illustrating the diabetic meal plan has also been included in this section. The last chapter discusses the role of Ayurveda, an ancient Indian herbal therapeutics, in the prevention of diabetes.

Section VI comprises a critical appraisal of various pharmacological modalities of management of diabetes that includes drugs and structurally diverse pharmacological agents that target different mechanisms in the underlying pathogenesis of diabetes. In addition to preclinical data, these chapters also discuss some of the key clinical studies that have formed the basis of therapeutic guidelines for treating diabetes. In addition, an extensive review of antidiabetic drugs for the adult population that takes into account various facets of the requirements of the elderly has been added. Finally, Section VII highlights the treatment of diabetes in dogs and cats and other animals.

In summary, this book covers a broad range of topics related to diabetes, including epidemiology, pathophysiology, complications, management and various treatment options that makes it an invaluable resource for professionals interested in diabetes.

The editors extend their sincere thanks and gratitude to all our eminent contributors and especially to Ms. Nancy Maragioglio and Ms. Carrie Bolger for their continued support, cooperation and fruitful suggestions.

Debasis Bagchi PhD, MACN, CNS, MAIChE
University of Houston College of Pharmacy, Houston, TX

Nair Sreejayan MPharm, PhD
University of Wyoming School of Pharmacy, Laramie, WY

References

1. WHO Diabetes Fact Sheet, http://www.who.int/mediacentre/factsheets/fs312/en/; January 2011. Accessed on June 28, 2011.

2. Type 1 diabetes and type 2 diabetes grow in prevalence. Available at, http://www.endocrineweb.com/news/type-1-diabetes/6222-type-1-diabetes-type-2-diabetes-grow-prevalence. Accessed June 28, 2011.

3. National Institute of Diabetes and Digestive and Kidney Diseases. National Diabetes Statistics. *National Diabetes Information Clearinghouse.* Available at, http://diabetes.niddk.nih.gov/dm/pubs/statistics/; 2007. Accessed June 28, 2011.

4. Pharma Times Online. One in three diabetes patients don't adhere to treatment, http://www.pharmatimes.com/Article/11-06-28/One_in_three_diabetes_patients_don_t_adhere_to_treatment.aspx. Accessed June 28, 2011.

5. U.S. Department of Health and Human Services, Centers for Disease Control and Prevention. *National diabetes fact sheet: national estimates and general information on diabetes and prediabetes in the United States.* 2011. Available at, http://www.cdc.gov/diabetes/pubs/pdf/ndfs_2011.pdf; 2011. Accessed June 28, 2011.

6. Park KS. The search for genetic risk factors of type 2 diabetes mellitus. *Diabetes Metab J* 2011;**35**:12–22.

7. Cooper ME, El-Osta A. Epigenetics: mechanisms and implications for diabetic complications. *Circ Res* 2010;**107**:1403–13.

Contributors

Kevin J. Acheson Nestlé Research Centre, Lausanne, Switzerland

Saleh Adi University of California, San Francisco, CA

Juan Pablo Arab Pontificia Universidad Católica de Chile, Santiago, Chile

Juan Pablo Arancibia Pontificia Universidad Católica de Chile, Santiago, Chile

Amin Ardestani University of Bremen, Germany

Harald Arnesen University of Oslo, Norway

Marco Arrese Pontificia Universidad Católica de Chile, Santiago, Chile

Sarah A. Bajorek University of California, San Diego, La Jolla, CA

Francisco Barrera Pontificia Universidad Católica de Chile, Santiago, Chile

Dawn Blatt Stony Brook University, NY

Meghan Brashear Pennington Biomedical Research Center, Louisiana State University System, Baton Rouge, LA

Jaya P. Buddineni University of Missouri School of Medicine, MO

Roberto Candia Pontificia Universidad Católica de Chile, Santiago, Chile

Francesco P. Cappuccio University of Warwick, Coventry, UK

Sonia Caprio Yale School of Medicine, New Haven, CT

Katarzyna Cypryk Medical University of Lodz, Lodz, Poland

Thanh L. Dinh Harvard Medical School, Boston, MA

Charles J. Everett Medical University of South Carolina, Charleston, SC

Christopher Federico Tulane University School of Medicine, New Orleans, LA

Evelyne Fleury-Milfort University of Southern California, Los Angeles, CA

Harry W. Flynn, Jr. University of Miami Miller School of Medicine, Miami, FL

Ivar L. Frithsen Medical University of South Carolina, Charleston, SC

Kei Fukami Kurume University School of Medicine, Fukuoka, Japan

Jose E. Galgani University of Chile, Santiago, Chile

Giovanni Ghirlanda Catholic University School of Medicine, Rome, Italy

Cosimo Giannini Yale School of Medicine, New Haven, CT

Kian-Peng Goh Khoo Teck Puat Hospital, Alexandra Health, Singapore

Andrea Gerard Gonzalez University of California, San Francisco, CA

Cheri L. Gostic Stony Brook University, NY

Deborah S. Greco Nestle Purina PetCare, St Louis, MO

Alok K. Gupta Pennington Biomedical Research Center, Louisiana State University System, Baton Rouge, LA

Yasuaki Hata Fukuoka Dental College, Fukuoka, Japan

Masashi Hosokawa Hokkaido University, Hokkaido, Japan

Ann N. Jessup The University of North Carolina at Chapel Hill, Chapel Hill, NC

William D. Johnson Pennington Biomedical Research Center, Louisiana State University System, Baton Rouge, LA

Andrew J. Krentz University of Bedfordshire, UK

Charlotte Ling Lund University, Malmö, Sweden

Kathrin Maedler University of Bremen, Germany

Raffaele Marfella Second University of Naples, Naples, Italy

Francesca Martini Catholic University School of Medicine, Rome, Italy

Nilanjana Maulik University of Connecticut Health Center, Farmington, CT

Ajay Menon University of Washington Seattle, WA

Michelle A. Miller University of Warwick, Coventry, UK

Kazuo Miyashita Hokkaido University, Hokkaido, Japan

Candis M. Morello University of California, San Diego, CA and Veterans Affairs of San Diego Healthcare System, San Diego, CA

Paulin Moszczynski Malopolska University, Brzesko, Poland

Beverly S. Mühlhäusler The University of Adelaide, Australia

Wadie I. Najm University of California, Orange, CA

Shintaro Nakao Fukuoka Dental College, and Kyushu University, Fukuoka, Japan

Show Nishikawa Hokkaido University, Hokkaido, Japan

Kerin O'Dea University of South Australia, Adelaide, SA, Australia

Giuseppe Paolisso Second University of Naples, Naples, Italy

Bhushan Patwardhan Symbiosis International University, Lavale, Pune, India

Jonathan Pinkney University of Plymouth, UK

Dario Pitocco Catholic University School of Medicine, Rome, Italy

Gabriella Pridjian Tulane University School of Medicine, New Orleans, LA

Amrutesh Puranik University of Minnesota, Minneapolis, MN

Erica L. Reineke University of Pennsylvania School of Veterinary Medicine, Philadelphia, PA

Arnoldo Riquelme Pontificia Universidad Católica de Chile, Santiago, Chile

Pamela Rojas University of Chile, Santiago, Chile

Jan A. Rutowski E. Szczeklic's Specialistic Hospital, Tarnow, Poland, and Scientific Committee of the EAHP in Brussels, Belgium

Juan A. Sanchez University of Connecticut Health Center, Farmington, CT

Nicola Santoro Yale School of Medicine, New Haven, CT

Stephen G. Schwartz University of Miami Miller School of Medicine, Naples, FL

Ingebjørg Seljeflot University of Oslo, Norway

Luan Shu University of Bremen, Germany

Alan J. Sinclair University of Bedfordshire, UK

James R. Sowers University of Missouri School of Medicine, and Harry S. Truman VA Medical Center, Columbia, MO

Elizabeth Stenhouse University of Plymouth, UK

Francesco Tecilazich Harvard Medical School, Boston, MA

Mahesh Thirunavukkarasu University of Connecticut Health Center, Farmington, CT

Julie Tomlinson University of Plymouth and Cornwall & Isles of Scilly Primary Care Trust, UK

Marius Trøseid University of Oslo, Norway

Belma Turan Ankara University, Ankara, Turkey

Jeff Unger Catalina Research Institute, Chino, CA

Guy Vassort INSERM U-1046, CHU Arnaud de Villeneuve, Montpellier, France

Aristidis Veves Harvard Medical School, Boston, MA

John B. Vincent The University of Alabama, Tuscaloosa, AL

Karen Z. Walker Monash University, Clayton, VIC, Australia

Adam Whaley-Connell University of Missouri School of Medicine, and Harry S. Truman VA Medical Center, Columbia, MO

Marzena Wojcik Medical University of Lodz, Lodz, Poland

Lucyna A. Wozniak Medical University of Lodz, Lodz, Poland

Sho-ichi Yamagishi Kurume University School of Medicine, Fukuoka, Japan

Francesco Zaccardi Catholic University School of Medicine, Rome, Italy

EPIDEMIOLOGY AND OVERVIEW

Type 1 Diabetes Mellitus: An Overview

Andrea Gerard Gonzalez, Saleh Adi

Department of Pediatrics, Division of Pediatric Endocrinology, University of California,
San Francisco, CA, USA

OUTLINE

INTRODUCTION

Diabetes mellitus (DM) is a group of heterogeneous disorders with distinct genetic, etiologic, and pathophysiologic mechanisms with the common elements of glucose intolerance and hyperglycemia, due to insulin deficiency, impaired insulin action, or both. The World Health Organization estimates that more than 220 million people worldwide have DM. The majority of these cases have type 2 DM. Currently, DM is classified on the basis of etiology and clinical presentation into four major types:[1]

(I) Type 1 DM: characterized by a gradual loss of insulin-producing β-cells, due to autoimmune destruction.

(II) Type 2 DM: caused predominantly by severe insulin resistance and subsequent β-cell failure.

(III) Gestational DM: defined as hyperglycemia with onset or first recognition during pregnancy.

(IV) Other Specific types: including monogenic forms of DM (neonatal DM and maturity onset diabetes of the young, or MODY), and DM that is attributable to

Nutritional and Therapeutic Interventions for Diabetes and Metabolic Syndrome
DOI: 10.1016/B978-0-12-385083-6.15001-6

3

diseases of exocrine pancreas, other endocrinopathies, and drug-induced DM.

This overview will focus on the autoimmune type 1 DM; definition and criteria for diagnosis, epidemiology, pathophysiology, clinical presentation, management, comorbidities, and new developments in the treatment and prevention of type 1 DM.

DEFINITION

Type 1 DM results from deficiency of insulin secretion due to a gradual autoimmune, T-cell mediated destruction of the β-cells in people with genetic predisposition to this disease. Recently, more evidence has accumulated that B-cell autoimmunity also has a major role in the pathogenesis of type 1 DM.[2] In 85–95% of cases of type 1 DM, at least one serum marker of autoimmunity is detected in the form of autoantibodies against insulin, islet cells, the protein tyrosine phosphatase IA2, the 65-kD form of glutamate decarboxylase (GAD-65), and the zinc transporter ZnT8.[3] This subgroup of type 1 DM (with positive antibodies) is designated as type 1A, while the remaining 5–15% of cases of phenotypic type 1 DM but no detectable antibodies are referred to as "idiopathic" or type 1B.[2–5] This does not necessarily mean that individuals with type 1B DM do not manifest markers of autoimmunity, but rather reflects our lack of knowledge of what these antibodies might be. Future discoveries of yet unidentified islet autoantigens may prove that in fact all cases of type 1 DM are autoimmune in nature. There have been limited efforts to further understand the pathophysiology behind this particular group of antibody-negative patients, with some data suggesting an increased incidence in individuals with African or Asian ancestry. This group tends to demonstrate a tendency for recurrent episodes of diabetic ketoacidosis (DKA) with varying degrees of insulin deficiency between episodes. This type of diabetes is strongly inherited and does not appear to have a genetic HLA-type association.[6] There are also reports of a more fulminant form of β-cell destruction primarily in Japanese patients, with T-cell infiltration of the islets but no measurable autoantibodies.[7–9]

Type 1 diabetes is generally thought of as "childhood or juvenile" diabetes, although it can be diagnosed at any age, with a peak incidence in the early teen years, around the time of puberty.[10] Worldwide, the incidence of T1DM has been steadily increasing at an average annual rate of 3%.[11,12]

EPIDEMIOLOGY

Worldwide, it is estimated that approximately 5.9%, or 246 million adults had diabetes in 2007. These estimates are expected to increase to some 380 million, or 7.1% of the adult population, by the year 2025. About 80% of these live in the developing countries where the largest increases will also take place.[13]

In the United States, the National Diabetes Fact Sheet estimates that 23.6 million children and adults had diabetes in 2007, accounting for 7.8% of the population. Of those, around 5.7 million were undiagnosed, making DM one of the most prevalent chronic diseases that carries an economic burden of around US$174 billion per year.[14] However, type 1 DM accounts for only 5–15% of these cases.

In the United States, approximately 30,000 new cases of type 1 DM are diagnosed each year; about two-thirds of them are in children under the age of 19 years.[12,15]

PATHOPHYSIOLOGY

The autoimmune trigger in type 1 DM is the result of certain environmental exposures in genetically susceptible individuals. This genetic susceptibility is strongly linked to specific HLA genes which encode the major histocompatibility complex (MHC) proteins. These proteins play a critical role in regulating immune responses and recognition of self *vs* non-self cells. Certain HLA types are associated with much higher risk for developing type 1 DM, with the HLA-DR3 and DR4, and HLA-DQ being the most common in people with type 1 DM, while other types (e.g., HLA-DR2) appear to be protective against developing autoimmunity against β-cells.[4,16] The inheritance of particular HLA alleles can account for over half of the genetic risk for developing type 1 DM.[16,17] Other genetic loci have been also identified.

While the genetics of type 1 DM continue to be carefully examined, identifying the environmental factors involved in developing type 1 DM remain largely uncertain.[18,19] The increasing incidence of type 1 DM over the past few decades adds further evidence that environmental factors are of importance since it is not likely that genetic changes could take place in such a short period of time. Most of the findings in this field have been based on strong associations between the incidence of type 1 DM and certain environmental elements, but no definitive studies have clearly demonstrated a cause and effect with any of these factors.[18,19] Examples of these associations have linked type 1 DM to dietary habits, vitamin deficiencies, exposure to certain viruses, and the so-called "hygiene hypothesis".[18–28] Population-based observational studies have found that children who were breastfed have a lower risk of type 1 DM than those who were not, and that exposure to cow's milk before the age of 6 months doubles the risk of developing type 1 DM, particularly in individuals with high-risk HLA types.[28,31] However, a recent report from Finland concluded that early exposure to cow's milk is not a risk factor for developing type 1 DM.[32] The EURODIAB Substudy-2 group suggested that rapid growth, rather than cow's milk or early introduction of solid foods, may explain the increased risk for type 1 DM.[33] Similar associations (although also controversial) have been found with intake of glutens, and foods rich in proteins, carbohydrates, and nitrosamine compounds.[34–36]

In animals, a number of viruses can cause a diabetes-like syndrome. In humans, epidemics of mumps, rubella and coxsackie viral infections have been associated with increases in the incidence of type 1 DM.[22–25,27,38,39] The viruses may act directly to destroy the β-cells, or by triggering a widespread immune response against several endocrine tissues including the β-cells.[37–41] Some investigators postulate that this is an example of molecular mimicry between these viruses and the antigenic determinants on the surface of the β-cells.[42]

There is increasing evidence that inadequate vitamin D increases the risk for type 1 and type 2 DM and other autoimmune conditions.[43–47] This is supported by epidemiological findings of higher incidence of type 1 DM at higher latitudes and in other conditions with decreased sun exposure,[43,51] and by the fact that vitamin D receptors are expressed in β-cells and in immune cells.[43,52–54] Furthermore, certain polymorphisms within the vitamin D receptor gene are associated with development of type 1 DM, at least in some populations.[55,56] In animal models, pharmacological doses of the active form, 1,25-dihydroxyvitamin D3, have been shown to modulate the immune system and delay the onset of diabetes.[22,59]

The hygiene hypothesis suggests that avoidance to pathogen exposure secondary to improved living conditions leads to inadequate maturation of the immune system. The hypothesis is based on the increased incidence of diseases like asthma or other atopic disorders in children, in addition to the fact that type 1 DM is more prevalent in developed societies.[27,61]

DIAGNOSIS

In general, DM is diagnosed when one or more of the following criteria are met [1,61]:

1. Symptoms of diabetes plus casual plasma glucose concentration $\geq$ 200 mg/dl (11.1 mmol/l); or
2. Fasting plasma glucose $\geq$ 126 mg/dl (7.0 mmol/l). Fasting is defined as no caloric intake for at least 8 h; or
3. Two-hour post load glucose $\geq$ 200 mg/dl (11.1 mmol/l) during an OGTT. The test should be performed as described by WHO,[62] using a glucose load containing the equivalent of 75 g anhydrous glucose dissolved in water or 1.75 g/kg of body weight to a maximum of 75 g.

Recently, both the WHO and the American Diabetes Association have added the 4th criterion of hemoglobin A1c $\geq$ 6.5% as being diagnostic of DM.[1]

As noted above, the presence of diabetes-related autoantibodies confirms the classification of type 1, while the presence of obesity, acanthosis nigricans, family history of type 2 DM, and other risk factors for insulin resistance such as the lack of physical activity or the ethnicity of Hispanic or African American origin, strongly point towards type 2 DM. However, type 1 DM can occur in obese individuals with one or more risk factors for insulin resistance, therefore screening for markers of autoimmunity is recommended in all cases of new onset DM.

CLINICAL PRESENTATION

Type 1 DM has four major clinical phases: preclinical diabetes, overt diabetes, partial remission phase (honeymoon), and the chronic phase.

In general, autoimmune destruction of the β-cells is a slow process that can take years before causing sufficient β-cell loss to cause insulin deficiency. Under normal physiological conditions, it is estimated that less than 50% of the β-cell mass is sufficient to maintain euglycemia in humans. Typically, in individuals who are "developing" type 1 DM, a transient state of insulin resistance occurs, mostly due to a viral or bacterial illness, leading to increased requirements for insulin production which cannot be met because of the ongoing loss of β-cells. This leads to hyperglycemia, which itself has a detrimental effect on β-cell function leading to further hyperglycemia and its manifestations, leading eventually to the diagnosis of DM. It is estimated that only between 10% and 40% of the insulin-producing β-cells are still functioning by the time someone develops clinical manifestations of DM.[63,64]

The symptoms and signs are related to the presence of hyperglycemia and the resulting effects of water and electrolyte imbalance. They generally include polyuria, polydipsia, polyphagia, weight loss and blurry vision. Onset of symptoms can be very variable from insidious to acute.[65]

It is also not uncommon that new onset diabetes presents with a more serious and life-threatening diabetic ketoacidosis (DKA) with severe dehydration. The occurrence of DKA is more commonly seen in children younger than 4 years of age, and is less common in adolescents and young adults.[64-66] Despite the increased awareness of diabetes in the public and among general practitioners, the incidence of initial DKA at diagnosis remains relatively high and varies between 15% and 29%.[64-68] Typically the patient is acidotic with acetone fruity odor, respiratory distress, abdominal pain, nausea, vomiting, and polyuria and polydipsia. Laboratory findings include hyperglycemia, glucosuria, ketonemia, and ketonuria. Without timely management, severe fluid and electrolyte depletion develops with signs of hypoperfusion and altered mental status that may lead to coma and death.[66,67]

Once the diagnosis is made, fluid resuscitation and insulin replacement can begin immediately. This reverses the metabolic derangements and hyperglycemia, which together with the recovery from the precipitating infectious process, leads to relative recovery of β-cell function and return to near-adequate insulin production to maintain euglycemia, heralding the honeymoon period.

This remission phase can last from a few months to 2 years in some cases.[69] However, the process of β-cell destruction continues, eventually resulting in a gradual decrease in insulin secretion and ensuing hyperglycemia, marking the chronic phase of type 1 DM.

MANAGEMENT

The cornerstone of type 1 DM management is providing insulin at all times. This can be achieved by administration of one to two doses of long-acting insulin, and frequent prandial rapid-acting insulin. A series of modified human insulins with altered dynamics of absorption after subcutaneous injection have been introduced since 1996 and are now standard in clinical care including the long-acting insulins Glargine and Detemir, and the rapid-acting insulins Lispro, Aspart, and Glulisine.[70–74] These "custom-designed" insulins provide excellent tools to try to mimic the physiologic patterns of endogenous insulin secretion and action, while minimizing the range of blood glucose excursions and the risk of hypoglycemia, two of the main obstacles to achieving more aggressive and optimal glucose control in patients with diabetes.[70,72,74]

In most practices, newly diagnosed patients are started on multiple daily injection (MDI) of subcutaneous insulin, while those who present with DKA are treated initially with intravenous insulin infusion then switched to MDI. It is widely accepted that replacement of insulin in all patients with type 1 DM should consist of a combination of "basal and bolus" insulin. Typically, the dose of long-acting, basal insulin is unchanged from day to day and should provide about half of the total daily insulin requirements. However, the dosing of rapid-acting insulin is different for each time, and follows certain formulas to calculate the insulin dose for each meal based on the blood glucose (BG) value and the carbohydrate content in each meal (and snack). Alternatively, a continuous subcutaneous insulin infusion (CSII) pump is used to provide frequent small doses of rapid-acting insulin as basal insulin in lieu of the long-acting insulin, and user-administered boluses of rapid-acting insulin for meals and high BG. Because of this, management of type 1 DM requires self-monitoring of BG and a certain degree of competency in carbohydrate counting. Type 1 DM is recognized as a primarily self-managed disease, and to achieve the recommended glycemic targets patients need to receive ongoing nutritional counseling and training in self-management of their insulin regimen. In most practices, clinic visits with a team of physicians, diabetes educators, and nutritionists are recommended every 3–4 months.

In addition, a series of devices are now available for the continuous measurement of glucose concentration in the subcutaneous interstitial fluids, which reflects, with some time lag, the glucose concentration in the blood. These continuous glucose monitors (CGMs) can be operated alone or can be integrated with an insulin pump. The current devices provide predictive alarms for high and low BG, as well as continuous readings of glucose concentrations. Intense studies are ongoing for the development of the "closed loop" in which a CGM will control the operation of an insulin pump in response to changes in BG levels. Recent studies have shown improved glycemic control with the use of CGMs in type 1 DM.[75–80] Using these tools, the goals of diabetes management in adults is to achieve a HgA1c of <7.0% with preprandial BG of 70–130 mg/dl (3.9–7.2 mmol/l) and a peak postprandial BG of <180 mg/dl (<10.0 mmol/l).[1] These goals should be invidualized in all patients and must be less stringent in children with type 1 DM.[1]

COMORBIDITIES

The same genetic factors that pre-dispose patients to type 1 DM make them more likely to develop other autoimmune diseases.[81−83] The most common of these are thyroid autoimmunity, celiac disease, gastric autoimmunity, and Addison's disease.

Autoimmune thyroid disease occurs in 17–30% of patients with type 1 DM. It is more common in females and is often associated with the presence of anti-thyroperoxidase (aTPO) and anti-thyroglobulin (aTG) antibodies.[82−84] The current recommendations are for screening for aTPO and aTG at or shortly after diagnosis of type 1 DM, and measurement of TSH concentrations after metabolic control has been established. If normal, TSH should be re-checked every 1–2 years, or if the patient develops symptoms of thyroid dysfunction, thyromegaly, or an abnormal growth rate.[1]

Celiac disease is an autoimmune enteropathy with a variable reported incidence of 1–10% in patients with type 1 DM, and is more common in children with the risk of developing celiac disease being about 10 times higher than the general population, especially in the first 5 years after diagnosis with type 1 DM.[87] Celiac disease can manifest with non-gastroenterologic signs, including poor growth, delayed puberty, amenorrhea, erratic blood glucose concentrations, and even psychiatric problems.[88−90] Therefore a high index of suspicion must be kept and periodic screening for serum levels of tissue transglutaminase (tTG) or anti-endomysial antibodies is recommended along with screening for thyroid disease in patients with type 1 DM.[1,84,88,91] Some studies suggest that celiac disease is more likely to develop in the first 5 years after diagnosis of type 1 DM[91] and is more likely in children diagnosed with type 1 DM before the age of 4 years than in those diagnosed as teenagers.[92]

Also associated with type 1 DM is antigastric parietal cell and antiadrenal autoimmunity. These, however, are more rare than thyroid and celiac disease, such that routine screening is not currently recommended. However, because of the potential higher risk of developing pernicious anemia and gastric carcinoid tumors and adenocarcinomas,[92] De Block *et al.* recently recommended periodic screening for antiparietal cell antibodies especially in adolescents with longer duration of diabetes, positive GAD-65 antibodies, and anti-TPO antibodies.[94,95]

COMPLICATIONS

Chronic hyperglycemia and poor control of type 1 DM can lead to several long-term complications including hyperlipidemia, cardiovascular disease, peripheral neuropathy, and renal disease. These complications are similar to those seen in type 2 DM and are discussed in other chapters in this book.

PREVENTION AND INTERVENTION TRIALS

As mentioned earlier, the pathophysiology of type 1 DM encompasses several stages, beginning by activation of the immune system in genetically susceptible individuals, which leads to β-cell injury, impaired insulin secretion, and eventually frank hyperglycemia and clinical diabetes. This process is relatively slow and can take up to 2 years or more. By the time the diagnosis of type 1 DM is made, only 10–50% of islet cell mass remains intact but continues to be gradually destroyed over time.[96−100] Therefore the principal challenge in any effort towards prevention of type 1 DM is the identification of at-risk individuals well before they lose a substantial β-cell mass. Currently, the best predictor of type 1 DM development is the presence of β-cell-directed autoantibodies, combined with carrying high-risk HLA alleles.[101] In such individuals, several interventions have been tried, with little success in preventing the progression to overt diabetes. However, in the past few years, significant efforts have shifted towards strategies that aim at modulating the autoimmune response to halt the destruction of pancreatic islets and preserving the remaining β-cells immediately after diagnosis of type 1 DM.[96–100] Such strategies fall into two main categories: the first is antigen-specific, with interventions aimed at inducing tolerance to the specific antigen that is targeted, and the second is non-antigen specific, which aims to alter the function of components of the immune system, specifically T-cells and B-cells.[97,100] Preliminary results have shown decreased insulin dependence at least in the first year after treatment and current extended phase 2 and 3 trials are being carried out.[102–104] Once these studies have shown sufficient safety and efficacy in newly diagnosed patients, they will then be tested in at-risk individuals before they lose significant β-cell mass and become clinically hyperglycemic.

More recently, the role of vitamin D in regulating the immune system has gained much attention.[21,43,105,106] A meta-analysis of recently published results suggested that vitamin D supplement given to children may reduce the risk for type 1 DM, particularly with doses of 2000 IU/day.[107]

In the meantime, much effort is focusing on stem cell therapy by generating new β-cells from autologous umbilical cord blood cells and gene-engineered dendritic cells.[108,109]

Other, more tertiary interventions such as whole-organ pancreatic transplant and transfer of isolated islet cells, combined with ongoing immune suppression, have both proven to be successful in terms of restoring glycemic level and insulin independence,[110,111] but they remain limited by the availability of viable donor organ.

In parallel, there is continued strong interest in linking an insulin pump with a CGM to create an artificial pancreas.

References

1. American Diabetes Association. Diagnosis and Classification of Diabetes Mellitus. *Diabetes Care* 2011;**34**:S11–61.

2. O'Neill Shannon K, Liu Edwin, Cambier John C. Change you can B(cell)eive in: recent progress confirms a critical role for B cells in type 1 diabetes. *Current Opinion in Endocrinology, Diabetes and Obesity* 2009;**16**(4):293–8.

3. Wenzlau JM, Juhl K, Yu L, Moua O, Sarkar SA, Gottlieb P, Rewers M, Eisenbarth GS, Jensen J, Davidson HW, Hutton JC. The cation efflux transporter ZnT8 (Slc30A8) is a major autoantigen in human type 1 diabetes. *Proc Natl Acad Sci USA* 2007;**23**;104(43):17040–5.

4. Zeitler P. Update on nonautoimmune diabetes in children. *J Clin Endocrinol Metab* 2009;**94**(7):2215–20.

5. Concannon P, Rich SS, Nepom GT. Genetics of type 1A diabetes. *N Engl J Med* 2009;**360**(16):1646–54.

6. Pörksen S, Laborie LB, Nielsen L. Louise Max Andersen M, Sandal T, de Wet H, Schwarcz E, Aman J, Swift P, Kocova M, Schönle EJ, de Beaufort C, Hougaard P, Ashcroft F, Molven A, Knip M, Mortensen HB, Hansen L, Njølstad PR; Hvidøre Study Group on Childhood Diabetes. Disease progression and search for monogenic diabetes among children with new onset type 1 diabetes negative for ICA, GAD- and IA-2 Antibodies. *BMC Endocr Disord* 2010;**23**:10–6.

7. Hanafusa T, Imagawa A. Fulminant type 1 diabetes: a novel clinical entity requiring special attention by all medical practitioners. *Nat Clin Pract Endocrinol Metab* 2007;**3**(1):36–45.

8. Imagawa A, Hanafusa T. Fulminant type 1 diabetes as an important exception to the new diagnostic criteria using HbA(1c)—response to the International Expert Committee. *Diabetologia* 2009;**52**(11):2464–5.

9. Zheng C, Zhou Z, Yang L, Lin J, Huang G, Li X, Zhou W, Wang X, Liu Z. Fulminant type 1 diabetes mellitus exhibits distinct clinical and autoimmunity features from classical type 1 diabetes mellitus in Chinese. *Diabetes Metab Res Rev* 2011;**27**(1):70–8.

10. Lévy-Marchal C, Patterson C, Green A. Variation by age group and seasonality at diagnosis of childhood IDDM in Europe. The EURODIAB ACE Study Group. *Diabetologia* 1995;**38**(7):823–30.

11. Onkamo P, Vaananen S, Karvonen M, Tuomilehto J. Worldwide increase in incidence of type 1 diabetes—the analysis of the data on published incidence trends. *Diabetologia* 1999;**42**:1395–403.

12. DIAMOND Project Group. Incidence and trends of childhood Type 1 diabetes worldwide 1990–1999. *Diabet Med* 2006;**23**:857–66.

13. International Diabetes Federation. *Diabetes Atlas*. 3rd ed. 2006;29–30.

14. National Diabetes Fact Sheet, www.cdc.gov/diabetes/pubs; 2007.

15. Dabelea D, Bell RA, et al. Writing Group for the SEARCH for Diabetes in Youth Study Group. Incidence of diabetes in youth in the United States. *JAMA* 2007;**297**(24):2716—24.

16. Pociot F, Akolkar B, Concannon P, Erlich HA, Julier C, Morahan G, Nierras CR, Todd JA, Rich SS, Nerup J. Genetics of type 1 diabetes: what's next? *Diabetes* 2010;**59**(7):1561—71.

17. Todd JA, Bell JI, McDevitt HO, et al. HLA-DQ beta gene contributes to susceptibility and resistance to insulin-dependent diabetes mellitus. *Nature* 1987;**329**:599.

18. Knip M, Veijola R, Virtanen SM, Hyöty H, Vaarala O, Akerblom HK. Environmental triggers and determinants of type 1 diabetes. *Diabetes* 2005; **54**(Suppl. 2):S125—36.

19. Peng H, Hagopian W. Environmental factors in the development of Type 1 diabetes. *Rev Endocr Metab Disord* 2006;**7**(3):149—62.

20. Fronczak CM, Baron AE, Chase HP. In utero dietary exposures and risk for islet autoimmunity in children. *Diabetes Care* 2003;**26**:3237—42.

21. Mathieu C, Bandenhoop K. Vitamin D and type 1 diabtes mellitus, state of the art. *Trends Endocrinol Metab* 2005;**16**:261—6.

22. Nejentsev S, Cooper JD, Godfrey L. Analysis of vitamin D receptor gene sequence variants in type 1 diabetes. *Diabetes* 2004;**53**:2709—12.

23. Hyoty H. Enterovirus infections and type 1 diabetes. *Ann Med* 2002;**34**:138—47.

24. Ginsber Fellner F, Witt ME, Fedun B. Diabetes mellitus and autoimmunity in patients with congenital rubella syndrome. *Rev Infect Dis* 1985; **7**(Suppl. 1):S170—6.

25. Viskari H, Ludvigsson J, Uibo R. Relationship between the incidence of type 1 diabetes and maternal enterovirus antibodies: time trends and geographical variation. *Diabetologica* 2005;**48**:1280—7.

26. Gale EA. A missing link in the hygiene hypothesis? *Diabetologica* 2002;**45**:588—94.

27. Bach JF. Infections and autoimmune diseases. *J Autoimmun* 2005;**25**:74—80.

28. Knip M, Virtanen SM, Seppä K, Ilonen J, Savilahti E, Vaarala O, Reunanen A, Teramo K, Hämäläinen AM, Paronen J, Dosch HM, Hakulinen T, Akerblom HK. Finnish TRIGR Study Group. Dietary intervention in infancy and later signs of beta-cell autoimmunity. *N Engl J Med* 2010;**363**(20):1900—8.

29. Wasmuth HE, Kolb H. Cow's milk and immune-mediated diabetes. *Proc Nutr Soc* 2000;**59**(4):573—9.

30. Norris JM. Infant and childhood diet and type 1 diabetes risk: recent advances and prospects. *Curr Diab Rep* 2010;**10**(5):345—9.

31. Rosenbauer J, Herzig P, Kaiser P, Giani G. Early nutrition and risk of Type 1 diabetes mellitus—a nationwide case-control study in preschool children. *Exp Clin Endocrinol Diabetes* 2007;**115**(8):502—8.

32. Savilahti E, Saarinen KM. Early infant feeding and type 1 diabetes. *Eur J Nutr* 2009;**48**(4):243—9.

33. EURODIAB Substudy 2 Study Group. Rapid early growth is associated with increased risk of childhood type 1 diabetes in various European populations. *Diabetes Care* 2002;**25**(10):1755—60.

34. Mueller DB, Koczwara K, Mueller AS, Pallauf J, Ziegler AG, Bonifacio E. Influence of early nutritional components on the development of murine autoimmune diabetes. *Ann Nutr Metab* 2009;**54**(3):208—17.

35. Visser J, Rozing J, Sapone A, Lammers K, Fasano A. Tight junctions, intestinal permeability, and autoimmunity: celiac disease and type 1 diabetes paradigms. *Ann NY Acad Sci* 2009 May;**1165**:195—205.

36. Frisk G, Hansson T, Dahlbom I, Tuvemo T. A unifying hypothesis on the development of type 1 diabetes and celiac disease: gluten consumption may be a shared causative factor. *Med Hypotheses* 2008;**70**(6):1207—9.

37. Richer MJ, Horwitz MS. Viral infections in the pathogenesis of autoimmune diseases: focus on type 1 diabetes. *Front Biosci* 2008;**13**:4241—57.

38. Cooke A. Infection and autoimmunity. *Blood Cells Mol Dis* 2009;**42**(2):105—7.

39. Richer MJ, Horwitz MS. Coxsackievirus infection as an environmental factor in the etiology of type 1 diabetes. *Autoimmun Rev* 2009;**8**(7):611—5.

40. Hober D, Sauter P. Pathogenesis of type 1 diabetes mellitus: interplay between enterovirus and host. *Nat Rev Endocrinol* 2010;**6**(5):279—89.

41. Dotta F, Galleri L, Sebastiani G, Vendrame F. Virus infections: lessons from pancreas histology. *Curr Diab Rep* 2010;**10**(5):357—61.

42. Christen U, Hintermann E, Holdener M, von Herrath MG. Viral triggers for autoimmunity: is the 'glass of molecular mimicry' half full or half empty? *J Autoimmun* 2010;**34**(1):38—44.

43. Bikle DD. Vitamin D regulation of immune function. *Vitam Horm* 2011;**86**:1—21.

44. Hyppönen E. Vitamin D and increasing incidence of type 1 diabetes—evidence for an association? *Diabetes Obes Metab* 2010 Sep;**12**(9):737—43.

45. Takiishi T, Gysemans C, Bouillon R, Mathieu C. Vitamin D and diabetes. *Endocrinol Metab Clin North Am* 2010;**39**(2):419—46.

46. Holick MF. Vitamin D: extraskeletal health. *Endocrinol Metab Clin North Am* 2010;**39**(2):381—400.

47. Baeke F, Takiishi T, Korf H, Gysemans C, Mathieu C. Vitamin D: modulator of the immune system. *Curr Opin Pharmacol* 2010;**10**(4):482—96.

48. Mathieu C, Van Etten E, Decallonne B, et al. Vitamin D and 1,25-dihydroxyvitamin D(3) as modulators in the immune system. *J Steroid Biochem Mol Biol* 2004;**89−90**:449−52.

49. Hypponen E, Laara E, Reunanen A, Jarvelin MR, Virtanen SM. Intake of vitamin D and risk of type 1 diabetes: a birth-cohort study. *Lancet* 2001;**358**:1500−3.

50. Chiu KC, Chu A, Go VL, Saad MF. Hypovitaminosis D is associated with insulin resistance and beta cell dysfunction. *Am J Clin Nutr* 2004;**79**:820−5.

51. Staples JA, Ponsonby AL, Lim LL, McMichael AJ. Ecologic analysis of some immune-related disorders, including type 1 diabetes, in Australia: latitude, regional ultraviolet radiation, and disease prevalence. *Environ Health Perspect* 2003;**111**(4):518−23.

52. Bruce D, Cantorna MT. Intrinsic requirement for the vitamin D receptor in the development of CD8alphaalpha-expressing T cells. *J Immunol* 2011;**186**(5): 2819−25.

53. Bhalla AK, Amento EP, Clemens TL, Holick MF, Krane SM. Specific high-affinity receptors for 1, 25-dihydroxyvitamin D3 in human peripheral blood mononuclear cells: presence in monocytes and induction in T lymphocytes following activation. *J Clin Endocrinol Metab* 1983;**57**:1308−10.

54. Lee S, Clark SA, Gill RK, Christakos S. 1,25-Dihydroxyvitamin D3 and pancreatic beta-cell function: vitamin D receptors, gene expression, and insulin secretion. *Endocrinology* 1994;**134**:1602−10.

55. Maestro B, Davila N, Carranza MC, Calle C. Identification of a vitamin D response element in the human insulin receptor gene promoter. *J Steroid Biochem Mol Biol* 2003;**84**:223−30.

56. Mimbacas A, Trujillo J, Gascue C, Javiel G, Cardoso H. Prevalence of vitamin D receptor gene polymorphism in a Uruguayan population and its relation to type 1 diabetes mellitus. *Genet Mol Res* 2007;**6**(3):534−42.

57. Eerligh P, Koeleman BP, Dudbridge F, Jan BG, Roep BO, Giphart MJ. Functional genetic polymorphisms in cytokines and metabolic genes as additional genetic markers for susceptibility to develop type 1 diabetes. *Genes Immun* 2004;**5**:36−40.

58. Mathieu C, Waer M, Laureys J, Rutgeerts O, Bouillon R. Prevention of autoimmune diabetes in NOD mice by 1,25 dihydroxyvitamin D3. *Diabetologia* 1994;**37**:552−8.

59. Zella JB, McCary LC, Deluca HF. Oral administration of 1,25-dihydroxyvitamin D3 completely protects NOD mice from insulin-dependent diabetes mellitus. *Arch Biochem Biophys* 2003;**417**:77−80.

60. D'Angeli MA, Merzon E, Valbuena LF, Tirschwell D, Paris CA, Mueller BA. Environmental factors associated with childhood-onset type 1 diabetes mellitus: an exploration of the hygiene and overload hypotheses. *Arch Pediatr Adolesc Med* 2010;**164**(8):732−8.

61. Craig ME, Hattersley A, Donaghue KC. Definition, epidemiology and classification of diabetes in children and adolescents. *Pediatr Diabetes* 2009; **10**(Suppl. 12):3−12.

62. World Health Organization. Definition, Diagnosis and Classification of Diabetes Mellitus and its Complications, *Part 1: Diagnosis and Classification of Diabetes Mellitus*. Geneva: WHO/NCD/NCS/99.2; 1999. Ref Type: Report.

63. Knip M, Korhonene S, Kulmala P, Veijola R. Prediction of type 1 diabetes in the general population. *Diabetes Care* 2010;**6**:1206−12.

64. Hekkala A, Knip M, Veijola R. Ketoacidosis at diagnosis of type 1 diabetes in children in northern Finland, temporal changes over 20 years. *Diabetes Care* 2007;**30**:861−6.

65. Maniatis AK, Goehrig SH, Gao D, Rewers A, Walravens P, Klingensmith GJ. Increased incidence and severity of diabetes ketoacidosis among uninsured children with newly diagnosed type 1 diabetes. *Pediatr Diabetes* 2005;**6**:79−83.

66. Neu A, Willasch A, Ehehalt S, Hub R, Ranke MB. DIARY Group Baden-Wuerttemberg. Ketoacidosis at onset of type 1 diabetes mellitus in children—frequency and clinical presentation. *Pediatr Diabetes* 2003;**4**(2):77−81.

67. Sundaram PC, Day E, Kirk JM. Delayed diagnosis in type 1 diabetes mellitus. *Arch Dis Child* 2009;**94**(2):151−2.

68. Rewers A, Klingensmith G, Davis C, Petitti DB, Pihoker C, Rodriguez B, Schwartz ID, Imperatore G, Williams D, Dolan LM, Dabelea D. Presence of diabetic ketoacidosis at diagnosis of diabetes mellitus in youth: the SEARCH for Diabetes in Youth Study. *Pediatrics* 2008;**121**(5):e1258−66.

69. Bowden SA, Duck MM, Hoffman RP. Young children (<5 yr) and adolescents (>12 yr) with type 1 diabetes mellitus have low rate of partial remission: diabetic ketoacidosis is an important risk factor. *Pediatr Diabetes* 2008;**9**:197−201.

70. Eckardt K, Eckel J. Insulin analogues: action profiles beyond glycaemic control. *Arch Physiol Biochem* 2008;**114**(1):45−53.

71. Hartman I. Insulin analogs: impact on treatment success, satisfaction, quality of life, and adherence. *Clin Med Res* 2008;**6**(2):54−67.

72. Freeman JS. Insulin analog therapy: improving the match with physiologic insulin secretion. *J Am Osteopath Assoc* 2009;**109**(1):26−36.

73. Jensen MG, Hansen M, Brock B, Rungby J. Differences between long-acting insulins for the treatment of type 2 diabetes. *Expert Opin Pharmacother* 2010;**11**(12):2027−35.

74. Brunton SA. Nocturnal hypoglycemia: answering the challenge with long-acting insulin analogs. *Med Gen Med* 2007;**9**(2):38.

75. Currie CJ, Poole CD, Papo NL. An overview and commentary on retrospective, continuous glucose monitoring for the optimisation of care for people with diabetes. *Curr Med Res Opin* 2009;**25**(10):2389−400.

76. Chetty VT, Almulla A, Odueyungbo A, Thabane L. The effect of continuous subcutaneous glucose monitoring (CGMS) versus intermittent whole blood finger-stick glucose monitoring (SBGM) on hemoglobin A1c (HBA1c) levels in Type I diabetic patients: a systematic review. *Diabetes Res Clin Pract* 2008;**81**(1):79−87.

77. Carchidi C, Holland C, Minnock P, Boyle D. New technologies in pediatric diabetes care. *MCN Am J Matern Child Nurs* 2011;**36**(1):32−9.

78. Davey RJ, Jones TW, Fournier PA. Effect of short-term use of a continuous glucose monitoring system with a real-time glucose display and a low glucose alarm on incidence and duration of hypoglycemia in a home setting in type 1 diabetes mellitus. *J Diabetes Sci Technol* 2010;**4**(6):1457−64.

79. Cooke D, Hurel SJ, Casbard A, Steed L, Walker S, Meredith S, Nunn AJ, Manca A, Sculpher M, Barnard M, Kerr D, Weaver JU, Ahlquist J, Newman SP. Randomized controlled trial to assess the impact of continuous glucose monitoring on HbA(1c) in insulin-treated diabetes (MITRE Study). *Diabet Med* 2009;**26**(5):540−7.

80. Satish Garg K, Mary Voelmle K, Christie Beatson R, Hayley Miller A, Lauren Crew B, Brandon Freson J, Rachel Hazenfield M. Use of continuous glucose monitoring in subjects with type 1 diabetes on multiple daily injections versus continuous subcutaneous insulin infusion therapy: A prospective 6-month study. *Diabetes Care* 2011;**34**:574−9.

81. Triolo TM, Armstrong TK, McFann K, Yu L, Rewers MJ, Klingensmith GJ, Eisenbarth GS, Barker JM. One-third of patients have evidence for an additional autoimmune disease at type 1 diabetes diagnosis. *Diabetes Care* 2011 Mar 23 [Epub ahead of print].

82. Barker JM. Clinical review: Type 1 diabetes-associated autoimmunity: natural history, genetic associations, and screening. *J Clin Endocrinol Metab* 2006;**91**(4):1210−7.

83. De Block CE, De Leeuw IH, Vertommen JJ, Rooman RP, Du Caju MV, Van Campenhout CM, Weyler JJ, Winnock F, Van Autreve J, Gorus FK. Belgian Diabetes Registry. Beta-cell, thyroid, gastric, adrenal and coeliac autoimmunity and HLA-DQ types in type 1 diabetes. *Clin Exp Immunol* 2001;**126**(2):236−41.

84. Kordonouri O, Maguire AM, Knip M, Schober E, Lorini R, Holl RW, Donaghue KC. Other complications and conditions associated with diabetes in children and adolescents. *Pediatric Diabetes* 2009;**10**(Suppl. 12):204−10.

85. Kordonouri O, Klinghammer A, Lang EB, Grüters-Kieslich A, Grabert M, Holl RW. Thyroid autoimmunity in children and adolescents with type 1 diabetes: a multicenter survey. *Diabetes Care* 2002;**25**(8):1346−50.

86. Kordonouri O, Hartmann R, Deiss D, Wilms M, Grüters-Kieslich A. Natural course of autoimmune thyroiditis in type 1 diabetes: association with gender, age, diabetes duration, and puberty. *Arch Dis Child* 2005;**90**(4):411−4.

87. Collin P, Kaukinen K, Valimaki M, Salmi J. Endocrinological disorders and celiac disease. *Endocr Rev* 2002;**23**:464−83.

88. Holmes GK. Screening for coeliac disease in type 1 diabetes. *Arch Dis Child* 2002;**87**(6):495−8.

89. Mohn A, Cerruto M, Lafusco D, Prisco F, Tumini S, Stoppoloni O, Chiarelli F. Celiac disease in children and adolescents with type I diabetes: importance of hypoglycemia. *J Ped Gastroent Nutr* 2001;**32**:37−40.

90. Barker JM, Liu E. Celiac disease: pathophysiology, clinical manifestations, and associated autoimmune conditions. *Adv Pediatr* 2008;**55**:349−65.

91. Larsson K, Carlsson A, Cederwall E, Jönsson B, Neiderud J, Jonsson B, Lernmark A, Ivarsson SA. Skåne Study Group. Annual screening detects celiac disease in children with type 1 diabetes. *Pediatr Diabetes* 2008;**9**:354−9.

92. Cerutti F, Bruno G, Chiarelli F, Lorini R, Meschi F, Sacchetti C. Diabetes Study Group of the Italian Society of Pediatric Endocrinology and Diabetology. Younger age at onset and sex predict celiac disease in children and adolescents with type 1 diabetes: an Italian multicenter study. *Diabetes Care* 2004;**27**(6):1294−8.

93. Kakkola A, Sjöblom SM, Haapiainen R, Sipponen P, Puolakkainen P, Jarvinen H. The risk of gastric carcinoma and carcinoid tumours in patients with pernicious anemia: a prospective follow-up study. *Scand J Gastroenterol* 1998;**33**:88−92.

94. De Block CE, De Leeuw IH, Van Gaal LF. Autoimmune gastritis in type 1 diabetes: A clinically oriented review. *J Clin Endocrinol Metab* 2008;**93**(2):363−71.

95. De Block CE, De Leeuw IH, Rooman RP, Winnock F, Du Caju MV, Van Gaal LF. Gastric parietal cell

antibodies are associated with glutamic acid decarboxylase-65 antibodies and the HLA DQA1*0501-DQB1*0301 haplotype in Type 1 diabetes mellitus. Belgian Diabetes Registry. *Diabet Med* 2000;**17**(8):618—22.

96. Zhang L, Eisenbarth GS. Prediction and prevention of Type 1 diabetes mellitus. *J Diabetes*. 2011 Mar;**3**(1):48—57.

97. Cernea S, Dobreanu M, Raz I. Prevention of type 1 diabetes: today and tomorrow. *Diabetes Metab Res Rev* 2010;**26**(8):602—5.

98. Rewers M, Gottlieb P. Immunotherapy for the prevention and treatment of type 1 diabetes: human trials and a look into the future. *Diabetes Care* 2009;**32**:1769—82.

99. Haller MJ, Atkinson MA, Schatz D. Type 1 diabetes mellitus: etiology, presentation, and management. *Pediatr Clin North Am* 2005;**52**:1553—78.

100. Sherr J, Sosenko J, Skyler JS, Herold KC. Prevention of type 1 diabetes: the time has come. *Nat Clin Pract Endocrinol Metab* 2008;**4**:334—43.

101. Verge CF, Gianani R, Kawasaki E, et al. Number of autoantibodies (against insulin, GAD or ICA512/IA2) rather than particular autoantibody specificities determines risk of type I diabetes. *J Autoimmun* 1996;**9**:379—83.

102. Herold KC, Gitelman SE, Masharani U, et al. A single course of anti-CD3 monoclonal antibody hOKT3γ1 (Ala-Ala) results in improvement in C-peptide responses and clinical parameters for at least 2 years after onset of type 1 diabetes. *Diabetes* 2005;**54**:1753-69.

103. Keymeulen B, Vandemeulebroucke E, Ziegler AG, et al. Insulin needs after CD3- antibody therapy in new-onset type 1 diabetes. *N Engl J Med* 2005;**352**:2598—608.

104. Herold KC, Gitelman S, Greenbaum C, et al. Immune Tolerance Network ITN007AI Study Group. Treatment of patients with new onset type 1 diabetes with a single course of anti-CD3 mAb teplizumab preserves insulin production for up to 5 years. *Clin Immunol* 2009;**132**:166—73.

105. Borges MC, Martini LA, Rogero MM. Current perspectives on vitamin D, immune system, and chronic diseases. *Nutrition* 2011;**27**(4):399—404.

106. Mathieu C, Gysemans C, Giulietti A, Bouillon R. Vitamin D and diabetes. *Diabetologia* 2005;**48**(7):1247—57.

107. Zipitis CS, Akobeng AK. Vitamin D supplementation in early childhood and risk of type 1 diabetes: a systematic review and meta-analysis. *Arch Dis Child* 2008;**93**(6):512—7.

108. Madsen OD. 2005 Stem cells and diabetes treatment. *APMIS* 2005;**113**:858—75.

109. Zhao Y, Mazzone T. Human cord blood stem cells and the journey to a cure for type 1 diabetes. *Autoimmun Rev* 2010;**10**(2):103—7.

110. Wen Y, Chen B, Ildstad ST. Stem cell-based strategies for the treatment of type 1 diabetes mellitus. *Expert Opin Biol Ther* 2011;**11**(1):41—53.

111. Krishna KA, Rao GV, Rao KS. Stem cell-based therapy for the treatment of Type 1 diabetes mellitus. *Regen Med* 2007;**2**(2):171—7.

2

Overview of Type 2 Diabetes

Jonathan Pinkney*, Julie Tomlinson[†], Elizabeth Stenhouse**

* Peninsula College of Medicine and Dentistry, University of Plymouth, UK [†] Peninsula College of Medicine and Dentistry, University of Plymouth and Cornwall & Isles of Scilly Primary Care Trust, UK ** Faculty of Health, University of Plymouth, UK

OUTLINE

DEFINITION AND DIAGNOSTIC CRITERIA

A diagnosis of type 2 diabetes (T2DM) requires both biochemical criteria and etiological considerations. The World Health Organization (WHO) has recommended fasting and 2-h oral glucose tolerance tests (OGTT) for the diagnosis of T2DM (Table 2.1),[1] and this classification of diabetes and impaired glucose regulation (IGR) is recognized by the American Diabetes Association (ADA).[2,3] Although the ADA revised their

TABLE 2.1 Values for Diagnosis of Diabetes and Other Categories of Hyperglycemia

Diagnosis	Glucose concentration, mmol.l^{-1} (mg.dl^{-1})		
	Venous	Capillary	Plasma venous
Diabetes Mellitus			
Fasting (or)	≥ 6.1 (≥ 110)	≥ 6.1 (≥ 110)	≥ 7.0 (≥ 126)
2-h post glucose load	≥ 10.0 (≥ 180)	≥ 11.1(≥ 200)	≥ 11.1(≥ 200)
Impaired Glucose Tolerance (IGT):			
Fasting (if measured) *and*	< 6.1 (< 110) *and*	< 6.1 (< 110) *and*	< 7.0 (< 126) *and*
2-h post glucose load	≥ 6.7 (≥ 120)	≥ 7.8 (≥ 140)	≥ 7.8 (≥ 140)
Impaired Fasting Glucose (IFG):			
Fasting	≥ 5.6 (≥ 100) *and*	≥ 5.6 (≥ 100) *and*	≥ 6.1 (≥ 110) *and*
and (if measured)	< 6.1 (< 110)	< 6.1 (< 110)	< 7.0 (< 126)
2-h post glucose load	< 6.7 (< 120)	< 7.8 (< 140)	< 7.8 (< 140)

For epidemiological or population screening purposes, the fasting or 2-h value after 75 g oral glucose load may be used alone. For clinical purposes, the diagnosis of diabetes should always be confirmed by repeating the test on another day unless there is an unequivocal hyperglycemia with acute metabolic decompensation or obvious symptoms.

Reproduced from: World Health Organization (1999) Definition, Diagnosis & Classification of Diabetes Mellitus and its complications: Part 1 Diagnosis & Classification of Diabetes. Geneva WHO.

diagnostic criteria in 2010, allowing the use of glycosylated hemoglobin (HbA1c) (Table 2.2), this suggestion remains controversial. An etiological classification of diabetes is described by the ADA,[3] and is summarized in Table 2.3. The main problems with this classification are that many individuals with "T2DM" are atypical, and so etiology may be hard to determine. Some individuals with T2DM exhibit features such as ketosis or islet autoimmunity, which leads to confusion with type 1 diabetes (T1D). Moreover, whereas once most children diagnosed with diabetes were considered to have T1D, now up to 45% of new cases in some populations of children

TABLE 2.2 American Diabetes Association Diagnostic Criteria for Diabetes

American diabetes association criteria for the diagnosis of diabetes
1 HbA1c 6.5%. The test should be performed in a laboratory using a method that is NGSP certified and standardized to the DCCT assay.* OR
2 FPG 126 mg/dl (7.0 mmol/l). Fasting is defined as no caloric intake for at least 8 h.* OR
3 Two-hour plasma glucose 200 mg/dl (11.1 mmol/l) during an Oral Glucose Tolerance Test. The test should be performed as described by the World Health Organization, using a glucose load containing the equivalent of 75 g anhydrous glucose dissolved in water.* OR
4 In a patient with classic symptoms of hyperglycemia or hyperglycemic crisis, a random plasma glucose 200 mg/dl (11.1 mmol/l).

* In the absence of unequivocal hyperglycemia, criteria 1−3 should be confirmed by repeat testing.
Reproduced from: American Diabetes Association. Standards of Medical Care in Diabetes. Diabetes Care (2011) 34: 9(Suppl. 1), S11.

TABLE 2.3 American Diabetes Association Etiological Classification of Diabetes

1. Type 1 diabetes (β-cell destruction, usually leading to absolute insulin deficiency): (a) Immune mediated. (b) Idiopathic

2. Type 2 diabetes (ranging from predominant insulin resistance with relative insulin deficiency to predominantly secretory defect with insulin resistance)

3. Other specific forms of diabetes:

    1. Genetic defects of β-cell function

    2. Genetic defects in insulin action

    3. Diseases of the exocrine pancreas

    4. Endocrinopathies

    5. Drug or chemical induced

    6. Infections

    7. Uncommon forms of immune-mediated diabetes

    8. Other genetic syndromes sometimes associated with diabetes

4. Gestational diabetes mellitus

Abbreviated from American Diabetes Association. Standards of Medical Care in Diabetes. Diabetes Care (2011) 34: 9(Suppl. 1), S62.

have T2DM,[4] resulting in diagnostic uncertainty. The etiological diagnosis of T2DM also requires exclusion of other forms of diabetes, including monogenic forms. Therefore, whilst the classification is useful to assess new patients with diabetes, it does not provide a watertight definition of T2DM. The etiological classification could be improved with better recognition of the heterogeneity and polygenic nature of the disease.

EPIDEMIOLOGY OF TYPE 2 DIABETES AND ITS COMPLICATIONS

Prevalence and Incidence

More than 220 million people worldwide have diabetes and 80% live in low- to middle-income countries.[5] The majority of these people have T2DM. In the US, 25.8 million people (8.3%) have diabetes, of which 90–95% have T2DM.[6] Of these, 18.8 million (73%) are diagnosed and 7 million (27%) are undiagnosed. Amongst the > 65 year age group, 10.9 million have diabetes, representing a prevalence of 26.9%. A further 50% of this age group (79 million) have prediabetes.[6] Similarly, in the UK, where T2DM accounts for 92% of all registered diabetics,[7] approximately 30% of people with diabetes remain undiagnosed in England and the actual prevalence was predicted to be 7.4% in 2010, rising to 8.5% by 2020 and 9.5% by 2030.[7] By 2025, 300 million people worldwide will have diabetes.[8] Thus, diabetes prevalence rates of 10–50% will be commonplace by 2030. Towards the end of the 20th century, especially high prevalences were observed in indigenous populations. Notably, in populations such as Native Americans,[9] Pacific Islanders[10] and Aboriginal Australians,[11] this high prevalence is linked to rapid transitions from traditional to modern lifestyles, major changes in diet and physical activity, and with excessive weight gain. Since much of that work, it has been apparent that the prevalence of diabetes is high and rising in most world populations.[8] In China, the increasing affluence and changing lifestyles have seen dramatic increases in T2DM prevalence, particularly in urban populations. The numbers of adults with diabetes is projected to rise from 53.1 million in 2009 to 76.1 million in 2016. This represents a prevalence of 3.9% (urban 5.2%, rural 2.9%) in 2009, increasing to 5.4% (urban 6.9%, rural 3.8%) in 2016.[12] In summary, T2DM poses a serious escalating public health problem, irrespective of gender, society, race, or age.

Complications

In 2005, there were 1.1 million deaths worldwide attributed to diabetes, almost half of which were below the age of 70 years and 55% were women. It is predicted that worldwide diabetes deaths will double between 2005 and 2030.[5] US data report diabetes as the seventh-highest leading cause of death, with heart disease listed as the highest and cerebrovascular disease as the third leading cause. However, only 35–40% of deceased people with diabetes have this condition listed on their death certificate. Furthermore, as a high percentage of diabetes remains undiagnosed, it is likely that diabetes as a cause of death is grossly underreported. Many of the cardiovascular deaths are likely to be associated with underlying diabetes.[13] Similarly, macrovascular disease is the commonest cause of premature death in people with T2DM, and has been shown to reduce life expectancy of middle-aged males with T2DM in England by about 8 years.[14,15] For individuals who develop uncomplicated T2DM in later life, there is likely to be less risk of progression of microvascular complications compared with individuals who develop this condition at a younger age, although risks vary between individuals. In general, younger patients with T2DM are likely to have high lifetime risks of both macrovascular and microvascular disease. A clear relationship between glycemic control and microvascular and macrovascular complications was shown in the UKPDS study.[16] A 1% reduction in HbA1c was associated with 21% reduction in risk of any diabetes-related end point or death. Specifically, myocardial infarction risk is reduced by 14% and microvascular disease risk by 37% by reducing HbA1c from 7.9% to 7.0%. Long-term follow-up of patients with tighter glycemic control showed lasting reductions in macrovascular and microvascular disease.[17] However, there has been controversy about tight glycemic targets. A meta-analysis of studies of intensive glycemic control suggested that risk reduction for major cardiovascular events was just 9%, accompanied by significant risk of hypoglycemia.[18] Furthermore, there is evidence that lower levels of HbA1c are associated with increased mortality.[19] Therefore, a current widespread view of glycemic control in T2DM is that this is best tailored to the individual. It has been suggested that younger patients with greater life expectancy merit more aggressive treatment than older patients with established cardiovascular complications and limited life expectancy.[2]

GENETIC RISK FACTORS FOR TYPE 2 DIABETES

An early breakthrough in unravelling the complexity of T2DM came from the analysis of DNA from families with autosomal dominant diabetes, so-called Maturity Onset Diabetes of the Young (MODY).[20] This family of disorders accounts for a few per cent of diabetes in some populations, and if not considered the diagnosis is missed.[21] Nearly 30 susceptibility genes have now been identified, mainly influencing aspects of insulin secretion.[22] Currently known genes appear to explain only a small fraction of inherited risk.[23] While the mechanisms causing associations with T2DM remain unclear for most of these genes, the majority of the genes are expressed in islet β-cells. Thus, whilst obesity is an important cause of insulin resistance, and is a powerful risk factor for T2DM,[24,25] genetic factors will protect some obese patients through β-cell compensation.

RISK FACTORS AND SCREENING FOR TYPE 2 DIABETES

The ADA[2] advocates screening in high-risk, asymptomatic individuals, so that early diagnosis and treatment can prevent and delay complications. Common risk factors for T2DM and features to prompt screening are shown in Table 2.4. There remains controversy regarding the optimal testing strategy, and several tests are currently recognized. The two main tests

TABLE 2.4 Criteria for Diabetes Screening in Asymptomatic Adult Individuals at High Risk of Type 2 Diabetes

Testing should be considered in all adults who are overweight (BMI $\geq$ 25 kg/m^2 or lower in high-risk ethnic groups) and have additional risk factors:

Physical inactivity

First degree relative with diabetes

High-risk ethnic group

Women with previous GDM or macrosomic baby

Blood pressure > 140/90 or treated hypertension

HDL cholesterol < 35 mg/dl (0.9 mmol/l) and/or triglycerides > 250 mg/dl (2.82 mmol/l)

Women with polycystic ovary syndrome

Previous IFG, IGT or HbA1c $\geq$ 5.7%

Other clinical condition associated with insulin resistance (e.g., acanthosis nigricans)

History of cardiovascular disease

In the absence of the above criteria testing should begin at age 45 years.

If results are normal testing should be repeated at intervals of at least 3 years, with consideration of more frequent testing based on initial results and risk status.

Modified from: American Diabetes Association. Standards of Medical Care in Diabetes. Diabetes Care (2011) 34: 9(Suppl. 1), S11.

are fasting plasma glucose (FPG) or the 2-h plasma glucose (2-h PG) level after a 75 g OGTT. The adoption of HbA1c as a diagnostic test has been more controversial[26] but was suggested by the ADA in 2010.[27] No current screening or diagnostic test is completely interchangeable, since FPG and 2-h PG identify different individuals,[28] many of whom are also missed with HbA1c.[29] In women with polycystic ovary syndrome (PCOS) for example, the diagnosis of T2DM is usually missed with an FPG.[30] The choice of test is also affected by whether the intention is to screen for IGR such as impaired fasting glucose (IFG) and impaired glucose tolerance (IGT), which are currently essential if "prediabetes" is to be identified by blood glucose measures. HbA1c also fails to identify many individuals with IGR.[31] Currently, screening has not been widely implemented in many risk groups, including those with obesity, women with PCOS or a history of gestational diabetes.

DIABETES IN PREGNANCY: IMPLICATIONS FOR MOTHER AND OFFSPRING

Gestational Diabetes Mellitus (GDM) has been widely defined as carbohydrate intolerance of variable severity with onset during pregnancy which returns to normal after delivery. Maternal hyperglycemia causes fetal hyperglycemia, fetal hyperinsulinemia and macrosomia, resulting in excess perinatal morbidity and mortality. Maternal risks include the need for induction of labor and caesarean section, and long-term risks of T2DM and possibly cardiovascular disease. The definition, diagnosis and importance of GDM have been controversial however. The Hyperglycemia and Adverse Pregnancy Outcomes Study (HAPO), found a clear association between maternal glucose levels below the threshold for diagnosis of diabetes and adverse outcomes in 25,000 pregnant women.[32] In 2010, after years

TABLE 2.5 Procedures for Screening and Diagnosis of GDM

Perform a 75 g oral glucose tolerance test (OGTT) with plasma glucose measurement fasting, at 1 and 2 h, at 24—28 weeks of gestation in women not previously diagnosed with overt diabetes.

The OGTT should be performed in the morning after an overnight fast of at least 8 h.

The diagnosis of GDM is made when any of the following glucose values are exceeded:

Fasting $\geq$ 92 mg/dl (5.1 mmol/l).

1 h $\geq$ 180 mg/dl (10.0 mmol/l).

2 h $\geq$ 153 mg/dl (8.5 mmol/l).

Reproduced from: American Diabetes Association. Standards of Medical Care in Diabetes. Diabetes Care (2011) 34: 9(Suppl. 1), S11.

of variation controversy, the International Association of Diabetes and Pregnancy Study Groups recommended the approach summarized in Table 2.5.[33] These criteria recognize that standard criteria for the diagnosis of diabetes are inadequate for identifying levels of hyperglycemia (i.e. GDM) that affect the fetus. This study influenced the US change from screening based on GDM risk factors (such as BMI > 30, previous GDM, a previous macrosomic baby, diabetes in a first degree relative, or maternal origin from a high-risk ethnic group)[2,34] to universal screening at 24—28 weeks' gestation.[2] However, the consequences of this are greatly increased screening of "low-risk" women.

Whether GDM requires active treatment was controversial for many years. The aim of treatment for women with GDM is to reduce maternal and neonatal morbidity with treatment options including diet and exercise, oral hypoglycemic agents and insulin. Recent studies show that pregnancy outcomes are improved by active treatment[35–37] but that a high proportion of women with maternal hyperglycemia maintain good glycemic control without drug therapy. A recent systematic review and meta-analysis of major trials concluded that there were few differences in most outcomes when comparing metformin with insulin, but that metformin led to less maternal weight gain.[38]

Maternal hyperglycemia has important long-term implications for both mother and child. The incidence of maternal T2DM after GDM is as high as 70% after 10 years.[39] Finally, maternal GDM also results in increased long-term metabolic risk in their adolescent offspring.[40] The consequences of GDM for the next generation are therefore an important emerging concern.

EVIDENCE FOR METABOLIC PROGRAMMING OF DIABETES IN EARLY LIFE

Neither traditional theories of genetic nor environmental causation account for increased risk of T2DM in adults who were of low birthweight for gestational age. Barker and Hales observed increased risks of IGT and T2DM in males who were of low birthweight.[41] These and other findings led them to formulate the concept of the "thrifty phenotype",[42] drawing on the earlier ideas of Neel.[43] The hypothesis of "thrifty" metabolism postulates that evolutionary pressure from scarcity of food led to the selection of highly efficient insulin secretion and action and that fuel starvation during intrauterine life leads to adaptation to ensure survival but also results in permanent "programming" of metabolism. Neel proposed that this evolutionarily thrifty metabolism had maladaptive consequences in the modern world, leading to T2DM.[43] This concept is supported by experimental data showing that transient nutritional deficiencies in early life lead to permanent metabolic programming.[44] The mechanism for programming of disease risk may involve inherited non-DNA, epigenetic modification through methylation and other chemical changes to DNA and histone proteins. If so, this could explain the well-known interethnic differences in the risk of diabetes.

EARLY INTERVENTION IN TYPE 2 DIABETES

T2DM is often present years before diagnosis.[45,46] Early diagnosis and treatment aim to reduce progression of cardiovascular disease and hyperglycemia. The need for targeted screening and early intervention in high-risk groups is not therefore in doubt.[2] A range of drug-based interventions have demonstrated improved metabolic control and slower disease progression[47,48] and data are emerging for the long-term effects of lifestyle intervention.[49] Clearly, the earlier these interventions are instituted, the greater the potential reduction of long-term health risks. The risk of T2DM can be reduced substantially by weight reduction and drug interventions in high-risk individuals with IGT[50,51] or obesity.[52] These studies have provided a powerful impetus for diabetes prevention programs. However, it remains to be determined whether public health programs can afford to target the vast numbers who now meet criteria for diabetes screening, such as sedentary individuals with BMI $> 25\,\text{kg/m}^2$.[2]

CLINICAL MANAGEMENT OF TYPE 2 DIABETES

Key aims of T2DM clinical management are to reduce associated health risks, control

symptoms and restore or maintain quality of life. This is achieved by a variety of interventions that include weight reduction through diet and exercise and using drug treatment to control risk factors for complications (i.e. levels of blood glucose, blood pressure and cholesterol). The underlying state of insulin resistance[53] and insulin secretory failure[54] provide the principles for these treatment options. Whilst the beneficial metabolic effects of weight loss are long established,[55] it is comparatively recently that large-scale research into lifestyle and weight loss interventions has been taken seriously.[49] Likewise, for selected patients with severe obesity, bariatric surgery offers a potential option.[56] Other requirements considered necessary for effective T2DM treatment include patient education programs, a multidisciplinary team approach and regular recall for screening and monitoring. Favorable effects on quality of life and cost-effectiveness of care are also essential.

TREATMENT GUIDELINES

Medical treatment priorities are to achieve blood glucose levels as near to normal as possible and to lower cholesterol and blood pressure to reduce microvascular and macrovascular complications.[2,57,58] The importance of tight glycemic control and treatment of hypertension is largely based on the findings of the UKPDS[59–61] and post-trial follow-up.[17] The ADA guidelines also include a significant focus on nutrition, exercise, weight loss and more recently the potential role of bariatric surgery in treating T2DM.[27] In the wake of recent trials,[27] however, there has been increasing recognition that targets for blood glucose lowering are best individualized, with less strict glycemic control being safer and more appropriate for older, frailer people with existing complications with relatively lower life expectancy. Based on some of these data, along with recent safety concerns related to tight glycemic control,[62] blood pressure and cholesterol targets will be the main focus of treatment for many.[63]

NUTRITION AND LIFESTYLE INTERVENTION

Over the years, the importance of nutrition and lifestyle modification to treat T2DM has often been neglected. Increasing Body Mass Index (BMI) is associated with worse glycemic control and increased complications.[64] However, definitive data are lacking and nutritional guidance and targets for physical activity have been controversial. The ADA clearly acknowledges the importance of nutrition and physical activity in the prevention and management of diabetes.[27] This consensus statement highlights both nutrient-specific and obesity-related issues. The aim of modest weight loss is to improve glycemic control and reduce cardiovascular risk, based upon data from the Diabetes Prevention Program[50] and the Look Ahead study.[49] The ADA highlights the importance of reduced dietary fats, trans fatty acids and cholesterol. Furthermore, despite evidence of short-term weight loss and improved glycemic control with low-carbohydrate diets (<130 g/day carbohydrate), the long-term performance and safety of these diets have been controversial.[27] Current ADA recommendations are to take at least 150 min/week of moderate-intensity aerobic physical activity, and unless contraindicated to perform resistance training three times per week.[27]

PHARMACOLOGICAL TREATMENTS

The mainstays of treatment have traditionally been insulin, sulfonylureas and metformin. The impact of improved glycemic control using these three treatments was described by the UKPDS.[59,60] The use of thiazolidinediones prompted treatment targeting insulin resistance. Pioglitazone was found to reduce macrovascular disease in high-risk patients,[65] however cardiovascular concerns were encountered with other members of this class. The most recent additions to hypoglycemic drug therapies are Glucagon-Like-Peptide-1 (GLP-1) agonists[66] and inhibitors of dipeptidyl peptidase-4 (DPP-4),[67] both of which enhance insulin secretion. Whilst drug options for achieving glycemic control have broadened, the optimum order and combination of these treatments remains debatable. Latterly, tight glycemic control as the prime objective in treating T2DM has been questioned.[18] The main comorbidity of T2DM is cardiovascur disease and therefore the treatment aim should be to reduce this risk. This is more readily achieved by treatments that target blood pressure and low-density lipoprotein (LDL) cholesterol.[63]

Weight-loss drugs and weight-neutral hypoglycemic agents are a significant consideration, however no firm recommendation is yet possible without long-term data. Unfortunately, antiobesity drugs such as sibutramine and rimonabant have proven unsafe, although orlistat has demonstrated a modest effect on T2DM.[68] Currently, GLP-1 agonists are promising for weight loss in T2DM.[66] It appears appropriate therefore to consider these drugs in conjunction with active weight management programs such as that described in the Look Ahead study,[49] although this remains to be explored. Whether the benefits of insulin, thiazolidinediones and sulfonylureas are offset by weight gain is unclear. The recognition of the benefits of weight loss in treating T2DM is an important factor in the mounting interest in bariatric surgery as a treatment for some patients. In summary, these trends indicate increasing acceptance of the significant need for targeting obesity in T2DM.

BARIATRIC SURGERY

Bariatric surgery came to prominence as a means to control T2DM in 1995[69] and has since attracted increasing attention.[56] A range of surgical procedures is increasingly used to enhance the control of T2DM in obese individuals. The main operations currently used include roux-en-Y gastric bypass (RYGB), adjustable gastric banding (AGB), biliopancreatic diversion (BPD), and recently sleeve gastrectomy (SG). These procedures appear to improve blood glucose levels through changes in gut hormones and afferent neural signalling. However, whilst these operations convey many benefits, their long-term role in treating T2DM has not been compared. A meta-analysis suggested T2DM "remission" in 78% of patients,[70] with different rates with each procedure, although patient selection makes most of the patients unrepresentative of the general diabetic population.[71] Another problem is the large number of uncontrolled retrospective studies. To date there has been only one small prospective randomized controlled trial comparing AGB versus medical treatment of T2DM, which achieved 72% normoglycemia 2 years after AGB *vs* 13% in the medical control arm.[72] A subsequent analysis[73] also suggested that AGB had a favorable health economic impact. However, diabetes relapse is also recognized after bariatric surgery.[74,75] In addition to this, it is obvious that long-term treatments for diabetes should be safe. Whilst the short-term safety of bariatric surgery is well described[76,77] more complex surgery leads to higher operative mortality and complication rates. Malabsorptive bariatric surgery also generates long-term micronutrient deficiencies that require close monitoring and replacement.[78] There is currently increasing interest in using bariatric surgery as a diabetes treatment for people with BMI below 35 kg/m^2, although the ADA has urged caution and recommends further research.[27]

ECONOMIC IMPACT OF TYPE 2 DIABETES

At the beginning of the 21st century, T2DM is one of the most serious economic challenges facing the world. Reliable economic data are difficult to obtain, and so the best cost estimates come from more developed healthcare systems. In the US, for example, the total direct costs of treating diabetes were estimated at $116 billion in 2007, with an additional $58 billion in lost productivity,[79] although these figures underestimated the full cost. Nevertheless, this still represented a colossal 12.8% of US Gross Domestic Product. Currently, T2DM poses the overwhelming economic burden, as a result of its prevalence and the costs of its complications.

In the UK, most routine management of diabetes is undertaken within primary care settings—91% of this is for T2DM. Between 1997 and 2007, prescribing costs for T2DM increased by 89%, with a 28% increase for diabetes-specific prescribing. There was a 112% increase in primary care appointments, and the overall costs of treating T2DM rose by 59%.[80] Recent analyses have found 12.6% of acute hospital admissions to be diabetes-related, and that diabetes accounts for 10.8% of hospital outpatient attendances.[81] The percentage of acute hospital expenditure attributable to diabetes rose from 8.7% to 12.3% between 1994 and 2004.[81] Thus we have seen substantial rises in both primary and secondary care costs attributable to T2DM.

FUTURE DIRECTIONS

Diabetes researchers of the 19th and early 20th centuries would be amazed at the advances described in this book, although some fundamental controversies remain and new challenges have arisen. The major new challenge is the worldwide explosion of T2DM related to obesity. Although clinical trials have demonstrated the feasibility of diabetes prevention,[50,51,82] it has been less clear how to achieve this cost-effectively. Public health programs on this scale require political and economic cooperation. Weight loss is now commonly seen as a key treatment priority and yet many diabetes clinics remain poorly equipped to offer good support for weight loss. The optimum drug treatment regimens remain unclear with the use of oral agents, the newer incretin mimetics, and insulins requiring longer-term studies. Basic research on the molecular genetics and the endocrinology of T2DM and obesity—especially the mechanisms of diabetes remission after bariatric surgery—may lead to new forms of treatment.

References

1. World Health Organisation. *Definition, diagnosis and classification of diabetes mellitus and its complications: report of a WHO consultation. Part 1, Diagnosis and classification of diabetes mellitus.* Geneva: World Health Organization, Department of Noncommunicable Disease Surveillance; 1999.
2. American Diabetes Association. Standards of Medical Care in Diabetes. *Diabetes Care* 2011;**34**(Suppl. 1):S11–61.
3. American Diabetes Association. Diagnosis and Classification of Diabetes Mellitus. *Diabetes Care* 2011;**34**(Suppl. 1):S62–9.
4. Pinhas-Hamiel O, Zeitler P. Clinical presentation and treatment of type 2 diabetes in children. *Pediatr Diabetes* 2007;**8**(Suppl. 9):16–27.
5. World Health Organization. Diabetes Fact Sheet 312, http://www.who.int/mediacentre/factsheets/fs312/en/; 2011.
6. Center for Disease Control. National Diabetes Factsheet, http://www.cdc.gov/diabetes /pubs/pdf/ndfs_2011.pdf; 2011.
7. Yorkshire and Humberside Public Health Observatory. APHO Diabetes Prevalence Model: Key findings for England, http://www.yhpho.org.uk/resource/view.aspx?RID=81090; 2010.
8. King H, Aubert RE, Herman WH. Global burden of diabetes, 1995-2025: prevalence, numerical estimates, and projections. *Diabetes Care* 1998;**21**:1414–31.
9. Knowler WC, Bennett PH, Hamman RF, Miller M. Diabetes incidence and prevalence in Pima Indians: a 19-fold greater incidence than in Rochester, Minnesota. *Am J Epidemiol* 1978;**108**:497–505.
10. Zimmet P, Taft P, Guinea A, Guthrie W, Thoma K. The high prevalence of diabetes mellitus on a Central Pacific Island. *Diabetologia* 1977;**13**:111–5.
11. Daniel M, Rowley KG, McDermott R, O'Dea K. Diabetes and impaired glucose tolerance in Aboriginal Australians: prevalence and risk. *Diabetes Res Clin Pract* 2002;**57**:23–33.
12. Pan C, Shang S, Kirch W, Thoenes M. Burden of diabetes in the adult Chinese population: A systematic literature review and future projections. *Int J Gen Med* 2010;**3**:173–9.
13. Xu J, Kochanek K, Murphy S, Tejada-Vera B. Deaths: Final data for 2007. In National Vital Statistics Reports, http://www.cdc.gov/nchs/data/nvsr/nvsr58/nvsr58_19.pdf; 2010.
14. Roper NA, Bilous RW, Kelly WF, Unwin NC, Connolly VM. Cause-specific mortality in a population with diabetes: South Tees Diabetes Mortality Study. *Diabetes Care* 2002;**25**:43–8.
15. Roper NA, Bilous RW, Kelly WF, Unwin NC, Connolly VM. Excess mortality in a population with diabetes and the impact of material deprivation: longitudinal, population based study. *BMJ* 2001;**322**:1389–93.
16. Stratton IM, Adler AI, Neil HA, Matthews DR, Manley SE, Cull CA, Hadden D, Turner RC, Holman RR. Association of glycaemia with macrovascular and microvascular complications of type 2 diabetes (UKPDS 35): prospective observational study. *BMJ* 2000;**321**:405–12.
17. Holman RR, Paul SK, Bethel MA, Matthews DR, Neil HA. 10-year follow-up of intensive glucose control in type 2 diabetes. *N Engl J Med* 2008;**359**:1577–89.
18. Turnbull FM, Abraira C, Anderson RJ, Byington RP, Chalmers JP, Duckworth WC, Evans GW, Gerstein HC, Holman RR, Moritz TE, Neal BC, Ninomiya T, Patel AA, Paul SK, Travert F, Woodward M. Intensive glucose control and macrovascular outcomes in type 2 diabetes. *Diabetologia* 2009;**52**:2288–98.
19. Currie CJ, Peters JR, Tynan A, Evans M, Heine RJ, Bracco OL, Zagar T, Poole CD. Survival as a function of HbA(1c) in people with type 2 diabetes: a retrospective cohort study. *Lancet* 2010;**375**:481–9.
20. Hattersley AT, Turner RC, Permutt MA, Patel P, Tanizawa Y, Chiu KC, O'Rahilly S, Watkins PJ, Wainscoat JS. Linkage of type 2 diabetes to the glucokinase gene. *Lancet* 1992;**339**:1307–10.
21. Shields BM, Hicks S, Shepherd MH, Colclough K, Hattersley AT, Ellard S. Maturity-onset diabetes of the young (MODY): how many cases are we missing? *Diabetologia* 2010;**53**:2504–8.
22. Staiger H, Machicao F, Fritsche A, Haring HU. Pathomechanisms of type 2 diabetes genes. *Endocr Rev.* 2009;**30**:557–85.
23. Bonnefond A, Froguel P, Vaxillaire M. The emerging genetics of type 2 diabetes. *Trends Mol Med* 2010;**16**:407–16.

24. Colditz GA, Willett WC, Rotnitzky A, Manson JE. Weight gain as a risk factor for clinical diabetes mellitus in women. *Ann Intern Med* 1995;**122**:481−6.

25. Chan JM, Rimm EB, Colditz GA, Stampfer MJ, Willett WC. Obesity, fat distribution, and weight gain as risk factors for clinical diabetes in men. *Diabetes Care* 1994;**17**:961−9.

26. World Health Organization / International Diabetes Federation. Definition and diagnosis of diabetes mellitus and intermediate hyperglyaemia. Geneva, http://www.who.int/diabetes/publications/Definition%20and%20diagnosis%20of%20diabetes_new.pdf; 2006.

27. American Diabetes Association. Standards of Medical Care in Diabetes - 2010. *Diabetes Care* 2010;**33**:S11.

28. DECODE Study Group on behalf of the European Diabetes Epidemiology Study Group. Will new diagnostic criteria for diabetes mellitus change phenotype of patients with diabetes? Reanalysis of European epidemiological data. *BMJ* 1998;**317**:371−5.

29. Pajunen P, Peltonen M, Eriksson JG, Ilanne-Parikka P, Aunola S, Keinanen-Kiukaanniemi S, Uusitupa M, Tuomilehto J, Lindstrom J. HbA(1c) in diagnosing and predicting Type 2 diabetes in impaired glucose tolerance: the Finnish Diabetes Prevention Study. *Diabet Med* 2010;**28**:36−42.

30. Tomlinson J, Millward A, Stenhouse E, Pinkney J. Type 2 diabetes and cardiovascular disease in polycystic ovary syndrome: what are the risks and can they be reduced? *Diabet Med* 2010;**27**:498−515.

31. Cosson E, Hamo-Tchatchouang E, Banu I, Nguyen MT, Chiheb S, Ba H, Valensi P. A large proportion of prediabetes and diabetes goes undiagnosed when only fasting plasma glucose and/or HbA1c are measured in overweight or obese patients. *Diabetes Metab* 2010;**36**:312−8.

32. Metzger BE, Lowe LP, Dyer AR, Trimble ER, Chaovarindr U, Coustan DR, Hadden DR, McCance DR, Hod M, McIntyre HD, Oats JJ, Persson B, Rogers MS, Sacks DA. Hyperglycemia and adverse pregnancy outcomes. *N Engl J Med* 2008;**358**: 1991−2002.

33. Metzger BE, Gabbe SG, Persson B, Buchanan TA, Catalano PA, Damm P, Dyer AR, Leiva A, Hod M, Kitzmiler JL, Lowe LP, McIntyre HD, Oats JJ, Omori Y, Schmidt MI. International association of diabetes and pregnancy study groups recommendations on the diagnosis and classification of hyperglycemia in pregnancy. *Diabetes Care* 2010;**33**:676−82.

34. National Institute for Health and Clinical Excellence. Diabetes in pregnancy. *Management of diabetes and its complications from pre-conception to the postnatal period*, http://www.nice.org.uk/nicemedia/pdf/CG063Guidance.pdf; 2008.

35. Crowther CA, Hiller JE, Moss JR, McPhee AJ, Jeffries WS, Robinson JS. Effect of treatment of gestational diabetes mellitus on pregnancy outcomes. *N Engl J Med* 2005;**352**:2477−86.

36. Landon MB, Spong CY, Thom E, Carpenter MW, Ramin SM, Casey B, Wapner RJ, Varner MW, Rouse DJ, Thorp Jr JM, Sciscione A, Catalano P, Harper M, Saade G, Lain KY, Sorokin Y, Peaceman AM, Tolosa JE, Anderson GB. A multicenter, randomized trial of treatment for mild gestational diabetes. *N Engl J Med* 2009;**361**:1339−48.

37. Rowan JA, Hague WM, Gao W, Battin MR, Moore MP. Metformin versus insulin for the treatment of gestational diabetes. *N Engl J Med* 2008;**358**:2003−15.

38. Waugh N, Royle P, Clar C, Henderson R, Cummins E, Hadden D, Lindsay R, Pearson D. Screening for hyperglycaemia in pregnancy: a rapid update for the National Screening Committee. *Health Technol Assess* 2010;**14**:1−183.

39. Kim C, Newton KM, Knopp RH. Gestational diabetes and the incidence of type 2 diabetes: a systematic review. *Diabetes Care* 2002;**25**:1862−8.

40. Vaarasmaki M, Pouta A, Elliot P, Tapanainen P, Sovio U, Ruokonen A, Hartikainen AL, McCarthy M, Jarvelin MR. Adolescent manifestations of metabolic syndrome among children born to women with gestational diabetes in a general-population birth cohort. *Am J Epidemiol* 2009;**169**:1209−15.

41. Hales CN, Barker DJ, Clark PM, Cox LJ, Fall C, Osmond C, Winter PD. Fetal and infant growth and impaired glucose tolerance at age 64. *BMJ* 1991;**303**:1019−22.

42. Hales CN, Barker DJ. Type 2 (non-insulin-dependent) diabetes mellitus: the thrifty phenotype hypothesis. *Diabetologia* 1992;**35**:595−601.

43. Neel JV. Diabetes mellitus: a thrifty genotype rendered detrimental by progress? *Am J Hum Genet.* 1962;**14**: 353−62.

44. Ozanne SE. Metabolic programming in animals. *Br Med Bull* 2001;**60**:143−52.

45. Singh BM, Jackson DM, Wills R, Davies J, Wise PH. Delayed diagnosis in non-insulin dependent diabetes mellitus. *BMJ* 1992;**304**:1154−5.

46. Ellis JD, Zvandasara T, Leese G, McAlpine R, Macewen CJ, Baines PS, Crombie I, Morris AD. Clues to duration of undiagnosed disease from retinopathy and maculopathy at diagnosis in type 2 diabetes: a cross-sectional study. *Br J Ophthalmol* 2010. ePub.

47. UK Prospective Diabetes Study (UKPDS) Group. Intensive blood-glucose control with sulphonylureas or insulin compared with conventional treatment and risk of complications in patients with type 2 diabetes (UKPDS 33). *Lancet* 1998;**352**:837−53.

48. United Kingdom Prospective Diabetes Study group. Tight blood pressure control and risk of macrovascular and microvascular complications in type 2 diabetes: UKPDS 38. *BMJ* 1998;**317**:703–13.

49. Pi-Sunyer X, Blackburn G, Brancati FL, Bray GA, Bright R, Clark JM, Curtis JM, Espeland MA, Foreyt JP, Graves K, Haffner SM, Harrison B, Hill JO, Horton ES, Jakicic J, Jeffery RW, Johnson KC, Kahn S, Kelley DE, Kitabchi AE, Knowler WC, Lewis CE, Maschak-Carey BJ, Montgomery B, Nathan DM, Patricio J, Peters A, Redmon JB, Reeves RS, Ryan DH, Safford M, Van Dorsten B, Wadden TA, Wagenknecht L, Wesche-Thobaben J, Wing RR, Yanovski SZ. Reduction in weight and cardiovascular disease risk factors in individuals with type 2 diabetes: one-year results of the look AHEAD trial. *Diabetes Care* 2007;**30**:1374–83.

50. Knowler WC, Barrett-Connor E, Fowler SE, Hamman RF, Lachin JM, Walker EA, Nathan DM. Reduction in the incidence of type 2 diabetes with lifestyle intervention or metformin. *N Engl J Med* 2002;**346**:393–403.

51. Tuomilehto J, Lindstrom J, Eriksson JG, Valle TT, Hamalainen H, Ilanne-Parikka P, Keinanen-Kiukaanniemi S, Laakso M, Louheranta A, Rastas M, Salminen V, Uusitupa M. Prevention of type 2 diabetes mellitus by changes in lifestyle among subjects with impaired glucose tolerance. *N Engl J Med* 2001;**344**:1343–50.

52. Torgerson JS, Hauptman J, Boldrin MN, Sjostrom L. XENical in the prevention of diabetes in obese subjects (XENDOS) study: a randomized study of orlistat as an adjunct to lifestyle changes for the prevention of type 2 diabetes in obese patients. *Diabetes Care* 2004;**27**:155–61.

53. Himsworth H. Diabetes Mellitus. It's differentiation into insulin-sensitive and insulin-insensitive types. *The Lancet* 1936:127–30.

54. DeFronzo RA. Lilly lecture 1987. The triumvirate: beta-cell, muscle, liver. A collusion responsible for NIDDM. *Diabetes* 1988;**37**:667–87.

55. Henry RR, Wallace P, Olefsky JM. Effects of weight loss on mechanisms of hyperglycemia in obese non-insulin-dependent diabetes mellitus. *Diabetes* 1986;**35**:990–8.

56. Pinkney JH, Sjostrom CD, Gale EA. Should surgeons treat diabetes in severely obese people? *Lancet* 2001;**357**:1357–9.

57. National Institute for Health and Clinical Excellence. Type 2 diabetes. *National clinical guideline for management in primary and secondary care (update)*, http://www.nice.org.uk/nicemedia/live/11983/40803/40803.pdf; 2009.

58. Ryden L, Standl E, Bartnik M, Van den Berghe G, Betteridge J, de Boer MJ, Cosentino F, Jonsson B, Laakso M, Malmberg K, Priori S, Ostergren J, Tuomilehto J, Thrainsdottir I, Vanhorebeek I, Stramba-Badiale M, Lindgren P, Qiao Q, Priori SG, Blanc JJ, Budaj A, Camm J, Dean V, Deckers J, Dickstein K, Lekakis J, McGregor K, Metra M, Morais J, Osterspey A, Tamargo J, Zamorano JL, Deckers JW, Bertrand M, Charbonnel B, Erdmann E, Ferrannini E, Flyvbjerg A, Gohlke H, Juanatey JR, Graham I, Monteiro PF, Parhofer K, Pyorala K, Raz I, Schernthaner G, Volpe M, Wood D. Guidelines on diabetes, pre-diabetes, and cardiovascular diseases: executive summary. The Task Force on Diabetes and Cardiovascular Diseases of the European Society of Cardiology (ESC) and of the European Association for the Study of Diabetes (EASD). *Eur Heart J* 2007;**28**:88–136.

59. UK Prospective Diabetes Study (UKPDS) Group. Intensive blood-glucose control with sulphonylureas or insulin compared with conventional treatment and risk of complications in patients with type 2 diabetes (UKPDS 33). *Lancet* 1998;**352**:837–53.

60. UK Prospective Diabetes Study (UKPDS) Group. Effect of intensive blood-glucose control with metformin on complications in overweight patients with type 2 diabetes (UKPDS 34). *Lancet* 1998;**352**:854–65.

61. UK Prospective Diabetes Study Group. Tight blood pressure control and risk of macrovascular and microvascular complications in type 2 diabetes: UKPDS 38. *BMJ* 1998;**317**:703–13.

62. Currie CJ, Peters JR, Tynan A, Evans M, Heine RJ, Bracco OL, Zagar T, Poole CD. Survival as a function of HbA(1c) in people with type 2 diabetes: a retrospective cohort study. *Lancet* 2010;**375**:481–9.

63. Yudkin JS, Richter B, Gale EA. Intensified glucose lowering in type 2 diabetes: time for a reappraisal. *Diabetologia* 2010;**53**:2079–85.

64. Daousi C, Casson IF, Gill GV, MacFarlane IA, Wilding JP, Pinkney JH. Prevalence of obesity in type 2 diabetes in secondary care: association with cardio-vascular risk factors. *Postgrad Med J* 2006;**82**:280–4.

65. Dormandy JA, Charbonnel B, Eckland DJ, Erdmann E, Massi-Benedetti M, Moules IK, Skene AM, Tan MH, Lefebvre PJ, Murray GD, Standl E, Wilcox RG, Wilhelmsen L, Betteridge J, Birkeland K, Golay A, Heine RJ, Koranyi L, Laakso M, Mokan M, Norkus A, Pirags V, Podar T, Scheen A, Scherbaum W, Schernthaner G, Schmitz O, Skrha J, Smith U, Taton J. Secondary prevention of macrovascular events in patients with type 2 diabetes in the PROactive Study (PROspective pioglitAzone Clinical Trial In macro-Vascular Events): a randomised controlled trial. *Lancet* 2005;**366**:1279–89.

66. Pinkney J, Fox T, Ranganath L. Pharmacology and clinical benefits of glucagon-like receptor-1 agonists in the treatment of type 2 diabetes. *Pharmacology and Clinical Risk*; 2010. In press.

67. Richter B, Bandeira-Echtler E, Bergerhoff K, Lerch CL. Dipeptidyl peptidase-4 (DPP-4) inhibitors for type 2 diabetes mellitus. *Cochrane Database Syst Rev* 2008. CD006739.

68. Hollander PA, Elbein SC, Hirsch IB, Kelley D, McGill J, Taylor T, Weiss SR, Crockett SE, Kaplan RA, Comstock J, Lucas CP, Lodewick PA, Canovatchel W, Chung J, Hauptman J. Role of orlistat in the treatment of obese patients with type 2 diabetes. A 1-year randomized double-blind study. *Diabetes Care* 1998;**21**:1288–94.

69. Pories WJ, Swanson MS, MacDonald KG, Long SB, Morris PG, Brown BM, Barakat HA, deRamon RA, Israel G, Dolezal JM, et al. Who would have thought it? An operation proves to be the most effective therapy for adult-onset diabetes mellitus. *Ann Surg* 1995;**222**:339–52. discussion 350–352.

70. Buchwald H, Estok R, Fahrbach K, Banel D, Jensen MD, Pories WJ, Bantle JP, Sledge I. Weight and type 2 diabetes after bariatric surgery: systematic review and meta-analysis. *Am J Med* 2009;**122**:248–56. e245.

71. Chipkin SR, Goldberg RJ. Obesity surgery and diabetes: does a chance to cut mean a chance to cure? *Am J Med* 2009;**122**:205–6.

72. Dixon JB, O'Brien PE, Playfair J, Chapman L, Schachter LM, Skinner S, Proietto J, Bailey M, Anderson M. Adjustable gastric banding and conventional therapy for type 2 diabetes: a randomized controlled trial. *JAMA* 2008;**299**:316–23.

73. Keating CL, Dixon JB, Moodie ML, Peeters A, Bulfone L, Maglianno DJ, O'Brien PE. Cost-effectiveness of surgically induced weight loss for the management of type 2 diabetes: modeled lifetime analysis. *Diabetes Care* 2009;**32**:567–74.

74. DiGiorgi M, Rosen DJ, Choi JJ, Milone L, Schrope B, Olivero-Rivera L, Restuccia N, Yuen S, Fisk M, Inabnet WB, Bessler M. Re-emergence of diabetes after gastric bypass in patients with mid- to long-term follow-up. *Surg Obes Relat Dis* 2010;**6**:249–53.

75. Chikunguwo SM, Wolfe LG, Dodson P, Meador JG, Baugh N, Clore JN, Kellum JM, Maher JW. Analysis of factors associated with durable remission of diabetes after Roux-en-Y gastric bypass. *Surg Obes Relat Dis* 2010;**6**:254–9.

76. Flum DR, Belle SH, King WC, Wahed AS, Berk P, Chapman W, Pories W, Courcoulas A, McCloskey C, Mitchell J, Patterson E, Pomp A, Staten MA, Yanovski SZ, Thirlby R, Wolfe B. Perioperative safety in the longitudinal assessment of bariatric surgery. *N Engl J Med* 2009;**361**:445–54.

77. Morino M, Toppino M, Forestieri P, Angrisani L, Allaix ME, Scopinaro N. Mortality after bariatric surgery: analysis of 13,871 morbidly obese patients from a national registry. *Ann Surg* 2007;**246**:1002–7. discussion 1007–9.

78. Mechanick JI, Kushner RF, Sugerman HJ, Gonzalez-Campoy JM, Collazo-Clavell ML, Guven S, Spitz AF, Apovian CM, Livingston EH, Brolin R, Sarwer DB, Anderson WA, Dixon J. American Association of Clinical Endocrinologists, The Obesity Society, and American Society for Metabolic & Bariatric Surgery Medical Guidelines for Clinical Practice for the perioperative nutritional, metabolic, and nonsurgical support of the bariatric surgery patient. *Surg Obes Relat Dis* 2008;**4**:S109–84.

79. American Diabetes Association. Economic costs of diabetes in the U.S. in 2007. *Diabetes Care* 2008;**31**:596–615.

80. Currie CJ, Gale EA, Poole CD. Estimation of primary care treatment costs and treatment efficacy for people with Type 1 and Type 2 diabetes in the United Kingdom from 1997 to 2007. *Diabet Med* 2010;**27**:938–48.

81. Morgan CL, Peters JR, Dixon S, Currie CJ. Estimated costs of acute hospital care for people with diabetes in the United Kingdom: a routine record linkage study in a large region. *Diabet Med* 2010;**27**:1066–73.

82. Pan XR, Li GW, Hu YH, Wang JX, Yang WY, An ZX, Hu ZX, Lin J, Xiao JZ, Cao HB, Liu PA, Jiang XG, Jiang YY, Wang JP, Zheng H, Zhang H, Bennett PH, Howard BV. Effects of diet and exercise in preventing NIDDM in people with impaired glucose tolerance. The Da Qing IGT and Diabetes Study. *Diabetes Care* 1997;**20**:537–44.

3

Pathogenesis of Type 2 Diabetes— A Comprehensive Analysis

Jeff Unger

Catalina Research Institute, Chino, CA, USA

INTRODUCTION

Effective clinical management of type 2 diabetes (T2DM) requires a comprehensive understanding of the mechanisms by which an individual progresses from euglycemia to abnormal glucose tolerance. Healthcare providers too often blame patients for being "non-compliant" with their treatment regimen as their glycated hemoglobin levels rise, their weight increases, and the long-term devastating complications of chronic hyperglycemia impact their quality of life and their longevity. However, diabetes is a chronic and progressive disorder affecting the lives of millions of individuals globally, many of whom are unaware that they may be the victims of microvascular and macrovascular complications. Successful management of diabetes requires an understanding of treatment strategies which directly target those pathophysiologic abnormalities fueling disease progression. Any hopes of preventing or curing T2DM will also necessitate a comprehensive and analytical insight into this multifactorial disorder.

From a historical perspective, the origin of diabetes was not determined until two German physicians, Oskar Minkowski and Joseph von Mehring, successfully removed the pancreas from a dog in 1889.[1] Within 48 h, the dog developed glycosuria, polyuria, marked thirst, and weight loss. Although the pancreas was obviously a prerequisite for diabetes, what was the mechanism that triggered the disorder? The pancreatic islets were known to have a dual function: the first involving the production and secretion of digestive enzymes and the second to produce the internal secretion related to regulated glucose levels. Eugen Opie in 1901 supplied another link by noting that damage to the islets of Langerhans directly limited one's ability to produce the pancreas' *internal secretion*.[1] Patients who were unable to produce the internal secretion developed diabetes. Over the next 110 years, researchers have continued to search for the molecular, genetic, environmental, and physiologic derivation of diabetes.

GENETICS OF TYPE 2 DIABETES

Type 2 diabetes is comprised of four distinct disorders. Five to ten per cent of patients have maturity-onset diabetes of youth (MODY),[2] 5–10% have latent adult-onset autoimmune diabetes while another 5–10% have rare diabetes secondary to rare genetic disorders.[3–5] The pathogenesis of T2DM in the remaining 70–85% of patients, those most often seen in clinical practice, is thought to be heterogeneous and ill defined. For example, the susceptibility genes which have been identified in Mexican Americans are different from those found in Finnish families with type 2 diabetes.[6,7]

The genome-wide association (GWA) study has detected a total of 18 polymorphisms which may increase one's risk of developing type 2 diabetes. Expression of these alleles in genetically predisposed individuals appears to be "activated" through environmental triggers such as body mass index, advancing age, acute illnesses, concurrent medications, gender, and serum vitamin D levels.[8,9]

Most experts believe that T2DM has a polygenic origin. A susceptible individual possesses several abnormal genes which lead to the appearance of both insulin resistance and loss of pancreatic β-cell function, the two primary elements associated with the disease origin. Intraabdominal obesity, insulin resistance, and diabetes are also under genetic control which explains why the incidence of diabetes in the US will rise as our aggregate body mass index increases.[10]

MODY is caused by a genetic mutation in a single gene, whereas T2DM is of polygenic origin. Patients with MODY 2 have a genetic mutation in their glucokinase gene.[2] Glucokinase is a key regulatory enzyme in the pancreatic β-cell, playing a crucial role in the regulation of insulin secretion and serving as an "intracellular continuous glucose sensor".[2] Normal functioning glucokinase levels will allow maintenance of one's blood glucose levels in the fasting state between 85 and 99 mg/dl. A mutation in the glucokinase (GCK) gene will cause the ambient glucose level to rise to greater than 100 mg/dl. Patients with GCK genetic mutations will experience mildly elevated fasting blood glucose levels (> 126 mg/dl) in the perinatal period. However, postprandial rises in blood glucose levels are slight. Several heterozygous activating GCK mutations that cause hypoglycemia have also been reported.[11]

Five other types of MODY have been identified involving mutations in transcription factor genes which control the way that insulin is produced by the pancreatic β-cells (HNF-1 alpha, HNF-1 beta, HNF-4 alpha, IPF-1, and

NEURO-D1). Each form of MODY produces a slightly different clinical form of diabetes.[11]

A typical MODY patient may present between 12 and 30 years of age with slowly advancing abnormal glucose tolerance. In some individuals with MODY, T2DM may increase such as during superimposed obesity, pregnancy, or periods of prolonged physical inactivity. These individuals are non-obese and both a parent and a grandparent will have diabetes. MODY patients are typically asymptomatic and may have been misdiagnosed with type 1 diabetes years prior due to their young age. Any young patient who appears to have type 1 diabetes, a strong family history of diabetes, but test GAD-65 (autoantibody) negative should undergo genetic testing to determine the presence of MODY. A HNF alpha + or glucokinase GCK gene + patient might respond to sulfonylurea therapy or plus lifestyle intervention.[12]

Other genetic influences for the development of T2DM may be entirely "non-specific". For example, genes which regulate appetite, energy expenditure, and intraabdominal fat accumulation may increase the likelihood of a patient becoming obese. These "diabetes-related genes" would enhance the progression of euglycemia towards impaired glucose tolerance and β-cell dysfunction under the influence of certain environmental factors (smoking, alcohol, reduction in serum vitamin D levels, increased BMI, loss of incretin response, etc). An individual with a specific mutation in the insulin receptor gene may develop insulin resistance sooner than a patient who does not have this genetic defect. Thus, the heterogeneous nature of T2DM often makes genetic determination of pathogenesis very complex.

MAINTENANCE OF NORMAL GLUCOSE HOMEOSTASIS

Several hormones (insulin, glucagon, amylin, leptin, epinephrine, resistin, GLP-1, and adiponectin) must interact in unity to maintain a normal metabolic environment. Insulin plays a crucial role in modulating the metabolism of fats and protein while being the primary regulator of cellular uptake and the use of glucose. Insulin regulates glucose homeostasis in the liver (hepatic glucose production), skeletal muscle (peripheral glucose disposal), and adipose tissue (endogenous glucose production).[13]

The brain and nervous system are insulin independent; autonomously regulating their use of glucose as a metabolic fuel. Glucose transport is mediated by a protein called glucose transporter 1 (GLUT-1) which actively carries glucose across neuronal cell membranes in the presence of either low or high plasma glucose levels in an insulin-independent manner.

Insulin activates the glucose transporter GLUT-4 in muscles and adipose tissue.[14] Glucose, ketone bodies or free fatty acids are their primary metabolic fuel. When large amounts of insulin are bound to receptors on cell surfaces, myocytes transport the glucose intracellularly as an energy source or store the excess glucose as muscle glycogen. Alternatively, glucose may be stored as fat in adipose tissue. Either way, insulin promotes the peripheral disposal of glucose from the plasma maintaining serum glucose levels in the narrow range of 85–140 mg/dl. When insulin levels are low, the cell switches to ketone/free fatty acid metabolism, reducing uptake of glucose and instead using circulating free fatty acids for energy. Glucose uptake by muscle and fat is regulated because these tissues are insulin responsive.

The gastrointestinal tract participates in glucose homeostasis by permitting glucose entry to the body during digestion. This process occurs episodically, delivering large amounts of glucose into the portal vein with meals. In patients with insulin resistance or impaired glucose tolerance, gastrointestinal absorption of glucose can stress already compromised glucose regulatory systems by overwhelming the other organs' abilities to dispose of elevated postprandial glucose. The result is postprandial hyperglycemia. Approximately 60% of the insulin response to an oral glucose load is due to the potentiating effect of gut-derived incretin hormones. The incretin effect has been attributed to peptide hormones that are released into the bloodstream from the intestinal K- and L-cells in response to a meal. Glucagon-like peptide-1 (GLP-1), secreted by the L-cells, helps regulate the rate of glucose appearance by inhibiting glucagon secretion, inhibiting hepatic glucose production, regulating gastric emptying, and reducing food intake by postulated centrally mediated mechanisms. GLP-1 stimulated insulin secretion modulates the rate of glucose disposal by insulin-sensitive tissues.

The levels of both GLP-1 and glucose-dependent insulinotropic polypeptide (GIP) increase within minutes of eating probably due to a combination of endocrine and neural signals which stimulate incretin release before digested food comes in contact with the L-cells of the small bowel and colon.[16] Plasma levels of GLP-1 are low (5—10 pmol/l) in the fasting state, and increase rapidly after eating, reaching 15—50 pmol/l. The circulating levels of both GLP-1 and GIP decrease rapidly because of enzymatic inactivation via dipeptidyl peptidase-4 (DPP-4), and renal clearance.[16] Approximately two-thirds of the insulin response to an oral glucose load is due to the potentiating effect of gut-derived incretin hormones.[17]

The pancreas regulates glucose homeostasis by secreting insulin from centrally positioned β-cells and glucagon from alpha-cells located on the periphery of the islet.[18] Insulin is secreted in response to high plasma glucose levels as well as GLP-1 stimulation following an oral meal stimulus. The secreted insulin suppresses hepatic production of glucose (glycogenolysis and gluconeogenesis), stimulates hepatic glucose uptake and storage, and regulates glucose uptake in muscle and, to a lesser extent,

adipose tissue. At low plasma glucose levels, pancreatic secretion of insulin is decreased. Low insulin levels facilitate hepatic glucose production and adipose tissue lipolysis.

Signaling occurs between the β- and alpha-cells so that glucose levels are tightly regulated, minimizing the likelihood of postprandial hypoglycemia. In the presence of falling plasma glucose levels, the alpha-cells will signal β-cells to cease insulin production and secretion as glucagon levels rise.[19] The secretion of glucagon will result in hepatic gluconeogenesis and a return of euglycemia. As β-cell function and mass deteriorates, the signaling between the alpha- and β-cell is disrupted, resulting in excess glucagon production.[20] Clinically, patients will experience elevations in fasting and postabsorptive glucose levels.

The liver performs two different functions, depending on the level of insulin. In the presence of low levels of insulin (25 mU/ml or less)—e.g., in the fasting state—the liver produces glucose from glycogenolysis and gluconeogenesis and releases it to maintain fasting plasma glucose levels. In the presence of moderate-to-elevated levels of insulin, the liver stops producing glucose and takes glucose from the plasma, storing it as glycogen for use when plasma glucose and insulin levels decrease. Following an overnight fast, the liver of a euglycemic individual produces glucose at a rate of approximately 2 mg/kg/min. A patient with diabetes will have basal hepatic glucose production levels of over 2.5 mg/kg/min resulting in an extra 25—30 g of glucose being delivered into the plasma each evening.[15] The overproduction of glucose by the liver in the fasting state occurs in the presence of fasting plasma insulin levels which are increased three-fold. The primary defect in T2DM appears to be related to peripheral glucose disposal rather than excessive hepatic glucose production.[15]

The role of the kidneys in maintaining normoglycemia through the filtration and reabsorption of glucose as well as gluconeogenesis is well established. Each day 180 l of plasma filters through the kidneys translating into a filtration load of approximately 180 g of glucose.[21] In healthy individuals, the kidneys efficiently reabsorb glucose from the glomerular filtrate with less than 0.5 g/day of glucose ultimately appearing in the urine. During periods of hyperglycemia, the amount of filtered glucose reabsorbed increases proportionately to the plasma glucose concentration until the resorptive capacity of the tubules is exceeded at which point the excess glucose is excreted in the urine. Glucose reabsorption in the renal tubules is driven by way of sodium glucose cotransporter 2 (SGLT2), a high-capacity, low-affinity transporter found in the brush border membrane of the S1 segment of the proximal tubule.[22] Thus, SGLT2 blockade will result in patients excreting glucose in their urine rather than reabsorbing glucose into plasma which is already exposed to chronic hyperglycemia.[23]

IMPAIRED GLUCOSE HOMEOSTASIS IN PATIENTS WITH TYPE 2 DIABETES

Unlike type 1 diabetes, the progression from prediabetes to T2DM occurs over a period of several years. As lean individuals gain weight and become obese over time, insulin sensitivity decreases significantly, but glucose tolerance remains relatively normal due to a compensatory increase in insulin secretion. The higher insulin output is accompanied by reduced insulin activity in the liver, adipose tissue, and skeletal muscles, resulting in diminished intracellular glucose disposal. Patients then progress through a spectrum of abnormal glucose states, including impaired fasting glucose (IFG) and impaired glucose tolerance (IGT) due to worsening of insulin resistance. However, the rise in plasma glucose concentrations is relatively modest because of a further compensatory increase in insulin secretion. A gradual decline in β-cell insulin secretion associated with an increase in hepatic glucose production lead to overt clinical diabetes manifested by fasting and postprandial hyperglycemia.

MECHANISTIC ACTIONS WHICH LEAD TO PROGRESSIVE β-CELL FAILURE AND TYPE 2 DIABETES

Multiple mechanistic anomalies have been implicated in the progression from euglycemia to clinical diabetes. The pancreas, liver, muscle, kidney, brain, gut, and adipose cells appear to be "team players" in driving susceptible individuals into chronic hyperglycemia. The individual pathways which appear to favor insulin resistance and β-cell destruction are discussed below.

β-Cell Failure and Apoptosis (Cell Death)

Pancreatic β-cell failure occurs much earlier in the natural history of T2DM and is more severe than previously thought. The San Antonio Metabolism (SAM) study evaluated patients with normal glucose tolerance, and type 2 diabetes. Patients received an oral glucose tolerance test with plasma glucose and insulin concentrations measured every 15 min to evaluate overall glucose tolerance and β-cell function.[24] An insulin clamp technique was used to measure insulin sensitivity. Patients with "impaired glucose tolerance" who had a 2-h postprandial glucose level of 180–199 mg/dl were found to have lost 80–85% of their β-cell function. Thus, by the time the diagnosis of clinical diabetes is made and therapeutic interventions are initiated, patients have already lost at least 80% of their β-cell function and are maximally insulin resistant. The SAM study provides insight as to the necessity of early and intensive pharmacologic management for patients with newly diagnosed type 2 diabetes. In post mortem analysis, Butler *et al.* determined that β-cell mass is significantly decreased in patients with T2DM and that the underlying mechanism for this is β-cell apoptosis (genetically mediated cell death).[25] Obese individuals in Butler's study had a 63% deficit in relative β-cell volume compared with nondiabetic obese individuals.[25] Thus, patients with prediabetes tend to lose β-cell function and mass prior to being clinically diagnosed with type 2 diabetes.

Several pathogenic mechanisms are known to promote β-cell failure including advanced age, genetic susceptibility, insulin resistance, elevated free fatty acids, and glucotoxicity.[15] Figure 3.1 depicts the multifactorial

mechanisms which target loss of β-cell function and mass.

Plasma glucose also influences the functionality and survivability of pancreatic β-cells. Short-term exposure of β-cells to increasing glucose concentrations initially induces proliferation of β-cell mass in a concentration-dependent manner.[26] However, the proliferative capacity of β-cells is suppressed following chronic exposure to increasing plasma glucose concentrations. For example, cultured human islets exposed to physiologic glucose concentrations ranging from 99 to 594 mg/dl undergo a linear acceleration of β-cell apoptosis suggesting that chronic hyperglycemia induces the demise of β-cells.[26]

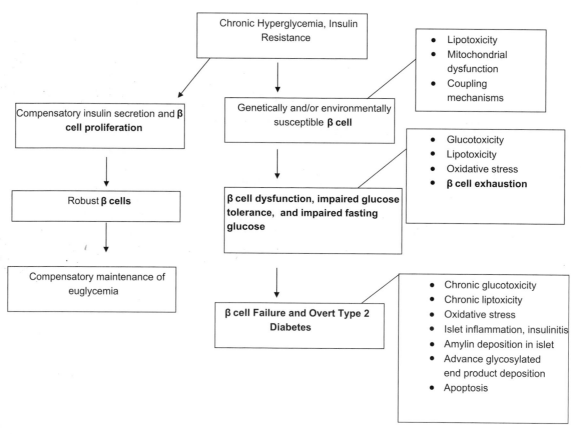

FIGURE 3.1 Theoretical mechanisms of β cell failure in type 2 diabetes.

Impaired glucose tolerance possibly in concert with elevated free fatty acids can induce oxidative stress. Intracellular oxidative stress occurs when the production of reactive oxygen species (byproducts of normal metabolism) exceeds the capacity of the cell's antioxidants to neutralize them. Oxidative stress can be minimized by optimization of metabolic control. Stress-induced pathways such as NF-κB, stress kinases, and hexosamines tend to promote not only β-cell apoptosis, but also pathways leading to long-term diabetes-related complications.[27]

Vitamin D (25-hydroxyvitamin D [25(OH)D]) may directly influence β-cell function. Increasing 25(OH)D levels from 10 to 30 ng/ml can improve insulin sensitivity by 60%. Subjects with hypovitaminosis D are at higher risk of insulin resistance and the metabolic syndrome.[28] Potential mechanisms underlying this association are supported by the following observations: (a) β-cells contain the vitamin D receptor and demonstrate activity of 1 alpha hydroxylase, an enzyme involved in vitamin D metabolism.[29] Vitamin D does not have significant biologic activity until it is metabolized to its hormonally active form, 1,25-dihydroxycholecalciferol. This occurs in a two-step process, first in the liver by hydroxylation with the enzyme 25 hydroxylase and second in one of many tissues with the enzyme 1 alpha hydroxylase.[30] (b) Vitamin D improves β-cell function by stimulating insulin release and restoring impaired insulin secretion in vitamin D deficient mice.[29] (c) Vitamin D is known to improve insulin action by stimulating expression of the insulin receptor and enhancing responsiveness for glucose transport.[28] The Nurses Health Study of 83,779 women with 20-year follow-up revealed 4,843 new cases of T2DM but showed that a "combined daily intake > 1000 mg calcium and > 800 mg of vitamin D was associated with a 33% lower risk of type 2 diabetes".[31]

The normal physiologic response to hyperglycemia and obesity-associated insulin resistance is compensatory insulin production and hypersecretion with the goal of maintaining plasma glucose levels in the range of 85–140 mg/dl. Type 2 diabetes will only develop in individuals who are unable to sustain this β-cell compensatory response. Longitudinal studies of subjects who develop T2DM show a rise in plasma insulin levels in normoglycemic and prediabetes phases which maintain glycemic control near normal despite insulin resistance. However, when fasting glycemia surpasses the upper limit of normal (85 mg/dl) β-cell failure is likely to occur.[32]

To summarize, hyperglycemia plays a central role among the factors which contribute to loss of β-cell function. Initially transient postprandial hyperglycemia may induce β-cell proliferation in insulin-resistant individuals. Over time this adaptive mechanism will fail as β-cell dysfunction and death ensues in genetically or environmentally predisposed individuals. Chronic glucotoxicity in patients with elevated free fatty acids, and inflammatory cytokine production, further weaken the β-cells' production and insulin secretory capacity. As glucose levels rise, oxidative stress becomes the dagger ultimately leading to the death and destruction of the islets' remaining functioning β-cells. Hyperglycemia has tissue-damaging effects on a subset of cell types such as capillary endothelial cells of the retina, mesangial cells in the renal glomerulus and peripheral neurons. Cells which are inefficient interstitial transporters of glucose will undergo oxidative stress which induces endothelial dysfunction, vascular inflammation, and activation of pathways which trigger microvascular complications.[27]

The progression to diabetes for patients with IGT is 6–10% per year, and for persons with both IFG and IGT, the cumulative incidence of diabetes within 6 years is estimated to be higher than 60%.[33] Progression rates from IFG or IGT to diabetes are dependent on multiple factors such as the severity and duration of the initial degree of hyperglycemia, racial and ethnic backgrounds, genetics, as well as other environmental influences.

Increased Lipogenesis and Free Fatty Acid Production

Free fatty acids (FFAs) have long been recognized as a potential mediator of insulin sensitivity, secretion, and hepatic glucose regulation in obesity.[34] Experimental elevation of plasma FFAs results in greater insulin resistance in skeletal muscle and activation of proinflammatory pathways which could promote macrovascular disease.[35] Fat cells secrete signaling molecules which tend to promote normal glucose homeostasis such as leptin and adiponectin. Adipocytes can also secrete proinflammatory cytokines which can adversely affect lipid and carbohydrate metabolism thereby promoting insulin resistance and progression to type 2 diabetes.[36] At the cellular level, FFAs inhibit insulin-mediated glucose uptake by interfering with the translocation of the glucose transport protein, GLUT-4, to the plasma membrane, effectively blocking glucose uptake by muscle cells and increasing peripheral insulin resistance. In hepatocytes, free fatty acids inhibit insulin-mediated suppression of glycogenolysis and gluconeogenesis resulting in an increase in hepatic glucose production.[37]

Several prospective epidemiologic studies have evaluated the link between elevated plasma concentrations of FFA and the development of diabetes. In the Pima study, subjects with plasma FFA levels in the highest decile had a 2.3-fold higher risk of developing diabetes than subjects in the lowest decile.[38] In the Paris Prospective Study, higher FFA levels were also associated with progression from normal glucose tolerance at baseline to clinical diabetes.[39]

Because insulin action promotes adipocyte stability, elevated plasma triglycerides and FFAs may be interpreted as representing defective fat storage in patients with type 2 diabetes.[40] Additionally, elevations in plasma FFA levels stimulate the hepatic production of triglyceride-rich lipoproteins which further impair peripheral insulin action.

Does the elevation in FFAs have a greater effect on the β-cells' ability to produce and secrete insulin or on the skeletal muscle cells' ability to uptake and utilize circulating glucose? A euglycemic hyperinsulinemic clamp study found a strong inverse association between fasting FFA concentrations and whole-body glucose disposal rate but no relationship between FFAs and fasting plasma insulin concentrations.[41] Thus, FFA appears to have a greater effect on peripheral insulin resistance resulting in reduced intracellular glucose transport than directly on β-cell toxicity. However, over time, as the β-cell is exposed to prolonged hyperglycemia, apoptosis will occur. Animal studies suggest that β-cell failure and death are preceded by an increase in plasma FFAs accompanied by an accumulation of triglyceride with the β-cell.[42]

The two main types of adipose tissue are subcutaneous and visceral adipose tissue (VAT). Eighty per cent of body fat is located in the subcutaneous adipose tissue, and 10% is located in VAT.[43] Visceral fat, which is prominent in obesity, produces higher levels of FFA, which explains the link between obesity and the progression to type 2 diabetes. Adipocytes in obese individuals are resistant to the antilipolytic effects of insulin. Both T2DM and obesity are characterized by an elevation in the mean day-long plasma FFA concentration as well as increased triglyceride levels within muscle, liver, and β-cells, further promoting insulin resistance.

In some studies, individuals whose first-degree relatives have T2DM tend to have elevated levels of circulating FFA.[44] FFA levels are also elevated in prediabetic states (impaired glucose tolerance and impaired fasting glucose) resulting in hyperinsulinemia, suggesting that FFAs may actually enhance β-cell production of insulin. FFAs are a potent insulin secretagogue and can compensate for most of the insulin resistance they produce. FFAs induce 30–50% of secreted basal insulin.[45] However, patients with a genetic predisposition to T2DM may be unable to compensate β-cell insulin secretion fully to overcome peripheral insulin resistance. Patients with impaired glucose tolerance and T2DM also are deficient in FFA-stimulated insulin secretion.[45] Obese patients with T2DM who are genetically predisposed to the disorder, develop slow, progressive β-cell failure and increased peripheral insulin resistance.

Finally, the consumption of a diet high in saturated fat can acutely increase plasma FFA levels in obese, insulin-resistant patients. Elevated free fatty acid levels for as little as 48 h markedly impairs both first and second phase insulin secretion in genetically predisposed individuals, further impairing insulin secretion and peripheral disposal.[46]

Hyperglucagonemia

Hyperglucagonemia is another primary feature of both prediabetes and diabetes. Under normal conditions, a postprandial increase in glucose concentration is associated with a corresponding reduction in glucagon. As plasma glucose levels decrease, glucagon levels increase, resulting in a 60% increase in hepatic glucose production and output through gluconeogenesis.[47] Glucagon secretion is regulated, in part, by endogenous insulin secretion. Insulin action results in the storage of glycogen within hepatocytes. Insulin resistance, insulinopenia, or an increase in glucagon output signals the liver to depolymerize glycogen, resulting in a rise in plasma glucose concentration. Glucagon secretion is substantially elevated in the fasting state and is not suppressed during the postabsorptive phase in patients with both

prediabetes and clinically apparent diabetes. Patients with T2DM appear to be hypersensitive to glucagon stimulation further promoting ambient hyperglycemia and insulin resistance.

In type 2 diabetes, the liver, brain, and skeletal muscles are resistant to insulin action. Excessive hepatic glucose production adds an extra 30 g of glucose to the systemic circulation of an 80-kg person each night. Patients will experience a significant rise in their fasting blood glucose levels due to the accelerated endogenous glucose production. β-cell insulin secretion becomes "inflated" in a feeble attempt to normalize fasting blood glucose levels. Unfortunately, even at secretion rates which exceed normal levels by three-fold, hepatic glucose production continues to increase. This leads leads credence to the belief that 90% of insulin resistance is secondary to defects in glucose uptake in the skeletal muscle tissue.[48]

The skeletal muscles are responsible for absorbing and processing glucose in the postabsortive state. Patients with T2DM exhibit defective insulin receptor binding and postreceptor signaling. As glucose clearance in the peripheral skeletal muscle is reduced, impaired glucose tolerance and chronic postabsorptive hyperglycemia replaces the normal euglycemic state. The combined decreased muscle glucose uptake and impaired suppression of hepatic glucose production contributes to insulin resistance; a metabolic state in which a given concentration of insulin produces a less than expected biological effect.

Defects in the insulin signal transduction system also play a paramount role in insulin resistance within skeletal muscles.[49] These defects lead to decreased glucose transport, impaired release of nitric oxide with endothelial dysfunction, and multiple anomalies in intramyocellular glucose metabolism. The mitogen-activated protein (MAP) kinase pathway retains its sensitivity to insulin, causing excessive stimulation of this inflammatory and atherogenesis-based system. This, in part, explains the strong association between high circulating plasma insulin levels, insulin resistance, and atherosclerotic cardiovascular disease in patients with type 2 diabetes.

Impaired Incretin Effect

The incretin effect refers to a phenomenon in which oral glucose administration elicits a much higher insulin secretory response than an intravenous infusion of glucose with similar glycemic rises.[56] In humans, the incretin effect is mediated by two peptide hormones, GLP-1 and GIP.

Contradicting information has been published regarding the secretion of GLP-1 in response to oral glucose in type 2 diabetic patients. Both elevated and reduced post-challenge responses have been described.[17,50] The plasma levels of DPP-4, which rapidly degrades GLP-1 following its meal-stimulated release from the small and large intestinal L-cells, are similar in euglycemic individuals and patients with diabetes.[17] As a consequence of the action of DPP-4, as well as rapid renal clearance, the half-life of GLP-1 is 1–2 min and that of GIP is approximately 7 min.[17] Basal (fasting) concentrations of GLP-1 are ~5 pmol/l while peak concentrations of ~15–40 pmol/l are observed 1 h after eating.[17] Although small reductions in postprandial GLP-1 secretion may occur in patients with type 2 diabetes, these observations do not appear to have a meaningful physiologic effect on glucose metabolism and insulin secretion.[51]

The effects of both GLP-1 and GIP are mediated by specific receptors present on β-cells and other target tissues. GLP-1 and GIP increase insulin secretion from β-cells in a glucose-dependent manner. In rodents, GLP-1 and GIP also enhance β-cell mass by increasing rates of proliferation and decreasing rates of apoptosis.[52] This effect, however, has not been observed in humans. GLP-1 suppresses glucagon secretion, slows gastric emptying

and enhances satiety. GIP has a direct effect on adipocytes to promote triglyceride storage.[52] Taken together, the incretin hormones provide a physiologic response to meals of variable sizes allowing for optimal metabolic control of nutrients.

In patients with type 2 diabetes, the incretin effect is reduced by approximately 50% compared with euglycemic subjects.[51] The defect appears to be secondary to impairments in incretin hormone action (resistance) rather than secretion because most studies have found comparable circulating concentrations of GLP-1 and GIP in response to nutrient challenges in subjects with T2DM and normal controls.[51] The glucodynamic effects observed in GLP-1-deficient patients may be overcome by infusing native GLP-1 subcutaneously to achieve "pharmacologic" plasma levels.[53]

GLP-1 resistance in some individuals may be secondary to a genetic defect affecting the receptor binding site. Defective GLP-1 receptor binding may result in loss of intracellular signaling, and reduced expression of hormonal action. A single nucleotide polymorphism (SNP) in which methionine is substituted for threonine at position 149 of GLPIR on the receptor binding site has been identified.[54] When present, this defect results in an altered insulin secretory response to GLP-1 infusion. Additional studies must assess if genetic polymorphisms play a role in GLP-1 and insulin resistance.

Glucose toxicity may downregulate GLP-1 receptor expression.[51] However, improvement in glucose control and reversal of glucose toxicity with both DPP-4 inhibitors and GLP-1 analogs can restore β-cell cell function and perhaps receptor responsiveness to endogenous GLP-1.[17]

The Kidney's Role in Promoting Insulin Resistance

The kidneys are normally so efficient at glucose reabsorption that no glucose appears in the urine in euglycemic individuals. Chronic hyperglycemia increases the plasma glucose exposure to the renal tubules exceeding the renal threshold of normal glucose absorption resulting in glycosuria. In patients with type 2 diabetes, the SGLT2 levels are significantly elevated, meaning that the renal absorption of glucose in the proximal tubules is paradoxically increased. This appears to be an adaptive response by the kidney to conserve glucose, which is required to meet the energy demands of the brain and cardiovascular system in the presence of severe insulin resistance. Thus, an individual with insulin resistance is incorrectly "marked" as developing intracellular starvation of nutrients. In an attempt to correct this pathological defect, the kidneys reabsorb excessive amounts of glucose hoping that this energy source will ease the burden of the brain, skeletal muscle, and cardiovascular system, all of which appear to be unable to transport glucose intracellularly. Unfortunately, the kidneys simply add to the ambient insulin resistance by increasing plasma glucose levels.

Impaired Neuroprotection

Few would argue that the current epidemic of diabetes is driven by the epidemic of obesity. Could the insulin resistance seen in peripheral tissues also extend into the central nervous system?

The direct administration of GLP-1 into the third cerebral ventricle of rats augments glucose-stimulated insulin secretion as the brain attempts to overcome a state of acute hyperglycemia.[55] In addition, when GLP-1 is directly administered into the arcuate nucleus of the hypothalamus, hepatic glucose production is reduced.[55] Food intake is reduced when GLP-1 was injected directly into the paraventricular nucleus.[55] Thus, GLP-1 receptor expression is based upon their unique location within the brain. Stimulation of those receptors within the arcuate nucleus lowers basal and postprandial glucose levels, whereas expression of GLP-1 receptors in the paraventricular nucleus will induce satiety.

Functional magnetic resonance imaging (MRI) has been used to evaluate the cerebral response to an ingested glucose load in obese subjects.[55] Following glucose ingestion, the ventromedial nuclei and the paraventricular nuclei demonstrated consistent inhibition. These are the key centers in the brain which regulate appetite. Whether the impaired functional MRI response in obese subjects contributes to or is a consequence of insulin resistance and weight gain is unclear. However, these results suggest that in patients with impaired glucose metabolism, the brain may not only be insulin resistant, but may have additional defects in GLP-1 expression and secretion.[55]

SUMMARY

The pathogenesis of T2DM is multifactorial. Genetically or environmentally "challenged" individuals begin the transformation from euglycemia towards clinically apparent T2DM as their skeletal muscles and hepatocytes exhibit evidence of insulin resistance. Initially, pancreatic β-cells attempt to compensate for the impaired glucose tolerance by overproducing insulin. Perhaps patients' appetites are increased at this early phase of prediabetes. As their meal portions increase, so does the secretion of GLP-1 resulting in β-cell hypertrophy. However, over time, other metabolic defects appear which tend to aggravate the existing state of hyperglycemia. Lipolysis is accelerated within the adipocytes resulting in release of FFA which not only worsen insulin resistance, but induce β-cell apoptosis. As glycemic control worsens further, the renal threshold for glucose excretion is exceeded. SGLT2 levels are elevated and the renal absorption of glucose is paradoxically increased as if the kidneys believed that the body required additional glucose to meet energy demands. Meanwhile, neuroprotective mechanisms within the central nervous system are also eliminated and the brain is unable to minimize hepatic glucose production or induce satiety. At the cellular level, defective receptor signaling and glucose transport has occurred. Glucose is unable to enter or provide fuel for skeletal muscle cells. Hyperglycemia tends to favor GLP-1 receptor resistance. As a result, meal-stimulated GLP-1 production by the intestinal L-cells can not induce insulin secretion by the pancreatic β-cells. Due to the theoretical communication between β-cells and alpha-cells, a defect in β-cell function may result in inappropriate glucagon production which would stimulate hepatic gluconeogenesis.

The indicators of β-cell responsiveness include glucose sensitivity, timing of insulin release following a glucose-mediated stimulus, as well as post- receptor signaling (glucose transport and insulin production). All of these factors are affected as one moves from normal glycemia towards prediabetes and into clinical diabetes.

References

1. Luft R, Minkowski Oskar. Discovery of the pancreatic origin of diabetes, 1889. *Diabetologia* 1989;**32**:399—401.
2. Fajans S. Maturity-onset diabetes of the young (MODY). *Diabetes Metab Rev* 1989;**5**:579—606.
3. Niskanen L, Tuomi T, Karjalainen J, Groop L, Uusitupa M. GAD antibodies in NIDDM: ten-year follow-up from the diagnosis. *Diabetes Care* 1995;**18**:1557—65.
4. Gerbitz K, Gempel K, Brdiczka D. Mitochondria and diabetes: genetic, biochemical, and clinical implications of the cellular energy circuit. *Diabetes* 1996;**45**:113—26.
5. Taylor SI. Molecular mechanisms of insulin resistance. Lessons from patients with mutations in the insulin-receptor gene. *Diabetes* 1992;**41**:1473—90.
6. Hanis C, Boerwinkle E, Chakraborty R, et al. A genome-wide search for human non-insulin-dependent (type 2) diabetes genes reveals a major susceptibility locus on chromosome 2. *Nat Genet* 1996;**13**:161—6.
7. Mahtani M, Widen E, Lehto M, et al. Mapping of a gene for type 2 diabetes associated with an insulin secretion defect by a genome scan in Finnish families. *Nat Genet* 1996;**14**:90—4.
8. Hamman R. Genetic and environmental determinants of noninsulin dependent diabetes mellitus (NIDDM). *Diabetes Metab Rev* 1992;**8**:287—338.
9. Bouchard C. Genetics and the metabolic syndrome. *Int J Obesity* 1995;**19**(Suppl):S52—9.
10. Hales C, Barker D. Type 2 (non-insulin-dependent) diabetes mellitus: the thrifty phenotype hypothesis. *Diabetologia* 1992;**35**:595—601.
11. Cuesta-Munoz AL, Tiinamaija T, Cobo-Vuilleumier N, et al. Clinical heterogeneity in monogenetic diabetes caused by nutations in the glucokinase gene (GCK-MODY). *Diabetes Care* 2010;**33**(2):290—2.
12. Owen KA, Thanabalasingham G, James TJ, et al. Assessment of high-sensitivity C-reactive protein levels as diagnostic discriminator of maturity-onset diabetes of the young due to HNF1A mutations. *Diabetes Care* 2010;**33**(9):1919—24.
13. Stefan N, Stumvoll M, Vozarova B, et al. Plasma adiponectin and endogenous glucose production in humans. *Diabetes Care* 2003;**26**(12):3315—9.
14. Unger RH. Lipotoxicity in the pathogenesis of obesity-dependent NIDDM: genetic and clinical implications. *Diabetes* 1995;**44**:863—70.
15. Unger J, Parkin C. Type 2 diabetes: An expanded view of pathophysiology and therapy. *Postgraduate Medicine* 2010;**122**(3):145—57.
16. Nauck MA, Baller B, Meier JJ. Gastric inhibitory polypeptide and glucagon-like peptide-1 in the pathogenesis of type 2 diabetes. *Diabetes* 2004;**53**(Suppl. 3):S190—6.
17. Unger J. Incretins: Clinical perspectives, relevance, and applications for the primary care physician in the treatment of patients with type 2 diabetes. *Mayo Clinic Proceedings* Dec. 2010;**85**(Suppl. 12):S38—49.
18. Baron AD, Schaeffer L, Shragg P, et al. Role of hyperglucagonemia in maintenance of increased rates of hepatic glucose output in type II diabetes. *Diabetes* 1987;**36**:274—83.
19. Dagogo-Jack S. Hypoglycemia in type 1 diabetes mellitus. Pathophysiology and prevention. *Treat Endocrinol* 2004;**3**(2):91—103.
20. Toft-Nielsen MB, Damholt MB, Madsbad S, et al. Determinants of the impaired secretion of glucagon-like peptide-1 in type 2 diabetic patients. *J Clin Endocrinol Metab* 2001;**86**:3717—23.
21. Wright EM, Hirayama BA, Loo DF. Active sugar transport in health and disease. *J Intern Med* 2007;**261**:32—43.
22. Wright EM. Renal NA (+) —glucose cotransporters. *Am J Physiol Renal Physiol* 2001;**280**:F10—8.
23. Brooks AM, Thacker SM. Dapagliflozin for the treatment of type 2 diabetes. *Ann Pharmacother* 2009;**43**:1286—93.
24. Abdul-Ghani M, Tripathy D, DeFronzo RA. Contributions of β-cell dysfunction and insulin resistance to the pathogenesis of impaired glucose tolerance

and impaired fasting glucose. *Diabetes Care* 2006;**29**:1130–9.

25. Butler AE, Janson J, Bonner-Weir S, et al. Beta-cell deficit and increased beta-cell apoptosis in humans with type 2 diabetes. *Diabetes* 2003;**52**(1):102–10.

26. Leahy JL, Cooper HE, Weir GC. Impaired insulin secretion associated with near normoglycemia: study in normal rats with 96-h in vivo glucose infusions. *Diabetes* 1987;**36**:459–64.

27. Unger J. Reducing oxidative stress in patients with type 2 diabetes mellitus. A primary care call to action. *Insulin* 2008;**3**:176–84.

28. Barengolts E. Vitamin D role and use in prediabetes. *Endocr Pract* 2010;**16**(3):476–85.

29. Bland R, Markovic D, et al. Expression of 25-hydroxy-vitamin D3-1 alpha hydroxylase in pancreatic islets. *J Steroid Biochem Mol Bio* 2004;**89-90**:121–5.

30. Gonzalez C. Vitamin D supplementation: an update. US Pharmacist. Medscape Today. Published 11/11/2010.

31. Pittas AG, Dawson-Hughes B, Li T, Willett WC, Van Dam RV, Manson JE, Hu FB. Vitamin D and calcium intake in relation to type 2 diabetes in women. *Diabetes Care* 2006;**29**(3):650–6.

32. Lillioja S. Impaired glucose tolerance in Pima Indians. *Diabet Med* 1996;**13**(9 Suppl. 6):S127–32.

33. Garber AJ, Handelsman Y, Einhorn D. Diagnosis and management of prediabetes in the continuum of hyperglycemia—When do the risks of diabetes begin? A consensus statement from the American College of Endocrinolgy and the American Association of Clinical Endocrinologists. *Endocr Pract* 2008;**14**(7):933–46.

34. Boden G. Role of fatty acids in the pathogenesis of insulin resistance and NIDDM. *Diabetes* 1997;**46**:3–10.

35. Arner P. Insulin resistance in type 2 diabetes: role of fatty acids. *Diabete Metab Res Rev* 2002;**18**(Suppl. 2):S5–9.

36. Mora S, Pessin JE. An adipocentric view of signaling and intracellular trafficking. *Diabete Metab Res Rev* 2002;**18**:345–56.

37. Saltiel AR, Kahn CR. Insulin signaling and the regulation of glucose and lipid metabolism. *Nature* 2001;**414**:799–806.

38. Paolisso G, Tataranni PA, Foley JE, et al. A high concentration of fasting plasma non-esterified fatty acids is a risk factor for the development of type 2 diabetes. *Diabetologia* 1995;**38**:1213–7.

39. Charles MA, Eschwege E, Thibult N, et al. The role of non-esterified fatty acids in the deterioration of glucose tolerance in Caucasian subjects: results of the Paris Prospective study. *Diabetologia* 1997;**40**:1101–6.

40. Mostaza JM, Vega GL, Snell P, Grundy SM. Abnormal metabolism of free fatty acids in hypertriglyceridaemic men: apparent insulin resistance of adipose tissue. *J Intern Med* 1998;**243**:265–74.

41. Baldeweg SE, Golay A, Natali A, et al. Insulin resistance, lipid and fatty acid concentrations in 867 healthy Europeans: European Group for the Study of Insulin Resistance (EGIR). *Eur J Clin Invest* 2000;**30**:45–52.

42. Lee Y, Hirosel T, Ohneda M, et al. Beta cell lipotoxicity of non-insulin dependent diabetes mellitus of obese rats: impairment in adipocyte-beta cell relationships. *Proc Natl Acad Sci USA* 1994;**91**:10878–82.

43. Arner P. Free fatty acids: do they play a central role in type 2 diabetes? *Diabetes Obes Metab* 2001;**3**(Suppl. 1):11–9.

44. Boden G, Chen X. Effects of fatty acids and ketone bodies on basal insulin secretion in type 2 diabetes. *Diabetes* 1999;**48**:577–83.

45. Boden G, Chen X, Iqbal N. Acute lowering of plasma fatty acids lowers basal insulin secretion in diabetic and nondiabetic subjects. *Diabetes* 1998;**47**:1609–12.

46. Groop LC, Bonadonna RC, Del Prato S, et al. Glucose and free fatty acid metabolism in non-insulin dependent diabetes mellitus. Evidence for multiple sites of insulin resistance. *J Clin Invest* 1989;**84**:205–15.

47. Guyton JR, Hall JE. Insulin, glucagon, and diabetes mellitus. In: Guyton JR, Hall JE, editors. *Textbook of Medical Physiology*. Philadelphia, PA: Elsevier Saunders; 2006. p. 961–77.

48. DeFronzo RA, Ferrannini E, Simonson DC. Fasting hyperglycemia in non-insulin-dependent diabetes mellitus: contributions of excessive hepatic glucose production and impaired tissue glucose uptake. *Metabolism* 1989;**38**(4):387–95.

49. Cusi K, Maezono K, Osman A, et al. Insulin resistance differentially affects the PI 3-kinase and MAP kinase-mediated signaling in human muscle. *J Clin Invest* 2000;**105**(3):311–20.

50. Nauck M, Stockmann F, Ebert R, et al. Reduced incretin effect in type 2 (non-insulin-dependent) diabetes. *Diabetologia* 1986;**29**(1):46–52.

51. Drucker DJ, Sherman SI, Gorelick FS, et al. Incretin-based therapies for the treatment of type 2 diabetes: Evaluation of the risks and benefits. *Diabetes Care* 2010;**33**:428–33.

52. Pratley R. GIP: An inconsequential incretin or not? *Diabetes Care* 2010;**7**(33):1691–2.

53. Russell-Jones D. Molecular, pharmacological and clinical aspects of liraglutide, a once-daily human GLP-1 analogue. *Mol Cell Endocrinol* 2009;**297**:137–40.

54. Sathananthan A, Man CD, Micheletto F, et al. Common genetic variation in GLPIR and insulin secretion in response to exogenous GLP-1 in nondiabetic subjects: a pilot study. *Diabetes Care* 2010;**33**(9):2123–5.

55. Mudaliar S, Henry RR. Incretin therapies: Effects beyond glycemic control. *European Journal of Medicine* 2009;(20):S319–28.

4

Managing the Broad Spectrum of Type 2 Diabetes

Evelyne Fleury-Milfort

Division of Endocrinology and Diabetes, Department of Medicine, Keck School of Medicine,
University of Southern California, Los Angeles, CA, USA

INTRODUCTION

Type 2 diabetes (T2DM) carries a tremendous healthcare burden. In individuals with this condition, there is a markedly increased incidence of myocardial infarction. The incidence of stroke is increased two- to three-fold, and peripheral vascular disease is very common. In 2007, the total direct medical cost for treating the disease was $116 billion. After adjusting for population age and sex differences, average medical expenditures among people with diabetes were 2.3 times higher than they would be in the absence of diabetes. The indirect cost for disability, work loss, premature mortality was $58 billion.[1]

T2DM encompasses a broad spectrum of chronic, heterogeneous, complex, and progressive metabolic defects resulting in hyperglycemia. The condition is characterized by insulin resistance and an initial compensatory hyperinsulinemia, followed by progressive loss of β-cell function. In the last two decades, clinical studies have broadened our understanding of the complex genetic defects involved in the development of T2DM. Within this new multifactorial pathophysiology, glucose intolerance is a continuum, and individuals with the condition move along this spectrum as a function of their insulin secretion/insulin resistance index. In addition, there is a continuous spectrum of glucose levels between those considered normal and those that are considered for the diagnosis of diabetes, with the levels for prediabetes in between. Consequently, the expression of different proportions of these pathogenic factors will cause a diverse array of presentations, as well as differences in the rate of progression in each patient. With this evolving understanding of the natural history of T2DM and the emergence of various agents targeting the spectrum of genetic defects, clinicians need to use a pathophysiologically-based paradigm for their clinical decision-making, taking into consideration the individual patient presentation and the characteristics of the available hypoglycemic agents.

EVOLVING PATHOPHYSIOLOGY OF TYPE 2 DIABETES

As described by De Fronzo,[2] there is an evolving body of evidence which supports that inherited components for pancreatic β-cell failure and insulin resistance in the tissues contribute to the glucose intolerance in individuals with T2DM. In the liver, this resistance is manifested by an overproduction of glucose during the fasting state and an impaired suppression of hepatic glucose production in response to insulin such as in the postprandial state. The muscle resistance is manifested by impaired glucose uptake following ingestion of carbohydrate resulting in postprandial hyperglycemia. To complicate matters, the insulin resistance itself places an increased demand on the β-cells and contributes further to their failure.

It is a well known fact that obesity is at an epidemic proportion in the US. In parallel, T2DM, which affects about 90% of people with diabetes, is also on the rise. According to the latest Centers for Disease Control and Prevention (CDC) data,[1] diabetes now affects 25.8 million people of all ages or 8.3% of the US population. Is the epidemic of diabetes being driven by the epidemic of obesity? Obesity, with or without diabetes, is characterized by insulin resistance and compensatory hyperinsulinemia. Food intake is found to be increased in obese patients despite the presence of hyperinsulinemia. It is now postulated that the insulin resistance found in the liver, muscle and fat tissues also extends to the brain.[2]

The insulin resistance in the tissues initially triggers a compensatory hyperinsulinemia. However, there is evidence that significant β-cell failure occurs at an early stage in the progression of T2DM. In the United Kingdom Prospective Diabetes Study (UKPDS), β-cell secretory capacity was found to be reduced by 50% by the time fasting hyperglycemia was present.[3] Progressive β-cell failure in type T2DM is caused by both genetic and acquired factors such as glucose toxicity (chronic hyperglycemia causing β-cell desensitization) and lipotoxicity due to elevated plasma free fatty acid.

Furthermore, in the last decade, the gut has been found to be a major endocrine organ and another contributor to the pathogenesis of T2DM. The functional effects of the incretin hormones glucagon-like peptide-1(GLP-1) and glucose-dependent insulinotrophic polypeptide, also called gastric inhibitory polypeptide (GIP), include increasing glucose-dependent insulin secretion, lowering glucagon secretion, inhibiting gastric emptying, reducing appetite, decreasing caloric intake, and improving β-cell function and insulin sensitivity.[4,5] People with T2DM are deficient in GLP-1 and have a resistance to the action of GIP. Abnormalities in GLP-1 have been shown to play an important role in the progressive β-cell failure of T2DM. Deficiency in GLP-1 response contributes to the rise in plasma glucagon secretion and impaired suppression of hepatic glucose production occurring postprandially.

ALTERING THE PROGRESSION OF TYPE 2 DIABETES

Mauricio, a 42-year-old male from South America, was referred to our practice after an abnormal fasting blood glucose of 116 mg/dl and an A1c of 6.1% on his last laboratory test. He has a 3-year history of hypertension and started on statin therapy a year ago after he was found to have elevated cholesterol. Mauricio has prediabetes, and he is joining a growing group. In 2005–2008, based on fasting glucose or A1c levels, 35% of US adults aged 20 years or older had prediabetes. When this percentage is applied to the entire US population in 2010, it yields an estimated 79 million Americans aged 20 years or older with prediabetes.[1] Individuals with prediabetes have either impaired fasting glucose [fasting plasma glucose levels 100–125 mg/dl (5.6–6.9 mmol/l)], impaired glucose tolerance [2-h plasma glucose values in the oral glucose tolerance test (GTT) of 140–199 mg/dl (7.8–11.0 mmol/l)], or an A1c of 5.7–6.4%. They have insulin resistance and have already lost 80% of their β-cell function.[6] At the time of diagnosis, about 10% have background retinopathy and another 10% have peripheral neuropathy.[7,8] Prediabetes is also associated with obesity (especially abdominal or visceral obesity), dyslipidemia with high triglycerides and/or low high-density lipoprotein (HDL) cholesterol, hypertension, risk of heart disease, and stroke. People with prediabetes are at increased risk of developing T2DM as in some individuals a progressive β-cell dysfunction appears after a period of long-standing insulin resistance.

NEED FOR EARLY INTERVENTION

Traditionally, clinicians just used to tell patients like Mauricio that they had "borderline" diabetes and simply advise them to "watch what they eat". This clinical inertia in the presence of a serious condition is no longer acceptable. Early lifestyle interventions focusing on weight loss have had some success in preventing or delaying the onset of T2DM in these insulin-resistant individuals. The Finnish Diabetes Prevention Study and the Diabetes Prevention Trial (DPT) both have shown that people with prediabetes who lose weight and increase their physical activity can prevent or delay T2DM and in some cases return their blood glucose levels to normal.[9,10] Based on these evidences, both the American Diabetes Association (ADA) and the American Association of Clinical Endocrinologists (AACE) recommend the implementation of aggressive lifestyle modification.[11,12] ADA specified that patients with prediabetes be advised and supported to achieve a weight loss of 7% of body weight and have moderate physical activity such as walking at least 150 min/week. Mauricio will be retested after he achieves his target weight loss and at least every year to evaluate the status of his glycemia. Although lifestyle modification may decrease hemoglobin A1c by 1–2%, follow-through tends to fail after 1 year. In view of this knowledge, should we start him on a medication?

Several studies have shown that the early use of pharmacologic agents such as metformin, β-glucosidase inhibitors, orlistat, and thiazolidinediones (TZDs), each of which has been shown to decrease the incidence of type 2 diabetes to various degrees. Sensitizers such as TZDs and biguanides decrease insulin resistance and facilitate β-cell rest. In the DPT, diabetes rates in patients with prediabetes treated with metformin declined by 31%.[13] If we consider that the ACT NOW trial (Actos Now for Prevention of Diabetes) showed a reduction of 81% with changes in the disposition index indicating both improved insulin sensitivity and β-cell function.[14] Similar results were obtained with the TRIPOD (Troglitazone in Prevention of Diabetes) and PIPOD (Pioglitazone in Prevention of Diabetes) studies of women with prior gestational diabetes.[15,16] More recent clinical studies suggest that incretin therapies may prove to be effective in the prevention of type 2 diabetes because of their beneficial effects on insulin secretion and β-cell function in humans and their effects in maintaining or improving β-cell function and mass in experimental animals.[17–20] In light of these evolving data, some argue for the use of pioglitazone to prevent the progression of prediabetes to diabetes. At this time, there is no medication approved for the management of prediabetes. Currently, ADA only recommends that metformin therapy for prevention of T2DM could be considered in individuals at the highest risk for developing diabetes, such as those with multiple risk factors (hypertension, hyperlipidemia), like Mauricio, especially if they demonstrate worsening of A1c or blood glucose despite lifestyle interventions.[11] The jury is still out since not all patients with diabetes progress to failure of the β-cell and diabetes and the persistence of the effect of these medications beyond the duration of treatment is not known. Before prescribing pharmacologic agents to high-risk patients with prediabetes, an individual assessment of risks and benefits should be done and discussed with each patient.

AGGRESSIVE MANAGEMENT AFTER DIAGNOSIS

Unfortunately, many patients arrive at our offices too late to delay or prevent the development of diabetes. This was the case for Linda, a 56-year-old Caucasian woman who has a 1-year history of hyperlipidemia, 8 years with hypertension and a BMI of 28. About 6 years ago, after being told for 2 years that she had "borderline diabetes", she was diagnosed with T2DM. When she came to our office, she was on glipizide 10 mg twice a day and metformin 500 mg twice a day. Her control was poor as evidenced by an A1c of 7.9%. She felt frustrated by her high blood sugar and weight gain in spite of walking for 30 min 3 days a week and trying to follow a low-calorie diet. As clinicians, we need to focus on early interventions to control glycemia as lower blood glucose at the time of initial therapy is associated with lower A1c levels over time as well as decreased long-term complications.[21]

HOW LOW DO WE GO FOR GLYCEMIC CONTROL?

The A1c reflects average blood glucose over the last 3 months and has strong predictive value for diabetes complications. Testing should be performed regularly, at initial assessment and every 3 months thereafter, as part of continuing care to determine if glycemic targets have been reached and maintained.

Tight blood sugar control has become a standard of treatment for most patients with diabetes based on results from National Institutes of Health (NIH) clinical trials, demonstrating that keeping A1c below 7% can prevent or delay devastating disease complications. More importantly, lowering A1c to below or around 7% has been shown to reduce microvascular and neuropathic complications of diabetes and, if implemented soon after the diagnosis of diabetes, is associated with long-term reduction in macro-vascular disease in what is called the legacy effect.[22]

The most recent glycemic goal recommended by the American Diabetes Association, is an A1c level of < 7%. The goal set by the AACE is an A1c level of < 6.5%.[23] Several recent clinical trials have aimed for A1c levels < 6.5% with a variety of interventions. However, this may have substantial negative clinical effects, in terms of mortality, morbidity, adherence to therapy, and quality of life. Results of clinical trials of intensive therapy such as Action to Control Cardiovascular Risk in Diabetes (ACCORD), Action in Diabetes and Vascular Disease: Preterax and Diamicron MR Controlled Evaluation (ADVANCE), and Veterans Affairs Diabetes Trial (VADT) have shown that intensive glycemic control was associated with a three- to four-fold increase in the incidence of hypoglycemia. In the ACCORD study, hypoglycemia was associated with excess mortality in both the intensively treated group and the conventionally treated group. The risk of hypoglycemia increases with advancing age and limited life expectancy; duration of diabetes; duration of insulin therapy; history of hypoglycemia; hypoglycemia unawareness; coexisting severe comorbidities; as well as other factors such as patient education, motivation, adherence, and use of other medications.[24-29]

Because additional analyses from randomized trials such as the UKPDS suggest a small but incremental benefit in microvascular outcomes with A1c values closer to normal, clinicians may reasonably strive for more stringent A1c goals for selected patients if it can be achieved without significant hypoglycemia or other adverse effects of treatment, but this goal must be customized for each individual patient. Such patients might include those with short duration of diabetes, long life expectancy, and no significant cardiovascular disease like Linda. Conversely, less stringent A1c goals may be appropriate for patients at high risk for hypoglycemia as described above.

TREATMENT OPTIONS

First of all, we need to evaluate her understanding of her condition, current self-care routine including lifestyle, food intake, physical activity, self-monitoring of blood sugar, and medication routine. She came with her most recent laboratory test results showing a normal serum creatinine level and liver function. Review of her meter download shows only fasting results with an average of 167 mg/dl. Since chronically elevated plasma glucose levels are believed to impair β-cell function, optimal glycemic control will be essential not only to prevent the long-term complications of diabetes but also to reverse the glucotoxic effect of her chronic hyperglycemia.

SELF-MANAGEMENT EDUCATION

We will also evaluate Linda's reported low-fat meal plan and exercise program, as well as work with her to enhance her self-management knowledge and skills. Diabetes self-management education (DSME) must be an essential element of diabetes care. Diabetes is treated at home and the patient is responsible for 90% of their care. DSME helps the patient initiate and maintain effective self-care behaviors and cope with their condition throughout a lifetime. Appropriate knowledge and skills helps the patient be a better partner in their care: as they make informed decisions they optimize their metabolic control, prevent and manage complications, and maximize their quality of life. To be effective, the DSME process must incorporate the needs, goals, and life experiences of the patient and should also address psychosocial issues since emotional well-being is associated with positive diabetes outcomes.

LIFESTYLE MODIFICATION

Linda is very motivated to participate in her care and had already started some lifestyle modification strategies which can and may help decrease her A1c by 1–2%. However, she will need a lot of support as follow-through tends to wax and wane and usually there is a high rate of weight regain in the long term.

As far as her blood glucose control, at this time, we only know her fasting blood sugar, which is elevated, and her A1c level. However, this does not give us a complete picture of her daily glycemia. The A1c represents the average blood glucose during the previous 3 months, it is insufficient to indicate the quality of control on a daily basis. Self-monitoring of blood glucose (SMBG) is an important element in adjusting or adding new intervention. The frequency of SMBG measurements is not clearly defined and is dependent on the medications used and the stability of the patient's glycemia. To better assess our patient's glycemic pattern on a day-to-day basis, we will ask Linda to test her blood sugar more often. For patients on non-insulin therapies, or medical nutrition therapy alone, ADA recommends self monitoring of blood sugar (SMBG) to guide to the success of therapy. Postprandial SMBG may be appropriate to achieve postprandial glucose targets. The A1c can serve as a check on the accuracy of the patient's meter, self-reported SMBG results as well as the adequacy of the SMBG testing schedule by using the correlation between A1c levels and mean plasma glucose levels published by the ADA and available on line at http://professional.diabetes.org/eAG.

At this time, Linda will be asked to test her blood sugar before meals and at bedtime. If she is unable or unwilling to test four times a day, we can ask her to test twice a day at varied times in order to have a more complete glycemic picture. To ensure her success, we will ensure that she is proficient at using her glucose monitor and understands how to use the data to adjust her exercise and food intake.

MEAL PLANNING

Which meal plan will be better for Linda? Weight management with medical nutrition therapy and increased physical activity are an integral part of the treatment strategies for patients with T2DM. Recent studies show that there may be a short-term advantage to low-carbohydrate diets as far as initial weight loss.[30] Several randomized controlled trials have found that people on low-carbohydrate diets (< 130 g/day of carbohydrate) lost more weight at 6 months than subjects on low-fat diets. The low-carbohydrate diets were associated with greater improvements in triglyceride and HDL cholesterol concentrations than low-fat diets; however, low-density lipoprotein (LDL) cholesterol was significantly higher. The difference in weight loss between groups was not significant at 1 year, and the total weight loss was modest with both diets.[31,32] Another study of overweight women randomized to one of four diets showed significantly more weight loss at 12 months with the Atkins low-carbohydrate diet than with higher carbohydrate diets.[33] In a 2-year dietary intervention study, Mediterranean and low-carbohydrate diets were found to be effective and safe alternatives to a low-fat diet for weight reduction in moderately obese participants.[34]

Since the superiority of one type of diet has not been established, I think that the best meal plan is the one the patient will adhere to. The best mix of carbohydrate, protein, and fat will vary depending on the individual circumstances and should be adjusted to meet the metabolic goals and patients' preferences. The total caloric intake must be appropriate to the weight management goal. ADA recommends either a low-carbohydrate, low-fat calorie-restricted, or the Mediterranean diets.[11] For

Linda, we will strive for a deficit of 500–700 calories per day and a slow weight loss of 1–2 lbs a week. Her meal plan will integrate the glycemic index and glycemic load that ADA now recognizes as possibly providing a modest additional benefit for glycemic control.[11] If she chooses a low-carbohydrate diet, lipid profiles will need to be monitored and her hypoglycemic agents adjusted. We will discuss with her that the goal of her effort is not for weight loss, but rather a modification of her lifestyle with changes in her eating and physical activity habits to achieve and maintain glycemic control and optimal health. The distinction is that when the focus is weight loss, patients tend to return to their previous eating habits after achieving the target weight loss, and maintenance becomes a problem.

PHYSICAL ACTIVITY

Another part of Linda's lifestyle intervention is physical activity. Exercise is not only an important component of weight management, but it is most helpful in maintenance of weight loss. Furthermore, exercise also appears to aid in the loss of visceral fat and is well known to ameliorate many of the known vascular disease risk factors associated with T2DM, favorably influencing levels of blood pressure, LDL cholesterol, HDL cholesterol, triglycerides, and blood glucose. The ADA recommends that people with diabetes and those at risk be advised to perform at least 150 min/week of moderate-intensity aerobic physical activity at 50–70% of maximum heart rate. In the absence of contraindications, patients should also be encouraged to perform resistance training three times per week as this type of activity has been found to also help decrease insulin resistance. Should Linda be referred for cardiac screening before starting the recommended exercise routine? A recent ADA consensus statement

on this issue concluded that routine screening is not recommended.[35] Clinicians should assess their patients for conditions that might contraindicate certain types of exercise or predispose to injury, such as uncontrolled hypertension, severe autonomic neuropathy, severe peripheral neuropathy or history of foot lesions, and unstable proliferative retinopathy and use their clinical judgment before advising exercise. High-risk patients should be encouraged to start with short periods of low-intensity exercise and increase the intensity and duration slowly. Since Linda is already walking for 30 min, 3 days a week, she will be encouraged to increase the frequency to 5 days a week and will be advised to gradually include resistance training to her routine.

PHARMACOLOGICAL TREATMENT

Now, let us look at Linda's pharmaceutical management. Although each patient is unique and the treatment should be customized based individual needs, several treatment algorithms have been created to guide clinicians in selecting appropriate care for their patients with T2DM. Recently DeFronzo[2] proposed an evidence-based treatment algorithm. It considers the pathophysiology of T2DM and combines lifestyle modification with a triple combination of metformin, TZD and incretin mimetic used early in therapy to correct and possibly reverse the progressive β-cell failure already started since prediabetes state. Both the ADA and the American Association of Clinical Endocrinologists (AACE) have also advocated guidelines for the treatment of T2DM. These algorithms recognize that the progressive nature of β-cell decline requires the intensification of therapy over time using a stepwise approach to achieve and maintain glycemic targets. However, these two algorithms differ in their focus and depth. The

ADA guidelines are more general and unstratified. The choice of the next agent that can be used is determined in part by target A1c achievement, with significant consideration given to the more effective glycemia-lowering agent, years of commercial availability of the agent, and medication cost. The AACE algorithms are stratified based on A1c levels, they are more specific, distinguish care between medication-naïve and patients already being treated and place more emphasis on the effects of the agents on the pathophysiological abnormalities in T2DM. Based on these algorithms, the following criteria can generally be used by the clinician in partnership with the patient to guide the choice of hypoglycemic agents: the expected hemoglobin A1c lowering potential, consideration of both fasting and postprandial glucose levels as end points, potential side effects such as hypoglycemia and weight gain, ease of use, safety and tolerability, effect on comorbidity, and cost of therapy.[36,37]

For Linda, if we use the A1c stratification-based AACE algorithm, with her A1c at 7.9%, she should be on dual therapy. Maximizing the metformin dose would be a good choice. This agent is an insulin sensitizer, especially at the level of the liver. It may decrease her A1c by up to 1.5%, has a positive effect on lipids, is weight neutral, or may lead to mild weight loss in some patients. Although it can have gastrointestinal (GI) side effects, metformin is generally well tolerated by most patients without severe complications when clinical indications are followed and is inexpensive. Another insulin sensitizer, a TZD, could also be considered. These agents increase the sensitivity of muscle, fat, and liver to endogenous and exogenous insulin, therefore having an additive effect in combination with metformin. They have been shown to improve blood lipids, may help preserve β-cells, appear to have a more durable effect on glycemic control, and have an expected A1c decrease of

0.5–1.4%. However, they are relatively costly, require liver function monitoring, and weight gain can be a major problem for patients like Linda who are overweight or obese. In addition, more recently, caution has been advised in using this class of agent on the basis that they are associated with increased incidence of fractures.[38,39] Their role has also become controversial following publication of several meta-analyses suggesting that this class of medications is associated with significant increases in congestive heart failure and several ischemic cardiovascular events.[40] The US Food and Drug Administration (FDA) has issued a black box warning for both rosiglitazone and pioglitazone that states that these agents should not be used in people with heart failure. Additional warnings were added to rosiglitazone's package insert, which identify the potential increased risk of myocardial ischemia. More recently in 2011, France has suspended the use of piogiltazone and Germany has recommended not to start the drug on new patients based on an epidemiological study conducted in France which suggest an increased risk of bladder cancer with pioglitazone. In the United States, the FDA has informed the public that the use of pioglitazone for more than a year may be associated with an increased risk of bladder cancer and recommended not to use the drug in patients with active bladder cancer and to use it with caution in patients with prior history of bladder cancer. The FDA decision was based on a review of data from a planned five-year interim analysis of an ongoing, ten-year epidemiological study (FDA website: www.fda/DrugsSafety/ucm259150.htm, accessed on 10/21/11). Since the significance of these actions on clinical practice is still being debated by the experts, it is important for the clinician and the patient, together, to weigh the potential risks and benefits of using the TZDs. As for Linda, she is already on a guanide and tolerating the medication well; we will maximize the metformin dosage, which will help reduce her elevated fasting glucose.

According to the AACE algorithm,[37] the second component that should be added to her regimen can be an incretin mimetic, a dipeptidyl peptidase-4 (DPP-4) inhibitor, glinide, or sulfonylurea in that order. Even though the glipizide may help decrease her A1c by 1—2%, a sulfonylurea or a glinide would not be the most appropriate choice for Linda because of the potential weight gain of about 2 kg and the risk of hypoglycemia, although less so with the glinide. These drugs, although they increase insulin secretion, on a long-term basis, they do not preserve β-cell function. As a result, after an initial beneficial response in terms of A1c reduction with the sulfonylureas, there is a progressive rise in the A1c after 1.5—2 years.

The addition of either an incretin mimetic like exenatide or liragutide or a DPP-4 inhibitor like sitagliptin and/or saxagliptin should be considered for Linda. The incretin mimetics mimic or enhance actions of the natural incretin hormones that help regulate metabolism and eating behavior as described earlier. They have been shown to bring about clinically significant reductions in A1c of about 1.5%, when initiated in drug-naïve patients as monotherapy, or when added to existing drug therapies such as metformin, sulfonylureas or TZDs.[41] The available evidence suggests that they have a more potent blood-glucose lowering effect than the DPP-4 inhibitors,[41,42] possibly because they cause pharmacological rather than physiological levels of GLP-1 receptor stimulation. Possible side effects which tend to abate over time include gastrointestinal disturbances, episodes of nausea, vomiting, or diarrhea. There have been a very small number of cases indicating a possible risk for pancreatitis associated with use of this category of agents. However, the relationship is not clear at this time.

Similar to the incretin mimetics, but through a different mechanism, the DPP-4 inhibitors enhance the incretin system to help regulate glucose by affecting the β- and alpha-cells in the pancreas. In the body, the incretin hormones GLP-1 and GIP are rapidly degraded by DPP-4. The DPP-4 inhibitors prolong the effects of GLP-1 and GIP, increasing glucose-mediated insulin secretion and suppressing glucagon secretion. The DPP-4 inhibitors lower A1c levels by 0.6—0.9%. They are weight neutral and relatively well tolerated. However, the potential for this class of agents to interfere with immune function is of concern. Stuffy or runny nose and sore throat, upper respiratory infection, and headache are the most common side effects. Used as monotherapy, their effect on A1c is relatively modest (with mean reductions typically about −0.7% in drug-naïve patients).[41] When combined with metformin, A1c reductions of up to 2.0% have been reported in previous drug therapy-naive patients.[43]

If she is willing to take injections, at this time, the best choice of second agent for a patient like Linda would be an incretin mimetic as this could have the possible added benefit of promoting weight loss and may help preserve the β-cells she has left. The dosing regimens of the GLP-1 receptor agonists are relatively simple, but administration is by injection using pen devices. Exenatide is given twice-daily and liraglutide is a once-daily treatment. It is to be noted that there is a black box warning for liraglutide regarding the occurrence of dose-dependent and treatment-duration-dependent thyroid C-cell tumors at clinically relevant exposures in both genders of rats and mice. It is unknown whether liraglutide causes thyroid C-cell tumors, including medullary thyroid carcinoma (MTC), in humans. Liraglutide is contraindicated in patients with a personal or family history of MTC and in patients with Multiple Endocrine Neoplasia syndrome type 2 (MEN 2). It is unknown whether monitoring with serum calcitonin or thyroid ultrasound will mitigate human risk of thyroid C-cell tumors. Patients should be counseled regarding the risk and symptoms of thyroid tumors.[44]

WHEN TO ADJUST TREATMENT

To avoid the complications of diabetes, we should avoid clinician inertia and monitor therapy every 2–3 months. Effectiveness of therapy is evaluated with assessment of A1c, logbook data for SMBG records, documented and suspected hypoglycemia, and other potential adverse events (weight gain, fluid retention, and hepatic, renal, or cardiac disease) as well as monitoring of comorbidities. Regimen must be modified until the goal for pre- and post-meals as well as A1c level has been achieved. It is important to recognize that, in some circumstances, some patients may not achieve the desired goals of treatment. When this situation arises, reevaluating the treatment regimen may require assessment of barriers including income, health literacy, diabetes distress, depression, and competing demands, including those related to family responsibilities and dynamics. Corrective strategies may include change in pharmacological therapy; reinforcement of lifestyle interventions, especially the relationship between food and blood sugar; frequent contact with the patient; referral to a social worker or mental health professional; or utilization of Continuous Glucose monitoring device to better evaluate glycemia. For patients on insulin or on short-acting repaglinide, providing an algorithm for self-titration based on SMBG may be appropriate.

After augmenting her metformin and adding the second agent, the effectiveness of Linda's new regimen will be evaluated in 2–3 months with a repeat A1c, as well as the assessment of her logbook data showing results of both pre- and post-meals. If her A1c is not at target, a third agent could be considered, based on the AACE algorithm. Using this approach, the third agent can be a TZD, glinide, or sulfonylurea, recommended in that order to minimize the risk of hypoglycemia. Additionally, the combination of metformin,

and incretin mimetic, may partially help to counteract the possible weight gain associated with these three new agents.[37]

INITIATING INSULIN THERAPY

The addition of a third agent is usually not preferred in the ADA guidelines.[36] Considering the pathophysiology of T2DM, adding a third agent at this point may not be more effective in lowering glycemia, and may be more costly. After a 6-year history of diabetes and 2 years of untreated prediabetes, as well as years of hyperglycemia treated with an SFU, it is clear that Linda has lost a great deal of her endogenous β-cell function. Generally, as patients become more deficient in insulin they will require insulin supplementation and later replacement in order to achieve and maintain glycemic goals. Unfortunately, insulin treatment remains underused in T2DM, and when it is used, it is often delayed and/or not appropriately titrated. The most common patient barriers are fear of beginning an injection regimen, including the implications of insulin therapy concerning progression of the disease; feelings of personal failure; time; cost; and complications such as hypoglycemia. Many clinicians tend to use scare tactics as a way to bring patients to follow treatment recommendations. In my own experience, much of the fear of insulin can be mitigated if patients are educated early about the progressive nature of T2DM and the eventual need for insulin at some stage. My approach is to tell them that insulin is a hormone that will eventually need to be supplemented and later replaced as their diabetes progresses.

For patients who reach this stage, insulin therapy is often implemented stepwise, based on their glycemic profile. A common cascade of insulin supplementation regimen includes: basal insulin, using a long-acting insulin analog (glargine, detemir), generally given once daily, or once daily premixed rapid-acting analog and protamine (NovoLog Mix, Humalog Mix) with the largest meal, along with secretagogues and sensitizers or incretins. Supplementation with basal insulin regimen offers the advantage of its simplicity and requiring only one daily injection usually given at bedtime. The dose is slowly titrated upward, based on fasting blood sugar. Such a regimen allows patients like Linda to improve glycemic control while becoming used to managing insulin self-injection. One drawback of this regimen is that it does not provide mealtime glucose control, so it works best in patients who have sufficient endogenous glucose production remaining to take care of mealtime insulin requirements. Eventually most patients on this regimen will require mealtime insulin. This is when short- or rapid-acting insulin is added at the largest meal to correct postprandial glucose excursions. The primary advantage of this approach is that patients can stay on the same regimen for a longer period, as both mealtime and fasting glucose are addressed. As patients become more insulin deficient, they can be transitioned to basal insulin with rapid-acting at breakfast and the largest meal, split-mixed regimen, or premixed insulin given twice daily with breakfast and dinner. When patients require coverage of more than one meal with prandial insulin the secretagogue, such as sulfonylurea or glinide, is no longer needed; however, insulin sensitizers such as metformin or TZDs can be continued to decrease insulin resistance. Later, when the secretory capacity of the β-cells worsens, the patient is moved to full insulin replacement.

The most efficient and physiological way to replace insulin is the basal-bolus regimen, also referred to as multiple daily injections. Several insulin replacement regimens can be initiated, such as split-mixed dosing with neutral protamine hagedorn insulin (NPH) and rapid-acting insulin, basal-bolus regimen, or using premeal rapid-acting insulin analogs—aspart (Novo-Log), lispro (Humalog), or glulisine (Apidra)—together with the long-acting insulin analog glargine (Lantus) or detemir (Levemir) at each meal. In this regimen, the dosage of rapid-acting insulin can be constant or the patient can be given a dosage algorithm or guidelines to cover their carbohydrate intake as well as supplemental dosages to cover blood sugars outside the target range. This option is good for patients interested in tighter control, in need of flexibility, willing and having the ability to test their blood sugar three to four times per day. Three-times-daily premixed insulin can be used effectively for patients who are unwilling or unable to take more than three daily injections and have stable activity levels as well as consistent intake of carbohydrates.

Each regimen has advantages and challenges. It is important to keep in mind that patients can be brought to target using either aggressive or conservative titration algorithms with any of these regimens. Both the ADA and the AACE have published guidelines for initiating and titrating insulin for patients with T2DM, including how to transition these patients to a basal-bolus regimen.[23,36,37] These should be used only as guides as the selection of a regimen needs to be tailored to the needs and abilities of individual patients, who should be involved in the selection process. When a patient begins insulin therapy, SMBG should be increased in frequency. For patients starting basal insulin therapy at bedtime or premixed insulin therapy before dinner, the morning fasting blood glucose levels should be monitored daily. For each additional injection of insulin, SMBG should be increased in frequency to ensure successful titration. SMBG should be carried out three or more times daily for patients on insulin replacement therapy with occasional postprandial and 2–3 a.m. testing done before visits or if A1c not consistent with premeal values. Advancement to insulin therapy is also an important opportunity to reinforce DSME with regard to lifestyle modification, meal planning, physical activity, weight management, and other important aspects of self-care such as prevention, identification, and treatment of hypoglycemia.

INSULIN DELIVERY DEVICES

Some of the patient barriers to initiation of insulin therapy have been fear of needles, difficulty managing with the syringe and vial system, and association of syringes with drug addiction. A range of devices are available, most of which have a very discreet appearance resembling a pen and are more acceptable and convenient for patients.

Some patients with T2DM using basal-bolus insulin therapy may benefit from use of an insulin pump (continuous subcutaneous insulin infusion). These battery-operated devices provide a more physiological delivery of insulin. They can be preprogrammed to deliver continuous microdoses of rapid-acting insulin by pulses termed "basal rate". Boluses of larger amounts of insulin are taken by the patient as needed to cover the carbohydrate in meals or snacks and to counteract hyperglycemia. An insulin pump can provide maximal flexibility with regard to mealtimes, size of meals, exercise, or travel. Several of these devices are available with various insulin delivery features.

CONCLUSIONS

T2DM is characterized by multiple genetic defects causing insulin resistance and progressive insulin deficiency. The evolving knowledge of the pathophysiology of diabetes is giving way to the development of various agents to address the spectrum of these defects. Treatment should be based on the pathophysiology of the disease and needs to consider factors such as expected hemoglobin A1c decrease, blood sugar control pre- and post-meal, patient tolerance, effect on weight and comorbidities, and cost of therapy. Clinicians must effectively use the available published guidelines as well as lifestyle intervention, DSME and regular monitoring to aggressively treat their patients with prediabetes and T2DM beginning at the onset of abnormal glycemia.

References

1. Centers for Disease Control and Prevention. *National Diabetes Fact Sheet: national estimates and general information on diabetes and prediabetes in the United States, 2011.* Atlanta, GA: U.S. Department of Health and Human Services, Centers for Disease Control and Prevention, http://diabetes.niddk.nih.gov/dm/pubs/statistics/#fast; 2011. Accessed on 2.12/11.
2. De Fronzo RA. From the triumvirate to the ominous octet: A new paradigm for the treatment of type 2 diabetes mellitus. *Diabetes* 2009;**58**:773—95.
3. UK Prospective Diabetes Study (UKPDS) Group. Intensive blood- glucose control with sulphonylureas or insulin compared with conventional treatment and risk of complications in patients with type 2 diabetes (UKPDS 33). *Lancet* 1998;**352**:837—53.
4. Flint A, Raben A, Astrup A, Holst JJ. Glucagon-like peptide 1 promotes satiety and suppresses energy intake in humans. *J Clin Invest* 1998;**101**:515—20.
5. Kieffer TJ, Habener JF. The glucagon-like peptides. *Endocr Rev* 1999;**20**:876—913.
6. Butler AE, Janson J, Bonner-Weir S, Ritzel R, Rizza RA, Butler PC. Beta cell deficit and increased beta cell apoptosis in humans with type 2 diabetes. *Diabetes* 2003;**52**:102—10.
7. Ziegler D, Rathmann W, Dickhaus T, Meisinger C, Mielck A. KORA Study Group. Prevalence of polyneuropathy in pre-diabetes and diabetes is associated with abdominal obesity and macroangiopathy: the MONICA/KORA Augsburg Surveys S2 and S3. *Diabetes Care* 2008;**31**:464—9.
8. Smith AG, Russell J, Feldman EL, Goldstein J, Peltier A, Smith S, Hamwi J, Pollari D, Bixby B, Howard J, Singleton JR. Lifestyle intervention for prediabetic neuropathy. *Diabetes Care* 2006;**6**:415—6.
9. Tuomilehto J, Lindström J, Eriksson JG, Valle TT, Hämäläinen H, Ilanne-Parikka P, Keinänen-Kiukaanniemi S, Laakso M, Louheranta A, Rastas M, Salminen V, Uusitupa M. Finnish Diabetes Prevention Study Group. Prevention of type 2 diabetes mellitus by

changes in lifestyle among subjects with impaired glucose tolerance. *N Engl J Med* 2001;**344**:1343—50.

10. Knowler WC, Barrett-Connor E, Fowler SE, Hamman RF, Lachin JM, Walker EA, Nathan DM. Diabetes Prevention Program Research Group. Reduction in the incidence of type 2 diabetes with lifestyle intervention or metformin. *N Engl J Med* 2002;**346**:393—403.

11. American Diabetes Aassociation. Standards of Medical Care. *Diabetes Care* 2011;**34**(Suppl. 1).

12. American College of Endocrinology and the American Association of Clinical Endocrinologists. Prediabetes Consensus Statement, *Endocr Pract* 2008;**14** (No. 7).

13. Knowler WC, Barrett-Connor E, Fowler SE, Hamman RF, Lachin JM, Walker EA, Nathan DM. Reduction in the incidence of type 2 diabetes with lifestyle intervention or metformin. *N Engl J Med* 2002;**346**:393—403.

14. Defronzo R, Banerji MA, Bray G, Buchana T, Clement S, Henry R, Kitabshi A, Mudaliar S, Musi N, Ratner RE, Reaven P, Schwenke D. Reduced insulin secretion/insulin resistance (disposition) index is the primary determinant of glucose intolerance in the pre-diabetic state: results from ACT NOW. Proc 68th Annual Meeting of the American Diabetes Association, 2008 (Abstract 151).

15. Xiang AH, Peters RK, Kjos SL, Marroquin A, Goico J, Ochoa C, Kawakubo M, Buchanan TA. Effect of pioglitazone on pancreatic beta cell function and diabetes risk in Hispanic women with prior gestational diabetes. *Diabetes* 2006;**55**:517—22.

16. Buchanan TA, Xiang AH, Peters RK, Kjos SL, Marroquin A, Goico J, Ochoa C, Tan S, Berkowitz K, Hodis HN, Azen SP. Preservation of pancreatic beta-cell function and prevention of type 2 diabetes by pharmacological treatment of insulin resistance in high-risk Hispanic women. *Diabetes* 2002;**51**:2796—803.

17. Drucker DJ. Enhancing incretin action for the treatment of type 2 diabetes. *Diabetes Care* 2003;**26**:2929—40.

18. Utzschneider KM, Tong J, Montgomery B, Udayasankar J, Gerchman F, Marcovina SM, Watson CE, Ligueros-Saylan MA, Foley JE, Holst JJ, Deacon CF, Kahn SE. The dipeptidyl peptidase-4 inhibitor vildagliptin improves beta cell function and insulin sensitivity in subjects with impaired fasting glucose. *Diabetes Care* 2008;**31**:108—13.

19. Mari A, Degn K, Brock B, Rungby J, Ferrannini E, Schmitz O. Effects of the long-acting human glucagon-like peptide-1 analog liraglutide on beta-cell function in normal living conditions. *Diabetes Care* 2007;**30**:2032—3.

20. Horton ES. Can newer therapies delay the progression of type 2 diabetes mellitus? *Endocr Pract* 2008;**14**:625—38.

21. Colagiuri S, Cull CA, Holman RR. Are lower fasting plasma glucose levels at diagnosis of type 2 diabetes associated with improved outcomes? U.K. Prospective Diabetes Study 61. *Diabetes Care* 2002;**25**:1410—7.

22. Holman RR, Paul SK, Bethel MA, Neil HA, Matthews DR. Long-term follow-up after tight control of blood pressure in type 2 diabetes. *N Engl J Med* 2008;**359**:1577—89.

23. Rodbard HW, Blonde L, Braithwaite SS, Brett EM, Cobin RH, Handelsman Y, Hellman R, Jellinger PS, Jovanovic LG, Levy P, Mechanick JI, Zangeneh F. American Association of Clinical Endocrinologists medical guidelines for clinical practice for the management of diabetes mellitus. *Endocr Pract* 2007;**13**(Suppl. 1):1—68.

24. Duckworth W, Abraira C, Moritz T, Reda D, Emanuele N, Reaven PD, Zieve FJ, Marks J, Davis SN, Hayward R, Warren SR, Goldman S, McCarren M, Vitek ME, Henderson WG, Huang GD, VADT Investigators. Glucose control and vascular complications in veterans with type 2 diabetes. *N Engl J Med* 2009;**360**:129—39.

25. Moritz T, Duckworth W, Abraira C. Veterans Affairs diabetes trial—corrections. *N Engl J Med* 2009;**361**:1024—5. 62.

26. Patel A, MacMahon S, Chalmers J, Neal B, Billot L, Woodward M, Marre M, Cooper M, Glasziou P, Grobbee D, Hamet P, Harrap S, Heller S, Liu L, Mancia G, Mogensen CE, Pan C, Poulter N, Rodgers A, Williams B, Bompoint S, de Galan BE, Joshi R, Travert F, ADVANCE Collaborative Group. Intensive blood glucose control and vascular outcomes in patients with type 2 diabetes. *N Engl J Med* 2008;**358**:2560—72.

27. Ismail-Beigi F, Craven T, Banerji MA, Basile J, Calles J, Cohen RM, Cuddihy R, Cushman WC, Genuth S, Grimm Jr RH, Hamilton BP, Hoogwerf B, Karl D, Katz L, Krikorian A, O'Connor P, Pop-Busui R, Schubart U, Simmons D, Taylor H, Thomas A, Weiss D, Hramiak I, ACCORD trial group. Effect of intensive treatment of hyperglycaemia on microvascular outcomes in type 2 diabetes: an analysis of the ACCORD randomized trial. *Lancet* 2010;**376**:419—30.

28. ACCORD Study Group, ACCORD Eye Study Group, Chew EY, Ambrosius WT, Davis MD, Danis RP, Gangaputra S, Greven CM, Hubbard L, Esser BA, Lovato JF, Perdue LH, Goff Jr DC, Cushman WC, Ginsberg HN, Elam MB, Genuth S, Gerstein HC, Schubart U, Fine LJ. Effects of medical therapies on retinopathy progression in type 2 diabetes. *N Engl J Med* 2010;**363**:233—44.

29. Action to Control Cardiovascular Risk in Diabetes Study Group, Gerstein HC, Miller ME, Byington RP, Goff Jr DC, Bigger JT, Buse JB, Cushman WC,

Genuth S, Ismail-Beigi F, Grimm Jr RH, Probstfield JL, Simons-Morton DG, Friedewald WT. Effects of intensive glucose lowering in type 2 diabetes. *N Engl J Med* 2008;**358**:2545−59.

30. Foster GD, Wyatt HR, Hill JO, McGuckin BG, Brill C, Mohammed BS, Szapary PO, Rader DJ, Edman JS, Klein SA. Randomized trial of a low-carbohydrate diet for obesity. *N Engl J Med* 2003;**348**:2082−90.

31. Stern L, Iqbal N, Seshadri P, Chicano KL, Daily DA, McGrory J, Williams M, Gracely EJ, Samaha FF. The effects of low-carbohydrate versus conventional weight loss diets in severely obese adults: one-year follow-up of a randomized trial. *Ann Intern Med* 2004;**140**:778−85.

32. Foster GD, Wyatt HR, Hill JO, Makris AP, Rosenbaum DL, Brill C, Stein RI, Mohammed BS, Miller B, Rader DJ, Zemel B, Wadden TA, Tenhave T, Newcomb CW, Klein S. Weight and metabolic outcomes after 2 years on a low-carbohydrate versus low-fat diet: a randomized trial. *Ann Intern Med* 2010;**153**:147−57.

33. Gardner CD, Kiazand A, Alhassan S, Kim S, Stafford RS, Balise RR, Kraemer HC, King AC. Comparison of the Atkins, Zone, Ornish, and LEARN diets for change in weight and related risk factors among overweight premenopausal women: the A TO Z Weight Loss Study: a randomized trial. *JAMA* 2007;**297**:969−77.

34. Shai I, Schwarzfuchs D, Henkin Y, Shahar DR, Witkow S, Greenberg I, Golan R, Fraser D, Bolotin A, Vardi H, Tangi-Rozental O, Zuk-Ramot R, Sarusi B, Brickner D, Schwartz Z, Sheiner E, Marko R, Katorza E, Thiery J, Fiedler GM, Bluher M, Stumvoll M, Stampfer MJ. Dietary Intervention Randomized Controlled Trial (DIRECT) Group. Weight loss with a low-carbohydrate, Mediterranean, or low-fat diet. *N Engl J Med* 2008;**359**:229−41.

35. Bax JJ, Young LH, Frye RL, Bonow RO, Steinberg HO, Barrett EJ. ADA. Screening for coronary artery disease in patients with diabetes. *Diabetes Care* 2007;2729−36.

36. Nathan DM, Buse JB, Davidson MB, Ferrannini E, Holman RR, Sherwin R, Zinman B. Medical management of hyperglycemia in type 2 diabetes: a consensus algorithm for the initiation and adjustment of therapy: a consensus statement of the American Diabetes Association and the European Association for the Study of Diabetes. *Diabetes Care* 2009;**32**:193−203.

37. Rodbard HW, Jellinger PS, Davidson JA, Einhorn D, Garber AJ, Grunberger G, Handelsman Y, Horton ES, Lebovitz H, Levy P, Moghissi ES, Schwartz SS. Glycemic Control Algorithm. *Endocr Pract* 2009;**15** No. 6.

38. Dormuth CR, Carney G, Carleton B, Bassett K, Wright JM. Thiazolidinediones and fractures in men and women. *Arch Intern Med* 2009;**169**:1395−402.

39. Outcome Progression Trial [ADOPT] Study Group. Rosiglitazone-associated fractures in type 2 diabetes: an analysis from A Diabetes Outcome Progression Trial (ADOPT). *Diabetes Care* 2008;**31**:845−51.

40. Nissen SE, Wolski K. An updated meta-analysis of risk for myocardial infarction and cardiovascular mortality. *Arch Intern Med* 2010;**170**(14):1191−201.

41. Amori RE, Lau J, Pittas AG. Efficacy and safety of incretin therapy in type 2 diabetes: systematic review and meta-analysis. *JAMA* 2007;**298**(2):194−206.

42. Defronzo RA, Fleck PR, Wilson CA, Mekki Q, on behalf of the Alogliptin Study Group. Efficacy and safety of the dipeptidyl peptidase-4 inhibitor alogliptin in patients with type 2 diabetes and inadequate glycemic control a randomized, double-blind, placebo-controlled study. *Diabetes Care* 2008;**31**:2315−7.

43. Goldstein BJ, Feinglos MN, Lunceford JK, Johnson J, Williams-Herman D, for the Sitagliptin Study Group. Effect of initial combination therapy with sitagliptin, a dipeptidyl peptidase-4 inhibitor, and metformin on glycemic control in patients with type 2 diabetes. *Diabetes Care* 2007;**30**:1979−87.

44. Liraglutide prescribing information at http://www.victoza.com/pdf/Victoza_ComboPI_1-4-11.pdf, accessed on 2/27/11.

Prediabetes: Prevalence, Pathogenesis, and Recognition of Enhanced Risk

Alok K. Gupta*, Ajay Menon†, Meghan Brashear*, William D. Johnson*

*Pennington Biomedical Research Center, Louisiana State University System, Baton Rouge, LA, USA
†University of Washington, Seattle, WA

Nutritional and Therapeutic Interventions for Diabetes and Metabolic Syndrome
DOI: 10.1016/B978-0-12-385083-6.00005-X

BACKGROUND

Type 2 diabetes, hypertension, dyslipidemia, and overweight or obese status are universally recognized chronic conditions which are, without reservation, afflicting an ever increasing proportion of the population at large.[1,2] All of these conditions individually, and in a variety of combinations with each other, also tend to increase the absolute risk for sudden catastrophic adverse cardiovascular events.[3-9] The treatment of each of these diseased states: glycemic control for diabetes, reduction in blood pressure for hypertension, appropriate correction of the disordered lipoprotein fraction in dyslipidemia and weight loss for the overweight and obese, substantially decrease the risks for a sudden catastrophic adverse cardiovascular event.[10,11] Despite rapid and meaningful strides made with the treatments for these chronic conditions (with the exception of obesity), the prevalence of these chronic conditions and the consequent occurrence of cardiovascular adverse events are still alarmingly high.[12]

There is also a curious phenomenon: two out of three of the sudden catastrophic cardiovascular adverse events which result in a death (myocardial infarction and cerebrovascular accident), occur in apparently healthy individuals with no known overt heart disease.[13,14] Thus, in order to prevent sudden death in healthy individuals, a more appropriate response would be to recognize the risk for developing chronic disease. It would also be prudent to intervene with the pre-disease states: prediabetes, prehypertension, or coexisting prediabetes and prehypertension and prevent their progression into full blown disease(s): type 2 diabetes or/ and hypertension. A high prevalence of prediabetes, prehypertension,[15] coexisting prediabetes and prehypertension[16] among the healthy adults in the US has recently been recognized. These pre-disease states, besides being at risk for conversion into a higher cardiovascular

disease risk state due to full blown chronic disease,[17-20] are by themselves being recognized as being on a pathway towards accelerated cardiovascular events.[15,16] Prediabetes which converts into type 2 diabetes at a variable rate of 6-29% within 4 years[19,20] has some perception of escalating the risk for cardiovascular disease.

In the present chapter we will describe the prevalence, pathogenesis and recognition of risk for one of these pre-disease states: prediabetes. At the beginning of each section we will detail our unpublished work in a representative sample of healthy adults in the US and will by the end of the chapter provide ample evidence supporting our assertion that these otherwise healthy adults with prediabetes are on an accelerated pathway for adverse cardiovascular events.

PREVALENCE

Methods

Study Sample

Analyses were conducted using the data from the United States National Health and Nutrition Examination Survey (US NHANES), years 1999 through 2006. NHANES uses a complex, multistage, probability sampling design, to select a representative sample of the non-institutionalized, civilian US population. Sample weights assigned to each participant allow for the development of good national prevalence estimates. The National Center for Health Statistics ethics review board approved the original survey protocols. An informed consent was obtained from all NHANES participants. Trained personnel conducted home interviews to obtain reliable demographic, socioeconomic, dietary, and health-related information. A mobile exam center was used to obtain anthropometric measurements and to secure a fasting blood draw. Medical personnel were utilized to obtain medical, dental, and physiological measurements, as well as the results from the laboratory tests. Details on these and other assessments can be accessed at the NHANES website.[21]

Sample Methods

Participants were required to come to a mobile examination clinic before 9 a.m. after fasting for at least 9 h. If they arrived having fasted for less than 8.5 h, they received an analytical sampling weight equal to zero, as part of the NHANES protocol. Blood was drawn from an antecubital vein of the left arm. Fasting plasma glucose (FPG) was assessed by the hexokinase method. Insulin, triglycerides (TG), and high-density lipoprotein cholesterol (HDL-C) were also assayed from the fasting serum samples. Homeostasis model assessment was used to measure insulin resistance (HOMA-IR) using the formula: fasting serum insulin (micro units per milliliter) × fasting plasma glucose (milligrams per deciliter)/405. Blood pressure was measured after the participant had rested quietly for 5 min. Three consecutive blood pressure readings were obtained. The average of these was recorded as resting blood pressure. Weight was measured with participants wearing minimal clothing. Height was measured using a fixed wall stadiometer, heels together, and arms by the side with the eyes in the Frankfort plane. Waist circumference was measured with the participant in a standing position at the end of normal expiration using a steel measuring tape placed at the high point of the iliac crest to the nearest 0.1 cm. Race or ethnicity was derived from questions about race and Hispanic origin (non-Hispanic White, Mexican American, non-Hispanic Black and "Other").

Diagnosis of Prediabetes

For purposes of this investigation, in keeping with the guidelines by the American Diabetes Association (ADA), normoglycemia, prediabetes and diabetes in healthy disease-free adults were defined as fasting serum glucose levels below 100 mg/dl, 100−125 mg/dl and equal to or greater than 126 mg/dl, respectively.[22]

Sample Description

This investigation is based on a subset of 5,574 participants from the 1999−2006 NHANES

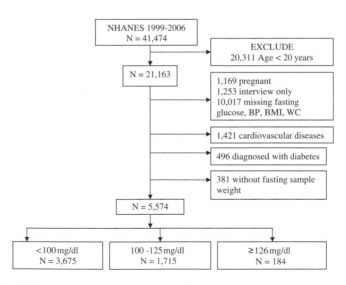

FIGURE 5.1 Schema for Data Inclusion into the Analytical Sample.

samples which included 41,474 participants (see Figure 5.1). There were 20,311 adults aged 20 years and older (21,163 participants under 20 years of age were excluded). Other exclusions included: 1,169 for an ongoing pregnancy, 1,253 for completing only the interview portion of the survey, 10,398 for not having had fasting blood glucose, body weight, body mass index or waist circumference measurements and 1,421 for having a history of coronary heart disease, congestive heart failure, angina, myocardial infarction, stroke or cancer. Finally, an additional 496 were not included for having a diagnosis of type 2 diabetes. Thus 14,737 were excluded from a subset of 20,311 adults. With a total of 35,900 of 41,474 participants not meeting the inclusion criteria, a final sample of disease-free healthy adults for this report was 5,574.

Statistical Analysis

Data are summarized as counts and percentages $\pm$ standard error of percentage for categorical variables and means $\pm$ standard error of mean for continuous variables. Prevalence (%) estimates the percentage of healthy US men and women with a condition at the time their data were collected and a mean estimates the average value of a characteristic in healthy US adults. All analyses were conducted using weighted procedures specific for sample survey data in order to account for the complex NHANES sampling design. The calculations were performed using the statistical software SAS® Version 9.1, SAS Institute, Inc, Cary, NC. Large sample z-tests were employed to assess statistical significance at $p \leq 0.05$.

RESULTS

Epidemiology of Prediabetes

United States (1999–2006: NHANES Study)

During the years 1999–2006, based on a representative sample of US adults (NHANES) evaluated after 8.5 h of fasting, the overall prevalence of normoglycemia, prediabetes, and undiagnosed type-2 diabetes in the disease-free adult population was $71.0 \pm 1.0\%$, $26.8 \pm 1.0\%$ and $2.3 \pm 0.2\%$, respectively, as shown in Table 5.1. The prevalence of prediabetes in adults increased 50% during 1999–2006 (22.1% in 1999–2000; 33.1% in 2005–2006; $p < 0.0001$). Men had higher prevalence than women (33.5% vs 20.1%; $p < 0.0001$). Prevalence increased with age (17.5% in 20–39 years vs 43.4% in 70+ years), BMI (14.6% for between 18.5 and $< 25 \text{ kg/m}^2$; 31.8% for between 25 and $< 30 \text{ kg/m}^2$; 35.4% for $> 30 \text{ kg/m}^2$; $p < 0.0001$) and waist circumference (males: 28.8% for $< 102 \text{ cm}$; 42.0% for $> 102 \text{ cm}$; $p < 0.0001$; and females: 8.2% for $< 88 \text{ cm}$; 30.2% for $> 88 \text{ cm}$; $p < 0.0001$). Non-Hispanic Black Americans (20.1%) had the lowest, while Mexican Americans (32.5%) had highest prevalence. Former smokers and those who consumed 5+ drinks per day had higher prevalence of prediabetes ($p < 0.0001$).

Australia (2002: ADOL Study)

A national sample (11,247 participants, ≥ 25 years in age living in 42 randomly selected areas from the six states and the Northern Territory) in a cross-sectional survey using the 75-g oral glucose tolerance test (75-g OGTT) to assess fasting and 2-h plasma glucose concentrations (World Health Organization diagnostic criteria: WHO) exhibited an overall prevalence of prediabetes at 16.4%. With men exhibiting an overall higher prevalence when compared to women, 5.7% had impaired fasting glucose (IFG), 8.0% had impaired glucose tolerance (IGT) and 2.6% had both. At the time of this publication (2002) this was the highest reported prevalence in a developed country.[23]

Europe (1999: DECODE Study)

In a pooled analysis using 75-g OGTT, prediabetes was assessed in 29,108 subjects aged ≥ 30 years. Total prevalence, IFG, IGT and both IFG

TABLE 5.1 Prevalence ± SEM (%) of Normoglycemia, Prediabetes and Undiagnosed Diabetes among Healthy Adults in the US Population

Data mean ± SEM	N	Glucose level		
		< 100 (mg/dl)	100−125 (mg/dl)	≥ 126 (mg/dl)
Overall	5,574	71.0% ± 1.0%	26.8% ± 1.0%	2.3% ± 0.2%
Survey year				
1999−2000	1,362	76.0% ± 1.6%	22.1% ± 1.7%	1.9% ± 0.4%
2001−2002	1,542	69.0% ± 1.4%	28.3% ± 1.5%	2.6% ± 0.3%
2003−2004	1,348	71.5% ± 2.5%	26.4% ± 2.6%	2.2% ± 0.4%
2005−2006	1,322	64.4% ± 2.9%	33.1% ± 2.6%	2.4% ± 0.5%
SEX				
Male	2,842	63.8% ± 1.4%	33.5% ± 1.4%	2.6% ± 0.3%
Female	2,732	78.0% ± 0.9%	20.1% ± 0.9%	1.9% ± 0.2%
AGE GROUP				
20−39 (y)	2,269	81.9% ± 1.0%	17.5% ± 1.0%	0.5% ± 0.2%
40−59 (y)	1,900	64.8% ± 1.6%	32.5% ± 1.6%	2.7% ± 0.5%
60−69 (y)	741	51.8% ± 2.5%	41.4% ± 2.5%	6.7% ± 1.2%
≥ 70 (y)	664	49.4% ± 2.8%	43.4% ± 3.0%	7.2% ± 1.4%
RACE/ETHNICITY				
Non-Hispanic White	2,720	70.8% ± 1.3%	27.0% ± 1.2%	2.2% ± 0.2%
Non-Hispanic Black	1,093	77.2% ± 1.7%	20.1% ± 1.5%	2.7% ± 0.4%
Mexican American	1,318	65.0% ± 1.8%	32.5% ± 1.6%	2.5% ± 0.4%
Other	443	69.6% ± 3.0%	28.2% ± 2.9%	2.2% ± 0.6%
SMOKING				
Never smoker	2,963	73.4% ± 1.2%	24.9% ± 1.1%	1.7% ± 0.3%
Former smoker	1,308	62.8% ± 2.0%	33.4% ± 1.9%	3.8% ± 0.6%
Current smoker	1,296	73.6% ± 1.8%	24.4% ± 1.8%	2.0% ± 0.4%
ALCOHOL CONSUMPTION				
1−4 drinks per day	3,064	72.0% ± 1.1%	25.8% ± 1.0%	2.2% ± 0.3%
5+ drinks per day	651	68.8% ± 3.0%	29.1% ± 3.0%	2.1% ± 0.6%
Non-drinker	1,594	68.4% ± 1.7%	29.1% ± 1.6%	2.5% ± 0.5%

and IGT were respectively at 18.8%, 6.9%, 8.8%, 3.1%.[24]

Hong Kong (1998)

Using the modified criteria published by ADA (1997) the overall total prevalence in 1,486 working Chinese subjects living in Hong Kong was of 8.1%. Men and women ranging from 18 to 66 years had IFG (0.9%), IGT (6.1%), or both IFG and IGT (1.1%).[25]

Mauritius (1999)

A group of 3,229 subjects, 25–77 years of age, had 266 subjects with IFG, 607 subjects with IGT and 118 with both translated to a total prevalence of prediabetes at 29%: with 6.7%, 18.7%, 3.6%, respectively, with IFG, IGT and both.[26]

Pima Indians in the United States (2000)

In an ethnic group with a very high prevalence of diabetes mellitus, 5,023 subjects over 15 years in age had a total prevalence of prediabetes, IFG, IGT and both IFG and IGT were at 15.1%, 1.9%, 10.7%, 2.5%, respectively.[27]

Sweden (1998)

A group of 1,843 subjects, 24–77 years of age, had a total prevalence of prediabetes at 37.6% with 9.7%, 20.3%, 7.6%, respectively, with IFG, IGT and both IFG and IGT.[28]

United States (1997)

In a representative sample of the population of 2,844 US subjects aged 40–74 years 19.9% had prediabetes, 4.4% IFG, 11.6% IGT and 3.9% both IFG and IGT.[29] A more recent study using 1,547 adult NHANES participants (> 18 years of age) from 2005 to 2006 without a diagnosis of type 2 diabetes, 19.4% had IFG, 5.4% had IGT, and 9.8% had both IFG and IGT. The overall prevalence of prediabetes was 34.6%.[30] This is in close agreement with our analyses which spanned the years 1999 to 2006 (Table 5.1).

The prevalence data from all over the world beginning with the US (1997), Sweden and Hong Kong (1998), Europe and Mauritius (1999), Pima Indians (2000) and Australia (2002), using the ADA criteria (1997: IFG 110–125 mg/dl) for their definition, place the prevalence of prediabetes in a range from 8.1–37.6%. Our most recent analyses (2010), using current ADA diagnostic criteria (2003: FPG 100–125 mg/dl), places the prevalence of prediabetes among healthy adults at an average of 26.8% during the years 1999–2006, with an alarming increase from 22.1% in 1999–2000 to 33.1% in 2005–2006. With one in every four seemingly healthy adults in the US currently in a state of prediabetes, understanding its pathophysiology, recognizing the associated risks, and devising modalities for intervention has become paramount.

PATHOGENESIS

Diagnosis

Diabetes mellitus: from the two Greek words (diabetes: "a siphon" or "a passer of"; and mellitus: "sweet") literally means "a passer of sweet urine". The Greeks thus diagnosed diabetes when the urine of the patient (because of its glucose content) attracted flies and bees. The ancient Chinese, using the same rationale, tested for diabetes by observing whether ants were attracted to an individual's urine. It was subsequently recognized that glucose begins to appear in the urine only after the blood glucose rises beyond a certain concentration: the glucose threshold in the kidneys.[31] The diagnosis for diabetes mellitus is therefore based upon: (1) Symptoms of diabetes plus casual plasma glucose concentration $\geq 200\,mg/dl$ (11.1 mmol; casual is defined as any time of day without regard to time since last meal). The classic symptoms of diabetes include polyuria, polydipsia, and unexplained weight loss. Or (2). FPG $\geq 126\,mg/dl$ (7.0 mmol/l; fasting is defined as no caloric intake for at least 8 h). Or

(3) 2-h post-load glucose ≥ 200 mg/dl (11.1 mmol/l) during an OGTT. (WHO criteria—the test is performed by using a glucose load containing the equivalent of 75 g anhydrous glucose dissolved in water).[32]

Prediabetes is a condition with blood glucose concentrations considerably below the renal threshold, and therefore cannot be recognized by testing for glucose in the urine. It is an asymptomatic clinical state where the FPG levels are ≥ 100 mg/dl (5.6 mmol/l) but < 126 mg/dl (7.0 mmol/l) and/or 2-h values during an oral glucose tolerance test (OGTT) of ≥ 140 mg/dl (7.8 mmol/l) but < 200 mg/dl (11.1 mmol/l). Thus, the current categories of glucose values are as follows: normal fasting glucose < 100 mg/dl (5.6 mmol/l); impaired fasting glucose (IFG)–glucose 100–125 mg/dl (5.6–6.9 mmol/l); provisional diagnosis of diabetes mellitus—glucose ≥ 126 mg/dl (7.0 mmol/l). The corresponding categories when the OGTT is used are the following: normal glucose tolerance—2-h post-load glucose < 140 mg/dl (7.8 mmol/l); IGT—2-h post-load glucose 140–199 mg/dl (7.8–11.1 mmol/l); provisional diagnosis of diabetes mellitus—2-h post-load glucose ≥ 200 mg/dl (11.1 mmol/l). The diagnosis of diabetes mellitus must be confirmed with a repeat OGTT.[32]

Pathophysiology

The traditional primary defects responsible for the development and progression of type 2 diabetes are pancreatic beta-cell dysfunction (leading to an impaired insulin secretion), hepatic and muscle insulin resistance (leading to an increased nocturnal glucose production by the liver and decreased peripheral glucose utilization by the muscles, respectively). These underlying deficits, impaired insulin secretion along with the hepatic and muscle insulin resistance, result in the distinct metabolic derangements which are the hallmarks for type 2 diabetes. A multitude of other factors, which

also appear to influence the gradually increasing insulin resistance, include an adipocyte insulin resistance (adipose tissue: increased lipolysis), increased glucagon secretion (pancreas: alpha-cell dysfunction), reduced incretin secretion/sensitivity (gastrointestinal: endocrine hormonal imbalance), enhanced glucose reabsorption (kidney: early glomerular functional alterations), and central nervous system insulin resistance (brain: neurotransmitter dysfunction). Beta-cell failure seen as the major determinant of the decreased insulin secretion is now known to occur much earlier in the natural history of type 2 diabetes.[33]

Prediabetes, an asymptomatic condition with subtle changes in fasting and/or post-meal serum glucose concentration/s, is an early stage in this continuum. IFG which manifests as fasting hyperglycemia (FPG 100–125 mg/dl) is due to an inadequate basal insulin secretion combined with an inappropriate insulin sensitivity of the liver, which fails to down regulate nocturnal hepatic glucose production. IGT, which is reflected as postprandial hyperglycemia (2-h post-load glucose 140–199 mg/dl), is due to an inadequate insulin response to serum glucose load primarily due to peripheral skeletal muscle insulin resistance.[34] Both prediabetes (a pre-disease state for diabetes) and type 2 diabetes are thus heterogeneous entities influenced by adipose tissue dysfunction, pancreatic alpha- and beta-cell impairment, gastrointestinal endocrine secretory imbalance, altered renal reabsorption, central nervous system neurotransmitter disruption, along with hepatic and muscle insulin resistance.

Adiposity Influences Prediabetes

Clinical measures of adiposity, body mass index (BMI) and waist circumference (WC) profoundly impact prediabetes.

As shown in Figure 5.2, a graduated increase in overall prevalence of prediabetes was observed with increasing BMI: lean (BMI < 18.5 kg/m^2) $13.9 \pm 4.8\%$, normal weight

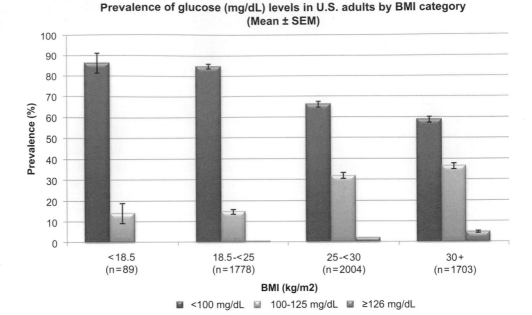

FIGURE 5.2   Prevalence of Glucose Levels in US Adults by BMI Category.

(BMI = 18.5−25 kg/m^2) 14.6 ± 0.6%, overweight (BMI 25−30 kg/m^2) 31.8 ± 1.4% and obese (BMI ≥ 30 kg/m^2) 36.4 ± 1.3%. Although not shown in the figure, prevalence of prediabetes in men increased across normal weight, overweight and obese categories: 22.3 ± 1.9%, 37.2 ± 1.7% and 41.1 ± 1.9%, respectively. Prevalence in women mirrored these increases at 8.5 ± 1.0%, 24.2 ± 1.7% and 32.5 ± 1.9%. The increases across BMI categories were also seen within age groups: 20−39 years (11.8 ± 1.4%, 20.2 ± 1.6%, 23.9 ± 1.8%), 40−59 years (15.3 ± 2.0%, 38.7 ± 2.3%, 42.2 ± 2.4%), 60−69 years (20.9 ± 3.9%, 43.6 ± 3.2%. 54.3 ± 3.7%), and 70+ years (31.4 ± 3.7%, 48.8 ± 4.0%, 52.8 ± 4.7%). Further, prevalence of prediabetes increased across BMI categories within all ethnic groups.

Waist circumference is a surrogate clinical measure for visceral adipose tissue which, when in excess, influences insulin sensitivity and predisposes to prediabetes. The prevalence

of normoglycemia, prediabetes, and unmedicated (undiagnosed) diabetes by gender and waist circumference category is given in Figure 5.3. In men with WC < 102 cm the prevalence of prediabetes was 28.8 ± 1.7%, while in those with WC > 102 cm prevalence was significantly higher at 42.0 ± 1.8% (p < 0.0001). Similarly, in women with WC < 88 cm prevalence was 8.2. ± 0.9% compared to 30.2 ± 1.5% in those with WC > 88 cm (p < 0.0001). Although not shown in the figure, the prevalence of prediabetes in men increased with WC within all age groups: 20−39 years 22.9 ± 2.0% for WC < 102 cm, 31.0 ± 2.5% for WC > 102 cm; 40−59 years 35.6 ± 2.8% for WC < 102 cm, 46.4 ± 2.9% for WC > 102 cm; 60−69 years 41.5 ± 5.4% for WC < 102 cm, 52.0 ± 4.2% for WC > 102 cm; and 70+ years 44.7 ± 4.9% for WC < 102 cm, 55.1 ± 6.0% for WC > 102 cm (all p < 0.0001). This pattern was also found in women: 20−39 years 3.5 ± 0.8% for WC < 88 cm, 16.4 ± 1.9% for WC > 88 cm;

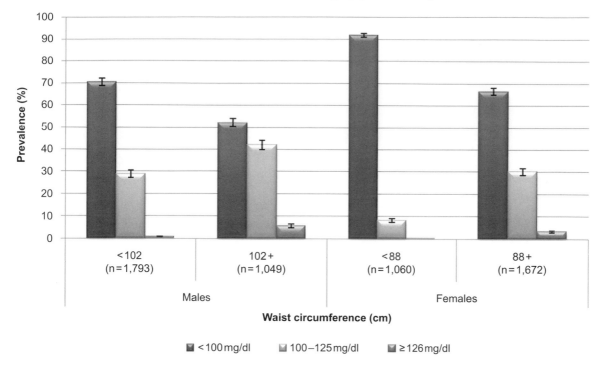

FIGURE 5.3 Prevalence of Glucose Levels in US Adults by Waist Circumference Category.

40–59 years 11.8 ± 1.7% for WC < 88 cm, 34.4 ± 2.5% for WC > 88 cm; 60–69 years 21.2 ± 5.1% for WC < 102 cm, 42.7 ± 4.0% for WC > 102 cm; and 70+ years 19.2 ± 5.1% for WC < 102 cm, 48.3 ± 4.8% for WC > 102 cm (all p < 0.0001). In males, Mexican Americans had a higher overall prevalence at 40%, regardless of the waist circumference, while in other ethnic groups the prevalence of prediabetes increased significantly with waist circumference > 102 cm. Among females in all ethnic groups the prevalence of prediabetes was two-fold or more greater in those with WC > 88 cm.

Prediabetes Alters Serum Lipoprotein Patterns, Glycemia, Resting Blood Pressure

Clinical measures for serum lipid profile are described in this section. The measures for glycemia, resting blood pressure and cardiovascular risk are detailed in the next section.

Prevalence of dysregulated TG and HDL-C levels in adults with normoglycemia, prediabetes, or undiagnosed diabetes is shown in Figure 5.4. The prevalence of high TG levels was 25% in adults with normal glucose vs 41% and 52%, respectively, in those with prediabetes and undiagnosed diabetes. Prevalence of low HDL-C levels was 42% in women with prediabetes and 36% in men with prediabetes. Prevalence of elevated cardiac risk ratios was about the same in adults with prediabetes as in those with unmedicated diabetes, which was significantly higher in both groups compared to adults with normal glucose levels.

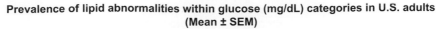

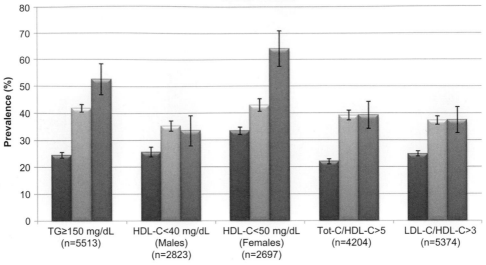

FIGURE 5.4 **Prevalence of Lipid Abnormalities Within a Glucose Category in Healthy US Adults.**

RECOGNITION OF ENHANCED RISK

Type 2 diabetes is widely recognized as a cardiovascular disease (CVD) risk equivalent.[35,36] Thus fasting serum glucose levels equal to, or greater than 126 mg/dl, are consistent with a diagnosis of diabetes and signify an elevated risk for early CVD. Although achieving tight glycemic control in diabetes has been thought to attenuate the magnitude of this CVD risk,[37] recent reports indicate that the risk remains elevated even when serum glucose concentrations are in the range of 100–125 mg/dl.[38] Persistent fasting serum glucose levels in this range, based on the recommendations of the ADA, result in a diagnosis of prediabetes.[36] This elevated latent risk for CVD in otherwise healthy adults with prediabetes can remain unrecognized as many as 15 years prior to the overt loss of glycemic control[39,40] associated with the clinical diagnosis of type 2 diabetes. Prediabetes has been associated with coronary artery calcification,[41] early carotid atherosclerosis,[42] as well as other vascular abnormalities. It is also an integral correlate of the metabolic syndrome,[43] a cluster of risk factors with underlying insulin resistance and compensatory hyperinsulinemia.[44] Metabolic syndrome in both men and women has been found to be significantly related to myocardial infarction and stroke.[45] Adults with prediabetes and/or the metabolic syndrome are at high risk for subsequently developing type 2 diabetes and consequently at risk for CVD.

The World Health Organization[46] (WHO), National Cholesterol Education Program, Adult Treatment Panel III[47] (NCEP ATP III) and International Diabetes Federation[48] (IDF) have all, over the years, proposed varying criteria for the diagnosis of metabolic syndrome. The WHO categorizes the five criteria into one related to glycemic parameters (which have changed after the initial description: the American Diabetes Association criteria changed for the diagnosis of type 2 diabetes) and the other four that relate to WC, fasting serum TG, HDL-C and microalbuminuria. The NCEP ATP III criteria focus on CVD risk and primary prevention. An adult with any three of the five criteria: fasting glucose > 110 mg/dl, WC > 102 cm in men, > 88 cm in women, TG > 150 mg/dl, HDL-C < 40 mg/dl in men, < 50 mg/dl in women, blood pressure > 130/85 mmHg, is diagnosed as having the metabolic syndrome.[47] The IDF definition includes fasting glucose > 100 mg/dl (instead of > 110 mg/dl) and ethnic group specific waist circumference cutoffs.[48]

Each one of the five components of the metabolic syndrome, notwithstanding its use for inclusion in the metabolic syndrome, is also a well recognized independent risk factor for CVD. The enlargement of waist circumference, a clinical marker for an expanding visceral adipose tissue compartment, has been linked with multiple untoward metabolic derangements, which increase cardiovascular morbidity and mortality.[49–51] High levels of fasting serum TG and low levels of HDL-C have similarly been associated with an elevated risk for untoward vascular events.[52–54] Fasting serum glucose levels which exceed 100 mg/dl are associated with an increased risk of developing CVD,[55] due to, among other things, abnormal circadian blood pressure variability.[56] At the population level, each blood pressure increment of 20/10 mmHg, over the usual or desirable systolic blood pressure/diastolic blood pressure of 120/80 mmHg, is associated with about a two-fold increase in death rate from cerebrovascular events (hemorrhage or ischemia) in addition to a two-fold increase in risk of developing ischemic heart disease or other vascular disease.[57] This incremental effect of blood pressure begins at levels in the proximity of 115/75 mmHg.[57] Each BMI increment of 5 kg/m^2, from an apparent optimum of about

22.5–25 kg/m^2, is associated with about a 30% higher overall mortality [hazard ratio per 5 kg/m^2 (HR) 1.29 995% CI 1.27–1.32], primarily from vascular events, including type 2 diabetes.[58] We therefore used these measures for CVD risk assignment in subjects with prediabetes.

MEANS FOR CARDIOMETABOLIC RISK FACTORS

Summary statistics (mean ± standard error of mean) for cardiometabolic risk factors are shown in Table 5.2 for disease-free adults with normoglycemia, prediabetes, or unmedicated diabetes. The means for both BMI and WC increased incrementally across glucose categories (all p < 0.0001). Adults with prediabetes on average were borderline obese (BMI 29.8 ± 0.2 kg/m^2) whereas those with unmedicated diabetes were obese (BMI 34.1 ± 1.1 kg/m^2); mean waist circumference was high for both genders (males 102.0 ± 0.6 cm; females 100.6. ± 1.0 cm).

Means for insulin, HOMA-IR and HbA1c all increased systematically across glucose categories (all p < 0.0001). Those with prediabetes tended to be insulin resistant with high mean fasting insulin (14 μU/ml) and HOMA-IR (3.7) but normal HbA1c.

Means for systolic blood pressure and pulse pressure both increased significantly across glucose categories (all p < 0.0001). Diastolic blood pressure was significantly higher in adults with prediabetes compared to those with normoglycemia (p < 0.0001). The difference between adults with prediabetes and undiagnosed diabetes, however, was not significant. Mean systolic blood pressure levels in adults with prediabetes were in the range for prehypertension (125/74 mmHg).

Means for fasting TG, Total-C and LDL-C levels all increased significantly across glucose categories (all p < 0.01); the means were high

TABLE 5.2 Mean ± SEM Cardiometabolic Risk Factors Among Healthy Adults in US Population

Data: Mean±SEM	N	Glucose level			p-value of normal vs. prediabetes	p-value of normal vs. undiagnosed diabetes
		<100 (mg/dl)	100–125 (mg/dl)	≥126 (mg/dl)		
Waist circumference (cm)						
Male	2,842	95.5 ± 0.4	102.0 ± 0.6	114.0 ± 2.9	<0.0001	<0.0001
Female	2,732	88.8 ± 0.5	100.6 ± 1.0	111.9 ± 2.0	<0.0001	<0.0001
Insulin (μU/ml)	5,500	9.5 ± 0.1	14.0 ± 0.4	21.5 ± 1.5	<0.0001	<0.0001
HbA1c (%)	5,564	5.2 ± 0.01	5.4 ± 0.01	7.3 ± 0.3	<0.0001	<0.0001
HOMA	5,500	2.1 ± 0.03	3.7 ± 0.1	8.9 ± 0.7	<0.0001	<0.0001
Body Mass Index (kg/m^2)	5,574	26.8 ± 0.1	29.8 ± 0.2	34.1 ± 1.1	<0.0001	<0.0001
Systolic BP (mmHg)	5,420	118.6 ± 0.4	125.6 ± 0.5	136.5 ± 2.7	<0.0001	<0.0001
Diastolic BP (mmHg)	5,390	71.8 ± 0.3	73.8 ± 0.3	74.0 ± 1.4	<0.0001	0.1481
Pulse Pressure (mmHg)	5,390	46.8 ± 0.5	51.6 ± 0.5	62.5 ± 2.6	<0.0001	<0.0001
Triglycerides (mg/dl)	5,513	125.4 ± 2.4	164.2 ± 3.4	262.4 ± 44.5	<0.0001	0.0031
Total-C (mg/dl)	4,204	197.7 ± 1.2	208.2 ± 1.4	215.4 ± 6.9	<0.0001	0.0094
LDL-C (mg/dl)	5,374	119.4 ± 0.8	126.6 ± 1.1	122.4 ± 3.2	<0.0001	0.3558
HDL-C (mg/dl)						
Male	2,823	47.7 ± 0.5	45.7 ± 0.5	45.1 ± 1.3	0.0039	0.0664
Female	2,697	58.0 ± 0.5	53.9 ± 0.9	47.0 ± 2.5	<0.0001	<0.0001
Total-C/HDL-C ratio						
Male	2,108	4.5 ± 0.1	4.9 ± 0.1	5.1 ± 0.3	<0.0001	0.0506
Female	2,096	3.7 ± 0.04	4.3 ± 0.1	5.3 ± 0.4	<0.0001	<0.0001
LDL-C/HDL-C ratio						
Male	2,706	2.7 ± 0.04	2.9 ± 0.05	2.7 ± 0.1	<0.0009	0.8043
Female	2,668	2.2 ± 0.03	2.5 ± 0.1	2.9 ± 0.2	<0.0001	0.0002

in adults with prediabetes (164 and 208 mg/dl, respectively). Means for atherogenic LDL-C increased significantly across glucose categories. Means for anti-atherogenic HDL-C decreased significantly for females (p < 0.0001) but for males, while the decrease was significant in prediabetes *vs* those with normal glucose levels (p < 0.004), the difference between prediabetes and undiagnosed diabetes was borderline significant. Means for cardiac risk ratios in females increased significantly across glucose levels (all p < 0.0002); in males the ratios were significantly higher for adults with prediabetes compared to normoglycemia but the differences between prediabetes and undiagnosed diabetes were either borderline significant or definitively not significant.

As shown in Table 5.3, the odds of having fasting glucose in the range 100–110 mg/dl were significantly higher than those of being normoglycemic for adults with elevated waist circumference, blood pressure (systolic and/or diastolic), triglycerides or lower HDL-C. Analogous odds were even higher for having fasting glucose in the range 111–125 mg/dl. The significantly higher odds were observed in the unadjusted models as well as in the models where the odds ratios were adjusted for age, race and gender.

DISCUSSION

The first novel finding from our study is that 26.8% of otherwise healthy disease free adults in the US (one in four disease-free adults) have fasting glucose levels in the range of 100–125 mg/dl. Although we do not have follow-up data to assess the persistence of these levels over time, we believe the quality of data in this cross sectional evaluation of the US population (NHANES) lends to the reliability of this estimate. Using fasting glucose in this range as a criterion for the diagnosis of prediabetes, we described the epidemiology of this predisease during 1999–2006 by

time, age, race/ethnicity, gender, smoking status and alcohol consumption. The overall prevalence is strikingly high, but even more concerning is the observed rapid increase over the 8-year period of surveillance.

It has been established that type 2 diabetes occurs as a sequelae of insulin resistance and while it is generally assumed, it has not been explicitly established that prediabetes, especially in disease-free adults, is associated with an adverse cardiometabolic profile. A second novel finding from this study is that prediabetes is strongly correlated with increased insulin resistance which by itself is a mediator for an adverse cardiometabolic profile. This is demonstrated by increased levels of fasting serum insulin and HOMA-IR, along with the implication of an increased risk for conversion to type 2 diabetes. Prediabetes is a reflection of early insulin resistance which is characterized by decreasing sensitivity of target tissues to the action of insulin, elevated blood glucose and insulin concentrations, along with an increased hepatic production of atherogenic lipids. Clinical markers include elevated plasma glucose concentration under fasting and/or post-meal conditions (IFG and/or IGT, respectively), increased serum TG and below-normal HDL-C concentrations.[59] A decrease in anti-atherogenic HDL-C is indicative of an impaired reverse cholesterol transport pathway,[60,61] which over time accelerates atherosclerosis. The increase of cardiac risk ratios: total-C/LDL-C and LDL-C/HDL-C above the desirable range attests to an elevated cardiovascular disease risk.[62]

An expanding visceral adipose tissue compartment[63] is an altered distribution pattern that is believed to impair adipose tissue function and increase CVD risk.[64] The altered adipose tissue secretions with auto-, para- and endocrine effects, appear to influence multiple metabolic pathways, including those that modulate glycemia and blood pressure control.[65] This altered adipose tissue[66–68] secretory activity can unhinge the anti-inflammatory

TABLE 5.3   Odds Ratios across Fasting Serum Glucose Levels for Healthy Adults with Disordered Cardiovascular Risk Factors

	Odds ratios (95% CI) and p-value				
	Glucose < 100 (mg/dl)	Glucose 100–110 (mg/dl)		Glucose 111–125 (mg/dl)	
Elevated waist circumference					
Unadjusted model	1.00	1.99	(1.70, 2.34)	3.62	(2.78, 4.72)
p value			< 0.0001		< 0.0001
Adjusted model	1.00	2.19	(1.84, 2.60)	3.27	(2.50, 4.26)
p value			< 0.0001		< 0.0001
Elevated Blood Pressure					
Unadjusted model	1.00	2.75	(2.21, 3.41)	6.44	(4.53, 9.14)
p value			< 0.0001		< 0.0001
Adjusted model	1.00	1.94	(1.54, 2.44)	2.88	(1.92, 4.33)
p value			0.0002		< 0.0001
Low HDL cholesterol					
Unadjusted model	1.00	1.37	(1.17, 1.60)	1.64	(1.23, 2.18)
p value			< 0.0001		0.0007
Adjusted model	1.00	1.63	(1.38, 1.92)	2.30	(1.67, 3.17)
p value			< 0.0001		< 0.0001
Elevated triglycerides					
Unadjusted model	1.00	2.08	(1.79, 2.41)	3.07	(2.29, 4.12)
p value			< 0.0001		< 0.0001
Adjusted model	1.00	1.69	(1.43, 2.00)	2.39	(1.71, 3.35)
p value			< 0.0001		< 0.0001
2+ risk factors					
Unadjusted model	1.00	2.25	(1.86, 2.72)	4.76	(3.57, 6.34)
p value			< 0.0001		< 0.0001
Adjusted model	1.00	2.08	(1.69, 2.55)	3.73	(2.79, 4.98)
p value			< 0.0001		< 0.0001

*Model 1 is unadjusted. Model 2 is adjusted for age categories, race, and gender.

and pro-inflammatory balance favoring inflammation, fostering dysglycemia (prediabetes), and disrupting blood pressure control (prehypertension). These result in a cascade of events which promote vascular changes,[66,67] and include adverse effects on blood pressure control, endothelial cell function, lipid profile, platelet function, and blood coagulation.[69] Prediabetes and prehypertension in disease-free obese adults correlates with an exacerbated systemic proinflammatory milieu.[70] We have shown that disease-free overweight subjects with prediabetes have circadian blood pressure variability abnormalities.[56] We have also shown that otherwise healthy obese subjects with prediabetes and a higher degree of systemic inflammation have both circadian blood pressure variability and endothelial function abnormalities.[71] Circadian blood pressure variability abnormalities[72,73] and endothelial dysfunction[74] are both early markers for an elevated cardiovascular disease risk.

A varying proportion of subjects (2.3–14.3%) with prediabetes (ADA 2003; IGT; 2-h OGTT 140–199 mg/dl) convert to type 2 diabetes over 1 year.[75–78] The Diabetes Prevention Program,[76] reporting a conversion rate of prediabetes with impaired glucose tolerance to type 2 diabetes of 11% per year, showed a 58% and 31% decrease in conversion in the diet/exercise and metformin-treated study arms, respectively. Women with gestational diabetes displayed conversion rates of 12.1% a year; when treated with troglitazone, they exhibited reduced yearly rates of 5.4%.[78] There is confusion in the follow-up data from large prospective studies like the Framingham Heart Study due to the changed ADA definition for impaired fasting glucose (from 110–125 mg/dl in 1997 to 100–125 mg/dl in 2003). The women with either definition for impaired fasting glucose (in contrast to men, who had no relationship between fasting serum glucose and CVD), had increased coronary heart disease, whereas those with fasting glucose in the earlier range (110–125 mg/dl) had risk similar to those with type 2 diabetes.[79]

The increased CVD risk in prediabetes is primarily due to systemic changes that occur with prediabetes itself,[56,70,71] not due to those that occur after conversion to type 2 diabetes which take place much later. The allocation of increased CVD risk in prediabetes in the context of diagnostic constructs for the metabolic syndrome: larger waist circumference, increased blood pressure, fasting serum TG, along with lower HDL-C levels is based on the independent CVD risk-enhancing association of each one of these factors.[49–55] The graded increases in odds ratios across fasting glucose levels 100–110 and 111–125 mg/dl for adults with disordered cardiovascular risk factors clearly demonstrate the need for close monitoring in otherwise disease-free subjects who have prediabetes. Primary prevention of disease (intervention to prevent disease from ever developing in susceptible individuals) is a goal that every physician aspires to. Conventional wisdom dictates a change in diet, an increase in exercise, and obtaining weight loss as the primary measures for intervention. Metformin added to the usual CVD risk-modifying therapies in overweight and obese individuals significantly reduced the occurrence of type 2 diabetes and decreased the rate of metabolic syndrome in those who did *vs* those who did not receive it.[80] Prediabetes by various estimates converts into type 2 diabetes at an annual rate of 2.3–14.3%; this conversion can be prevented with diet, exercise, and metformin.[80,81] Prediabetes is thus a key target for primary prevention.

CONCLUSION

These data highlight the high prevalence of prediabetes in otherwise healthy adults. Prediabetes, a precursor for the development of subsequent type 2 diabetes, is due to a multitude of subtle derangements in the adipose tissue, pancreas, gastrointestinal tract, kidney, liver, muscle and brain. The measurable clinical and laboratory changes in prediabetes by themselves are early correlates for an adverse cardiometabolic profile. Interventions designed to prevent progression from prediabetes to type 2 diabetes can attenuate this increased risk and may even provide primary prevention for cardiovascular disease.

References

1. Colin Mathers D, Dejan Loncar. Projections of Global Mortality and Burden of Disease from 2002 to 2030. *PLoS Med* 2006;3(11):e442.
2. Heidenreich PA, Trogdon JG, Khavjou OA, Butler J, Dracup K, Ezekowitz MD, Finkelstein EA, Hong Y,

Johnston SC, Khera A, Lloyd-Jones DM, Nelson SA, Nichol G, Orenstein D, Wilson PW, Woo YJ, on behalf of the American Heart Association Advocacy Coordinating Committee, Stroke Council, Council on Cardiovascular Radiology and Intervention, Council on Clinical Cardiology, Council on Epidemiology and Prevention, Council on Arteriosclerosis, Thrombo. *Forecasting the Future of Cardiovascular Disease in the United States: A Policy Statement From the American Heart Association* Circulation 2011;**123**:933—44.

3. Stratmann B, Tschoepe D. Atherogenesis and atherothrombosis—focus on diabetes mellitus. *Best Pract Res Clin Endocrinol Metab* 2009;**23**(3):291—303.

4. Yamagishi S, Nakamura K, Matsui T, Takenaka K, Jinnouchi Y, Imaizumi T. Cardiovascular disease in diabetes. *Mini Rev Med Chem* 2006;**6**(3):313—8.

5. Messerli FH, Williams B, Ritz E. Essential hypertension. *Lancet* 2007;**370**;18(9587):591—603.

6. Whitworth JA. Blood pressure and control of cardiovascular risk. *Vasc Health Risk Manag* 2005;**1**(3):257—60.

7. Arsenault BJ, Boekholdt SM, Kastelein JJ. Lipid parameters for measuring risk of cardiovascular disease. *Nat Rev Cardiol* 2011;**8**(4):197—206.

8. Gelber RP, Gaziano JM, Orav EJ, Manson JE, Buring JE, Kurth T. Measures of obesity and cardiovascular risk among men and women. *J Am Coll Cardiol* 2008;**52**(8):605—15.

9. Bonora E. The metabolic syndrome and cardiovascular disease. *Ann Med* 2006;**38**(1):64—80. Review.

10. Bestermann W, Houston MC, Basile J, Egan B, Ferrario CM, Lackland D, Hawkins RG, Reed J, Rogers P, Wise D, Moore MA. Addressing the global cardiovascular risk of hypertension, dyslipidemia, diabetes mellitus, and the metabolic syndrome in the southeastern United States, part II: treatment recommendations for management of the global cardiovascular risk of hypertension, dyslipidemia, diabetes mellitus, and the metabolic syndrome. *Am J Med Sci* 2005;**329**(6):292—305.

11. Daviglus ML, Lloyd-Jones DM, Pirzada A. Preventing cardiovascular disease in the 21st century: therapeutic and preventive implications of current evidence. *Am J Cardiovasc Drugs* 2006;**6**(2):87—101.

12. Roger V, Go A, Lloyd-Jones D, et al. Heart disease and stroke statistics—2011 update. A report from the American Heart Association Statistics Committee and Stroke Statistics Subcommittee. *Circulation* 2011;**123**:e1—192.

13. Myerburg RJ, Kessler KM, Castellanos A. Sudden cardiac death: epidemiology, transient risk, and intervention assessment. *Ann Intern Med* 1993;**119**:1187—97.

14. Rosamond W, Flegal K, Friday G, Furie K, Go A, Greenlund K, Haase N, Ho M, Howard V, Kissela B, Kittner S, Lloyd-Jones D, McDermott M, Meigs J, Moy C, Nichol G, O'Donnell CJ, Roger V, Rumsfeld J, Sorlie P, Steinberger J, Thom T, Wasserthiel-Smoller S, Hong Y, American Heart Association Statistics Committee, Stroke Statistics Subcommittee. Heart disease and stroke statistics—2007 update: A report from the American Heart Association Statistics Committee and Stroke Statistics Subcommittee. *Circulation* 2007;**115**(5):e69—171.

15. Gupta AK, McGlone M, Greenway FL, Johnson WD. Prehypertension in disease-free adults: a marker for an adverse cardiometabolic risk profile. *Hypertens Res* 2010;**33**(9):905—10.

16. Gupta AK, Brashear MM, Johnson WD. Coexisting prehypertension and prediabetes in healthy adults: a pathway for accelerated cardiovascular events. *Hypertens Res* 2011;**34**(4):456—61.

17. Vasan RS, Larson MG, Leip EP, Kannel WB, Levy D. Assessment of frequency of progression to hypertension in non-hypertensive participants in the Framingham Heart Study: a cohort study. *Lancet* 2001;**358**(9294):1682—6.

18. De Marco M, de Simone G, Roman MJ, Chinali M, Lee ET, Russell M, Howard BV, Devereux RB. Cardiovascular and metabolic predictors of progression of prehypertension into hypertension. The Strong Heart Study. *Hypertension* 2009;**54**:974—80.

19. Edelstein SL, Knowler WC, Bain RP, Andres R, Barrett-Connor EL, Dowse GK, Haffner SM, Pettitt DJ, Sorking JD, Muller DC, Collins VR, Hamman RF. Predictors of progression from impaired glucose tolerance to NIDDM: An analysis of six prospective studies. *Diabetes* 1997;**46**:701—10.

20. Tuomilehto J, Lindstrom J, Eriksson JG, Valle TT, Hamalainen H, Ilanne-Parikka P, Keinanen-Kiukaanniemi S, Laakso M, Louheranta A, Rastas M, Salminen V, Uusitupa M. Prevention of type 2 diabetes mellitus by changes in lifestyle among subjects with impaired glucose tolerance. *N Engl J Med* 2001;**344**:1343—50.

21. United States Department of Health and Human Services. The National Health and Nutrition Examination Survey. http://www.cdc.gov/nchs/nhanes.htm. Accessed 13 December 2010.

22. Diagnosis and classification of diabetes mellitus. *Diabetes Care* 2008;**31**(Suppl. 1):S55—60.

23. Dunstan DW, Zimmet PZ, Welborn TA, Cameron AJ, de Court, Sicree RA, Dwyer T, Colagiuri S, Jolley D, Knuiman M, Atkins R, Shaw JE. The rising prevalence of diabetes and impaired glucose tolerance: The Australian Diabetes, Obesity and Lifestyle Study. *Diabetes Care* 2002;**25**:829—34.

24. Is fasting glucose sufficient to define diabetes? Epidemiological data from 20 European studies. The DECODE-study group. European Diabetes Epidemiology Group. Diabetes Epidemiology: Collaborative Analysis of Diagnostic Criteria in Europe. *Diabetologia* 1999 Jun;**42**(6):647—54.

25. Ko GT, Chan JC, Woo J, Cockram CS. Use of the 1997 American Diabetes Association diagnostic criteria for diabetes in a Hong Kong Chinese population. *Diabetes Care* 1998;**21**:2094—7.

26. Shaw JE, Zimmet PZ, de Courten M, Dowse GK, Chitson P, Gareeboo H, Hemraj F, Fareed D, Tuomilehto J, Alberti KG. Impaired fasting glucose or impaired glucose tolerance. What best predicts future diabetes in Mauritius? *Diabetes Care* 1999;**22**:399—402.

27. Gabir MM, Hanson RL, Dabelea D, Imperatore G, Roumain J, Bennett PH, Knowler WD. Plasma glucose and prediction of microvascular disease and mortality: evaluation of 1997 American Diabetes Association and 1999 World Health Organization criteria for diagnosis of diabetes. *Diabetes Care* 2000;**23**:1113—8.

28. Larsson H, Berglund G, Lindgarde F, Ahren B. Comparison of ADA and WHO criteria for diagnosis of diabetes and glucose intolerance [letter]. *Diabetologia* 1998;**41**:1124—5.

29. Harris MI, Eastman RC, Cowie CC, Flegal KM, Eberhardt MS. Comparison of diabetes diagnostic categories in the U.S. population according to the 1997 American Diabetes Association and 1980-1985 World Health Organization diagnostic criteria. *Diabetes Care* 1997;**20**:1859—62.

30. Karve A, Hayward RA. Prevalence, diagnosis, and treatment of impaired fasting glucose and impaired glucose tolerance in nondiabetic U.S. adults. *Diabetes Care* 2010 Nov;**33**(11):2355—9.

31. Lawrence RD. Renal threshold for glucose: Normal and in diabetics. *Br Med J* 1940;**1**(4140):766—8.

32. American Diabetes Association. Diagnosis and classification of diabetes mellitus. *Diabetes Care* 2011;**34**(Suppl. 1):S62—9.

33. DeFronzo RA. Pharmacologic therapy for type 2 diabetes mellitus. *Ann Intern Med* 1999;**131**:281—303.

34. Weyer C, Bogardus C, Pratley RE. Metabolic characteristics of individuals with impaired fasting glucose and/or impaired glucose tolerance. *Diabetes* 1999;**48**:2197—203.

35. Juutilainen A, Lehto S, Ronnemaa T, Pyorala K, Laakso M. Type 2 diabetes as a coronary heart disease equivalent: an 18-year prospective population-based study in Finnish subjects. *Diabetes Care* 2005;**28**:2901—7.

36. Whiteley L, Padmanabhan S, Hole D, Isles C. Should diabetes be considered a coronary heart disease risk equivalent?: results from 25 years of follow-up in the Renfrew and Paisley survey. *Diabetes Care* 2005;**28**:1588—93.

37. The Diabetes Control and Complications Trial Research Group. The effect of intensive treatment of diabetes on the development and progression of long term complications in the diabetes control in insulin dependent diabetes mellitus. *N Engl J Med* 1993;**329**(14):977—86.

38. Nielson C, Lange T, Hadjokas N. Blood glucose and coronary artery disease in nondiabetic patients. *Diabetes Care* 2006;**29**:998—1001.

39. Schnell O, Standl E. Impaired glucose tolerance, diabetes, and cardiovascular disease. *Endocr Pract* 2006;**12**(Suppl. 1):16—9.

40. Barr EL, Zimmet PZ, Welborn TA, Jolley D, Magliano DJ, Dunstan DW, Cameron AJ, Dwyer T, Taylor HR, Tonkin AM, Wong TY, McNeil J, Shaw JE. Risk of cardiovascular and all-cause mortality in individuals with diabetes mellitus, impaired fasting glucose, and impaired glucose tolerance: The Australian Diabetes, Obesity, and Lifestyle Study (AusDiab). *Circulation* 2007;**116**:151—7.

41. Meigs JB, Larson MG, D'Agostino RB, Levy D, Clouse ME, Nathan DM, Wilson PW, O'Donnell CJ. Coronary artery calcification in type 2 diabetes and insulin resistance: the Framingham offspring study. *Diabetes Care* 2002;**25**:1313—9.

42. Diamantopoulos EJ, Andreadis EA, Tsourous GI, Katsanou PM, Georgiopoulos DX, Nestora KC, Raptis SA. Early vascular lesions in subjects with metabolic syndrome and prediabetes. *Int Angiol* 2006;**25**:179—83.

43. Kim SH, Reaven GM. The metabolic syndrome: one step forward, two steps back. *Diab Vasc Dis Res* 2004;**1**:68—75.

44. Reaven GM. Insulin resistance, the insulin resistance syndrome, and cardiovascular disease. *Panminerva Med* 2005;**47**:201—10.

45. Ninomiya JK, L'Italien G, Criqui MH, Whyte JL, Gamst A, Chen RS. Association of the metabolic syndrome with history of myocardial infarction and stroke in the Third National Health and Nutrition Examination Survey. *Circulation* 2004;**109**:42—6.

46. Alberti KG, Zimmet PZ. Definition, diagnosis and classification of diabetes mellitus and its complications. Part 1: diagnosis and classification of diabetes mellitus provisional report of a WHO consultation. *Diabet Med* 1998;**15**:539—53.

47. Executive Summary of the Third Report of the National Cholesterol Education Program (NCEP) Expert Panel on Detection. Evaluation, and Treatment

of High Blood Cholesterol in Adults (Adult Treatment Panel III). *JAMA* 2001;**285**:2486—97.

48. The IDF consensus worldwide definition of the metabolic syndrome. Part 1. Worldwide definition for use in clinical practice. Internet, www.idf.org (Accessed 13 December 2010).

49. Fox CS, Massaro JM, Hoffmann U, Pou KM, Maurovich-Horvat P, Liu CY, Vasan RS, Murabito JM, Meigs JB, Cupples LA, D'Agostino Sr RB, O'Donnell CJ. Abdominal visceral and subcutaneous adipose tissue compartments: association with metabolic risk factors in the Framingham Heart Study. *Circulation* 2007;**116**(1):39—48.

50. St-Pierre J, Lemieux I, Perron P, Brisson D, Santuré M, Vohl MC, Després JP, Gaudet D. Relation of the hypertriglyceridemic waist phenotype to earlier manifestations of coronary artery disease in patients with glucose intolerance and type 2 diabetes mellitus. *Am J Cardiol* 2007;**99**(3):369—73.

51. Haffner SM. Abdominal adiposity and cardiometabolic risk: do we have all the answers? *Am J Med* 2007;**120**(9 Suppl. 1):S10—6. discussion S16—7. Review.

52. Patsch JR, Miesenbock G, Hopferwieser T, Muhlberger V, Knapp E, Dunn JK, Gotto Jr AM, Patsch W. Relation of triglyceride metabolism and coronary artery disease: studies in the postprandial state. *Arterioscler Thromb* 1992;**12**:1336—45.

53. Castelli WP, Doyle JT, Gordon T, Hames CG, Hjortland MC, Hulley SB, Kagan A, Zukel WJ. HDL cholesterol and other lipids in coronary heart disease. *Circulation* 1977;**55**:767—72.

54. Manninen V, Tenkanen L, Koskinen P, Huttunen JK, Manttari M, Heinonen OP, Frick MH. Joint effects of serum triglyceride and LDL cholesterol and HDL cholesterol concentrations on coronary heart disease risk in the Helsinki heart study: implications for treatment. *Circulation* 1992;**85**:37—45.

55. Nielson C, Lange T, Hadjokas N. Blood glucose and coronary artery disease in nondiabetic patients. *Diabetes Care* 2006;**29**:998—1001.

56. Gupta AK, Greenway FL, Cornelissen G, Pan W, Halberg F. Prediabetes is associated with abnormal circadian blood pressure variability. *J Hum Hypertens* 2008;**22**(9):627—33.

57. Lewington S, Clarke R, Qizilbash N, Peto R, Collins R. Prospective Studies Collaboration. Age-specific relevance of usual blood pressure to vascular mortality: a meta-analysis of individual data for one million adults in 61 prospective studies. *Lancet* 2002;**360**(9349):1903-13.

58. Whitlock G, Lewington S, Sherliker P, Clarke R, Emberson J, Halsey J, Qizilbash N, Collins R, Peto R. Body-mass index and cause-specific mortality in

900 000 adults: collaborative analyses of 57 prospective studies. Prospective Studies Collaboration. *Lancet* 2009;**373**(9669):1083—96.

59. Festa A, Williams K, Hanley AJ, Otvos JD, Goff DC, Wagenknecht LE, Haffner SM. Nuclear magnetic resonance lipoprotein abnormalities in prediabetic subjects in the Insulin Resistance Atherosclerosis Study. *Circulation* 2005;**111**(25):3465—72.

60. Toth PP. Reverse cholesterol transport: high-density lipoprotein's magnificent mile. *Curr Atheroscler Rep* 2003;**5**:386—93 (Review).

61. Gupta AK, Ross EA, Myers JN, Kashyap ML. Increased reverse cholesterol transport in athletes. *Metabolism* 1993;**42**(6):684—90.

62. Malone DC, Boudreau DM, Nichols GA, Raebel MA, Fishman PA, Feldstein AC, Ben-Joseph RH, Okamoto LJ, Boscoe AN, Magid DJ. Association of Cardiometabolic Risk Factors and Prevalent Cardiovascular Events. *Metab Syndr Relat Disord* 2009;**7**(6):585—93.

63. Després JP. Cardiovascular disease under the influence of excess visceral fat. *Crit Pathw Cardiol* 2007;**6**:51—9.

64. Rajala MW, Scherer PE. Minireview: the adipocyte at the crossroads of energy homeostasis, inflammation, and atherosclerosis. *Endocrinology* 2003;**144**:3765—73.

65. Moreno-Aliaga MJ, Campion J, Milagro FI, Berjon A, Martinez JA. Adiposity and proinflammatory state: the chicken or the egg? *Adipocytes* 2005;**1**:1—16.

66. Fantuzzi G. Adipose tissue, adipokines, and inflammation. *J Allergy Clin Immunol* 2005;**115**:911—9.

67. Vettor R, Milan G, Rossato M, Federspil G. Review article: adipocytokines and insulin resistance. *Aliment Pharmacol Ther* 2005;**22**(Suppl. 2):3—10.

68. Xu H, Barnes GT, Yang Q, Tan G, Yang D, Chou CJ, Sole J, Nichols A, Ross JS, Tartaglia LA, Chen H. Chronic inflammation in fat plays a crucial role in the development of obesity-related insulin resistance. *J Clin Invest* 2003;**112**:1785—8.

69. Kougias P, Chai H, Lin PH, Yao Q, Lumsden AB, Chen C. Effects of adipocyte-derived cytokines on endothelial functions: implication of vascular disease. *J Surg Res* 2005;**126**:121—9.

70. Alok Gupta K, Johnson William D. Prediabetes and prehypertension in disease free obese adults correlate with an exacerbated systemic proinflammatory milieu. *Journal of Inflammation* 2010;**7**:36.

71. Gupta AK, Cornelissen G, Greenway FL, Dhoopati V, Halberg F, Johnson WD. Abnormalities in circadian blood pressure variability and endothelial function: pragmatic markers for adverse cardiometabolic profiles in asymptomatic obese adults. *Cardiovasc Diabetol* 2010;**9**:58.

72. Halberg F, Cornélissen G, Katinas G, Tvildiani L, Gigolashvili M, Janashia K, Toba T, Revilla M, Regal P,

Sothern RB, Wendt HW, Wang ZR, Zeman M, Jozsa R, Singh RB, Mitsutake G, Chibisov SM, Lee J, Holley D, Holte JE, Sonkowsky RP, Schwartzkopff O, Delmore P, Otsuka K, Bakken EE, Czaplicki J. International BIOCOS Group. Chronobiology's progress: season's appreciations 2004-2005. Time, frequency, phase, variable, individual, age- and site-specific chronomics. *J Appl Biomed* 2006;**4**:1—38.

73. Halberg F, Cornélissen G, Katinas G, Tvildiani L, Gigolashvili M, Janashia K, Toba T, Revilla M, Regal P, Sothern RB, Wendt HW, Wang ZR, Zeman M, Jozsa R, Singh RB, Mitsutake G, Chibisov SM, Lee J, Holley D, Holte JE, Sonkowsky RP, Schwartzkopff O, Delmore P, Otsuka K, Bakken EE, Czaplicki J. International BIOCOS Group. Chronobiology's progress: part II, chronomics for an immediately applicable biomedicine. *J Appl Biomed* 2006;**4**:73—86.

74. Corrado E, Rizzo M, Coppola G, Muratori I, Carella M, Novo S. Endothelial dysfunction and carotid lesions are strong predictors of clinical events in patients with early stages of atherosclerosis: a 24-month follow-up study. *Coron Artery Dis* 2008;**19**(3):139—44.

75. Edelstein SL, Knowler WC, Bain RP, Andres R, Barrett-Connor EL, Dowse GK, Haffner SM, Pettitt DJ, Sorking JD, Muller DC, Collins VR, Hamman RF. Predictors of progression from impaired glucose tolerance to NIDDM: An analysis of six prospective studies. *Diabetes* 1997;**46**:701—10.

76. Tuomilehto J, Lindstrom J, Eriksson JG, Valle TT, Hamalainen H, Ilanne-Parikka P, Keinanen-Kiukaanniemi S, Laakso M, Louheranta A, Rastas M, Salminen V, Uusitupa M. Prevention of type 2 diabetes mellitus by changes in lifestyle among subjects with impaired glucose tolerance. *N Engl J Med* 2001;**344**:1343—50.

77. Buchanan TA, Xiang AH, Peters RK, Kjos SL, Marroquin A, Goico J, Ochoa C, Tan S, Berkowitz K, Hodis HN, Azen SP. Preservation of pancreatic beta-cell function and prevention of type 2 diabetes by pharmacological treatment of insulin resistance in high-risk Hispanic women. *Diabetes* 2002;**51**:2796—803.

78. Azen SP, Peters RK, Berkowitz K, Kjos S, Xiang AN, Buchanan TA, for the TRIPOD Study Group. TRIPOD (TRoglitazone In the Prevention Of Diabetes): A randomized, placebo-controlled trial of troglitazone in women with prior gestational diabetes mellitus. *Controlled Clin Trials* 1998;**19**:217—31.

79. Levitz YS, Pencina MJ, D'Agostino RB, Meigs JB, Murabito JM, Vasan RS, Fox CS. Impact of impaired fasting glucose on cardiovascular disease: the Framingham Heart Study. *J Am Coll Cardiol* 2008;**51**(3):264—70.

80. Andreadis EA, Katsanou PM, Georgiopoulos DX, Tsourous GI, Yfanti GK, Gouveri ET, Diamantopoulos EJ. The effect of metformin on the incidence of type 2 diabetes mellitus and cardiovascular disease risk factors in overweight and obese subjects—the Carmos study. *Exp Clin Endocrinol Diabetes* 2009;**117**(4):175—80.

81. Chiasson JL. Prevention of Type 2 diabetes: fact or fiction? *Expert Opin Pharmacother* 2007;**8**(18):3147—58 (Review).

6

Obesity and Type 2 Diabetes in Youths: New Challenges to Overcome

Nicola Santoro, Cosimo Giannini, Sonia Caprio

Department of Pediatrics, Yale School of Medicine, New Haven, CT, USA

OBESITY: THE 21ST CENTURY EPIDEMIC

Two-thirds of the adult population in the US and in many other developed countries are currently overweight or obese.[1] Obesity has been estimated to decrease life expectancy by as little as 0.8[2] to as much as 7 years,[3,4] being the second leading cause of preventable, premature death in the US after smoking,[5] while in high-income countries smoking, alcohol consumption, and obesity are the most important causes of cancer.[6]

Along with adult obesity, the prevalence of childhood obesity has doubled or tripled between the early 1970s and the late 1990s in Australia, Brazil, Canada, Chile, Finland, France, Germany, Greece, Japan, the UK, and the US.[7] The increase in childhood obesity prevalence seems not to spare even the developing countries undergoing a rapid nutritional transition.[8] Overweight children are more

Nutritional and Therapeutic Interventions for Diabetes and Metabolic Syndrome
DOI: 10.1016/B978-0-12-385083-6.00006-1

prone to become overweight adults, especially at higher Body Mass Index (BMI)[9] or if they have an obese parent.[10] Almost half of overweight adults were overweight during childhood, and two-thirds of children in the highest BMI quartile transitioned into the highest BMI quartile as young adults.[11] Obesity during adolescence has been shown to be associated with many adverse health consequences,[6,12,13] and dietary habits, physical inactivity, rates and degree of obesity become worse with the transition into adulthood.[14] Adolescents with a higher BMI experienced 30% higher rates of mortality as young and middle-aged adults, although the persistence of higher BMIs into adulthood accounted for much of the association.[15] In addition, it has been observed[16] that being an obese adolescent was associated with an increased risk of multiple comorbidities in adulthood, even if obesity doesn't persist.

METABOLIC COMPLICATIONS OF OBESITY IN CHILDREN AND ADOLESCENTS

Many of the metabolic and cardiovascular complications of obesity are already present during childhood; this may be a consequence of the insulin resistance, which is the most common abnormality of obesity.[8] Insulin resistance, in fact, represents one of the most important pathogenetic determinants of the metabolic complications of obesity. The clustering of some complications occurring in obese patients defines the so-called metabolic syndrome (MS).

The metabolic syndrome in children is commonly defined by the co-occurrence of three or more of the following features: severe obesity (usually with a waist circumference higher than the 90th sex- and age-specific percentile), dyslipidemia [increase of triglycerides and decrease of high-density lipoproteins

(HDL)], hypertension and alterations of glucose metabolism such as impaired glucose tolerance (IGT) and type 2 diabetes (T2D).[17]

Weiss et al. have well demonstrated how the increase of insulin resistance parallels the increase in the risk of metabolic syndrome in obese children and adolescents.[17] In this latter study, a strong loading of insulin resistance to obesity and glucose metabolism factor and moderate loading to the dyslipidemia factor have been observed.[17] In vivo studies showed that hyperinsulinemia stimulates the synthesis of triglycerides by increasing the transcription of genes for lipogenic enzymes in liver.[18] Moreover, recent reports showed that the forkhead transcription factor FoxO1 acts in the liver to integrate hepatic insulin action to very-low-density lipoprotein (VLDL) production. Augmented FoxO1 activity in insulin-resistant livers promotes hepatic VLDL overproduction and predisposes to the development of hypertriglyceridemia.[19]

Although obesity is the most important cause of insulin resistance among the obese children and adolescents, it has not to be forgotten that a transient physiological insulin-resistant state occurs in children during puberty, maybe due to the increase in growth hormone and insulin-like growth factor 1,[20] and that this state may worsen the insulin resistance present in obese children, accelerating the progression to metabolic syndrome and type 2 diabetes.

Along with insulin resistance, the metabolic syndrome in children is associated with a proinflammatory state,[17] which in turn, seems to be related with a worsening in the risk of coronary artery disease (CAD). The relationship between inflammatory markers and individual components of the metabolic syndrome is still unclear. In fact, it is not known yet if the proinflammatory state is a result of the metabolic syndrome and insulin resistance, or if the increase of inflammatory cytokines derived from adipocytes may be partly responsible for insulin resistance and metabolic syndrome.

Some studies have been focused on the contribution of proinflammatory adipocytokines such as TNF-alpha and IL-6 molecules produced by adipose tissue (or macrophages resident in adipose tissue). In a multiethnic cohort of obese and lean children, IL-6 levels have been shown to increase with the degree of obesity; results concerning the association between TNF-alpha, childhood obesity, and its metabolic complications are more unclear.[20,21] In particular, studies dealing with TNF-alpha in obese children show contrasting results, with some of them showing a positive association with body fat and others showing a decrease of TNF-alpha in obese prepubertal children.[22,23] Conversely, the effect of TNF-alpha on insulin resistance has been well demonstrated. In fact, this cytokine induces lipolysis in adipose tissue, inhibits insulin signaling, and affects the expression of some genes that are important for adipocyte function. TNF-alpha may also enhance the release of free fatty acids from adipose tissue, which affects whole-body energy homeostasis and overall insulin sensitivity.[24] Furthermore, a recent report demonstrated a positive correlation between IL-6, TNF-alpha and adipocyte diameter studied by a needle biopsy of subcutaneous abdominal fat in obese children.[25]

Along with the increase of cytokines affecting insulin sensitivity and CAD risk, the adipose tissue of obese children reduces the production of the adiponectin, a cytokine exclusively expressed by adipocytes that can be found in high concentrations in human blood.[26] It exerts several beneficial actions such as antiatherogenetic, antidiabetogenic, and anti-inflammatory, hence protecting against the development of type 2 diabetes and CAD.[26,27] Interestingly, adiponectin is decreased in obesity and the decreased adiponectin levels are associated with parameters of metabolic syndrome in obese children.[28,29] In summary, the co-occurrence of the insulin resistance and an adverse proinflammatory state drives the obese child to develop a worse metabolic asset, with a consequent occurrence of the most frightened complication of childhood obesity: type 2 diabetes. In the Figure 6.1 we show our personal data on 1,589 obese children and adolescents (mean age 13.2 ± 3.0; mean z-score BMI 2.30 ± 058). The

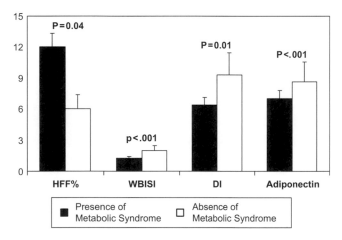

FIGURE 6.1 **Metabolic Pattern According to Presence/Absence of Metabolic Syndrome.** Obese children and adolescents showing the features of the Metabolic Syndrome (MS), as defined by Weiss *et al.*,[17] have a clear precocious metabolic derangement, characterized by the marked hepatic fat content (HFF%), the reduced insulin sensitivity (WBISI) and secretion (DI) and the reduced levels of adiponectin. Hepatic fat content data based on MRI measurements were available only for 139 subjects. HFF% (hepatic fat fraction), DI (disposition index), WBISI (whole body insulin sensitivity index).

513 (32%) subjects with features of metabolic syndrome clearly show a higher hepatic fat content (HFF%), a lower insulin sensitivity as evaluated by the whole body insulin sensitivity index (WBISI), a lower disposition index (DI), and lower levels of adiponectin.

TYPE 2 DIABETES IN CHILDREN AND ADOLESCENCE: A NEW FRIGHTENING EPIDEMIC?

According to the American Diabetes Association (ADA), the criteria for type 2 diabetes are defined as fasting plasma glucose levels higher than 126 mg/dl or plasma glucose levels higher than 200 mg/dl 2 h after an oral glucose tolerance test (OGTT), while impaired glucose tolerance (IGT) is defined as when plasma glucose levels are higher than 140 mg/dl 2 h after the loading during the OGTT.[30] Along with IGT another prediabetic state (also defined as category at risk of diabetes) has been identified: impaired fasting glucose (IFG). IFG is defined as serum fasting glucose levels between 100 and 125 mg/dl. Epidemiological studies indicate that IFG and IGT are two distinct categories of individuals[31] and only a small number of subjects meet both criteria, showing that these categories overlap only to a very limited extent in children, as already reported in adults.[31]

Moreover, after years of debate, ADA published revised recommendations to use hemoglobin A_{1c} (HbA1c) to diagnose diabetes and also to identify subjects at risk of developing diabetes in the future.[30] In particular, a cut-off point of 6.5% has been suggested to diagnose type 2 diabetes. This cut-off point was chosen on the basis of cross-sectional and longitudinal studies conducted in adult subjects showing that a cut-off point of 6.5% identifies about one-third of cases of undiagnosed diabetes and that subjects with HbA1c higher than that cut-off have a long-term higher prevalence of microvascular complications.[30] Subjects with HbA1c between 5.7% and 6.4% have been defined as "at increased risk of diabetes" (Table 6.1).

According to a recent report by the SEARCH for Diabetes in Youth Study Group,[32] incidence rates of type 2 diabetes among children and adolescents are higher among racial and ethnic minorities than non-Hispanic whites.[32] The prevalence of type 2 diabetes in the US in children is estimated to be around 5%, while the prevalence of IGT has been estimated to be around 15%.[33] These prevalence rates are 10- to 20-times higher than those observed in European children, independently of the ethnicity/race.[34] Also the prevalence of IFG among children in the US seems to be about 10-times higher than that observed in European obese children.[35] In a cross-sectional survey among school-leaving students (mean age 15.5 years) of below-average socio-economic status and above-average weight in Dusseldorf (Germany), the combined prevalence of type 2 diabetes and impaired glucose regulation was reported to be 25/1000.[36] It has recently been argued that these data seem to underestimate

TABLE 6.1 Criteria for Diagnosis of Prediabetes and Diabetes

Criteria for diagnosis of increased risk for diabetes (prediabetes)	Criteria for diagnosis of diabetes
HbA1c 5.7−6.4%	HbA1c $\geq$ 6.5%
Fasting plasma glucose $\geq$ 100 mg/dl: IFG	Fasting plasma glucose $\geq$ 126 mg/dl
	2 h plasma glucose $\geq$ 200 mg/dl
2 h plasma glucose $\geq$ 140 mg/dl: IGT	Random plasma glucose $\geq$ 200 mg/dl in patients with symptoms

the effective prevalence of type 2 diabetes in Europe.[37] Not only the environment, but mostly genetic background may account for these differences.

PATHOGENESIS OF TYPE 2 DIABETES IN OBESE CHILDREN AND ADOLESCENTS

The glucose metabolism is tightly regulated from a multitude of factors; the most important among them being insulin. The insulin resistance, occurring in obese children, is just the consequence of a progressive resistance of the principal tissues (muscle, liver, adipose tissue) to insulin action.

The β-cells respond to insulin resistance occurring in obese children and adolescents by producing a vigorous state of hyperinsulinemia, which will maintain normal values of glucose levels. However, in the long run, the β-cell function may deteriorate in some, and the insulin secretion will not be sufficient to maintain glucose levels within the normal range. In addition, insulin resistance itself, by placing an increased demand on the β-cell to hypersecrete insulin, influences the progressive β-cell failure of type 2 diabetes.[38]

To understand the dynamics of the events leading to the development of type 2 diabetes, a few steps need to be taken into account and clearly highlighted. First: what leads an obese child to develop insulin resistance? and second: why the beta cell reduces progressively its ability to compensate the resistance?

ROLE OF ECTOPIC FAT DEPOSITION IN THE PATHOGENESIS OF INSULIN RESISTANCE

Ectopic fat deposition usually describes the anomalous deposition of the excess fat in organs and tissues that usually do not accumulate it, such as the liver and the skeletal muscle.

Although it remains unclear whether hepatic steatosis is a consequence or a cause of derangements in insulin sensitivity, the presence of steatosis is an important marker of multiorgan insulin resistance[39]; moreover, insulin resistance is directly related to percentage of liver fat.[39]

The intrahepatic fat accumulation induced by insulin resistance causes the development of non-alcoholic fatty liver disease (NAFLD) that is a clinical pathological condition of emerging importance in obese children.[40] NAFLD encompasses the entire spectrum of liver conditions, ranging from asymptomatic steatosis with elevated or normal aminotransferases to steatohepatitis (non-alcoholic steatohepatitis, NASH) and advanced fibrosis with cirrhosis.[41,42]

The association between NAFLD and a metabolic derangement has been clearly demonstrated by Burget et al.[40] In this latest study, as surrogate of liver injury, alanine aminotransferase (ALT) levels were measured in 392 obese adolescents. Elevated ALT (>35 U/l) levels were found in 14% of participants, with a predominance in White/Hispanic individuals. After adjusting for potential confounders, rising ALT levels were associated with deterioration in insulin sensitivity and glucose tolerance as well as increasing free fatty acid and triglyceride levels. Furthermore, increased hepatic fat accumulation (assessed using fast magnetic resonance imaging) was found in 32% of obese adolescents and was associated with decreased insulin sensitivity and adiponectin levels, and with increased triglycerides and visceral fat.[40]

These results demonstrate that in obese children and adolescents, hepatic fat accumulation is associated with the components of metabolic syndrome, such as insulin resistance, dyslipidemia and altered glucose metabolism.

Recent studies have shown that patterns of fat partitioning are probably one major link between insulin resistance, NAFLD and insulin resistance in obese children.[43] In a multiethnic cohort study, 118 obese adolescents were stratified into tertiles based on the proportion of abdominal fat in the visceral depot. Abdominal fat and intramyocellular lipid (IMCL) were measured by magnetic resonance imaging and by proton magnetic resonance spectroscopy, respectively. A high proportion of visceral fat was associated with muscle and hepatic steatosis, insulin resistance, high triglycerides and low HDL and adiponectin levels. As the proportion of visceral fat increased across tertiles, percentage subcutaneous fat decreased. Notably, the risk for the metabolic syndrome was five times greater in the adolescents with this particular fat partitioning profile compared with those with lower visceral accumulation.[44]

That is why it has been suggested that obese adolescents with a high proportion of visceral fat and relatively low subcutaneous fat have a phenotype reminiscent of partial lipodystrophy. Those who fit this profile are not necessarily the most severely obese, yet they suffer from severe metabolic complications of obesity and are at high risk of having metabolic syndrome.[43,44]

In conclusion, it is unclear whether hepatic steatosis is a consequence or a cause of the metabolic derangements in insulin sensitivity (metabolic syndrome). However, it is clear that liver steatosis represents a major metabolic concern in obese children, and that is why it should be deeply and precociously investigated and identified in order to prevent further metabolic complications.

THE β-CELL IN THE STORM OF INSULIN RESISTANCE

The β-cells respond to insulin resistance occurring in obese children and adolescents by producing a vigorous state of hyperinsulinemia, which will maintain normal values of glucose levels. In the long run, however, β-cell function may deteriorate in some, and the insulin secretion will be not sufficient to maintain glucose levels within the normal range.

Surely, different genetic predisposition plays an important role in the development of type 2 diabetes. This idea is supported both by genome wide association scan studies[45] (GWAS) and by clinical studies clearly showing that subjects, who develop IGT or type 2 diabetes, have a compromising insulin secretion even before developing IGT or type 2 diabetes. When estimating insulin secretion in the context of the 'resistant milieu' of the IGT subjects, and thus using the disposition index (DI), it has been found that IGT subjects had a significantly lower DI than the NGT group. The lower DI indicates that the secretion of insulin is not able to compensate for the increased resistance, resulting in a marked decrease in insulin-stimulated glucose metabolism in the IGT subjects.[46] More recently, Cali' et al. showed that obese adolescents with normal glucose tolerance who successively progress to IGT manifest a primary defect in β-cell function.[47] These data are in agreement with those reported by Lyssenko et al. on MPP and Botnia studies in adults, showing that impaired insulin secretion and action, particularly insulin secretion adjusted for insulin resistance (disposition index) are strong predictors of future diabetes.[45] Moreover, the progression of obese children with insulin resistance to type 2 diabetes seems to be faster than in adults.[48] An accurate case report by Gungor et al. suggested that, despite relatively robust initial insulin secretion, the deterioration in β-cell function in youth with type 2 diabetes may be much more accelerated (~15% per year) than that observed in adults.[48]

However, because type 2 diabetes in youth is a recent phenomenon, longitudinal long-term follow-up data are lacking. Findings from the SEARCH study showed that youths with type 2 diabetes and relatively short diabetes duration (1.5 years in mean) have a higher prevalence of CAD risk factors compared with non-diabetics of similar age, sex, and race.[49] In the same study it has also been suggested that adiposity and glycemic control account for much of the association between type 2 diabetes and an unfavorable CAD risk factor profile in youth.[49]

Type 2 diabetes is progressive, and one main factor responsible for this is a continued decline in β-cell function.[38] Several studies[38] have demonstrated that diabetes and prediabetes do not develop until the β-cell fails to compensate appropriately to the peripheral insulin resistance state. The ability of the β-cell to secrete sufficient insulin to adequately respond to the peripheral insulin resistance state depends on multiple factors, including β-cell mass[38] and secretory capacity,[38] influenced by genetic[45] and environmental factors.[45] In fact, although the progressive loss of β-cell function could be due to different metabolic derangements (insulin resistance, lipotoxicity), several studies have suggested that β-cell dysfunction also depends on a pre-existing and perhaps

genetically determined risk, which is crucial for β-cell dysfunction to occur (Figure 6.2).[38,45]

THERAPY OF TYPE 2 DIABETES IN YOUTHS

As for adults with type 2 diabetes, treatment goals for youths with the disease include glycemic control as close to normoglycemia as possible while avoiding episodes of hypoglycemia, and reducing other risk factors for long-term complications of diabetes (e.g., hypertension, dyslipidemia, and albuminuria).[30] Treatment initiated at the time of diagnosis will vary according to clinical presentation, which can range from asymptomatic hyperglycemia to diabetic ketoacidosis. In particular, non-pharmacological measures (diet and physical exercise) represent the first step in approaching youths with type 2 diabetes. If results achieved are not within the guideline

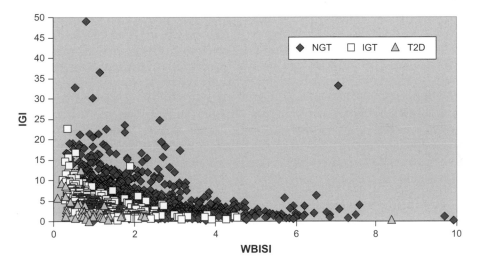

FIGURE 6.2 **The Parabolic Relationship Between Insulin Sensitivity and the β-Cell Secretion According to Glucose Tolerance.** In particular, obese children and adolescents showing a normal glucose tolerance (NGT—black diamonds) have lower insulin secretion and better insulin sensitivity than obese subjects with impaired glucose tolerance (IGT—white squares) and type 2 diabetes (T2D—grey triangles). This graph has been obtained by using personal data on 1,589 obese children and adolescents (mean age 13.2 ± 3.0; mean z-score BMI 2.30 ± 058). Of them, 40 showed type 2 diabetes, 335 IGT and 1,214 were NGT.

targets for the specific age range, introduction of approved drugs are needed. Insulin and metformin represent the two pharmacological approaches approved for children and adolescents with type 2 diabetes, though other oral hypoglycemic agents have been proposed.

Insulin therapy is essentially suggested when a child presents with severe hyperglycemia (2 h glucose > 200 mg/dl, HbA1c $> 8.5\%$ and/or ketosis), in order to rapidly achieve metabolic control.

Metformin represents the main therapy for young people with type 2 diabetes; it gained approval for its use in pediatrics based on a randomized, double-blind, placebo-controlled trial that evaluated the efficacy and safety of the medication, at doses up to 1000 mg twice daily in 82 children aged 10–16 years. The participants were treated for up to 16 weeks. Interestingly the results showed that metformin significantly improved glycemic control and HbA1c values with no cases of lactic acidosis and minimal side effects.[50] Therefore, metformin treatment is prescribed in non-ketotic patients starting with a low dose followed by a progressive increase of it during a phase of a 1- to 3-week period to the final therapeutic dose of 1000 mg twice a day. The presence of renal impairment or hepatic or cardiopulmonary insufficiency, or if a patient is undergoing evaluation with radiographic contrast materials (because it may precipitate lactic acidosis) represent important contraindications for its adoption. The most frequently encountered side effect is mild gastrointestinal discomfort which rarely necessitates drug discontinuation.[50]

There are no other oral hypoglycemic agents that have been approved for use in the pediatric population, though rosiglitazone, a potent insulin sensitizer, was evaluated in juvenile-onset type 2 diabetes. The study included 195 obese type 2 diabetes children (age range 8–17 years), in a 24-week double-blind, randomized, metformin-controlled, parallel group design.

Participants were randomized to rosiglitazone, maximum dose of 4 mg twice a day, or metformin, maximum dose 1000 mg twice a day. Results from this study showed that the median reductions in HbA1c from baseline (rosiglitazone group: -0.25%, p $= 0.027$; metformin group: -0.55%, p < 0.0001) and from screening (rosiglitazone group: -0.5%, p $= 0.011$; metformin group: -0.5%, p $= 0.0037$) to week 24 were statistically significant in both groups.[51]

Sulfonylurea (e.g., glimepiride, glyburide, glipizide), which increases both basal and meal-stimulated insulin secretion, has been used in the treatment of type 2 diabetes in adults for more than half a century. Results from a single-blind, 26-week active-controlled, multinational study randomized 263 obese youths with type 2 diabetes to receive glimepiride (1–8 mg once daily) or metformin (500–1000 mg twice daily) for 24 weeks are available.[52] In this study, no significant difference in HbA1c reduction between the two groups was shown. However, there was a difference in weight gain (kg) (glimepiride: change from baseline +2.2 8 0.6 and metformin: +0.7 8 0.64).[52] During the last few years, novel and promising treatment opportunities have been developed. In particular, recent studies in adults with type 2 diabetes including GLP-1 analogs (exenetide) or amylin analogs (pramlintide) may prove to be beneficial in youth.

Relevant pediatric trials are also underway in order to clarify the effectiveness of some of the available drugs available for the treatment of type 2 diabetes in youth. In particular, the Treatment Options for type 2 Diabetes in Adolescents and Youth (TODAY) is a 15-center clinical trial sponsored by the National Institute of Diabetes and Digestive and Kidney Diseases (start date, 2003; projected end date, 2011), that is examining the comparative efficacy of three approaches to the treatment of type 2 diabetes in youth ages 10–17 years: metformin alone, metformin plus rosiglitazone or metformin plus an intensive lifestyle intervention called the TODAY Lifestyle Program (TLP).

CONCLUSIONS AND FUTURE PERSPECTIVES

Given the relatively recent occurrence of type 2 diabetes in childhood, long-term follow-up studies are not available yet. However, it is reasonable to think that the metabolic derangement observed in obese children will have dramatic repercussions on their health earlier than that observed in adults, with a consequent worsening of the prognosis in terms of morbidity and mortality when they are still young. To date, we know that the physician has few arrows with which to fight this disease. The majority of drugs needed to treat insulin resistance, hypercholesterolemia, hypertension or even type 2 diabetes are now off-label, although more and more studies dealing with pharmacological treatment of obesity and its complications in pediatrics are coming up. The weight loss achieved by diet and physical exercise is still the most powerful and useful weapon against obesity and its metabolic complications. Several genetic studies and programs dealing with childhood obesity, insulin resistance and type 2 diabetes are now ongoing all over the world. These studies have been designed to find genes associated with these conditions and to discover how their alterations determine the occurrence of the disease. Hopefully, they will help us achieve new objectives crossing the border that now does not allow us to give a strong and definitive answer to these diseases.

References

1. Berrington de Gonzalez A, Hartge P, Cerhan JR, Flint AJ, Hannan L, MacInnis RJ, Moore SC, Tobias GS, Anton-Culver H, Freeman LB, Beeson WL, Clipp SL, English DR, Folsom AR, Freedman DM, Giles G, Hakansson N, Henderson KD, Hoffman-Bolton J, Hoppin JA, Koenig KL, Lee IM, Linet MS, Park Y, Pocobelli G, Schatzkin A, Sesso HD, Weiderpass E, Willcox BJ, Wolk A, Zeleniuch-Jacquotte A, Willett WC, Thun MJ. Body-mass index and mortality among 1.46 million white adults. N Engl J Med 2010;363:2211–9.
2. Reuser M, Bonneux L, Willekens F. The burden of mortality of obesity at middle and old age is small. A life table analysis of the US Health and Retirement Survey. Eur J Epidemiol 2008;23:601–7.
3. Muennig P, Lubetkin E, Jia H, Franks P. Gender and the burden of disease attributable to obesity. Am J Public Health 2006;96:1662–8.
4. Peeters A, Barendregt J, Willekens F, Mackenbach JP, Mamun AA, Bonneux L. Obesity in adulthood and its consequences for life expectancy: a life-table analysis. Ann Intern Med 2003;138:24–32.
5. Mokdad AH, Marks JS, Stroup DF, Gerberding JL. Actual causes of death in the United States, 2000. JAMA 2004;291:1238–45.
6. Danaei G, Vander Hoorn S, Lopez AD, Murray CJ, Ezzati M. Causes of cancer in the world: comparative risk assessment of nine behavioural and environmental risk factors. Lancet 2005;366:1784–932.
7. Han JC, Lawlor DA, Kimm SY. Childhood obesity. Lancet 2010;375:1737–48.
8. Cali AMG, Caprio S. Obesity in children and adolescents. J Clin Endocrinol Metab 2008;93:S31–6.
9. Guo SS, Chumlea WC. Tracking of body mass index in children in relation to overweight in adulthood. Am J Clin Nut 1999;70:145S–8S.
10. Whitaker RC, Wright JA, Pepe MS, Seidel KD, Dietz WH. Predicting obesity in young adulthood from childhood and parental obesity. N Engl J Med 1997;337:869–73.
11. Deshmukh-Taskar P, Nicklas TA, Morales M, Yang SJ, Zakeri I, Berenson GS. Tracking of overweight status from childhood to young adulthood: the Bogalusa Heart Study. Eur J Clin Nutr 2006;60:48–57.
12. Dietz WH. Health consequences of obesity in youth: childhood predictors of adult disease. Pediatrics 1998;101:518–25.
13. Dietz WH, Robinson TN. Overweight children and adolescents. N Engl J Med 2005;352:2100–9.
14. Harris KM, Gordon-Larsen P, Chantala K, Udry JR. Longitudinal trends in race/ethnic disparities in leading health indicators from adolescence to young adulthood. Arch Pediatr Adolesc Med 2006;160:74–81.
15. Engeland A, Bjorge T, Tverdal A, Sogaard AJ. Obesity in adolescence and adulthood and the risk of adult mortality. Epidemiology 2004;15:79–85.

16. Must A, Jacques PF, Dallal GE, Bajema CJ, Dietz WH. Long-term morbidity and mortality of overweight adolescents. A follow-up of the Harvard Growth Study of 1922 to 1935. *N Engl J Med* 1992;**327**:1350–5.

17. Weiss R, Dziura J, Burgert TS, Tamborlane WV, Taksali SE, Yeckel CW, Allen K, Lopes M, Savoye M, Morrison J, Sherwin RS, Caprio S. Obesity and the metabolic syndrome in children and adolescents. *N Engl J Med* 2004;**350**:2362–74.

18. Assimacopoulos-Jeannet F, Brichard S, Rencurel F, Cusin I, Jeanrenaud B. *In vivo* effects of hyperinsulinemia on lipogenic enzymes and glucose transporter expression in rat liver and adipose tissues. *Metabolism* 1995;**44**:228–33.

19. Kamagate A, Dong HH. FoxO1 integrates insulin signaling to VLDL production. *Cell Cycle* 2008;**7**:3162–70.

20. Caprio S, Plewe G, Diamond MP, Simonson DC, Boulware SD, Sherwin RS, Tamborlane WV. Increased insulin secretion in puberty: a compensatory response to reductions in insulin sensitivity. *J Pediatr* 1989;**114**:963–7.

21. Körner A, Kratzsch J, Gausche R, Schaab M, Erbs S, Kiess W. New predictors of the metabolic syndrome in children—role of adipocytokines. *Pediatr Res* 2007;**61**:640–5.

22. Nemet D, Wang P, Funahashi T, Matsuzawa Y, Tanaka S, Engelman L, Cooper DM. Adipocytokines, body composition, and fitness in children. *Pediatr Res* 2003;**53**:148–52.

23. Dixon D, Goldberg R, Schneiderman N, Delamater A. Gender differences in TNF-alpha levels among obese vs nonobese Latino children. *Eur J Clin Nutr* 2004;**58**:696–9.

24. Ruan H, Lodish HF. Insulin resistance in adipose tissue: direct and indirect effects of tumor necrosis factor-alpha. *Cytokine Growth Factor Rev* 2003;**14**:447–55.

25. Maffeis C, Silvagni D, Bonadonna R, Grezzani A, Banzato C, Tatò L. Fat cell size, insulin sensitivity, and inflammation in obese children. *J Pediatr* 2007;**151**:647–52.

26. Hara K, Yamauchi T, Kadowaki T. Adiponectin: an adipokine linking adipocytes and type 2 diabetes in humans. *Curr Diab Rep* 2005;**5**:136–40.

27. Kadowaki T, Yamauchi T. Adiponectin and adiponectin receptors. *Endocr Rev* 2005;**26**:439–51.

28. Böttner A, Kratzsch J, Müller G, Kapellen TM, Blüher S, Keller E, Blüher M, Kiess W. Gender differences of adiponectin levels develop during the progression of puberty and are related to serum androgen levels. *J Clin Endocrinol Metab* 2004;**89**:4053–61.

29. Reinehr T, Roth C, Menke T, Andler W. Adiponectin before and after weight loss in obese children. *J Clin Endocrinol Metab* 2004;**89**:3790–4.

30. American Diabetes Association. Standards of Medical Care in Diabetes. *Diabet Care* 2011;**34**:S11–61.

31. Meyer C, Pimenta W, Woerle HJ, Van Haeften T, Szoke E, Mitrakou A, Gerich J. Different mechanisms for impaired fasting glucose and impaired postprandial glucose tolerance in humans. *Diabetes Care* 2006;**29**:1909–14.

32. The Writing Group for the SEARCH for Diabetes in Youth Study Group. Incidence of diabetes in youth in the United States. *JAMA* 2007;**297**:2716–24.

33. Sinha R, Fisch G, Teague B, Tamborlane WV, Banyas B, Allen K, Savoye M, Rieger V, Taksali S, Barbetta G, Sherwin RS, Caprio S. Prevalence of impaired glucose tolerance among children and adolescents with marked obesity. *N Engl J Med* 2002;**346**:802–10.

34. Invitti C, Gilardini L, Viberti G. Impaired glucose tolerance in obese children and adolescents. *N Engl J Med* 2002;**347**:290–2.

35. Gilardini L, Girola A, Morabito F, Invitti C. Fasting glucose is not useful in identifying obese white children with impaired glucose tolerance. *J Pediatr* 2006;**149**:282.

36. Herder C, Schmitz-Beuting C, Rathmann W, Haastert B, Schmitz-Beuting J, Schäfer M, Scherbaum WA, Schneitler H, Martin S. Prevalence of impaired glucose regulation in German school-leaving students. *Int J Obes (Lond)* 2007;**31**:1086–8.

37. Reinehr T, Kiess W, Kapellen T, Wiegand S, Holl RW. APV and DPV Wiss Study Group and German Competence Net Obesity Children with diabetes mellitus type 2 in Europe: an underserved population. *Arch Dis Child* 2010;**95**:954.

38. Defronzo RA. From the Triumvirate to the Ominous Octet: a new paradigm for the treatment of type 2 diabetes mellitus. *Diabetes* 2009;**58**:773–95.

39. Fabbrini E, Sullivan S, Klein S. Obesity and nonalcoholic fatty liver disease: biochemical, metabolic, and clinical implications. *Hepatology* 2010;**51**:679–89.

40. Burgert TS, Taksali SE, Dziura J, Goodman TR, Yeckel CW, Papademetris X, Constable RT, Weiss R, Tamborlane WV, Savoye M, Seyal AA, Caprio S. Alanine aminotransferase levels fatty liver in childhood obesity: Associations with insulin resistance, adiponectin, and visceral fat. *J Clin Endocrinol Metab* 2006;**91**:2487–94.

41. Manco M, Marcellini M, Devito R, Comparcola D, Sartorelli MR, Nobili V. Metabolic syndrome and liver histology in paediatric non-alcoholic steatohepatitis. *Int J Obes (Lond)* 2008;**32**:381–7.

42. Angulo P. Nonalcoholic fatty liver disease. *N Engl J Med* 2002;**346**:1221–31.

43. Taksali SE, Caprio S, Dziura J, Dufour S, Cali A, Goodman TR, Papademetris X, Burgert TS, Pierpont BM, Savoye M, Shaw M, Seyal AA, Weiss R. High visceral and low abdominal subcutaneous fat

stores in the obese adolescent. *Diabetes* 2008;**57**: 367–71.

44. Cali AMG, Caprio S. Ectopic fat deposition and the metabolic syndrome in obese children and adolescents. *Horm Res* 2009;**71**:2–7.

45. Lyssenko V, Jonsson A, Almgren P, Pulizzi N, Isomaa B, Tuomi T, Berglund G, Altshuler D, Nilsson P, Groop L. Clinical risk factors, DNA variants, and the development of type 2 diabetes. *N Engl J Med* 2008;**359**: 2220–32.

46. Weiss R, Caprio S. The metabolic consequences of childhood obesity. *Best Pract Res Clin Endocrinol Metab* 2005;**19**:405–19.

47. Cali AM, Dalla Man C, Cobelli C, Dziura D, Seyal A, Shaw M, Allen K, Chen S, Caprio S. Primary defects in beta-cell function further exacerbated by worsening of insulin resistance mark the development of impaired glucose tolerance in obese adolescents. *Diabetes Care* 2009;**32**:456–61.

48. Gungor N, Arslanian S. Progressive beta cell failure in type 2 diabetes mellitus of youth. *J Pediatr* 2004;**44**:656–9.

49. West NA, Hamman RF, Mayer-Davis EJ, D'Agostino Jr RB, Marcovina SM, Liese AD, Zeitler PS, Daniels SR, Dabelea D. Cardiovascular risk factors among youth with and without type 2 diabetes: differences and possible mechanisms. *Diabetes Care* 2009;**32**:175–80.

50. Jones KL, Arslanian S, Peterokova VA, Park JS, Tomlinson MJ. Effect of metformin in pediatric patients with type 2 diabetes: a randomized controlled trial. *Diabetes Care* 2002;**25**:89–94.

51. Dabiri GJK, Krebs J, Sun Y, Mudd P, Weston W, Cobitz A, Freed M, Porter LE. Benefits of rosiglitazone in children with T2DM. *Diabetes* 2005;**8**:74–87.

52. Gottschalk M, Danne T, Vlajnic A, Cara JF. Glimepiride versus metformin as monotherapy in pediatric patients with type 2 diabetes: a randomized, single-blind comparative study. *Diabetes Care* 2007;**30**:790–4.

Diabetes Pathophysiology: A Nutritional Perspective

Kevin J. Acheson

Department of Nutrition & Health, Nestlé Research Centre, Lausanne, Switzerland

OUTLINE

"Until we have a cure, normalizing blood sugars is the best solution we have, because that is exactly what a cure will do. Why wait?"
R.K. Bernstein, 8th December 2008.

INTRODUCTION

Before the discovery of insulin by Banting and Best in 1921, diet was the only means by which the symptoms of diabetes could be alleviated. More than 2000 years ago the Susruta Samhita writings indicate that diabetics produced sweet urine and that two forms of the disease were apparent; one in older individuals and the other in the young who did not live long after diagnosis of the disease.[1] In the intervening period up until the 20th century, a number of observations on the treatment of diabetes were reported, such as that of Dr John Rollo who published *An Account of Two Cases of Diabetes Mellitus* in 1797, in which he describes treating an obese diabetic with a diet rich in protein and fat and low in carbohydrate, which resulted in weight loss and reversal of glycosuria[1]; and later in the 19th century, Apollinaire Bouchardat proposed that his patients self-monitored their glycosuria, with simple chemical reagents, while encouraging physical labor and a diet low in starchy foods and sugars.[2]

For individuals diagnosed with diabetes before the discovery of insulin, the prognosis

Nutritional and Therapeutic Interventions for Diabetes and Metabolic Syndrome
DOI: 10.1016/B978-0-12-385083-6.00007-3

89

was poor, with a life expectancy of less than one year for 68% of cases diagnosed at the Massachusetts General Hospital between 1824 and 1898,[3] improving to 6 years when dietary restriction was introduced as treatment.[4] While undernutrition worked more or less well for obese diabetics, it was less effective in non-obese individuals and children who developed diabetes; however, it did succeed in keeping some of them alive until they received insulin, which prolonged and completely changed their lives.

With the use of insulin diabetics were able to consume a diet similar to that of non-diabetics and Adlersberg observed, 25 years after the discovery of insulin, that its use had led to neglect of the dietary treatment of diabetes and emphasized that many mild and moderately severe cases of type 2 diabetes could be satisfactorily maintained without insulin by the proper application of dietotherapy.[5] Indeed Joslin writing about the same time comments "Insulin is so good that doctors and patients take advantage of it disregarding diet and exercise".[6] Certainly, since then diet composition and quantity have changed and this has been accompanied by an increase in the prevalence of diabetes. In 2010, the estimated prevalence for global diabetes was 285 million and it is predicted to rise to 438 million in 2030.[7] While this alarming increase is associated with a variety of factors such as rapid social and cultural changes, aging populations, increased urbanization and unhealthy lifestyles, the International Diabetes Federation believes that the majority of type 2 diabetes cases can be prevented and that the non-preventable forms of diabetes can be treated.[7]

Lifestyle change, which includes diet and physical activity, is still believed to be the best first choice treatment for weight management[8] and although the success rate over the long term is considered to be poor, it is still regarded as the primary strategy for the prevention of cardiovascular disease and type 2 diabetes[9]

as well as weight loss in obesity and for improving metabolic control in type 2 diabetics.[10–14]

DIETARY TREATMENT FOR DIABETES AT THE TURN OF THE 20TH CENTURY

In the years immediately preceding the discovery of insulin, dietary restriction was the only therapy available to medicine for diabetics, and was focused upon preventing glycosuria and reducing blood sugar concentrations into the range observed in non-diabetic individuals. Dietary restriction was typified by the "Starvation diet" developed by Frederick Allen and described by Hill and Eckman in "The Starvation Treatment of Diabetes".[15] Upon admission the patient was kept on an ordinary diet to determine the severity of the disease, after which he received a very-low-calorie diet providing 800 kcal per day, composed of whiskey and black coffee, until glycosuria was no longer detected. Low-carbohydrate foods were then slowly re-introduced into the diet in sufficient quantities to prevent the reappearance of glycosuria. In general, for adults, protein was introduced into the diet until it provided approximately 1 g per kilogram body weight per day and total energy amounted to ~30 kcal per kilogram per day. So although this treatment was called the "starvation diet", the diet established to keep the patient free of glycosuria was not very different from present day protein recommendations nor was it more draconian than calorie-restricted diets used for weight control today.

Other physicians of the time, Elliot Joslin and Louis Newburgh, promoted Allen's "Starvation diet" with slight[3] or more substantial modifications.[16] Newburgh[16] preferred to provide his patients with 900 kcal per day composed of 9% protein, 85% fat and 6% carbohydrate, which was consumed until glycosuria and ketonuria were absent and blood glucose concentrations had returned to normal. Thereafter the energy content of the diet was increased, mainly by increasing the fat content of the diet (~85%), until the patient's energy requirements were met and nitrogen balance was established. Although Newburgh's diet initially produced hyperlipidemia, blood lipids decreased with time to attain normolipidemic values.[17] Newburgh believed that his high-fat diet was more appropriate for diabetics than that of Allen's, since besides preventing glycosuria and ketonuria, it also enabled his patients to consume sufficient energy to perform physical work and earn a living.[18] However, Alderberg observed that excessive amounts of fat impaired carbohydrate tolerance and, with others, introduced more liberal or "high-carbohydrate" diets as a therapy for diabetics, *provided* that they were treated with insulin. Without insulin, higher-carbohydrate diets caused unfavorable effects on blood sugar and glycosuria,[5] but this could be overcome by resorting to the "protein trick", in which proteins were substituted for the carbohydrate component of the diet to subsequently liberate glucose more slowly via gluconeogenesis. As glycosuria became negative and blood sugar levels improved, dietary protein was gradually replaced by carbohydrates sufficient to prevent glycosuria.[5]

When describing the diet used by his patients at the George F. Baker Clinic in 1941, 20 years after the discovery of insulin, Joslin indicated that the average carbohydrate intake for all patients and all ages was 156 g[6] or 625 kcal/day, which for an individual consuming 2,500 kcal/day corresponds to only 25% of his daily energy intake. He further comments, "With the carbohydrate in the diet as high as 150 grams, the chances of a diabetic not being able to obtain enough calories in the form of protein and fat seem slight".[6] However, in the 70 intervening years since this statement was made the carbohydrate component of the diabetic diet has increased considerably from 5–25%, to recommendations varying from 40% to 65%[19,20] of daily energy requirements. Is this due to improvements in medical nutrition and pharmaceutical therapy for diabetics or is it as Joslin feared that "Insulin is so good that it covers up a multitude of therapeutic sins."?[6]

DIETARY RECOMMENDATIONS

At the beginning of the 20th century, fat provided approximately 35% of the daily energy intake of the American diet and increased to ~40% during the 1950s and 1960s, at which time saturated, monounsaturated, and polyunsaturated fatty acids provided ~16%, 17%, and 4% of total energy intake, respectively.[21] Recommendations to reduce total fat and the saturated fatty acid components of the diet began in the 1960s[22] and subsequent decreases in the diet were observed.[21,23–25] These recommendations were introduced as a means of lowering serum cholesterol, for the prevention of heart disease,[26] and were later adopted by the American Medical Association and other medical and dietetic institutions. Despite reports indicating declines in mortality from coronary heart and cardiovascular diseases since then,[27–29] these have been confounded by the increasing prevalence of obesity and diabetes,[27] which has occurred during the same period of time, due to concomitant increases in energy and carbohydrate intake.[24,30,31]

Although the process for dietary recommendations has changed from "expert opinion" to "evidence-based", the recommendations for a healthy diet have remained relatively unchanged for the last 40 years.[8,19,32] The latest 2010 Dietary Guidelines Advisory Committee indicate that in an environment where the majority of the American population is overweight or obese, saturated fats should provide at most 10% and preferably less than 7% of total energy intake by substituting with mono- or polyunsaturated fatty acids; dietary cholesterol should be < 300 mg/day, preferably < 200 mg/day, and *trans*-fatty acids should be avoided. Since protein recommendations have not changed the primary energy source remains carbohydrates that should be provided by fiber-rich fruits, vegetables, whole grain, and legumes, with the addition of reduced-fat and fat-free milk and milk products. Added sugar, sugar-sweetened beverages, and refined grain products should be reduced as much as possible to help with calorie control.[32]

At the present time relatively high-carbohydrate, low-fat diets are recommended as a healthy diet for the population in general[32] as well as for individuals susceptible to heart disease,[27] cancer,[33] hypertension,[27,34] and diabetes.[35] However, in spite of these recommendations there is considerable evidence that high-carbohydrate, low-fat diets promote the insulin resistance syndrome[36–39] and that they are not favorable for patients with mild or moderately severe type 2 diabetes.[40] In some individuals high-carbohydrate diets promote the conversion of less atherogenic large low-density lipoprotein (LDL) into the more atherogenic small, dense LDL[41] and fructose, once considered the ideal sweetener for diabetics, has now been shown to predict smaller LDL particle size in schoolchildren.[42] These arguments, together with more recent evidence that low-carbohydrate diets have health benefits for weight management,[43–46] diabetes[47,48] and cardiovascular disease[44,49–52] have led an increasing number of researchers to question present-day dietary guidelines.[53–55]

While it is very possible that a large proportion of the population does not follow the recommended guidelines,[56–59] one might expect that type 2 diabetics and others who suffer the metabolic consequences of an inappropriate diet would be more committed to lifestyle changes to avoid resorting to pharmacological therapy. Although the use of oral hypoglycemics and insulin reduce hyperglycemia in the short and medium term, the fact that some individuals are able to reduce, or completely discontinue, their medications by dietary changes alone[47,48,60–62] should be sufficient motivation for greater efforts to be made to treat susceptible individuals with the most appropriate diet to prevent the onset and progression of the disease.

GLUCOSE CONTROL

A number of large cohort, long-term clinical trials have documented that tight glycemic control has benefits not only in preventing the onset and progression of type 2 diabetes,[63–65] but that it also prevents or delays morbidities of type 1 and type 2 diabetes such as retinopathy, nephropathy, neuropathy, foot ulcers, and cardiovascular disease.[63–67] In consequence, the effective treatment of hyperglycemia is the priority of diabetes associations worldwide[68] to maintain blood glucose concentrations as near to normal as possible. Other studies have implicated high postprandial glucose concentrations in cardiovascular risk as well as the microvascular complications of diabetes[69–71] and recommend that targeting both chronic and acute glucose fluctuations is necessary.[70] But in spite of this diabetics continue to receive recommendations to consume a diet rich in carbohydrates. When saturated fats and dietary cholesterol were associated with cardiovascular disease in the 1960s, the response was to decrease saturated fats and cholesterol in the diet. However, it is perhaps surprising that when studies provide irrefutable evidence that hyperglycemia, which in large part is the result of consuming dietary carbohydrate, is responsible for the progression of type 2 diabetes and the debilitating complications associated with type 1 and type 2 diabetes, the response is to maintain a high-carbohydrate diet!

Nevertheless, an increasing number of health professionals believe that glucose control is far easier if dietary carbohydrate is restricted. Of note is Dr Richard Bernstein, a former engineer and type 1 diabetic since the age of 12, who with deteriorating health and dissatisfied with the American Diabetes Association's recommended treatment, bought a blood glucose analyzer and tested the effects of different foods and diet on his blood glucose control throughout the day.[72] He soon realized that glycemia was easier to control, and could be more tightly controlled with less insulin when his diet contained restricted amounts of carbohydrate. With his change in diet, insulin treatment, and increased physical activity, his symptoms of diabetic complications regressed and when he wanted to share his experiences with the medical community they were met with indifference. Surprised and frustrated by this lack of interest, he amazingly entered medical school at the age of 45 and after graduating opened his own diabetes clinic in New York, where he has been treating type 1 and type 2 diabetics ever since. As recommended above, Bernstein has been tightly controlling chronic and acute glucose fluctuations in his patients for a number of years, by means of a low-carbohydrate diet, and has observed that microvascular complications can be avoided.[72] Over the years some of his experiences such as blood glucose self-monitoring have become accepted, but a diet without fruit will always be an anathema for the dietetic establishment.

Although low-carbohydrate diets are often associated with weight loss, Nuttall's group in Minneapolis have been investigating the dietary management of blood glucose control in type 2 diabetics without medication or weight loss, in the hope that such diets will be more acceptable to type 2 diabetics.[73,74] In a series of studies, blood glucose control was compared in mild, untreated type 2 diabetics after 5 weeks on a conventional, high-carbohydrate (55% carbohydrate, 15% protein, 30% fat), weight-maintenance diet and after diets in which carbohydrate provided 40%,[75] 30%,[76] and 20%[73] of energy intake in a randomized, crossover design. As the proportion of carbohydrate

in the diets decreased, the mean 24-h integrated glucose response and HbA1c at the end of each dietary intervention also decreased in a proportional manner. Such results, observed in weight maintenance conditions, demonstrate the close relationship between dietary carbohydrates and blood glucose control in untreated type 2 diabetics and indicate that carbohydrate reduction, even over periods as short as 5 weeks, can provide benefits during the dietary treatment of type 2 diabetes.

Interestingly the "Joslin Clinical Nutrition Guidelines for overweight and obese adults with type 2 diabetes, prediabetes or those at high risk for developing type 2 diabetes — 03/29/2007", recommends a diet with a macronutrient composition of ~40% energy from carbohydrate, 30—35% fat, and 20—30% protein[77] and their "Why WAIT" program, albeit over 12 weeks, provides a diet with an energy composition of 40% carbohydrate, 30% fat, and 30% protein.[78] Not only has the carbohydrate content of the diet been reduced, but it has been replaced by increasing the protein component of the diet. However, in spite of doubling the protein composition of the diet from 15 to 30%, the absolute amount of protein consumed does not change that much due to the overall reduction in daily energy intake.[78] Although the "Why WAIT" program imposes an energy reduction of at least 500 kcal per day, the rationale behind the low-carbohydrate diet is that energy reduction occurs unconsciously, since for the majority of individuals it is difficult to consume excessive amounts of fat and protein in the absence of carbohydrate.

LOW-CARBOHYDRATE DIETS

Low-carbohydrate diets were studied for a number of years, before being popularized by "Dr Atkins Diet Revolution" published in 1972.[79] It was perhaps very unfortunate that in popularizing his diet plan, Atkins highlighted the consumption of unlimited amounts of protein and saturated fats, which in the 1970s was very much the antithesis of dietary guidelines that had been established for the prevention of heart disease.[26] In fact his diet program was not very different to the diets previously described for diabetics by Joslin and Allen,[3,15] except that after the initial phase of weight loss, instead of adjusting the amount of dietary carbohydrates to prevent glycosuria, they were modulated to prevent weight gain. However, since his diet plan contravened conventional nutrition wisdom at that time it was relegated to a "fad-diet" for weight control.

The resistance to changing established dietary guidelines is considerable, for a number of reasons which include the following critiques:-

1. If carbohydrates are reduced, dietary protein and/or fat must increase.
2. If dietary fat increases this could be detrimental for cardiovascular disease, and non-alcoholic liver disease.
3. If dietary protein increases it could impair kidney function.
4. Reduction of carbohydrates will reduce the intake of fruits and vegetables and their associated vitamins, minerals and phytonutrients.
5. Reduction of carbohydrates will decrease fiber intake.
6. They are not consistent with national guidelines![80]

Before the publication of Atkins' book there were reports in the scientific literature, albeit with small numbers of subjects studied over short periods of time, describing low-carbohydrate diets, which again, unfortunately, were sometimes referred to as "high-fat" diets. However, their findings do help reject Critiques 1—3, listed above. As Yudkin explains,[81] when carbohydrates are reduced to approximately 50 g/d, with no conscious restriction of protein or fat intake, consumption of dietary fat is self-limiting and its *ad libitum* intake was found to be the same or less than that consumed when his subjects consumed their habitual diet.[82] Similarly, protein intake did not increase on the low-carbohydrate diet when compared with the subjects' habitual diets.[82,83] Interestingly, Yudkin's results are confirmed by those of Samaha *et al.* (Table 7.1) whose subjects consumed a low-carbohydrate diet for 6 months.[45]

Hamdy and Carver also observed that protein intake did not increase by much in their "Why WAIT" program.[78] In the absence of disproportionate increases in fat and protein intake on low-carbohydrate diets, one would not expect them to cause microvascular problems or kidney dysfunction. In a more recent publication Hamdy and Horton[84] discuss the potential effects of moderate increases in protein intake on kidney function.

Yudkin's group also investigated potential claims that a low-carbohydrate diet would lead to vitamin and mineral deficiencies (Critique 4) when energy intake was decreased by 30—50%.[82,83] They demonstrated that nutrient intake was as good, if not better, on the low-carbohydrate diet than on their subjects'

TABLE 7.1 Protein and Fat Consumption do not Increase on an Ad Libitum Low-Carbohydrate Diet

	Energy intake (kcal/d)	Protein (%)	Carbohydrate (%)	Fat (%)	Protein (g)	Carbohydrates (g)	Fat (g)
Baseline	2090	17	49	33	89	256	77
6 months	1630	22	37	41	90	151	74

Mean values taken from Samaha *et al.*,[45] Table 3.

habitual diets (due to the restriction of nutrient-poor foods) and certainly better than if each of the macronutrients had been decreased by ~30%, as in the case of an energy-restricted, equilibrated diet.[82]

Regarding Critique 5, two popular low-carbohydrate diets, "*Dr. Atkins Diet Revolution*"[79] and "*Dr. Bernstein's Diabetes Solution*"[72] both recommend the consumption of green leafy vegetables, which are low in available carbohydrate and relatively high in fiber. Consequently, even when on the initial weight loss phase of the Atkins program during which dietary carbohydrates are reduced to 20 g, if all of the available carbohydrate (referred to as "Sugars, total" in the USDA Nutrient Database)[85] was supplied by boiled spinach, one would need to consume 465 g spinach, providing 112 g total dietary fiber. Although this example will be criticized as being unrealistic, it does demonstrate that by judicious selection of green leafy vegetables it is possible to cover an individual's recommended dietary fiber intake, while consuming an exceptionally low-carbohydrate diet.

To suggest that a popular diet is inadequate because it is not consistent with national guidelines to reduce chronic disease risk is based on the premise that the national guidelines are perfect and unquestionable,[80] however, it is for precisely this reason that the national guidelines are being questioned (Critique 6).[53–55]

Since the publication of a number of intervention trials in 2003 demonstrating certain advantages for obese and diabetic individuals consuming a low-carbohydrate diet,[43–45] more evidence in favor of low-carbohydrate diets has been published. Although this evidence is not always clear-cut it does appear to be having some influence on the nutritional guidelines recommended by a number of medical associations and institutions, which rely more and more on results from randomized, controlled clinical trials.

In a meta-analysis of randomized control trials comparing low-carbohydrate diets, without energy restriction against low-fat, energy-restricted diets, Nordmann et al.[86] concluded that low-carbohydrate diets were at least as effective as low-fat diets for weight loss, with the caveat that favorable changes in triglycerides and high-density lipoprotein (HDL)-cholesterol should be weighed against potentially unfavorable increases in LDL-cholesterol. However, the atherogenic potential of LDL-cholesterol appears to depend more upon particle size than its concentration.[87] Although two studies investigating the effect of three popular diets, the Atkins, Ornish, and Zone diets, on weight loss and metabolic risk factors over 1 year observed disparate results[88,89] with respect to weight loss on the Atkins diet, the authors of both studies comment in favor of low-carbohydrate diets for weight loss[89] and improvement of cardiovascular risk factors.[88,89] Dansinger et al.[88] comment that their study was designed to investigate dietary adherence under uncontrolled conditions rather than to identify the most appropriate diet for weight loss and reduction of cardiovascular risk. Since the attrition rates were high (35–50%) and adherence to the diets decreased over time, they concluded that sustained adherence to a diet, rather than diet type, predicted weight loss and reduction of cardiac risk factors.

Further support for low-carbohydrate diets was provided by the results of the OmniHeart trial[90] which demonstrated that the macronutrient composition of the diet, even under weight maintenance conditions, could have significant effects on improving blood pressure and cardiovascular risk factors. They observed that consuming a carbohydrate diet, similar to the DASH (Dietary Approaches to Stop Hypertension) diet, providing 15% protein, 58% carbohydrate, and 27% fat energy for 6 weeks, resulted in decreased blood pressure as well as lower total cholesterol, LDL-cholesterol, and HDL-cholesterol concentrations. Although HDL-cholesterol decreased, the decrease was much less than that of LDL-cholesterol. However, two other weight maintenance diets consumed over the same period of time and designed to replace 10% of carbohydrate energy with either protein (i.e. 25% protein, 48% carbohydrate, and 27% fat) or unsaturated fat (15% protein, 48% carbohydrate, and 37% fat) lowered systolic and diastolic blood pressure further, improved blood lipid concentrations and further reduced estimated cardiovascular risk. The authors discuss the potential of hypocaloric diets rich in protein or monounsaturated fats to facilitate weight loss and the possibility that the DASH diet could be improved by partial substitution of carbohydrate with protein from plant and animal sources or with monounsaturated fats. Indeed, under controlled hypocaloric conditions, both low-fat, high-protein and high-monounsaturated fat, standard-protein diets induced similar weight loss, ~10 kg, in overweight and obese individuals over a 12-week period, with concomitant improvements in insulin sensitivity and cardiovascular disease risk factors.[91] In a subsequent analysis, critical of the nutritional adequacy of popular diets when compared with the Harvard group's modified DASH diets, they suggest that guidelines can now be fine-tuned to optimize for disease prevention.[80]

In the past, Reaven proposed substituting unsaturated for saturated fats to reduce low-density lipoprotein-cholesterol concentrations[92] and provided evidence to support this by assigning insulin-resistant obese individuals to a 16-week energy-restricted diet similar to that recommended by the ADA (American Diabetes Association) composed of 15% protein, 60% carbohydrate, and 25% fat or another diet in which 20% of carbohydrate energy was substituted for by mono- and polyunsaturated fats such that the final composition was 15% protein, 40% carbohydrate, and 45% fat.[93] Weight loss was slightly, but not significantly, greater on the lower 40%-carbohydrate diet, which one might expect if the subjects adhered to their energy-restricted diet, and improved insulin sensitivity correlated with weight loss.

Throughout the day insulin and triglyceride concentrations were significantly less, fasting triglyceride and E-selectin concentrations were reduced, and greater increases in HDL-cholesterol concentrations and LDL particle size were observed after the lower carbohydrate diet, indicating that although weight loss was similar on the two diets, reducing the carbohydrate content of the diet and replacing it with unsaturated fats improves cardiovascular disease risk factors.

Other short-term studies have observed that an isocaloric high-protein diet increases satiety.[94] In the same study, increasing the protein content of an *ad libitum* diet from 15% to 30%, by replacing fat and keeping carbohydrate at 50% energy for 12 weeks, decreased spontaneous energy intake with concomitant reductions in body weight and body fat.[94] Increasing the protein content of a weight-maintenance diet, after a period of weight loss, was also found to improve weight maintenance when compared with a diet rich in carbohydrates over a 12-week period.[95] More extreme diets, such as the Very Low Carbohydrate Ketogenic Diet (VLCKD), evaluated over a similar time-frame, have also demonstrated better body weight and fat losses, improved insulin sensitivity and glucose control as well as decreased leptin concentrations, in overweight and obese subjects with atherogenic dyslipidemia, when compared with a low-fat diet.[96] Although anti-inflammatory effects were observed on both diets, they were greater on the VLCKD.[97] When such a diet was extended to 6 months and compared with a low-glycemic index diet, it was associated with greater weight loss, better improvements in metabolic control and more frequent reduction or discontinuation of diabetes medication.[62]

Although these short-term studies provide evidence that dietary carbohydrate restriction has a number of health benefits, longer trials have demonstrated mixed results.[98] Comparison of three diets—low-carbohydrate unrestricted energy, Mediterranean restricted energy and low-fat restricted energy—for weight loss in moderately obese subjects over 2 years demonstrated significant decreases in body weight, blood pressure, and waist circumference with all diets; however, they were greater on the low-carbohydrate and Mediterranean diets than on the low-fat diet.[46] Concomitant improvements in lipid profiles and other markers were also more favorable on the low-carbohydrate and Mediterranean diets.[46] However, Sacks et al,[98] found that weight loss of overweight subjects consuming reduced-calorie diets with different fat, protein and carbohydrate contents over 2 years, occurred regardless of the macronutrient composition of the diet. Unfortunately, in spite of intensive participant instruction throughout this trial, adherence to the diets was poor and the requisite differences between groups for energy intake and macronutrient composition were not attained.

CONCLUSIONS

Where the dietary treatment of weight loss and diabetes control is concerned, almost everyone has their own hypothesis for their prevention and cure, and it is possible to find arguments in the scientific literature for or against any particular one. However, from this non-exhaustive review, and other literature that has not been cited, there is ample evidence to show that low-carbohydrate diets in combination with physical exercise and/or strength training can prevent the onset of type 2 diabetes and prevent or retard the progression of the debilitating morbidities associated with type 1 and type 2 diabetes. Although Bernstein's question *"Why wait?"* in the quote at the beginning of the chapter has nothing to do with the acronym chosen by the Joslin Diabetes Center's "Why WAIT" program, it is reassuring that at least one diabetes organization is not *waiting* to explore how short-term, moderate carbohydrate

reduction can improve the metabolic control and quality of life of type 2 diabetics, while at the same time reducing the direct and indirect costs of the disease.

References

1. Witters LA, Luciano M, Williams C, Yang J. Diabetes Detectives. *Dartmouth Medicine* 2008;**33**:36−57.
2. Chast F, Slama G. [Apollinaire Bouchardat and diabetes]. *Hist Sci Med* 2007;**41**:287−301.
3. Joslin EP. The treatment of diabetes mellitus. *Can Med Assoc J* 1916;**6**:673−84.
4. Joslin EP. The treatment of diabetes mellitus. *Can Med Assoc J* 1924;**14**:808−11.
5. Aldersberg D. The use of high protein diets in the treatment of diabetes mellitus. *Am J Dig Dis* 1948;**15**:109−15.
6. Joslin EP. The diabetic. *Can Med Assoc J* 1943;**48**:488−97.
7. *International Diabetes Federation Diabetes Atlas.* 4th ed. Brussels: International Diabetes Federation; 2009.
8. Dietary Guidelines for Americans. *United States Department of Agriculture, Center for Nutritional Policy and Promotion,* www.cnpp.usda.gov/dietaryguidelines.htm; 2010.
9. Rosenzweig JL, Ferrannini E, Grundy SM, Haffner SM, Heine RJ, Horton ES, Kawamori R. Primary prevention of cardiovascular disease and type 2 diabetes in patients at metabolic risk: an endocrine society clinical practice guideline. *J Clin Endocrinol Metab* 2008;**93**:3671−89.
10. Hamman RF, Wing RR, Edelstein SL, Lachin JM, Bray GA, Delahanty L, Hoskin M, Kriska AM, Mayer-Davis EJ, Pi-Sunyer X, Regensteiner J, Venditti B, Wylie-Rosett J. Effect of weight loss with lifestyle intervention on risk of diabetes. *Diabetes Care* 2006;**29**:2102−7.
11. Ratner RE. An update on the Diabetes Prevention Program. *Endocr Pract* 2006;**12**(Suppl. 1):20−4.
12. Wadden TA, West DS, Delahanty L, Jakicic J, Rejeski J, Williamson D, Berkowitz RI, Kelley DE, Tomchee C, Hill JO, Kumanyika S. The Look AHEAD study: a description of the lifestyle intervention and the evidence supporting it. *Obesity (Silver Spring)* 2006;**14**:737−52.
13. Wadden TA, West DS, Neiberg RH, Wing RR, Ryan DH, Johnson KC, Foreyt JP, Hill JO, Trence DL, Vitolins MZ. One-year weight losses in the Look AHEAD study: factors associated with success. *Obesity (Silver Spring)* 2009;**17**:713−22.
14. Wolf AM, Conaway MR, Crowther JQ, Hazen KY, Nadler L, Oneida B, Bovbjerg VE. Translating lifestyle

intervention to practice in obese patients with type 2 diabetes: Improving Control with Activity and Nutrition (ICAN) study. *Diabetes Care* 2004;**27**:1570–6.

15. Hill LW, Eckman RS. *The starvation treatment of diabetes.* Boston: W.M. Leonard; 1916.

16. Newburgh LH, Marsh PL. The use of a high fat diet in the treatment of (1920).

17. Lusk G. Diabetes Mellitus. In: Lusk G, editor. *The elements of the Science of Nutrition.* New York: Johnson Reprint Corporation; 1976. p. 650–82.

18. Beeuwkes AM, Johnston MW. Louis Harry Newburgh—A biographical sketch (June 17, 1883–July 17, 1956). *J. Nutr* 1965;**85**:3–7.

19. Katsilambros N, Liatis S, Makrilakis K. Critical review of the international guidelines: what is agreed upon—what is not? *Nestle Nutr Workshop Ser Clin Perform Programme* 2006;**11**:207–18.

20. Zivkovic AM, German JB, Sanyal AJ. Comparative review of diets for the metabolic syndrome: implications for nonalcoholic fatty liver disease. *Am J Clin Nutr* 2007;**86**:285–300.

21. Stephen AM, Wald NJ. Trends in individual consumption of dietary fat in the United States, 1920–1984. *Am J Clin Nutr* 1990;**52**:457–69.

22. Kritchevsky D. History of recommendations to the public about dietary fat. *J Nutr* 1998;**128**:449S–52S.

23. Heini AF, Weinsier RL. Divergent trends in obesity and fat intake patterns: the American paradox. *Am J Med* 1997;**102**:259–64.

24. Marantz PR, Bird ED, Alderman MH. A call for higher standards of evidence for dietary guidelines. *Am J Prev Med* 2008;**34**:234–40.

25. Willett WC. Is dietary fat a major determinant of body fat? *Am J Clin Nutr* 1998;**67**:556S–62S.

26. Stamler J, Beard RR, Connor WE, et al. Report of Inter-Society Commission for Heart Disease Resources. Prevention of Cardiovascular Disease. Primary prevention of the atherosclerotic diseases. *Circulation* 1970;**42**:A55–95.

27. Gidding SS, Lichtenstein AH, Faith MS, Karpyn A, Mennella JA, Popkin B, Rowe J, Van HL, Whitsel L. Implementing American Heart Association pediatric and adult nutrition guidelines: a scientific statement from the American Heart Association Nutrition Committee of the Council on Nutrition, Physical Activity and Metabolism, Council on Cardiovascular Disease in the Young, Council on Arteriosclerosis, Thrombosis and Vascular Biology, Council on Cardiovascular Nursing, Council on Epidemiology and Prevention, and Council for High Blood Pressure Research. *Circulation* 2009;**119**:1161–75.

28. U.S. Department of Health and Human Services National Center for Health Statistics. *Health United*

States. Hyattsville, MD: DHHS Publication No. (PHS) 96; 1995.

29. Stamler J. Diet and coronary heart disease. *Biometrics* 1982;**38**(Suppl):95–118.

30. Austin GL, Ogden LG, Hill JO. Trends in carbohydrate, fat, and protein intakes and association with energy intake in normal-weight, overweight, and obese individuals: 1971–2006. *Am J Clin Nutr* 2011;**93**:836–43.

31. Woolf SH, Nestle M. Do dietary guidelines explain the obesity epidemic? *Am J Prev Med* 2008;**34**:263–5.

32. US Department of Agriculture and US Department of Health and Human Services. Report of the Dietary Guidelines Advisory Committee on the dietary guidelines for Americans, 2010. June 15, 2010.

33. Kushi LH, Byers T, Doyle C, Bandera EV, McCullough M, McTiernan A, Gansler T, Andrews KS, Thun MJ. American Cancer Society Guidelines on Nutrition and Physical Activity for cancer prevention: reducing the risk of cancer with healthy food choices and physical activity. *CA Cancer J Clin* 2006;**56**:254–81.

34. Appel LJ, Brands MW, Daniels SR, Karanja N, Elmer PJ, Sacks FM. Dietary approaches to prevent and treat hypertension: a scientific statement from the American Heart Association. *Hypertension* 2006;**47**:296–308.

35. Bantle JP, Wylie-Rosett J, Albright AL, Apovian CM, Clark NG, Franz MJ, Hoogwerf BJ, Lichtenstein AH, Mayer-Davis E, Mooradian AD, Wheeler ML. Nutrition recommendations and interventions for diabetes: a position statement of the American Diabetes Association. *Diabetes Care* 2008;**31**:S61–78.

36. Abbasi F, McLaughlin T, Lamendola C, Kim HS, Tanaka A, Wang T, Nakajima K, Reaven GM. High carbohydrate diets, triglyceride-rich lipoproteins, and coronary heart disease risk. *Am J Cardiol* 2000;**85**:45–8.

37. Jeppesen J, Hein HO, Suadicani P, Gyntelberg F. Relation of high TG-low HDL cholesterol and LDL cholesterol to the incidence of ischemic heart disease. An 8-year follow-up in the Copenhagen Male Study. *Arterioscler Thromb Vasc Biol* 1997;**17**:1114–20.

38. Jeppesen J, Schaaf P, Jones C, Zhou MY, Chen YD, Reaven GM. Effects of low-fat, high-carbohydrate diets on risk factors for ischemic heart disease in postmenopausal women. *Am J Clin Nutr* 1997;**65**:1027–33.

39. Reaven GM. Diet and Syndrome X. *Curr Atheroscler Rep* 2000;**2**:503–7.

40. Garg A, Grundy SM, Unger RH. Comparison of effects of high and low carbohydrate diets on plasma lipoproteins and insulin sensitivity in patients with mild NIDDM. *Diabetes* 1992;**41**:1278–85.

41. Krauss RM. Dietary and genetic effects on low-density lipoprotein heterogeneity. *Annu Rev Nutr* 2001;**21**:283–95.

42. Aeberli I, Zimmermann MB, Molinari L, Lehmann R, l'Allemand D, Spinas GA, Berneis K. Fructose intake is a predictor of LDL particle size in overweight schoolchildren. *Am J Clin Nutr* 2007;**86**:1174—8.

43. Brehm BJ, Seeley RJ, Daniels SR, D'Alessio DA. A randomized trial comparing a very low carbohydrate diet and a calorie-restricted low fat diet on body weight and cardiovascular risk factors in healthy women. *J Clin Endocrinol Metab* 2003;**88**:1617—23.

44. Foster GD, Wyatt HR, Hill JO, McGuckin BG, Brill C, Mohammed BS, Szapary PO, Rader DJ, Edman JS, Klein S. A randomized trial of a low-carbohydrate diet for obesity. *N Engl J Med* 2003;**348**:2082—90.

45. Samaha FF, Iqbal N, Seshadri P, Chicano KL, Daily DA, McGrory J, Williams T, Williams M, Gracely EJ, Stern L. A low-carbohydrate as compared with a low-fat diet in severe obesity. *N Engl J Med* 2003;**348**:2074—81.

46. Shai I, Schwarzfuchs D, Henkin Y, Shahar DR, Witkow S, Greenberg I, Golan R, Fraser D, Bolotin A, Vardi H, Tangi-Rozental O, Zuk-Ramot R, Sarusi B, Brickner D, Schwartz Z, Sheiner E, Marko R, Katorza E, Thiery J, Fiedler GM, Bluher M, Stumvoll M, Stampfer MJ. Weight loss with a low-carbohydrate, Mediterranean, or low-fat diet. *N Engl J Med* 2008;**359**:229—41.

47. Boden G, Sargrad K, Homko C, Mozzoli M, Stein TP. Effect of a low-carbohydrate diet on appetite, blood glucose levels, and insulin resistance in obese patients with type 2 diabetes. *Ann Intern Med* 2005;**142**:403—11.

48. Nielsen JV, Joensson EA. Low-carbohydrate diet in type 2 diabetes: stable improvement of bodyweight and glycemic control during 44 months follow-up. *Nutr Metab (Lond)* 2008;**5**:14.

49. Foster GD, Wyatt HR, Hill JO, Makris AP, Rosenbaum DL, Brill C, Stein RI, Mohammed BS, Miller B, Rader DJ, Zemel B, Wadden TA, Tenhave T, Newcomb CW, Klein S. Weight and metabolic outcomes after 2 years on a low-carbohydrate versus low-fat diet: a randomized trial. *Ann Intern Med* 2010;**153**:147—57.

50. Layman DK, Evans EM, Erickson D, Seyler J, Weber J, Bagshaw D, Griel A, Psota T, Kris-Etherton P. A moderate-protein diet produces sustained weight loss and long-term changes in body composition and blood lipids in obese adults. *J Nutr* 2009;**139**:514—21.

51. Samaha FF, Foster GD, Makris AP. Low-carbohydrate diets, obesity, and metabolic risk factors for cardiovascular disease. *Curr Atheroscler Rep* 2007;**9**:441—7.

52. Stern L, Iqbal N, Seshadri P, Chicano KL, Daily DA, McGrory J, Williams M, Gracely EJ, Samaha FF. The effects of low-carbohydrate versus conventional weight loss diets in severely obese adults: one-year follow-up of a randomized trial. *Ann Intern Med* 2004;**140**:778—85.

53. Accurso A, Bernstein RK, Dahlqvist A, Draznin B, Feinman RD, Fine EJ, Gleed A, Jacobs DB, Larson G, Lustig RH, Manninen AH, McFarlane SI, Morrison K, Nielsen JV, Ravnskov U, Roth KS, Silvestre R, Sowers JR, Sundberg R, Volek JS, Westman EC, Wood RJ, Wortman J, Vernon MC. Dietary carbohydrate restriction in type 2 diabetes mellitus and metabolic syndrome: time for a critical appraisal. *Nutr Metab (Lond)* 2008;**5**:9.

54. Hite AH, Feinman RD, Guzman GE, Satin M, Schoenfeld PA, Wood RJ. In the face of contradictory evidence: report of the Dietary Guidelines for Americans Committee. *Nutrition* 2010;**26**:915—24.

55. Layman DK. Dietary guidelines should reflect new understandings about adult protein needs. *Nutr Metab (Lond)* 2009;**6**:12.

56. King DE, Mainous III AG, Carnemolla M, Everett CJ. Adherence to healthy lifestyle habits in US adults, 1988—2006. *Am J Med* 2009;**122**:528—34.

57. Mellen PB, Gao SK, Vitolins MZ, Goff Jr DC. Deteriorating dietary habits among adults with hypertension: DASH dietary accordance, NHANES 1988—1994 and 1999—2004. *Arch Intern Med* 2008;**168**:308—14.

58. Millen BE, Quatromoni PA, Franz MM, Epstein BE, Cupples LA, Copenhafer DL. Population nutrient intake approaches dietary recommendations: 1991 to 1995 Framingham Nutrition Studies. *J Am Diet Assoc* 1997;**97**:742—9.

59. Reeves MJ, Rafferty AP. Healthy lifestyle characteristics among adults in the United States, 2000. *Arch Intern Med* 2005;**165**:854—7.

60. Nielsen JV, Jonsson E, Nilsson AK. Lasting improvement of hyperglycaemia and bodyweight: low-carbohydrate diet in type 2 diabetes—a brief report. *Ups J Med Sci* 2005;**110**:69—73.

61. Westman EC, Yancy WS, Haub MD, Volek JS. Insulin resistance from a low carbohydrate, high fat diet perspective. *Metab Syndr Relat Disord* 2005;**3**:14—8.

62. Westman EC, Yancy Jr WS, Mavropoulos JC, Marquart M, McDuffie JR. The effect of a low-carbohydrate, ketogenic diet versus a low-glycemic index diet on glycemic control in type 2 diabetes mellitus. *Nutr Metab (Lond)* 2008;**5**:36.

63. Intensive blood-glucose control with sulphonylureas or insulin compared with conventional treatment and risk of complications in patients with type 2 diabetes (UKPDS 33). UK Prospective Diabetes Study (UKPDS) Group. *Lancet* 1998;**352**:837—53.

64. Effect of intensive blood-glucose control with metformin on complications in overweight patients with type 2 diabetes (UKPDS 34). UK Prospective Diabetes Study (UKPDS) Group. *Lancet* 1998;**352**:854—65.

65. Ohkubo Y, Kishikawa H, Araki E, Miyata T, Isami S, Motoyoshi S, Kojima Y, Furuyoshi N, Shichiri M. Intensive insulin therapy prevents the progression of diabetic microvascular complications in Japanese patients with non-insulin-dependent diabetes mellitus: a randomized prospective 6-year study. *Diabetes Res Clin Pract* 1995;**28**:103–17.

66. The effect of intensive treatment of diabetes on the development and progression of long-term complications in insulin-dependent diabetes mellitus. The Diabetes Control and Complications Trial Research Group. *N Engl J Med* 1993;**329**:977–86.

67. Nathan DM, Cleary PA, Backlund JY, Genuth SM, Lachin JM, Orchard TJ, Raskin P, Zinman B. Intensive diabetes treatment and cardiovascular disease in patients with type 1 diabetes. *N Engl J Med* 2005;**353**:2643–53.

68. Nathan DM, Buse JB, Davidson MB, Heine RJ, Holman RR, Sherwin R, Zinman B. Management of hyperglycemia in type 2 diabetes: A consensus algorithm for the initiation and adjustment of therapy: a consensus statement from the American Diabetes Association and the European Association for the Study of Diabetes. *Diabetes Care* 2006;**29**:1963–72.

69. Ceriello A, Hanefeld M, Leiter L, Monnier L, Moses A, Owens D, Tajima N, Tuomilehto J. Postprandial glucose regulation and diabetic complications. *Arch Intern Med* 2004;**164**:2090–5.

70. Heine RJ, Balkau B, Ceriello A, Del PS, Horton ES, Taskinen MR. What does postprandial hyperglycaemia mean? *Diabet Med* 2004;**21**:208–13.

71. Middelbeek RJ, Horton ES. The role of glucose as an independent cardiovascular risk factor. *Curr Diab Rep* 2007;**7**:43–9.

72. Bernstein RK. New York: Dr. Bernstein's Diabetes Solution. Little, Brown and Company; 2007.

73. Gannon MC, Nuttall FQ. Effect of a high-protein, low-carbohydrate diet on blood glucose control in people with type 2 diabetes. *Diabetes* 2004;**53**:2375–82.

74. Gannon MC, Nuttall FQ. Control of blood glucose in type 2 diabetes without weight loss by modification of diet composition. *Nutr Metab (Lond)* 2006;**3**:16.

75. Gannon MC, Nuttall FQ, Saeed A, Jordan K, Hoover H. An increase in dietary protein improves the blood glucose response in persons with type 2 diabetes. *Am J Clin Nutr* 2003;**78**:734–41.

76. Nuttall FQ, Schweim K, Hoover H, Gannon MC. Effect of the LoBAG30 diet on blood glucose control in people with type 2 diabetes. *Br J Nutr* 2008;**99**:511–9.

77. *Joslin Clinical Nutrition Guidelines for overweight and obese adults with type 2 diabetes, prediabetes or those at high risk for developing type 2 diabetes – 03/29/2007*, www.joslin.org/joslin_clinical_guidelines.html; 2007.

78. Hamdy O, Carver C. The Why WAIT program: improving clinical outcomes through weight management in type 2 diabetes. *Curr Diab Rep* 2008;**8**:413–20.

79. Atkins RC. *Dr. Atkins Diet revolution*. New York: David McKay; 1972.

80. de Souza RJ, Swain JF, Appel LJ, Sacks FM. Alternatives for macronutrient intake and chronic disease: a comparison of the OmniHeart diets with popular diets and with dietary recommendations. *Am J Clin Nutr* 2008;**88**:1–11.

81. Yudkin J, Carey M. The treatment of obesity by the "highfat" diet. The inevitability of calories. *Lancet* 1960;**2**:939–41.

82. Stock AL, Yudkin J. Nutrient intake of subjects on low carbohydrate diet used in treatment of obesity. *Am J Clin Nutr* 1970;**23**:948–52.

83. Evans E, Stock AL, Yudkin J. The absence of undesirable changes during consumption of the low carbohydrate diet. *Nutr Metab* 1974;**17**:360–7.

84. Hamdy O, Horton ES. Protein Content in Diabetes Nutrition Plan. *Curr Diab*; 2011. Rep published online 05 January 2011.

85. USDA Agriculture Research Service, Nutrient Data Laboratory. The USDA National Nutrient Database for Standard Reference (2011).

86. Nordmann AJ, Nordmann A, Briel M, Keller U, Yancy Jr WS, Brehm BJ, Bucher HC. Effects of low-carbohydrate vs low-fat diets on weight loss and cardiovascular risk factors: a meta-analysis of randomized controlled trials. *Arch Intern Med* 2006;**166**:285–93.

87. Krauss RM. Dietary and genetic probes of atherogenic dyslipidemia. *Arterioscler Thromb Vasc Biol* 2005;**25**:2265–72.

88. Dansinger ML, Gleason JA, Griffith JL, Selker HP, Schaefer EJ. Comparison of the Atkins, Ornish, Weight Watchers, and Zone diets for weight loss and heart disease risk reduction: a randomized trial. *JAMA* 2005;**293**:43–53.

89. Gardner CD, Kiazand A, Alhassan S, Kim S, Stafford RS, Balise RR, Kraemer HC, King AC. Comparison of the Atkins, Zone, Ornish, and LEARN diets for change in weight and related risk factors among overweight premenopausal women: the A TO Z Weight Loss Study: a randomized trial. *JAMA* 2007;**297**:969–77.

90. Appel LJ, Sacks FM, Carey VJ, Obarzanek E, Swain JF, Miller III ER, Conlin PR, Erlinger TP, Rosner BA, Laranjo NM, Charleston J, McCarron P, Bishop LM. Effects of protein, monounsaturated fat, and carbohydrate intake on blood pressure and serum lipids: results of the OmniHeart randomized trial. *JAMA* 2005;**294**:2455–64.

91. Luscombe-Marsh ND, Noakes M, Wittert GA, Keogh JB, Foster P, Clifton PM. Carbohydrate-restricted diets high in either monounsaturated fat or protein are equally effective at promoting fat loss and improving blood lipids. *Am J Clin Nutr* 2005;**81**:762—72.

92. Reaven GM. Diet and Syndrome X. *Curr Atheroscler Rep* 2000;**2**:503—7.

93. McLaughlin T, Carter S, Lamendola C, Abbasi F, Yee G, Schaaf P, Basina M, Reaven G. Effects of moderate variations in macronutrient composition on weight loss and reduction in cardiovascular disease risk in obese, insulin-resistant adults. *Am J Clin Nutr* 2006;**84**:813—21.

94. Weigle DS, Breen PA, Matthys CC, Callahan HS, Meeuws KE, Burden VR, Purnell JQ. A high-protein diet induces sustained reductions in appetite, ad libitum caloric intake, and body weight despite compensatory changes in diurnal plasma leptin and ghrelin concentrations. *Am J Clin Nutr* 2005;**82**:41—8.

95. Claessens M, van Baak MA, Monsheimer S, Saris WH. The effect of a low-fat, high-protein or high-carbohydrate ad libitum diet on weight loss maintenance and metabolic risk factors. *Int J Obes (Lond)* 2009;**33**:296—304.

96. Volek JS, Phinney SD, Forsythe CE, Quann EE, Wood RJ, Puglisi MJ, Kraemer WJ, Bibus DM, Fernandez ML, Feinman RD. Carbohydrate restriction has a more favorable impact on the metabolic syndrome than a low fat diet. *Lipids* 2009; **44**:297—309.

97. Forsythe CE, Phinney SD, Fernandez ML, Quann EE, Wood RJ, Bibus DM, Kraemer WJ, Feinman RD, Volek JS. Comparison of low fat and low carbohydrate diets on circulating fatty acid composition and markers of inflammation. *Lipids* 2008;**43**:65—77.

98. Sacks FM, Bray GA, Carey VJ, Smith SR, Ryan DH, Anton SD, McManus K, Champagne CM, Bishop LM, Laranjo N, Leboff MS, Rood JC, de Jonge L, Greenway FL, Loria CM, Obarzanek E, Williamson DA. Comparison of weight-loss diets with different compositions of fat, protein, and carbohydrates. *N Engl J Med* 2009;**360**:859—73.

8

Diabetes Mellitus: A Nursing Perspective

Ann N. Jessup

School of Nursing, The University of North Carolina at Chapel Hill, Chapel Hill, NC

INTRODUCTION/OVERVIEW

Diabetes mellitus is defined as "a group of metabolic diseases characterized by hyperglycemia resulting from defects in insulin secretion, insulin action, or both", and may be further classified into various types depending on symptomatology and presentation.[1] The two most common types, type 1 and type 2, are characterized, respectively, by autoimmune destruction of pancreatic β-cells with subsequent complete loss of insulin production, and by a relative decrease in insulin production combined with insulin resistance. Genetics and obesity are considered to play a significant role in the development of type 2 diabetes, and while there is a genetic contribution to type 1 diabetes

the increased association with a positive family history is stronger for type 2 diabetes. Type 2 diabetes is also associated with chronic activation of the innate immune system, which is associated with obesity.[2] In addition to diabetes types 1 and 2, there are many other potential causes of diabetes or altered insulin production, ranging from genetic defects or illnesses that affect the pancreas or metabolism to the use of certain drugs that may lead to an increase in blood glucose.[1]

According to the Centers for Disease Control and Prevention, approximately 26.8 million people in the US currently have a diagnosis of diabetes. This number includes 7 million who have diabetes but have not been diagnosed as yet.[3] All races are affected, but diabetes is

Nutritional and Therapeutic Interventions for Diabetes and Metabolic Syndrome
DOI: 10.1016/B978-0-12-385083-6.00008-5

more prevalent in people of non-Caucasian ethnicity. On a global scale, diabetes is thought to affect 220 million people and death rates from diabetes are projected to double in relation to 2005 rates by 2030.[4] In addition, 79 million people aged 20 years and older, or approximately 35% of the US population, have blood glucose or HgbA1c levels consistent with prediabetes, placing them at risk for developing diabetes.[3] Type 2 diabetes is also a growing problem in children and adolescents; 215,000 youth less than 20 years of age have been diagnosed with diabetes.[3] Although type 1 diabetes remains the most commonly diagnosed type of diabetes in children,[5] type 2 diabetes in youth has become more prevalent over the last 20 years.[6] This is especially concerning when one considers that these children and adolescents will potentially be exposed to the effects of elevated blood glucose for a longer portion of their lives, leading to a greater potential for development of complications related to diabetes.

No matter the cause or classification of diabetes, the effects of increased blood glucose over time can lead to devastating effects on almost every system of the body.[7] Diabetes is the leading cause of new cases of blindness and kidney failure.[3] It is so closely associated with heart disease that it is considered a cardiovascular disease equivalent, meaning that a person with diabetes is as much at risk for having a myocardial infarction as someone without diabetes who has already had one myocardial infarction. Peripheral and autonomic neuropathies are commonly noted in patients with diabetes. Peripheral neuropathies and poor circulation from vascular disease may also lead to foot ulcers and non-trauma related amputations, of which diabetes is the number one cause. In addition to the many physiological complications of diabetes, people with diabetes may also suffer from associated depression.[3] Studies such as the Diabetes Control and Complications Trial[8] and the UK

Prospective Diabetes Study[9,10] have demonstrated the beneficial effects of maintaining glycemic control in the prevention of complications such as retinopathy, nephropathy, and neuropathy. Early research on the effects of intensive glycemic control on cardiovascular complications did not show significant effects, but a recent meta-analysis has shown more encouraging results for prevention of macrovascular issues.[11] Cardiovascular events overall were reduced slightly (HR 0.91, 95% CI 0.84–0.99), and the risk of myocardial infarction was reduced by 15% (HR 0.85, 95% CI 0.76–0.94). The authors, however, cautioned against using very intensive control across the board because of the risk of hypoglycemic events. Considering the prevalence of diabetes and the risk for major complications, primary prevention of diabetes as well as education and proper management of patients who have been diagnosed is of utmost importance. The potential for contribution by nursing professionals is great.

NURSING PERSPECTIVE

Registered nurses comprise the largest group of healthcare providers, making up almost one-third of healthcare professionals,[12] and can therefore impact the care of people with diabetes in multiple ways. Nursing professionals, whether functioning at the registered nurse or nurse practitioner level, provide health promotion, disease prevention, and care for a wide variety of health concerns for people across the age spectrum. Nurses may provide nursing care on an individual basis, or function as part of a multidisciplinary team of healthcare providers. The American Nurses Association defines nursing as, "the protection, promotion, and optimization of health and abilities, prevention of illness and injury, alleviation of suffering through the diagnosis and treatment of human response, and advocacy in the care of individuals, families, communities, and populations".[14] People with diabetes may have healthcare needs in all of these areas.

Nurses are trained with an emphasis on holistic care, which has been defined as being, "patient led and patient focused in order to provide individualized care, thereby, caring for the patient as a whole person rather than in fragmented parts".[13] The American Nurses Association states "Nurses are educated to be attuned to the whole person, not just the unique presenting health problem".[14] In other words, all of a person's needs, including the physical, psychological and spiritual needs, and their own healthcare goals are important and must be considered when assessing for problems and planning or evaluating care. The components of an individual's environment such as their family, workplace, school, neighborhood, must also be considered. This is similar to the approach used by the Social Ecological Model, which may also be used to address the multifaceted needs of people with diabetes.[15] With regard to nursing and holism, Potter and Frisch suggest "Holistic assessment and care are inseparable from the nursing process".[16] The nursing emphasis on holistic care transfers easily into efforts to address the needs of patients with diabetes who have a variety of healthcare needs, from health promotion and disease prevention to management of their diabetes-related issues.

Registered nurses and nurse practitioners provide healthcare for people with diabetes in a wide variety of settings, such as hospitals, primary care offices, public health departments, and schools or daycares. Just as the types of healthcare settings are different, the types of care provided can vary according to a person's needs. The care provided by nurses may range from providing complete care for those patients and families who can not provide required care, to the encouragement of autonomy and responsibility for self-care and health promotion. This is illustrated by the nursing theorist Dorothea

Orem,[17] who proposed that nurses assess patient needs related to their ability to provide self-care, and then plan nursing care on the identified deficits. For example, some patients may require extensive nursing care in order to successfully deal with their health concerns and other patients may only need supportive and educational assistance. Practice by nurses in diabetes care may range from primary prevention of type 2 diabetes and education, to the screening measures used in secondary prevention, and further, to tertiary prevention to prevent further complications by promoting careful glycemic control and management of any existing complications.

PREVENTION AND MANAGEMENT OF DIABETES BY NURSING PROFESSIONALS

In primary prevention, education is ideally used to prevent illnesses such as diabetes, and should be provided well before any evidence of disease is apparent. A recent review of the evidence regarding lifestyle change for prevention of type 2 diabetes indicated there is a strong rationale for optimal nutrition and physical activity, and other lifestyle changes like smoking cessation.[18] The authors point out the benefits of overall lifestyle change that decreases obesity for people with prediabetes, and note that research has demonstrated the benefits of even moderate amounts of weight loss in preventing the progression from prediabetes to type 2 diabetes. Nurses and nurse practitioners often begin teaching about healthy lifestyles including proper nutrition and physical activity when providing care for pediatric patients. Education by nurses on subjects related to prevention of type 2 diabetes continues across the lifespan in various healthcare settings such as primary care offices, occupational health and public health departments. Methods for prevention of type 1 diabetes are not as clearly defined, but research is underway to investigate intervention possibilities for primary, secondary, and tertiary prevention.[19] An example of primary prevention would be the identification of possible triggers and ways of preventing them from affecting children and young adults who are at increased genetic risk.

Secondary prevention for type 2 diabetes involves screening those at increased risk based on various factors, and may often be done by nurses or nurse practitioners depending on the healthcare setting. The American Diabetic Association (ADA)[7] recommends screening with fasting glucose, HgBA1c, or an oral glucose tolerance test with 75 g glucose for adults who are classified as overweight by having a body mass index greater than $25\,kg/m^2$ and have associated risk factors, which are detailed in the ADA recommendations. If the patient's history and exam does not indicate increased risk for type 2 diabetes, the ADA recommends testing by one of the recommended methods beginning at age 45, and then testing every 3 years or more often if risks change.

Once a patient is diagnosed with diabetes there is a need for tertiary prevention, or proper management of glycemic control to prevent further illness or the complications associated with diabetes. One way that nurses may assist in this type of prevention is by offering Diabetes Self Management Education (DSME). DSME has been defined by Funnell *et al.* as "the ongoing process of facilitating the knowledge, skill, and ability necessary for diabetes self-care. This process incorporates the needs, goals, and life experiences of the person with diabetes and is guided by evidence-based standards".[20] Funnell and her colleagues describe 10 standards that provide guidelines for DSME, from organizational structure for the DSME program to key curriculum components, evaluation and quality assurance. The recommended components of the DSME curriculum cover a broad range of topics such as the pathophysiology of diabetes, lifestyle change and prescribed medical treatments, monitoring and understanding the mean of blood glucose levels, complications that may present and how to prevent them, dealing with day-to-day stressors and how lifestyle changes may best be put into action. In addition to DSME for management of issues related to diabetes, the American Association of Diabetes Educators also advocates for DSME for people with prediabetes, and calls for Medicare coverage for the education in hopes of preventing progression to diabetes.[21]

DSME is described as being based on an "empowerment"[20] model. Anderson and Funnell[22] describe empowerment as "a process when the purpose of an educational intervention is to increase one's ability to think critically and act autonomously" and "an outcome when an enhanced sense of self-efficacy occurs as a result of the process". Healthcare providers can use empowerment strategies to assist the patient with diabetes to make an informed and autonomous decision about their healthcare and lifestyle goals and choices. Holistic practice by nursing professionals fits well with the use of empowerment. For example, Potter and Frisch[16] describe holistic nursing care as a practice where goals are made and evaluated jointly by patient and healthcare provider. Corser and Xu[23] present a framework for integration of DSME into a primary care setting, and suggest that nurses are well suited to coordinate the DSME because of their holistic focus.

The value of a nursing contribution to care is also reflected in the national standards for DSME, as they recommend a team approach to care and advise, "At least one of the instructors will be a registered nurse, dietitian, or pharmacist". Professionals with specialized training and certification as a Certified Diabetes Educator (CDE) or Advance Diabetes Manager (ADM) are well prepared to provide DSME. Both certifications may be earned by nurses, and require advanced education and completion of practice hours. The CDE is initially trained as a healthcare provider, for example a nurse, pharmacist, physician, or dietitian. For the most part, CDE practice tends to be more related to the provision of education, but some educators may provide clinical management in collaboration with physician care.[24] The ADM certification is offered by the American Association of Diabetes Educators, and is available to masters-prepared nurses, dietitians, and pharmacists. This type of certification allows the healthcare provider to provide more in-depth clinical management, beyond education alone.[24] According to the American Association of Diabetes Educators website (http://www.diabeteseducator.org/Professional Resources/Certification/BC-ADM/), the ADM may provide management services such as "medication adjustment, medical nutrition therapy, exercise planning, counseling for behavior management and psychosocial issues … treatment and monitoring of acute and chronic complications".

In addition to DSME, nurses may also provide diabetes case management, or facilitate nurse or nurse practitioner run clinics. Nurse practitioners may participate in case management or in more medically focused interventions based on national evidence-based guidelines.[7,25] Welch and associates recommend a team approach and describe case management as "a collaborative process that assesses, plans, implements, coordinates, monitors, and evaluates the options and services required to meet the client's health and human service needs".[26] Results of their meta-analysis of studies that examined diabetes care by case management multidisciplinary teams led by nurses indicated a significant decrease in HgbA1c, in comparison to the care provided by one healthcare professional alone. The effect was stronger for patients whose HgbA1c was higher than 8% than for patients with lower A1c levels. Carey and Courteney[27] reviewed studies that examined diabetes care provided by nurses around the globe in the US, Korea, Hong Kong, and the UK, and found that nurses participate in a variety of activities related to diabetes care such as "education, individualized care, patient safety, promotion of self-care, acquisition of physical skills and psychological support". Although they recommended further rigorous research with larger samples overall and longer follow-up periods, results of their review indicated significant positive changes such as improved self-care, self-efficacy, and glycemic control with nurse-led interventions for patients with diabetes as compared to control groups who received usual care.

Nurse practitioners also provide and coordinate care for patients with diabetes. They are initially trained as registered nurses, and then receive further graduate-level training to prepare them for a wider scope of practice that includes the diagnosis and management of a variety of common acute and chronic healthcare concerns and problems, depending on their area of concentration. Their practice is therefore based in the nursing philosophy of holistic care, but they are able to expand upon the care provided by registered nurses. Rules and regulations governing nurse practitioners in the US vary somewhat by state of practice, but all nurse practitioners are nationally certified by organizations such as the American Nurses Credentialing Center or the American Academy of Nurse Practitioners (AANP) among others, depending on practice specialty. According to the AANP Standards of Practice (http://www.aanp. org/NR/rdonlyres/FE00E81B-FA96-4779-972B-6162F04C309F/0/2010StandardsOfPractice.pdf) "The nurse practitioner's practice model emphasizes … patient and family education … [and] … facilitation of patient participation in self care", both of which may contribute to the nurse practitioner's ability to provide effective diabetes care. Nurse practitioners intervene at the prevention and health promotion level, or follow comprehensive evidence-based guidelines[7,25] to provide assessment, screening, diagnosis, and the management and follow-up of patients with diabetes, especially those with type 2 diabetes. In addition, Dancer and Courtney[28] describe how the Chronic Care Model may be used to improve the care of patients with diabetes, and how nurse practitioners may participate in this approach by expanding the focus of care provided to not only include individual patient care but to also address patient needs and concerns within the broader healthcare system and community. This is important, as the health of people with diabetes may be affected by a variety of influences.

RESEARCH

In addition to provision of care for patients with diabetes, nursing professionals also participate in the advancement of knowledge related to prevention and management of diabetes. Skelly, Leeman, Carlson, Soward, and Burns[29] describe a conceptual framework for an approach to helping elderly African American patients with diabetes based on the symptoms they experience. Using this framework, patients are taught to use self-management that is tailored to their understanding of symptoms from their own lived experience with diabetes. Symptoms are interpreted in the light of the influence of a patient's family, culture, spiritual, or faith-based practices. The researchers state "This approximates a 'real-world' situation where people with diabetes are required to assess their health status and take appropriate action". Another nurse researcher (J.S. Harrell) has served as one of a team of primary investigators in the Studies to Treat or Prevent Pediatric Type 2 Diabetes. Research in one arm of this large, multisite, national study aimed to reduce factors such as obesity that might place youth at a higher risk for developing Type 2 diabetes. A multi-faceted intervention was put into place to increase the availability of healthy foods and water and decrease unhealthy foods,

change the approach to physical education classes, and provide behavioral interventions designed to encourage a healthier lifestyle. The rates of obesity and overweight in participants overall were no different in the control or intervention groups at the end of the study, but there was a significant decrease in obesity in intervention group subjects who were heavier at baseline; these subjects were 21% less likely to be obese at the end of the 2-year study (p = 0.04). In addition, the overall intervention group had significantly lower body mass index z-scores and mean insulin levels, and fewer students with elevated waist circumference (p = 0.04 for each comparison). Still other nurse researchers have helped to lay the groundwork for DSME by researching the use of empowerment techniques to encourage self-care by patients with diabetes.[30] Anderson, Funnell, Aiken and colleagues examined the effects of a self-management intervention based on empowerment techniques for patients with type 2 diabetes, and noted better quality of life measures, self-efficacy, satisfaction with care and HgbA1c values when compared to a control group. The knowledge created by these and other nurse researchers can contribute to better management and care for patients with diabetes.

CONCLUSION

In conclusion, diabetes is a prevalent disease that can lead to multiple types of serious complications. Nursing professionals, both registered nurses and nurse practitioners, are well suited to provide preventative care and management of diabetes, and to conduct research that may improve future care. The holistic approach used by nurses to assess and treat the whole person ensures attention to the overall spectrum of interventions needed for the care of patients and families with this multifaceted disease.

References

1. American Diabetes Association. Diagnosis and classi-fication of diabetes mellitus. *Diabetes Care* 2011;**34**(S1):S62–9.

2. Wellen KE, Hotamisligil GS. Inflammation, stress and diabetes. *Journal of Clinical Investigation* 2005;**115**:1111–9.

3. World Health Organization, Diabetes Fact Sheet No. 312. January. Available at: http://www.who.int/mediacentre/factsheets/fs312/en/index.html; 2011.

4. Centers for Disease Control and Prevention. National diabetes fact sheet: national estimates and general information on diabetes and prediabetes in the United States, 2011. Atlanta, GA: U.S. Department of Health and Human Services, Centers for Disease Control and Prevention; 2011.

5. Duncan GE. Prevalence of diabetes and impaired fasting glucose levels among US adolescents. National Health and Nutrition Examination Survey, 1999–2002. *Archives of Pediatric and Adolescent Medicine* 2006;**160**:523–8.

6. D'Adamo E, Caprio S. Type 2 Diabetes in youth: Epidemiology and pathophysiology. *Diabetes Care* 2011;**34**(S2):S161–5.

7. American Diabetes Association. Standards of medical care in diabetes 2011. *Diabetes Care* 2011;**34**(S1):S11–61.

8. The Diabetes Control and Complications Trial Research Group. DCCT: The effect of intensive treat-ment of diabetes on the development and progression of long-term complications in insulin-dependent dia-betes mellitus. *The New England Journal of Medicine* 1993;**329**:977–86.

9. UK Prospective Diabetes Study (UKPDS) Group. UKPDS: Effect of intensive blood-glucose control with metformin on complications in overweight patients with type 2 diabetes (UKPDS 34). *Lancet* 1998;**352**:854–65.

10. UK Prospective Diabetes Study (UKPDS) Group. UKPDS: Intensive blood-glucose control with sul-phonylureas or insulin compared with conventional treatment and risk of complications in patients with type 2 diabetes (UKPDS 33). *Lancet* 1998;**352**:837–53.

11. Turnbull FM, Abraira C, Anderson RJ, Byington RP, Chalmers JP, Duckworth WC, Evans GW, Gerstein HC, Holman RR, Moritz TE, Neal BC, Ninomiya T, Patel AA, Paul SK, Travert F, Woodward M. Intensive glucose control and macro-vascular outcomes in type 2 diabetes. *Diabetologia* 2009;**52**:2288–98.

12. Bureau of Labor Statistics. Career Guide to Industries. *Edition: Health Care* Available at: http://www.bls.gov/oco/cg/cgs035.htm; 2010-11.

13. M'Evoy L, Duffy A. Holistic Practice – a concept analysis. *Nurse Education in Practice* 2008;**8**:412–9.

14. American Nurses Association – What is Nursing? Available at: http://www.nursingworld.org/EspeciallyForYou/StudentNurses/WhatisNursing.aspx.

15. Whittemore R, Melkus GD, Grey M. Applying the social ecological theory to type 2 diabetes prevention and management. *Journal of Community Health Nursing* 2004;**21**:87–99.

16. Potter PJ, Frisch N. Holistic assessment and care: Presence in the process. *Nursing Clinics of North America* 2007;**42**:213–28.

17. Orem DE. *Nursing: Concepts of Practice.* 6th ed. St Louis, MO: Mosby; 2001.

18. Psaltopoulou T, Illias I, Alevizaki M. The role of diet and lifestyle in primary, secondary, and tertiary dia-betes prevention: A review of meta-analyses. *The Review of Diabetic Studies* 2010;**7**:26–35.

19. Wherrett DK, Daneman D. Prevention of type 1 dia-betes. *Endocrinology and Metabolism Clinics of North America* 2009;**38**:777–90.

20. Funnell MM, Brown TL, Childs BP, Haas LB, Hosey GM, Jensen B, Maryniuk M, Peyrot M, Piette JD, Reader D, Siminerio LM, Weinger K, Weiss MA. National standards for diabetes self-management education. *Diabetes Care* 2011;**34**(S1):S89–96.

21. Fillman DS. A new focus for diabetes educators in prediabetes. *Diabetes Educator* 2010;**36**:684–6.

22. Anderson RM, Funnell MM. Patient empowerment: Myths and misconceptions. *Patient Education and Counseling* 2010;**79**:277–82.

23. Corser W, Xu Y. Facilitating patients' diabetes self-management: A primary care intervention framework. *Journal of Nursing Care and Quality* 2009;**24**:172–8.

24. Valentine V, Kulkarni K, Hinnen D. Evolving roles: From diabetes educators to advanced diabetes managers. *Diabetes Spectrum* 2003;**16**:27–31.

25. Nathan DM, Buse JB, Davidson MB, Ferrannini El, Holman RR, Sherwin R, Zinman B. Medical management of hyperglycemia in type 2 diabetes: A consensus algorithm for the initiation and adjust-ment of therapy: A consensus statement of the American Diabetes Association and the European Association for the Study of Diabetes. *Diabetes Care* 2009;**32**:193–203.

26. Welch G, Garb J, Zagarins S, Lendel I, Gabbay RA. Nurse diabetes case management interventions and blood glucose control: Results of a meta-analysis. *Diabetes Research and Clinical Practice* 2010;**88**:1–6.

27. Carey N, Courtenay M. A review of the activity and effects of nurse-led care in diabetes. *Journal of Clinical Nursing* 2007;**16**:296–304.

28. Dancer S, Courtney M. Improving diabetes patient outcomes: Framing research into the chronic care model. *Journal of the American Academy of Nurse Prac-titioners* 2010;**22**:580–5.

29. Skelly AH, Leeman J, Carlson J, Soward A, Burns D. Conceptual model of symptom-focused diabetes care for African Americans. *Journal of Nursing Scholarship* 2008;**40**:261—7.

30. The HEALTHY Study Group. A school-based intervention for diabetes risk reduction. The HEALTHY Study Group. *New England Journal of Medicine* 2010;**363**:443—53.

31. Anderson RM, Funnell MM, Aikens JE, Krein SL, Fitzgerald JT, Nwankwo R, Tannas CL, Tang TS. Evaluating the efficacy of an empowerment-based self-management consultant intervention: Results of a two-year randomized controlled trial. *Therapeutic Patient Education* 2009;**1**:3—11.

9

Roles of Environmental Pollution and Pesticides in Metabolic Syndrome and Diabetes: The Epidemiological Evidence

Ivar L. Frithsen, Charles J. Everett

Department of Family Medicine, Medical University of South Carolina, Charleston, SC, USA

OUTLINE

INTRODUCTION

The pathophysiology of diabetes is discussed in other chapters; the etiology of diabetes involves a combination of genetic, lifestyle, and environmental factors. "Environmental factor" is a broad term that could encompass anything from dietary components to chemical exposures; here the focus will be on environmental pollutants or contaminants. Various pollutants have been linked to a spectrum of diseases from asthma to certain cancers. There is evidence in the form of basic science research, animal models, and epidemiologic studies that environmental contaminants may play a role in the development of diabetes. We will focus

Nutritional and Therapeutic Interventions for Diabetes and Metabolic Syndrome
DOI: 10.1016/B978-0-12-385083-6.00009-7

on epidemiologic evidence linking certain environmental contaminants to diabetes.

Human studies of environmental contaminants are always observational and focus on long-term or acute high-level exposures; or chronic low-level exposures as found in the general population. Since randomized studies are not feasible, the majority of the epidemiologic studies of environmental contaminants and diabetes are cross-sectional with some longitudinal research. Since it would not be possible to include every environmental contaminant in this chapter, several have been chosen that are representative of the current evidence.

Dioxins, furans, polychlorinated biphenyls (PCBs) and some pesticides are part of a group of chemicals known as persistent organic pollutants (POPs). These chemicals are environmentally persistent; although many are now either banned or their production tightly regulated, they will be present in the environment for decades to come. These compounds are some of the most widely studied in terms of health effects from environmental exposures and there is an extensive body of evidence examining the link to diabetes. Pesticides are some of the most widely applied chemicals produced by humans and exposure is essentially universal either from ingestion of treated foods or from other environmental sources. Bisphenol-A or BPA is included as there has been widely publicized debate recently about the potential health effects from this chemical that is used in a variety of everyday products. Air pollution and toxic metals are also included to demonstrate the diversity of compounds studied to determine their role in the development of diabetes.

This chapter should not be considered to be a systematic review of each contaminant described; rather studies that are representative of the current evidence will be presented as an overview to this complex area of research. For some pollutants comprehensive reviews have been published recently; articles published after those reviews are noted in those cases.

DIOXINS, FURANS AND POLYCHLORINATED BIPHENYLS

POPs are ubiquitous in the environment and the majority of the worldwide population is exposed to these chemicals. Current exposure is mainly chronic low level from dietary sources with the highest concentrations being found in animal products because POPs bioaccumulate in the food chain. In the past, high-level exposures have been from accidents or were occupationally related. Recent reviews have examined the relationship between type 2 diabetes and POPs and PCBs.[1-3] Here we describe the recent epidemiologic studies (2008—2010) examining the association of glucose metabolism with dioxins, furans, and PCBs.

Metabolic Syndrome and Insulin Resistance

A cross-sectional study in Japan examined the association of 29 dioxins, furans, and dioxin-like PCBs with metabolic syndrome. Toxic equivalent factors were used to calculate toxic equivalents (TEQs) for each class of chemical analyzed. Metabolic syndrome was defined as body mass index (BMI) ≥ 25 kg/m^2 and glycohemoglobin (HbA1c) $\geq 5.6\%$. Dioxin TEQs, furan TEQs, dioxin-like PCB TEQs, and total TEQs were all associated with metabolic syndrome among non-diabetic participants with increasing odds ratios from the first quartile to the fourth quartile of total TEQs.[4]

A Belgian cross-sectional study examined the association of four serum PCBs with insulin resistance. Insulin resistance was calculated using the homeostasis model assessment for insulin resistance (HOMA-IR) with the following equation: insulin [mU/l] $\times$ glucose [mmol/l]/22.5. The sum of PCBs measured had a significant negative correlation with HOMA-IR.[5] However, a separate study found adiponectin had a significant negative correlation with PCB 153 among obese women.

Adiponectin plasma levels have been shown to be reduced in insulin-resistant patients, and in type 2 diabetics.[6]

In a cross-sectional study of Greenland Inuits, dioxin-like PCB congeners and non-dioxin-like PCB congeners (13 PCBs in all) were evaluated for associations with impaired glucose tolerance, insulin resistance and insulin secretion. Impaired glucose tolerance was measured with a 75-g oral glucose tolerance test (OGTT) and insulin secretion was measured with the homeostasis model assessment of β-cell function (HOMA-B) calculated by the equation: (fasting insulin [pmol/l]× 3.33)/(fasting glucose) [mmol/l]-3.5. No association with insulin resistance markers or impaired glucose tolerance was found, but a significant negative association with indices of insulin secretion was found.[7]

A Taiwanese cross-sectional study of 40 pregnant women living in an area with high levels of POP exposure examined associations between insulin sensitivity and 29 POPs. Multiple comparisons were made in this study using insulin sensitivity based on the inverse of HOMA-IR and quantitative insulin-sensitivity check index (QUICKI) methods; TEQs and concentrations of POPs were used. Analysis was performed using PCBs as a class and individual PCB congeners. TEQs of PCBs 123, 126, and 169, and sum of PCBs TEQ were negatively associated with insulin sensitivity in age- and pre-pregnancy BMI-adjusted correlations using inverse HOMA-IR, but not with the QUICKI method.[8] In Slovakia, subjects from a heavily polluted area and an area with normal exposures were included in a cross-sectional study of 17 POPs. This study found fasting glucose (≥ 5.6 mmol/l) and fasting insulin (> 10 mIU/ml) were significantly associated with elevated PCBs.[9]

A Taiwanese cross-sectional study of non-diabetics living near a highly contaminated area examined the relationships of 17 polychlorinated dibenzo-p-dioxins and dibenzofurans (PCDD/F) with insulin resistance (HOMA-IR) and insulin

secretion (HOMA-B). In an adjusted logistic regression PCDD/F were significantly associated with HOMA-IR, but not HOMA-B.[10] A cross-sectional examination of National Health and Nutrition Examination Survey (NHANES) 2003–2004 data evaluated associations between metabolic syndrome and six biomarkers of brominated flame retardants. This study found that polybrominated biphenyl (PBB) 153 was significantly associated with metabolic syndrome (with values $\geq 75^{th}$ percentile being significant), while the polybrominated diphenyl ether (PBDE) 153 showed a quadratic relationship (with values $\geq 75^{th}$ percentile not being significantly associated with metabolic syndrome).[11]

Diabetes Cross-Sectional Studies

A study in a First Nation Community in Northern Ontario, Canada examined associations between diabetes and several PCBs and p,p'—DDE (p,p'-dichlorodiphenyltrichloroethylene). Both wet weight and lipid-standardized PCBs were tested and found to be associated with diabetes. Among this population, an important source of PCB exposure is from fish consumption, yet consumption of trout and white fish was negatively associated with diabetes.[12]

A study examined the association of diabetes and 111 POPs among Great Lakes sport fish consumers who were surveyed and had blood collected in 2004–2005. Undiagnosed diabetes was assessed using HbA1c $> 6.3\%$ and HbA1c $> 6.1\%$. The sum of PCB congeners was not associated with diagnosed diabetes or with diagnosed diabetes plus undiagnosed diabetes (either definition) in adjusted analyses. The sum of dioxin-like PCBs was associated with HbA1c $> 6.3\%$ in some adjusted analyses, but not when further adjusted for p,p'-DDE.[13]

A Slovakian study examined the association of prediabetes and diabetes with PCBs, pesticides and pesticide metabolites in a heavily polluted area. Prediabetes was defined as impaired fasting glucose (fasting plasma glucose

5.6–7.0 mmol/l) and/or impaired glucose tolerance (2-h glucose 7.8–11.1 mmol/l). Diabetes was defined as fasting plasma glucose > 7.0 mmol/l or 2-h glucose > 11.1 mmol/l. Elevated odds ratios for prediabetes and diabetes were noted in higher PCB quintiles. Stepwise logistic regressions showed that PCBs were a significant factor for prediabetes; and p,p'-DDT (p,p'-dichlorodiphenyltrichloroethane) was a significant factor for diabetes.[14] A population-based study in Japan evaluated associations between 29 POPs and diabetes. Dioxins, furans, and dioxin-like PCB congeners were expressed as TEQs. The highest quartile of total TEQ had an elevated odds ratio for diagnosed plus undiagnosed diabetes in an adjusted logistic regression.[15]

Brominated flame retardants (six POPs) were evaluated for associations with diabetes using NHANES 2003–2004 data. Diabetes was defined as taking insulin or an oral agent; fasting glucose ≥ 7.0 mmol/l; or non-fasting glucose ≥ 11.1 mmol/l. Four PBDEs and a PBB were not associated with diabetes, but PBDE 153 showed a significant quadratic relationship (with values ≥ 75th percentile not associated with diabetes).[11] Data from NHANES 1999–2006 was used to analyze the association of 266 environmental contaminants and diabetes. Diabetes was defined as fasting glucose ≥ 7.0 mmol/l. Persons with diagnosed diabetes and fasting glucose < 7.0 mmol/l were characterized as not having diabetes. In adjusted logistic regression models, non-dioxin-like PCB 170 was significantly associated with diabetes. One standard deviation of change of PCB 170 had an odds ratio of 2.2 (p < 0.001) for fasting glucose ≥ 7.0 mmol/l.[16]

Diabetes Longitudinal Studies

A case-control design was used to reanalyze data from the Air Force Health Study to assess the effects of spraying Agent Orange and other 2,3,7,8-tetrachlorodibenzo-p-dioxin (TCDD)-contaminated herbicides in Vietnam from 1962 to 1971. The study followed veterans from their time of service through December 31, 2004 for development of diabetes either by medical diagnosis or a 2-h postprandial glucose ≥ 11.1 mmol/l. TCDD was measured in blood collected in 1987–2002 to define a "background" exposure (≤ 10 ppt TCDD in 1987). Vietnam veterans exposed to more TCDD than the "background" concentration, whose calendar period of service was in 1969 or earlier, and/or consisted of ≥ 90 days of spraying, were more likely to develop diabetes than the comparison group.[17]

A Taiwanese study with 24 years of follow-up analyzed a cohort of Yucheng "oil disease" victims with matched controls. The participants of this study were accidentally exposed to high levels of PCBs and polychlorinated dibenzofurans (PCDFs) by ingestion of contaminated rice-bran oil. In age-adjusted logistic regressions there was no increased risk of developing diabetes among men in the Yucheng group compared to controls, but women in the Yucheng group did have an increased risk of developing diabetes. Chloracne is a dermatologic condition associated with exposure to high levels of PCBs and dioxins. Chloracne diagnosis among those in the Yucheng cohort, and age ≥ 30 years, was associated with diabetes in age and BMI adjusted analysis among women, but not men.[18]

An additional cohort study of Great Lakes sport fish consumers followed participants from 1994–1995 to 2004–2005. A total of 101 PCB congeners and DDE were measured. The sum of PCB congeners was analyzed along with PCB 118 by itself. The sum of the PCBs and PCB 118 were not associated with incident diabetes in age-, gender-, and BMI-adjusted analyses. In participants with biomarker analyses in both 1994–1995 and 2001–2005 there was no difference in mean PCB 132/153 annual percent change between those with diabetes at any time during the study, and those without diabetes.[19]

A Swedish case-control study examined the association of PCB 153 and p,p'-DDE with type 2 diabetes among women 50–59 years old at baseline. Serum concentrations of PCB 153 and p,p'-DDE were used rather than lipid-adjusted values. A majority of the cases (56%) were diagnosed with diabetes within 1 year after baseline examination. In the overall analysis PCB 153 and p,p'-DDE were not associated with development of diabetes. It was only in the subset of cases who were diagnosed with diabetes at least 7 years after the baseline exam that there was a significant difference in p,p'-DDE, but not PCB 153.[20]

Data from the Coronary Artery Risk Development in Young Adults (CARDIA) cohort was used to conduct a longitudinal case-control study examining the association between incident diabetes and 22 PCB congeners and nine other POPS. Follow-up was over a 20-year period. In adjusted logistic regressions, only the second quartiles of PCB congeners 74, 178, 180, and 187 were significantly associated with incident diabetes. The third and fourth quartiles of all of the PCB congeners were not significantly associated with incident diabetes.[21]

For these environmental contaminants there is conflicting evidence as to the association with glucose metabolism. One cross-sectional study utilizing toxic equivalency factors found an association between metabolic syndrome and furans, dioxins, and dioxin-like PCBs. Another study found an association of certain PCBs with insulin resistance using one method, but not another method. Some studies examine multiple contaminants, but find associations with one or two congeners. The strongest evidence is from the longitudinal studies, yet the results from these studies vary as well with some failing to find a consistent dose–response relationship. Some evidence was presented to refute the claim that metabolic alterations of diabetics cause them to accumulate higher levels of POPs (reverse causality). This is representative of the body of evidence published prior to 2008.

PESTICIDES

Pesticides are some of the most common environmental contaminants humans are exposed to from ingestion, inhalation or dermal absorption. The majority of pesticide exposure is from the food we eat since most food products are treated with pesticides at some point during production and trace amounts remain. Other common sources of pesticide exposures include contaminated drinking water, personal or pet insecticides, and home treatment for indoor/outdoor insects, mold or weeds. Pesticides have been shown to cause a wide range of morbidity from skin irritation to cancer and neurological disorders. The strongest associations linking environmental contaminants to diabetes are found in the body of evidence relating to pesticides.

Metabolic Syndrome and Insulin Resistance

Articles on pesticide exposure and diabetes, published before 2008, have been reviewed by Everett and Matheson.[22] Some of the most notable of these studies were from the NHANES 1999–2002.[23,24] One other NHANES study found serum β-hexachlorocyclohexane $\geq 75^{th}$ percentile was significantly associated with metabolic syndrome and impaired fasting glucose. In the same study, p,p'-DDE $\geq 75^{th}$ percentile was associated with impaired fasting glucose. Another NHANES study focused on HOMA-IR. HOMA-IR $\geq 90^{th}$ percentile (≥ 5.06) was associated with oxychlordane and $trans$-nonachlor $\geq 75^{th}$ percentile.

In a cross-sectional study of Greenland Inuits, 11 chlorinated pesticides or their metabolites were studied. No association with insulin resistance markers or impaired glucose tolerance was found, but a significant negative association with indices of insulin secretion was found.[7] A South Korean cross-sectional study examined associations with metabolic syndrome and eight organochlorine pesticides. The definition of metabolic syndrome was altered to include waist circumference ≥ 90 cm for men and ≥ 80 cm for women. Beta-hexachlorocyclohexane and heptachlor epoxide were positively associated with metabolic syndrome. As serum concentration of heptachlor epoxide increased, HOMA-IR increased significantly in subjects with metabolic syndrome even after adjusting for BMI.[25] A Belgian study examined associations of insulin resistance using HOMA-IR with p,p'-DDE and β-hexachlorocyclohexane. Beta-hexachlorocyclohexane was positively associated with HOMA-IR.[5]

The Agricultural Health Study is an ongoing study of farmers, other licensed pesticide applicators and their families in Iowa and North Carolina (US). Researchers used data from this study to determine if pesticide exposure was associated with gestational diabetes. Exposure was categorized as agricultural, indirect, residential, or no exposure. Agricultural exposure during the first trimester was significantly associated with gestational diabetes. Indirect exposure and residential exposure were not significantly different from no exposure. Specifically, gestational diabetes was significantly associated with the reporting of ever-use of the herbicides 2,4,5-T; 2,4,5-TP/silvex, atrazine, and butylate; the organophosphate insecticides diazinon and phorate; and the carbamate carbofuran in logistic regressions.[26]

Cross-Sectional Studies of Type 2 Diabetes

Two early NHANES studies evaluating the association of pesticides and pesticide metabolites with type 2 diabetes have been reviewed previously.[22] In these studies both diagnosed and undiagnosed diabetes were evaluated.

Undiagnosed diabetes was presumed when fasting glucose was ≥ 7.0 mmol/l, non-fasting glucose was ≥ 11.1 mmol/l, or non-fasting glycohemoglobin (HbA1c) was $> 6.1\%$. In one study, β-hexachlorocyclohexane, oxychlordane, *trans*-nonachlor, and p,p'-DDE were associated with total diabetes (diagnosed plus undiagnosed).[24]

In another NHANES study, p,p'-DDT was associated with total diabetes. Diabetics have been hypothesized to accumulate pesticides and pesticide metabolites, due to impaired elimination of the compounds from the body. When participants with poor liver and poor kidney function were excluded from the analysis, p,p'-DDT was still significantly associated with type 2 diabetes. This study also found the number of years since diagnosis of diabetes was not correlated with serum p,p'-DDT concentration using regression analysis.[23]

A study of participants in the Hispanic Health and Nutrition Examination Survey (HHANES), 1982–1984, evaluated associations of seven organochlorine pesticides and pesticide metabolites with type 2 diabetes. Whole weight *trans*-nonachlor, oxychlordane, β-hexachlorocyclohexane, p,p'-DDT and p,p'-DDE were associated with self-reported diabetes. When the pesticides were lipid adjusted, only p,p'-DDT remained significant. Participants who reported ever having worked in a pesticide processing plant, or ever doing farm work were more likely to report diabetes. Ever working as a pesticide applicator was not associated with self-reported diabetes.[27]

A study of Canadian First Nation Community members investigated the association of self-reported diabetes with p,p'-DDE. Both wet weight p,p'-DDE $\geq 75^{th}$ percentile and lipid-standardized values were associated with prevalent diabetes.[12] A cross-sectional study of Great Lakes sport fish consumers was based on data collected in 2004–2005. Serum DDE was associated with diagnosed diabetes or undiagnosed diabetes (HbA1c $> 6.3\%$) in fully adjusted analyses. DDE quartiles remained significant when further adjusted for PCBs and PBDEs.[13]

A study using the NHANES 1999–2004 investigated eight organochlorine pesticides and pesticide metabolites and their association with total diabetes (diagnosed diabetes and undiagnosed diabetes determined by HbA1c $\geq$ 6.5%) and pre-diabetes (HbA1c 5.7–6.4%). Beta-hexachlorocyclohexane, p,p'-DDE, p,p'-DDT, oxychlordane, *trans*-nonachlor, and heptachlor epoxide were associated with total diabetes in fully adjusted analyses. When further adjusted for all of the other significant pesticides, only oxychlordane and heptachlor epoxide remained associated with total diabetes. Four or more of the pesticides and pesticide metabolites elevated (out of 6) had an odds ratio of 4.99 (95% CI 1.97–12.61) compared to none elevated. Both p,p'-DDT and heptachlor epoxide were associated with prediabetes. When further adjusted for the other significant pesticide, only heptachlor epoxide remained associated with pre-diabetes. However, when p,p'-DDT and heptachlor epoxide were analyzed together the odds ratio was higher than the odds ratio for either alone. This study suggests that two to six pesticides or pesticide metabolites are associated with diabetes.[28]

A South Korean study tested associations between 10 organochlorine pesticides and type 2 diabetes. Both wet weight and lipid-standardized values for the organochlorine pesticides were evaluated. Wet weight tertiles of hexachlorobenzene, β-hexachlorocyclohexane, mirex, p,p'-DDE, p,p'-DDD, and p,p'-DDT were significantly associated with prevalent type 2 diabetes. Similarly, lipid-standardized tertiles of oxychlordane, *trans*-nonachlor, hexachlorobenzene, β-hexachlorocyclohexane, p,p'-DDE, p,p'-DDT, and o,p'-DDT were associated with diabetes.[29]

A Slovakian study evaluated associations of four organochlorine pesticides with diabetes and prediabetes. Both fasting plasma glucose (FPG) and an oral glucose tolerance test were used to determine diabetes (FPG > 7.0 mmol/l, 2-h glucose > 11.1 mmol/l) and prediabetes (FPG 5.6–7.0 mmol/l and/or impaired glucose tolerance: 2-h glucose 7.8–11.1 mmol/l). Both p,p'-DDE and p,p'-DDT were associated with prevalent diabetes; and p,p'-DDE, p,p'-DDT, hexachlorobenzene, and β-hexachlorocyclohexane were associated with prediabetes. In a fully adjusted model, p,p'-DDT was significantly associated with diabetes, but not prediabetes.[14]

Data from NHANES 1999–2006 were used to assess 266 environmental factors and their association with diabetes. Only participants who were fasting were included in their study, and fasting glucose $\geq$ 7.0 mmol/l was used to identify those with diabetes. Persons with diagnosed diabetes and fasting glucose < 7.0 mmol/l were characterized as non-diabetics. Heptachlor epoxide was found to be associated with diabetes in this study. Also found to be associated were PCB 170, γ-tocopherol (a form of vitamin E), and β-carotenes. This study was the first to attempt to be all-inclusive with respect to environmental factors that may be associated with type 2 diabetes.[16]

Longitudinal Studies of Type 2 Diabetes

A quasi-longitudinal study of US workers occupationally exposed to pesticides was conducted between 1971 and 1978. The age-adjusted geometric mean serum DDT/DDE concentration in 1971–1973 was 29% higher in people who developed diabetes between 1971 and 1977 than non-diabetics. While serum DDT/DDE concentrations were not lipid adjusted in this study, total cholesterol concentration was not significantly different between the diabetes group and the control group.[30]

Incident diabetes has been studied using data from the Agricultural Health Study. Participants enrolled at baseline (1993–1997) were contacted 5 years later for a follow-up interview (1999–2003). Diabetics at baseline were excluded; participants who developed diabetes by the follow-up interview and non-diabetics were evaluated for exposure to 49 pesticides. Ever-use of the organochlorines chlordane and heptachlor; organophosphates coumaphos, phorate, terbufos, and trichlorfon; and the herbicides alachlor and cyanazine was associated with incident diabetes in logistic regressions. In addition, a dose—response relationship with cumulative days of use was found for the organochlorine heptachlor, the organophosphates chlorpyrifos, diazinon, and trichlorfon, and the herbicides alachlor and cyanazine.[31]

A study of Great Lakes sport fish consumers with follow-up from 1994—1995 to 2005 was performed to examine a link between contaminants and diabetes. Those with diabetes in 1994—1995 were excluded. DDE was significantly associated with incident diabetes in this study. In participants with repeat measures, diabetics were no different than non-diabetics in annual percent change in DDE.[19]

A case-control study of Swedish women compared cases of incident diabetes with matched controls. Concentrations of p,p'-DDE were measured in stored blood samples. Within one year of the baseline examination, 56% of the cases were diagnosed with diabetes. In the overall analysis, p,p'-DDE was not associated with incident diabetes; however, when the 39 cases diagnosed seven or more years following baseline were compared to their matched controls, p,p'-DDE $\geq 75^{th}$ percentile was associated with incident diabetes.[20]

A case-control study nested within the Coronary Artery Risk Development in Young Adults (CARDIA) cohort compared cases of incident diabetes with matched controls. Eight organochlorine pesticides, and pesticide metabolites, were measured in stored blood collected in 1987—1988. Subjects were followed from 1987—1988 to 2005—2006. In age-, sex-, race-, and BMI-adjusted analyses, oxychlordane and $trans$-nonachlor $\geq 75^{th}$ percentiles were associated with incident diabetes. However, when

further adjusted for triglycerides and total cholesterol, only the second quartile of $trans$-nonachlor remained significantly elevated when compared to the first quartile.[21]

Cross-sectional studies have found associations between specific pesticides and metabolic syndrome, decreased insulin secretion, insulin resistance, gestational diabetes, prediabetes, and diabetes. Other cross-sectional studies failed to find the same associations in some cases. One study found that farm workers were more likely to report diabetes, but not pesticide applicators. The results of the Agricultural Health Study and other longitudinal studies suggest several pesticides are associated with incident diabetes. Some evidence to refute reverse causality was presented. This is representative of previously reported evidence linking pesticides and diabetes.

BISPHENOL-A

BPA is an endocrine disrupter that is found in many consumer products; human exposure is believed to be mainly from food product packaging containing BPA. Various polycarbonate plastic products contain BPA and are widely used since they are clear and essentially shatterproof. Items ranging from baby bottles to sports equipment may contain BPA; some countries have banned the use of BPA in baby bottles. Epoxy resins produced with BPA are used as aluminum can liners; in Japan these liners were replaced due to health concerns about BPA.

Two studies using NHANES data from different study periods were performed. The first examined data from NHANES 2003—2004 and found that an increase in one standard deviation of urinary BPA was associated with increased prevalent diabetes.[32] The next study examined a larger data set that included pooled data from 2003—2006. Although the pooled data analysis resulted in a similar finding of an association between increased urinary BPA and diabetes, the result was not significant when 2005—2006 data were examined separately.[33]

AIR POLLUTION

The United States Environmental Protection Agency lists six common substances as criteria air pollutants because they are known to have deleterious health affects in humans.[34] These substances are; particulate matter (PM), carbon monoxide (CO), nitrogen oxides (NO_x), sulfur oxides (SO_x), ozone, and lead. There is a large body of evidence linking air pollution to cardiovascular disease, and diabetics are more susceptible to air pollution related cardiovascular morbidity.[35,36] Tobacco smoke contains some of the criteria air pollutants and there have been conflicting results in studies examining an association between tobacco smoke and glucose metabolism. Tobacco smoke has been shown to be associated with type 1 diabetes in children, the metabolic syndrome in adolescents, glucose intolerance in young adults, and type 2 diabetes in middle-aged men.[37—40] Smoking was not found to be associated with diabetes in other studies that focused on middle-aged women or adults.[41,42] A prospective cohort study showed a positive dose—response relationship between smoking and diabetes while also demonstrating a decrease in diabetes risk for smokers who quit.[43]

A population level study revealed a relationship between statewide levels of diabetes and total state air emissions in the US; a US county-level study also found similar results.[44,45] A large cohort study in Canada showed a positive association between estimated long-term NO_2 exposure and diabetes in women, but not in men.[42] Air pollution has been found to be associated with markers of inflammation and insulin resistance among children; and has been associated with type 1 diabetes in children.[40,46] A large prospective population-based study of German women found that there was an association between incident diabetes and air pollution exposure.[47] These studies show conflicting results of an association between diabetes and tobacco smoke, and some evidence of an association between diabetes and air pollution from ecological studies. However, there are no prospective studies using individual level exposure assessments showing a link between air pollution and diabetes or altered glucose metabolism.

TOXIC METALS

Human exposures to toxic metals can be the result of naturally occurring contamination, but often are the result of industrial activity and waste incineration. Metals can contaminate drinking water, are found in foods, and can be airborne; exposure is via ingestion, dermal absorption, and inhalation. Toxic metals have been shown to cause a wide range of human morbidity from cancer to neurological disorders. Several studies have examined the association between toxic metals and diabetes; the largest body of evidence is related to lead, cadmium and arsenic.

A cross-sectional study of males from Pakistan examined the concentrations of lead, cadmium, and arsenic among diabetics and controls while also examining the effect of smoking. This study found that diabetics and smokers had higher lead, cadmium, and arsenic levels than controls; diabetics who smoke had the highest levels.[48] A cross-sectional study comparing lead-exposed workers to matched controls in the United Arab Emirates found a positive correlation between blood lead levels and fasting glucose.[49] A prospective study of male US military veterans to examine the effect of lead levels on renal function found that longitudinal decline in renal function is dependent on circulating and stored lead levels; this finding was more pronounced among diabetics.[50] A cross-sectional study from India found that diabetics had higher tooth lead levels than controls; there was no significant difference in tooth concentrations of copper, iron, chromium, zinc, or nickel.[51]

An examination of NHANES data revealed a positive association between cadmium and both impaired fasting glucose and diabetes in a dose-dependent manner.[52] A cross-sectional study of island inhabitants off the coast of Australia found no difference in urinary cadmium levels between diabetics and non-diabetics. This study found that diabetics with albuminuria had higher levels of urinary cadmium than diabetics without albuminuria in a dose-dependent manner.[53] A cross-sectional study of a cadmium-exposed population in Thailand found no association of elevated urinary cadmium levels and diabetes.[54] A cross-sectional study of Swedish women found that diabetes-associated renal disease was potentiated by increased cadmium levels.[55]

An ecological study of a six-county area in Michigan with elevated arsenic exposure from drinking water found increased diabetes-associated mortality.[56] A cross-sectional study of pregnant women living near a superfund site in the US found that elevated serum arsenic levels (but not hair arsenic levels) were positively associated with impaired glucose tolerance.[57] Two examinations of NHANES data found positive associations between low levels of urine inorganic arsenic and diabetes; a separate analysis of the data used in the original study with different control measures failed to find an association.[58–60] A case-control study from Mexico found a dose-dependent association of arsenic and diabetes.[61] A prospective cohort study in Taiwan evaluated the association of diabetes with arsenic exposure from artesian wells using an exposure estimate (cumulative arsenic exposure or CAE) that was based on well water arsenic levels and duration of residence in a particular area. This study found an association between CAE and incident diabetes based on results of glucose tolerance testing.[62]

An ecologic study using information from the National Health Insurance Database in Taiwan found a higher prevalence of diabetes among residents living in areas known to have elevated arsenic levels in the drinking water.[63] A cross-sectional study of Wisconsin residents living in an area with artesian wells known to have high levels of arsenic was performed to evaluate association with several diseases; subjects all had arsenic levels determined from well water samples. This study included only those residents who had been drinking well water for at least 20 years prior to the study and found no association with higher arsenic levels and diabetes.[64] A cross-sectional study from Bangladesh found no association between diabetes and elevated arsenic levels, based on exposure estimates and urinary arsenic levels.[65]

The majority of the evidence linking toxic metal exposure to diabetes is cross-sectional, thereby limiting any inference regarding a causal relationship. The only large prospective study used an exposure estimate that was based on residence in certain villages with highly contaminated drinking water. Therefore, there are no prospective studies based on individually measured exposure assessments that link any heavy metals to diabetes or altered glucose metabolism.

SUMMARY AND FUTURE RESEARCH

There are several factors that contribute to the development of type 2 diabetes such as obesity, sedentary lifestyle and family history that are widely accepted in the medical community. However, the role of environmental contaminants or pollutants in diabetes is not yet well understood. The strongest body of epidemiological evidence is that linking certain POPs to diabetes. Some of these chemicals such as DDT, heptachlor and PCBs are no longer produced as they have been recognized as hazardous to humans and/or the environment. However, they are now dispersed essentially over the entire planet and by virtue of their environmental persistence will be cause for concern over many years to come. Therefore, it remains an important area of research to investigate the health effects of these substances, yet greater urgency should be on the evaluation of substances that are still in widespread production such as BPA.

There are some areas of weakness in the current epidemiologic evidence linking environmental contaminants to diabetes. Studies that examine large numbers of contaminants to find only one or two associations should be viewed with caution. Some studies have used different values as the cut-off for diabetes that are not generally accepted, such as hemoglobin A1c of 6.1% where the American Diabetes Association guidelines use 6.5% as their cut-off.[66] Self-reporting of diabetes or exposures, the use of exposure estimates, and the use of population level data are all issues that limit the conclusions that can be drawn from the current body of evidence. Many studies have been on populations subject to high-level exposures that the general population is not subject to. Finally, reporting bias is likely present as negative studies are less likely to be published or even submitted for publication.

Despite these weaknesses, there is now sufficient epidemiologic evidence showing an association between several environmental contaminants and diabetes to warrant large-scale prospective epidemiologic studies. Future research should focus on the effect of low-level exposures that are typical for the majority of the population. Another important factor for future research is to examine any cumulative or synergistic effects of multiple concurrent exposures. One such study used a novel approach they termed environment-wide association study or EWAS to examine the association of 266 environmental factors and diabetes. The authors of that study have suggested this method will be expanded in the future to include the ability to combine EWAS results with genetics research.[16]

The main goal of diabetes treatment is to prevent long-term complications that include both microvascular- and macrovascular-induced morbidity. Future studies should therefore focus on the role of environmental contaminants in disease progression such as renal disease. One example of an important study to explore disease progression first examined the effect of arsenic on renal function in diabetics, then went on to validate that effect in a rat model.[67] More studies that integrate various research disciplines will allow for a greater understanding of the role of environmental contaminants in diabetes. In conclusion, further research should be comprised of large, prospective studies with emphasis on individual level exposure assessments verified through biologic sampling.

Acknowledgments

Portions of this article were previously published in Everett *et al.* (2011) and reproduced with permission from the Royal Society of Chemistry.[3] Portions of this article also published in Everett and Matheson (2011) and reproduced with permission from Elsevier.[22]

References

1. Carpenter DO. Environmental contaminants as risk factors for developing diabetes. *Rev Environ Health* 2008;23:59–74.
2. Wang CX, Xu SQ, Lv ZQ, Li YY, Wang YJ, Chen T. Exposure to persistent organic pollutants as potential risk factors for developing diabetes. *Sci China Chem* 2010;53:980–94.
3. Everett CJ, Frithsen I, Player M. Relationship of polychlorinated biphenyls with type 2 diabetes and hypertension. *J Environ Monit* 2011;13:241–51.
4. Uemura H, Arisawa K, Hiyoshi M, Kitayama A, Takami H, Sawachika F, Dakeshita S, Nii K, Satoh H, Sumiyoshi Y, Morinaga K, Kodama K, Suzuki T, Nagai M, Suzuki T. Prevalence of metabolic syndrome

associated with body burden levels of dioxin and related compounds among Japan's general population. *Environ Health Perspect* 2009;**117**:568–73.

5. Dirinck E, Jorens PG, Covaci A, Geens T, Roosens L, Neels H, Mertens I, Van Gaal L. Obesity and persistent organic pollutants: Possible obesogenic effect of organochlorine pesticides and polychlorinated biphenyls. *Obesity*; 2010. DOI: 10.1038/oby.2010.133.

6. Mullerova D, Kopecky J, Matejkova D, Muller L, Rosmus J, Racek J, Sefrna F, Opatrna S, Kuda O, Matejovic M. Negative association between plasma levels of adiponectin and polychlorinated biphenyl 153 in obese women under non-energy-restrictive regime. *Int J Obes Relat Metab Disord* 2008;**32**:1875–8.

7. Jorgensen ME, Borch-Johnsen K, Bjerregaard P. A cross-sectional study of the association between persistent organic pollutants and glucose intolerance among Greenland Inuit. *Diabetologia* 2008;**51**:1416–22.

8. Chen J, Wang S, Liao P, Chen H, Ko Y, Lee C. Relationship between insulin sensitivity and exposure to dioxins and polychlorinated biphenyls in pregnant women. *Environ Res* 2008;**107**:245–53.

9. Langer P, Kocan A, Tajtakova M, Susienkova K, Radikova Z, Koska J, Ksinantova L, Imrich R, Huckova M, Drobna B, Gasperikova D, Trnovec T, Klimes I. Multiple adverse thyroid and metabolic health signs in the population from the area heavily polluted by organochlorine cocktail (PCB, DDE, HCB, dioxin). *Thyroid Res* 2009;**2**:3.

10. Chang JW, Chen HL, Su HJ, Liao PC, Guo HR, Lee CC. Dioxin exposure and insulin resistance in Taiwanese living near a highly contaminated area. *Epidemiology* 2010;**21**:56–61.

11. Lim JS, Lee D-H, Jacobs Jr DR. Association of brominated flame retardants with diabetes and metabolic syndrome in the U.S. population, 2003–2004. *Diabetes Care* 2008;**31**:1802–7.

12. Philibert A, Schwartz H, Mergler D. An exploratory study of diabetes in a first nation community with respect to serum concentrations of p, p'-DDE and PCBs and fish consumption. *Int J Environ Res Public Health* 2009;**6**:3179–89.

13. Turyk M, Anderson HA, Knobeloch L, Imm P, Persky VW. Prevalence of diabetes and body burdens of polychlorinated biphenyls, polybrominated diphenyl ethers, and p,p'-diphenyldichloroethene in Great Lakes sport fish consumers. *Chemosphere* 2009;**75**:674–9.

14. Ukropec J, Radikova Z, Huckova M, Koska J, Kocan A, Sebokova E, Drobna B, Trnovec T, Susienkova K, Labudova V, Gasperikova D, Langer P, Klimes I. High prevalence of prediabetes and diabetes in a population exposed to high levels of an organochlorine cocktail. *Diabetologia* 2010;**53**:899–906.

15. Uemura H, Arisawa K, Hiyoshi M, Satoh H, Sumiyoshi Y, Morinaga K, Kodama K, Suzuki T, Nagai M, Suzuki T. Associations of environmental exposure to dioxins with prevalent diabetes among general inhabitants in Japan. *Environ Res* 2008;**108**:63–8.

16. Patel CJ, Bhattacharya J, Butte A. An environment-wide association study (EWAS) on type 2 diabetes mellitus. *PLoS ONE* 2010;**5**:e10746.

17. Michalek JE, Pavuk M. Diabetes and cancer in veterans of Operation Ranch Hand after adjustment for calendar period, days of spraying, and time spent in Southeast Asia. *J Occup Environ Med* 2008;**50**:330–40.

18. Wang S-L, Tsai P-C, Yang C-Y, Leon Guo Y. Increased risk of diabetes and polychlorinated biphenyls and dioxins: A 24-year follow-up study of the Yucheng cohort. *Diabetes Care* 2008;**31**:1574–9.

19. Turyk M, Anderson H, Knobeloch L, Imm P, Persky V. Organochlorine exposure and incidence of diabetes in a cohort of Great Lakes sport fish consumers. *Environ Health Perspect* 2009;**117**:1076–82.

20. Rignell-Hydbom A, Lidfeldt J, Kiviranta H, Rantakokko P, Samsioe G, Agardh C-D, Rylander L. Exposure to p,p'-DDE: A risk factor for type 2 diabetes. *PLoS ONE* 2009;**4**:e7503.

21. Lee D-H, Steffes MW, Sjodin A, Jones RS, Needham LL, Jacobs Jr DR. Low dose of some persistent organic pollutants predicts type 2 diabetes: A nested case-control study. *Environ Health Perspect* 2010;**118**:1235–42.

22. Everett CJ, Matheson EM. Pesticide exposure and diabetes. In: Nriagu J, editor. *Encyclopedia of Environmental Health*. Elsevier, Burlington 2011;**4**:407–11.

23. Everett CJ, Frithsen IL, Diaz VA, Koopman RJ, Simpson Jr WM, Mainous III AG. Association of a polychlorinated dibenzo-p-dioxin, a polychlorinated biphenyl, and DDT with diabetes in the 1999–2002 National Health and Nutrition Examination Survey. *Environ Res* 2007;**103**:413–8.

24. Lee D-H, Lee I-K, Steffes M, Jacobs Jr DR. Extended analyses of the association between serum concentrations of persistent organic pollutants and diabetes. *Diabetes Care* 2007;**30**:1596–8.

25. Park S-K, Son H-K, Lee S-K, Kang J-H, Chang Y-S, Jacobs Jr DR, Lee D-H. Relationship between serum concentrations of organochlorine pesticides and metabolic syndrome among non-diabetic adults. *J Prev Med Pub Health* 2010;**43**:1–8.

26. Saldana TM, Basso O, Hoppin JA, Baird DD, Knott C, Blair A, Alavanja MCR, Sandler DP. Pesticide exposure and self-reported gestational diabetes mellitus in the Agricultural Health Study. *Diabetes Care* 2007;**30**:529–34.

27. Cox S, Niskar AS, Narayan KMV, Marcus M. Prevalence of self-reported diabetes and exposure to organochlorine pesticides among Mexican Americans: Hispanic Health and Nutrition Examination Survey, 1982–1984. *Environ Health Perspect* 2007;**115**:1747–52.

28. Everett CJ, Matheson EM. Biomarkers of pesticide exposure and diabetes in the 1999–2004 National Health and Nutrition Examination Survey. *Environ Int* 2010;**36**:398–401.

29. Son H-K, Kim S-A, Kang J-H, Chang Y-S, Park S-K, Lee S-K, Jacobs Jr DR, Lee D-H. Strong associations between low-dose organochlorine pesticides and type 2 diabetes. *Environ Int* 2010;**36**:410–4.

30. Morgan DP, Lin LI, Saikaly HH. Morbidity and mortality in workers occupationally exposed to pesticides. *Arch Environ Contam Toxicol* 1980;**9**:349–82.

31. Montgomery MP, Kamel F, Saldana TM, Alavanja MCR, Sandler DP. Incident diabetes and pesticide exposure among licensed pesticide applicators: Agricultural Health Study, 1993–2003. *Am J Epidemiol* 2008;**167**:1235–46.

32. Lang IA, Galloway TS, Scarlett A, Henley WE, Depledge M, Wallace RB, Melzer D. Association of urinary bisphenol A concentration with medical disorders and laboratory abnormalities in adults. *JAMA* 2008;**300**:1303–10.

33. Melzer D, Rice NE, Lewis C, Henley WE, Galloway TS. Association of urinary bisphenol A concentration with heart disease: Evidence from NHANES 2003/06. *PLoS ONE* 2010;**5**:e8673.

34. U.S. Environmental Protection Agency. Air Pollutants. URL, www.epa.gov/air/airpollutants.html. Accessed February 26, 2011.

35. Filho M, Pereira L, Arbex F, Arbex M, Conceição G, Santos U, Lopes A, Saldiva P, Braga A, Cendon S. Effect of air pollution on diabetes and cardiovascular diseases in Sao Paolo, Brazil. *Braz J Med Biol Res* 2008;**41**:526–32.

36. O'Neill M, Veves A, Zanobetti A, Sarnat J, Gold D, Economides P, Horton E, Schwartz J. Diabetes enhances vulnerability to air pollution-associated vascular reactivity and endothelial function. *Circulation* 2005;**111**:2913–20.

37. Weitzman M, Cook S, Auinger P, Florin T, Daniels S, Nguyen M, Winickoff J. Tobacco smoke exposure is associated with metabolic syndrome in adolescents. *Circulation* 2005;**112**:862–9.

38. Wannamethee S, Shaper A, Perry I. Smoking as a modifiable risk factor for type 2 diabetes in middle aged men. *Diabetes Care* 2001;**24**:1590–5.

39. Houston T, Person S, Pletcher M, Liu K, Iribarren C, Kiefe C. Active and passive smoking and development of glucose intolerance among young adults in a prospective cohort: CARDIA study. *Br Med J* 2006;**332**:1064.

40. Hathout E, Beeson W, Ischander I, Rao R, Mace J. Air pollution and type 1 diabetes in children. *Pediatric Diabetes* 2006;**7**:81–7.

41. Pradhan A, Manson J, Rifai N, Buring J, Ridker P. C-reactive protein, interleukin 6, and risk of developing type 2 diabetes mellitus. *JAMA* 2001;**286**:327–34.

42. Brook R, Jerrett M, Brook J, Bard R, Finkelstein M. The relationship between diabetes mellitus and traffic-related air pollution. *J Occup Environ Med* 2008;**50**:32–8.

43. Will J, Galuska D, Ford E, Mokdad A, Calle E. Cigarette smoking and diabetes mellitus: Evidence of a positive association from a large prospective cohort study. *Int J Epidemiol* 2001;**30**:540–6.

44. Lockwood A. Diabetes and air pollution. *Diabetes Care* 2002;**25**:1487–8.

45. Pearson J, Bachireddy C, Shyamprasad S, Goldfine A, Brownstein J. Association between fine particulate matter and diabetes prevalence in the U.S. *Diabetes Care* 2010;**33**:2196–201.

46. Kelishadi R, Mirghaffari N, Poursafa P, Gidding S. Lifestyle and environmental factors associated with inflammation, oxidative stress and insulin resistance in children. *Atherosclerosis* 2009;**203**:311–9.

47. Krämer U, Herder C, Sugiri D, Strassburger K, Schikowski T, Ranft U, Rathmann W. Traffic-related air pollution and incident type 2 diabetes: Results from the SALIA Cohort Study. *Environ Health Perspect* 2010;**118**:1273–9.

48. Afridi HI, Kazi TG, Kazi N, Jamali MK, Arain MB, Jalbani N, Baig JA, Sarfraz RA. Evaluation of status of toxic metals in biological samples of diabetes mellitus patients. *Diabetes Res Clin Pract* 2008;**80**:280–8.

49. Bener A, Obineche E, Gillett M, Pasha M, Bishawi B. Association between blood levels of lead, blood pressure and risk of diabetes and heart disease in workers. *Int Arch Occup Environ Health* 2001;**74**:375–8.

50. Tsaih S, Korrick S, Schwartz J, Antonio A, Sparrow D, Hu H. Lead, diabetes, hypertension, and renal function: the normative aging study. *Environ Health Perspect* 2004;**112**:1178–82.

51. Nagaraj G, Sukumar A, Nandlal B, Vellaichamy S, Thanasekaran K, Ramanathan A. Tooth element levels indicating exposure profiles in diabetic and hypertensive subjects from Mysore, India. *Biol Trace Elem Res* 2009;**131**:255–62.

52. Schwartz G, Il'Yasova D, Ivanova A. Urinary cadmium, impaired fasting glucose and diabetes in NHANES III. *Diabetes Care* 2003;**26**:468–70.

53. Haswell-Elkins M, Satarug S, O'Rourke P, Moore M, Ng J, McGrath V, Walmby M. Striking association

between urinary cadmium and albuminuria among Torres Strait Islander people with diabetes. *Environ Res* 2008;**106**:379–83.

54. Swaddiwudhipong W, Mahasakpan P, Limpatanachote P, Krintratun S. Correlations of urinary cadmium with hypertension and diabetes in persons living in cadmium-contaminated villages in northwestern Thailand: A population study. *Environ Res* 2010;**110**:612–6.

55. Åkesson A, Lundh T, Vahter M, Bjellerup P, Lidfeldt J, Nerbrand C, Samsioe G, Strömberg U, Skerfving S. Tubular and glomerular kidney effects in Swedish women with low environmental cadmium exposure. *Environ Health Perspect* 2005;**113**:1627–31.

56. Meliker JR, Wahl RL, Cameron LL, Nriagu JO. Arsenic in drinking water and cerebrovascular disease, diabetes mellitus, and kidney disease in Michigan: A standardized mortality ratio analysis. *Environmental Health: A Global Access Science Source* 2007;**6**:4–11.

57. Ettinger A, Zota A, Amarasiriwardena C, Hopkins M, Schwartz J, Hu H, Wright R. Maternal arsenic exposure and impaired glucose tolerance during pregnancy. *Environ Health Perspect* 2009;**117**:1059–64.

58. Navas-Acien A, Silbergeld E, Pastor-Barriuso R, Guallar E. Arsenic exposure and prevalence of type 2 diabetes in US adults. *JAMA* 2008;**300**:814–22.

59. Steinmaus C, Yuan Y, Smith A. Low-level population exposure to inorganic arsenic in the United States and diabetes mellitus. *Epidemiology* 2009;**20**:807–15.

60. Navas-Acien A, Silbergeld E, Pastor-Barriuso R, Guallarb E. Rejoinder: arsenic exposure and prevalence of type 2 diabetes. *Epidemiology* 2009;**20**:816–20.

61. Coronado-Gonzalez J, Del Razo L, Garcia-Vargas G, Sanmiguel-Salazar F, Escobedo-de la Pena J. Inorganic arsenic exposure and type 2 diabetes mellitus in Mexico. *Environ Res* 2007;**104**:383–9.

62. Tseng C, Tai T, Chong C, Tseng C, Lai M, Lin B, Chiou H, Hsueh Y, Hsu K, Chen C. Long-term arsenic exposure and incidence of non-insulin-dependent diabetes mellitus: a cohort study in arseniasis-hyper-endemic villages in Taiwan. *Environ Health Perspect* 2000;**108**:847–51.

63. Wang S, Chiou J, Chen C, Tseng C, Chou W, Wang C, Wu T, Chang L. Prevalence of non-insulin-dependent diabetes mellitus and related vascular diseases in southwestern arseniasis-endemic and nonendemic areas in Taiwan. *Environ Health Perspect* 2003;**111**:155–9.

64. Zierold K, Knobeloch L, Anderson H. Prevalence of chronic diseases in adults exposed to arsenic-contaminated drinking water. *Am J Public Health* 2004;**94**:1936–7.

65. Chen Y, Ahsan H, Slavkovich V, Peltier G, Gluskin R, Parvez F, Liu X, Graziano J. No association between arsenic exposure from drinking water and diabetes mellitus: a cross-sectional study in Bangladesh. *Environ Health Perspect* 2010;**118**:1299–305.

66. American Diabetes Association. Standards of Medical Care in Diabetes—2011. *Diabetes Care* 2011;**34**:S11–61.

67. Wang JP, Wang SL, Lin Q, Zhang L, Huang D, Ng JC. Association of arsenic and kidney dysfunction in people with diabetes and validation of its effects in rats. *Environ Int* 2009;**35**:507–11.

10

Preventing Diabetes with Diet and Exercise

Karen Z. Walker*, *Kerin O'Dea†*

* Department of Nutrition and Dietetics, Monash University, Clayton, VIC, Australia † Sansom Institute
for Health Research, Division of Health Sciences, University of South Australia,
Adelaide, SA, Australia

INTRODUCTION

As individuals proceed through the prediabetic stages of impaired fasting glucose (IFG) or impaired glucose tolerance (IGT)[1] they are often unaware that diabetes prevention remains possible at this stage.[2] Although type 2 diabetes has genetic antecedents (as yet not clearly defined), lifestyle factors are the predisposing triggers and these are amenable to change.[3] The most important lifestyle trigger is obesity: the result of a poor diet with excessive energy intake[4] and/or low physical activity.[5] A population-based approach to preventing type 2 diabetes will therefore target overweight, sedentary individuals with prediabetes. Here we review studies examining diabetes prevention in such high-risk individuals, and discuss diet and exercise programs that can be implemented.

DIET AND EXERCISE INTERVENTIONS TO PREVENT DIABETES

Major studies in quite ethnically diverse populations have convincingly demonstrated that diabetes can be prevented through diet and lifestyle intervention in high-risk groups (Table 10.1). In Da Qing, Chinese individuals with IGT were randomized to an exercise intervention, a dietary intervention, or to exercise and diet combined. After 6 years, 68% [95% confidence interval (CI), 60–75%] of people in the control group developed diabetes. In contrast, diabetes was found in only 41% (95% CI, 33–49%) of the exercise group ($P < 0.05$); 44% (95% CI, 35–52%) of the diet group and 46% (95% CI, 37–55%) of the diet plus exercise group.[6] Although this study indicated little

TABLE 10.1 Diabetes Prevention in Ethnically Diverse Groups

Study	Population (% female)	Follow-up (years)	Intervention	Reduction in diabetes incidence[a]
Da Qing Diabetes Prevention Study[6]	577 Chinese with IGT (44%)	6	• Diet • Exercise • Diet *plus* exercise • Control	56% 59% 51% -
Finnish Diabetes Prevention Study (DPS)[7]	522 Finns with IGT (67%)	3.2	• Intensive lifestyle change • Control	58% -
Diabetes Prevention Program (DPP)[8]	3,234 Americans with IGT (68%)	2.8	• Intensive lifestyle program • Control	58% -
Indian Diabetes Prevention Programme (IDPP)[9]	531 Indians with IGT (21%)	2.5	• Lifestyle intervention • Control	28.5% -
Taranomon Hospital Trial[10]	102 Japanese with IGT (0%)	4.0	• Intensive diet *plus* exercise • Standard recommendations	68% -
The Tehran Lipid and Glucose Study (TLGS)[12]	1,754 Iranians[b] (60%)	3.6	• Lifestyle intervention • Control	39% -
PREDIMED-Reus[13]	418 Spaniards[b] (58%)	4.0	• Lifestyle intervention[c] • Control	52% -

[a] *All interventions showed significant differences from the control group.*
[b] *Normoglycemic at baseline.*
[c] *Pooled data.*

additional benefit in combining diet with exercise, other major studies usually combine these two approaches.

In the Finnish Diabetes Prevention Study (DPS) participants with IGT were randomly assigned to intensive lifestyle intervention or to a control group who received only general dietary advice. Those in the intervention group received individualized dietary counseling for the first year, and were encouraged to increase physical activity and were also offered circuit-type resistance training. After 3.2 years, diabetes incidence in the intervention group was reduced by 58%.[7] In the US Diabetes Prevention Program (DPP), participants with IGT again received an intensive lifestyle program, aided by a 16-week behavior modification curriculum in which goals were set for weight loss ($\geq 7\%$ initial body weight), moderate intensity physical activity (> 150 min/week) and for a high-carbohydrate, low-fat (HCLF) diet. After 2.8 years, this intensive intervention reduced diabetes incidence by 58% (95% CI: 48−66%).[8]

In the Indian Diabetes Prevention Programme (IDPP), participants with IGT also received aid for lifestyle modification which after 30 months decreased the incidence of diabetes by 28.5% (95% CI, 20.5−37.3, $P = 0.018$). No added benefit accrued by combining lifestyle change with medication (metformin).[9] In a Japanese study conducted in men with IGT, intensive lifestyle intervention included advice to lower body mass index (BMI) (< 22 kg/m^2), to reduce intake of saturated fat and alcohol, to increase vegetable consumption and to walk for 30−40 min daily. After 4 years, diabetes incidence had fallen 68% relative to the control group given standard advice.[10]

The five prevention studies[6−10] outlined above were carried out in individuals with IGT. In people with IFG where genetic inheritance, smoking, and male gender have a stronger effect on outcome than dietary factors, the impact of lifestyle change may not be as great.[11]

Nevertheless, studies in individuals who were normoglycemic at baseline also indicate the beneficial impact of lifestyle change. The Tehran Lipid and Glucose Study (TLGS) followed 2,993 individuals who received nutritional education classes based on American Heart Association guidelines plus advice to increase physical activity and to stop smoking. After 3.6 years, the incidence of diabetes was reduced by 39%.[12] In another study, 418 older Spanish individuals at the Reus center of the PREvención con DIeta MEDiterránea (PREDIMED) trial followed *ad libitum* Mediterranean diets high in nuts (30 g/day) or olive oil or a control HCLF diet. After 4 years, both Mediterranean diets reduced diabetes incidence (in pooled data, by 52%) relative to controls. Notably, this occurred without change in body weight or physical activity.[13]

The benefits of lifestyle interventions can continue well beyond the intervention period. Twenty years after the Da Qing Study commenced, there was a 43% lower incidence of type 2 diabetes among those who had participated in the diet *plus* exercise intervention *vs* the control group (HR 0.57; 95% CI, 0.41−0.81).[14] Similarly, a 7-year follow-up of the DPS found that incidence of type 2 diabetes remained 43% lower in the intervention group than in controls ($P = 0.0001$).[15] Successful continued risk reduction was associated with weight loss, improved diet (reduced consumption of total and saturated fat, increased intake of dietary fiber) and increased physical activity. The US-based DPP Outcomes Study (DPPOS) also reported continued benefit after lifestyle intervention. After 10 years the intensive lifestyle group still had 34% less diabetes than the control group.[16]

The efficacy of lifestyle change in diabetes prevention has been confirmed by meta-analysis of 17 randomized controlled trials in 8,084 people with IGT.[17] A pooled hazard ratio of 0.51 (95 % CI, 0.44−0.60) was obtained for lifestyle change *vs* 0.70 (95% CI, 0.62−0.79) for those who received standard advice only. One case of diabetes could be prevented if only

6.4 people (95% CI, 5.0—8.4) received lifestyle intervention.[17]

WEIGHT LOSS AND EXERCISE BOTH CONTRIBUTE TO REDUCING DIABETES RISK

Genetically susceptible individuals who become obese are highly likely to progress to type 2 diabetes. For obese Americans enrolled in the lifestyle arm of the DPP, weight loss proved the dominant predictor of reduced diabetes incidence. After adjustment for changes in diet and activity, for every kilogram of weight lost, there was a 16% reduction in the risk of developing diabetes.[18] In high-risk individuals, a weight loss of 5—7% total body weight may be sufficient to prevent progression to diabetes.[19] Weight loss interventions must be sustained to achieve the continued negative energy balance that promotes loss of body fat. In one small closely supervised study, 36 overweight individuals undertook aerobic exercise or a calorie-controlled diet, or combined diet *plus* exercise for 6 months. Each treatment resulted in similar loss of body fat.[20] Exercise *plus* diet, while not increasing fat loss more than either treatment alone, brought the additional benefits of improved blood pressure, low-density lipoprotein (LDL)-cholesterol, and insulin sensitivity.[20]

Studies in Finnish cohorts have shown that while maintenance of normal body weight (BMI < 25 kg/m^2) has the strongest influence on progression to type 2 diabetes, adequate exercise, lack of smoking habit, moderate alcohol consumption and adequacy of serum Vitamin D levels are inversely associated with risk.[21] Notably, physical inactivity acts as a risk factor independently from obesity.[22] Thus in the US Nurses' Health Study, the relative risk of type 2 diabetes in physically inactive women of normal body weight (BMI < 25 kg/m^2) was twice that of active women of normal weight.[23]

WHAT TYPE OF DIET BEST ENCOURAGES WEIGHT LOSS?

When the same energy intake deficit is maintained, diets that differ widely in macronutrient balance can promote similar weight loss. Recently, 811 overweight adults were randomized to four very different hypocaloric (-3.2 MJ/day) diets where macronutrient content ranged from 20% total energy (%E) to 40%E for total fat and 35%E to 65%E for carbohydrate. After 2 years, average weight loss remained around 4 kg regardless of diet.[24] The overriding importance of the energy restriction rather than the macronutrient balance appeared clear. It is only when people are prescribed diets where they are allowed to eat to appetite without counting calories, that food choice and macronutrient balance can freely exert effects on satiety, total energy intake, and achieved weight loss.[25]

Important dietary elements impacting on weight loss in the *ad libitum* context are energy density, protein content, and the glycemic index (GI) of carbohydrate foods. Higher weight loss occurs when an *ad libitum* diet is composed predominantly of low-energy dense foods such as fresh or cooked vegetables.[26] *Ad libitum* diets with high protein content are also more satiating, leading to lower total energy intake.[27] Carbohydrate foods with low GI will moderate rates of glucose absorption and insulin secretion and this may also have long-term effects on energy intake.[28]

Given the varied factors involved, there is considerable room to individualize diets to suit client preference. Approaches discussed below include the widely recommended HCLF diet, as well as high-protein (LCHP) diets and Mediterranean-style diets.

High-Carbohydrate, Low-Fat Diets

Most trials for diabetes prevention have employed HCLF calorie-restricted diets. Good outcomes here are largely governed by the degree of success in limiting total energy intake. If calories are not strictly counted, it becomes increasingly important to optimize the quality of the dietary carbohydrate. Carbohydrate foods for HCLF diets should comprise wholegrain cereal foods and other fibre-rich food sources. Complex carbohydrate foods of low GI are of particular utility in aiding satiety as well as moderating glycemic excursions.[28] Conversely, refined carbohydrates, high in fructose or sucrose, should be avoided as these increase liver and serum triglycerides and promote insulin resistance and visceral obesity.[29]

Low-Carbohydrate, High-Protein Diets

High-protein foods like eggs and lean meat are relatively satiating[27] and increase body thermogenesis and energy expenditure.[30] Interest has thus grown in the use of LCHP diets for weight loss. After 6 months, obese women following an *ad libitum* LCHP diet where carbohydrate was restricted to 20–60 g/day lost an average of 8.5 kg as compared with a 3.9-kg loss in women following a HCLF diet.[25] An *ad libitum* diet high in both protein ($>30\%$E) and dietary fibre (>35 g/day) has also been reported to produce successful weight loss in women.[31] Comparison of LCHP and HCLF diets by meta-analysis clearly indicated that after 6 months better weight loss is achieved via LCHP diets. This difference, however, was attenuated when diets were followed for one year.[32]

The early benefit of LCHP diets in promoting weight loss must be balanced with other concerns. One is the potential for an adverse change in blood lipids if the increased consumption of animal protein also leads to an increased consumption of saturated fat. After one year, LCHP diets have been associated with a 0.37 mmol/l increase in LDL-cholesterol relative to HCLF diets.[32] This has implications for health as diets high in both animal fat and animal protein are associated with increased mortality.[33]

One further concern is that the higher protein intake in a LCHP diet may impose a metabolic burden on the liver and kidneys. A recent study in obese but otherwise healthy people found that over one year, an energy-restricted LCHP diet (35%E as protein, 124 g/day) induced good weight loss without change in estimated glomerular filtration rate.[34] Nevertheless, change to kidney function may occur slowly, taking years to develop in susceptible people. When American women with normal renal function at baseline were followed for an 11-year period, no association was evident between protein intake and change in renal function. In contrast, for women with mild renal insufficiency at baseline, renal function declined with high protein intake.[35] One mechanism whereby such slow kidney damage can occur on LCHP diets is through enhanced formation of endogenous advanced glycation endproducts (AGE).[36] Given the importance of diabetes as a risk factor for end-stage kidney disease, further investigation of whether high-protein diets adversely affect kidney function long-term remains warranted.

People tend to adhere reasonably well to LCHP diets.[32] If this diet type is selected, considerable attention must be given to the selection of lean, high-quality protein foods that are low in saturated fat, and in maintaining this choice long-term. Protein intake in absolute terms will be necessarily lower during the period of energy restriction than it is during the phase of weight maintenance. In this maintenance phase, consideration should be given to reducing protein intake to avoid any potential risk of long-term kidney damage.

Mediterranean Diets

Traditional Mediterranean diets are based on a high intake of a wide range of fruit and vegetables, nuts and legumes, and unrefined cereals. The predominant fat is olive oil.[37] Fish and dairy foods are eaten regularly, while red meat and poultry are consumed only occasionally. Wine is drunk in moderation only with meals.[38] This dietary intake pattern protects against the development of diabetes.[13] Accordingly, Spaniards who strictly followed a Mediterranean diet had an 83% lower risk of diabetes [odds ratio: 0.17 (95% CI: 0.04—0.72)] than other Spaniards.[39] US participants in the Multi-Ethnic Study of Atherosclerosis (MESA) who followed a Mediterranean-style diet also had a 15% lower risk of diabetes (after adjusting for other known confounders) than those with non-Mediterranean diets.[40] It is also relevant that a recent review reports no evidence of any adverse effects from Mediterranean diets on glycemic control.[41]

As the Mediterranean diet has a relatively high total fat content (albeit of mainly mono-unsaturated fat), concerns have been raised whether it will promote weight gain. Yet Mediterranean-style meals generally are high in vegetables and other unrefined plant foods that through their bulk, effectively lower average meal energy density and make it harder to over-consume.[42] Data from EPIC-PANACEA involving 373,803 people from 10 European countries showed that people adhering strongly to a Mediterranean dietary pattern were 10% less likely to become overweight or obese than people not following this eating pattern.[43] Additionally, no evidence has emerged from intervention studies to suggest that a Mediterranean diet prescription will result in weight gain.[44]

If a Mediterranean diet is chosen, care must be taken that the main fats eaten are mono- and polyunsaturates and that the traditional Mediterranean dietary pattern is adhered to. In particular, the high and varied intake of fresh fruits and vegetables (to provide beneficial phytonutrients and to lower meal energy density) and a daily intake of legumes (for their beneficial effects on glycemic control) are key components.

Weight Loss on Mediterranean Diets

Relatively few studies compare Mediterranean diets with alternate diets for weight loss.

When overweight US adults followed hypo-caloric Mediterranean or HCLF diets for 18 months, each group exhibited similar weight loss at 12 months. At 18 months, however, the group on the HCLF diet regained weight, while those on the Mediterranean diet maintained their weight loss.[45]

Another study has compared a hypocaloric Mediterranean diet with both HCLF and a LCHP diets over a 2-year period.[46] After 2 years, similar weight loss was achieved on both the LCHP and after the Mediterranean diet (−4.7 kg and −4.4 kg, respectively), while those on the HCLF diet fared less well (−2.9 kg). Interestingly, in women, the Mediterranean diet promoted much better weight loss (−6.2 kg) than the low-fat diet (−0.1 kg), a striking difference not observed in men (−4.0 kg vs −3.4 kg, respectively, $P < 0.001$).[46]

Other Potentially Beneficial Dietary Patterns

There are other phytonutrient-rich dietary patterns, high in fresh fruit and vegetables and low in meat, refined grains, sugar, saturated fat, and salt that potentially may prevent the development of type 2 diabetes. One example is the Okinawan diet traditional for people in the Rykuyu Islands of Japan. Their diet and high physical activity promotes a very high life expectancy and low diabetes incidence.[47] The diet is based on high vegetable intake (sweet potato, okra, pumpkin and seaweeds), high intake of soy products (tofu and miso-paste), moderate serves of omega-3-rich fish and the infrequent consumption of meat or dairy foods. The Okinawan diet thus has a high monounsaturated:saturated fat ratio and is based on a low-GI staple carbohydrate (sweet potato). In addition water-rich foods [mushrooms, burdock, *konnyaku* (jelly) and *daikon* (radish)] help lower meal energy density. The potential of diets of this type for diabetes prevention needs further exploration.

Rate of Weight Loss

Regardless of the type of dietary regimen chosen, the degree of energy restriction needs to be moderate and sustainable until the weight loss goal is achieved. An energy deficit sufficient to induce weight loss of up to 0.45 kg per week is recommended. More drastic loss only induces deleterious loss of muscle mass and muscle strength.[48]

THE ROLE OF EXERCISE

Exercise increases the insulin-mediated glucose disposal to muscle,[49] aids weight maintenance[50] and may promote beneficial anti-inflammatory effects.[51] Yet many people in developed countries spend most of their waking life sitting and engage in minimal leisure time activity or regular exercise.[52] This very sedentary behavior increases diabetes risk.[53] Even without weight loss, regular exercise will reduce diabetes risk in sedentary people. For example, 495 participants from the DPP who exercised but failed to lose weight showed a 44% lower incidence of diabetes during follow-up.[18]

While the importance of regular exercise for diabetes prevention is well recognized, the optimal exercise prescription is less clear. Aerobic exercise (running, brisk walking, swimming, cycling) improves both vascular function[54] and the metabolic profile.[55] In most large diabetes-prevention trials[6,8–10] recommendations for regular aerobic exercise were associated with diabetes risk reduction ranging from 28.5 to 68%.[22] Highly sedentary individuals about to engage in aerobic exercise can be encouraged by the finding that prolonged moderate-intensity exercise can be as effective in metabolic improvement as higher-intensity regimens.[56] Where weight loss is not an issue, 30 min of brisk walking at least five times per week (150 min/week) appears sufficient to maintain health.[57] The major barriers to engagement in physical activity are reported to be lack of time, tiredness, and competition with other priorities. These barriers are similar for both normoglycemic adults and those with abnormal glucose metabolism.[58]

Regular resistance training (RT) increases muscle mass through the enlargement (hypertrophy) of muscle fibers.[51] This has positive effects not only on energy expenditure and the maintenance of a healthy body weight, but also on insulin sensitivity.[59] In the DPS, a combined regimen of aerobic plus resistance exercise together with a low-fat, high-fibre diet achieved a diabetes risk reduction of 58%.[15] RT should be undertaken at least twice a week and include eight to 10 exercises for the major muscle groups, each with at least one set of 10–15 repetitions.[60] Regular training is important to gain the full anti-inflammatory impact.[51] Sporadic acute bouts can be pro-inflammatory particularly if recovery between bouts is not well promoted.[61]

Exercise and Body Weight

All individuals in the general community should participate in moderate-intensity physical activity for at least 30 min per day on most if not all days in the week.[48] Increasing exercise levels without dietary change has only modest effects on weight loss (−0.5 to −4 kg) while adopting a hypocaloric diet has more substantial effects (in the order of −2.8 to −13.6 kg).[62] Adding exercise to a hypocaloric diet then has a very modest (around 1.1 kg) additional impact.[62] In contrast to its modest effects on weight loss, regular exercise is critical for successful weight maintenance. In this phase, at least 280 min of physical activity per week appear to be required with the expenditure of around 8.4 MJ (2,000 kcals) per week.[48]

CONCLUSION

Diabetes can clearly be prevented by lifestyle change. There is choice of several dietary patterns that can be tailored to individual preference in order to promote weight loss or weight maintenance. The impact of dietary interventions should be aided by regular aerobic and resistance exercise.

References

1. Crandall JP, Knowler WC, Kahn SE, Marrero D, Florez JC, Bray GA, Haffner SM. The prevention of type 2 diabetes. *Nat Clin Pract Endocrinol Metab* 2008;**4**:382—93.

2. Geiss LS, James C, Gregg EW, Albright A, Williamson DF, Cowie CC. Diabetes risk reduction behaviors among U.S. adults with prediabetes. *Am J Prev Med* 2010;**38**:403—9.

3. Laaksonen MA, Knekt P, Rissanen H, Härkänen T, Virtala E, Marniemi J, Aromaa A, Heliövaara M, Reunanen A. The relative importance of modifiable potential risk factors of type 2 diabetes: a meta-analysis of two cohorts. *Eur J Epidemiol* 2010;**25**:115—24.

4. Astrup A, Dyerberg J, Selleck M, Stender S. Nutrition transition and its relationship to the development of obesity and related chronic diseases. *Obes Rev* 2008;**9**(Suppl. 1):48—52.

5. Qin L, Knol MJ, Corpeleijn E, Stolk RP. Does physical activity modify the risk of obesity for type 2 diabetes: a review of epidemiological data. *Eur J Epidemiol* 2010;**25**:5—12.

6. Pan XR, Li GW, Hu YH, Wang JX, Yang WY, An ZX, Hu ZX, Lin J, Xiao JZ, Cao HB, Liu PA, Jiang XG, Jiang YY, Wang JP, Zheng H, Zhang H, Bennett PH, Howard BV. Effects of diet and exercise in preventing NIDDM in people with impaired glucose tolerance. The Da Qing IGT and Diabetes Study. *Diabetes Care* 1997;**20**:537—44.

7. Tuomilehto J, Lindström J, Eriksson JG, Valle TT, Hämäläinen H, Ilanne-Parikka P, Keinänen-Kiukaanniemi S, Laakso M, Louheranta A, Rastas M, Salminen V, Uusitupa M, Finnish Diabetes Prevention Study Group. Prevention of type 2 diabetes mellitus by changes in lifestyle among subjects with impaired glucose tolerance. *N Engl J Med* 2001;**344**:1343—50.

8. Knowler WC, Barrett-Connor E, Fowler SE, Hamman RF, Lachin JM, Walker EA, Nathan DM, Diabetes Prevention Program Research Group. Reduction in the incidence of type 2 diabetes with lifestyle intervention or metformin. *N Engl J Med* 2002;**346**:393—403.

9. Ramachandran A, Snehalatha C, Mary S, Mukesh B, Bhaskar AD, Vijay V, Indian Diabetes Prevention Programme (IDPP). The Indian Diabetes Prevention Programme shows that lifestyle modification and metformin prevent type 2 diabetes in Asian Indian subjects with impaired glucose tolerance (IDPP-1). *Diabetologia* 2006;**49**:289—97.

10. Kosaka K, Nodaa M, Kuzuyab T. Prevention of type 2 diabetes by lifestyle intervention: a Japanese trial in IGT males. *Diabetes Res Clin Pract* 2005;**67**:152—62.

11. Faerch K, Borch-Johnsen K, Holst JJ, Vaag A. Pathophysiology and aetiology of impaired fasting glycaemia and impaired glucose tolerance: does it matter for prevention and treatment of type 2 diabetes? *Diabetologia* 2009;**52**:1714—23.

12. Harati H, Hadaegh F, Momenan AA, Ghanei L, Bozorgmanesh MR, Ghanbarian A, Mirmiran P, Azizi F. Reduction in incidence of type 2 diabetes by lifestyle intervention in a middle eastern community. *Am J Prev Med* 2010;**38**:628—36. e621.

13. Salas-Salvadó J, Bulló M, Babio N, Martínez-González MA, Ibarrola-Jurado N, Basora J, Estruch R, Covas MI, Corella D, Arós F, Ruiz-Gutiérrez V, Ros E, For the PREDIMED Study investigators. Reduction in the incidence of type 2-diabetes with the Mediterranean diet: Results of the PREDIMED-Reus Nutrition Intervention Randomized Trial. *Diabetes Care*; 2010. 2010 Oct 13. [Epub].

14. Li G, Zhang P, Wang J, Gregg EW, Yang W, Gong Q, Li H, Li H, Jiang Y, An Y, Shuai Y, Zhang B, Zhang J, Thompson TJ, Gerzoff RB, Roglic G, Hu Y, Bennett. PH. The long-term effect of lifestyle interventions to prevent diabetes in the China Da Qing Diabetes Prevention Study: a 20-year follow-up study. *Lancet* 2008;**371**:1783—9.

15. Lindström J, Ilanne-Parikka P, Peltonen M, Aunola S, Eriksson JG, Hemiö K, Hämäläinen H, Härkönen P, Keinänen-Kiukaanniemi S, Laakso M, Louheranta A, Mannelin M, Paturi M, Sundval IJ, Valle TT, Uusitupa M, Tuomilehto J, Finnish DPSG. Sustained reduction in the incidence of type 2 diabetes by lifestyle intervention: follow-up of the Finnish Diabetes Prevention Study. *Lancet* 2006;**368**:1673—9.

16. Diabetes Prevention Program Research Group. 10-year follow-up of diabetes incidence and weight loss in the Diabetes Prevention Program Outcomes Study. *Lancet* 2009;**374**:1677—86.

17. Gillies CL, Abrams KR, Lambert PC, Cooper NJ, Sutton AJ, Hsu RT, Khunti K. Pharmacological and lifestyle interventions to prevent or delay type 2 diabetes in people with impaired glucose tolerance: systematic review and meta-analysis. *BMJ* 2007;**334**: 299. Epub.

18. Hamman RF, Wing RR, Edelstein SL, Lachin JM, Bray GA, Delahanty L, Hoskin M, Kriska AM, Mayer-Davis EJ, Pi-Sunyer X, Regensteiner J, Venditti B,

Wylie-Rosett J. Effect of weight loss with lifestyle intervention on risk of diabetes. *Diabetes Care* 2006;**29**:2102–7.

19. Curtis J, Wilson C. Preventing type 2 diabetes mellitus. *J Am Board Fam Pract* 2005;**18**:37–43.

20. Larson-Meyer DE, Redman L, Heilbronn LK, Martin CK, Ravussin E. Caloric restriction with or without exercise: the fitness versus fatness debate. *Med Sci Sports Exerc* 2010;**42**:152–9.

21. Laaksonen MA, Knekt P, Rissanen H, Härkänen T, Virtala E, Marniemi J, Aromaa A, Heliövaara M, Reunanen A. The relative importance of modifiable potential risk factors of type 2 diabetes: a meta-analysis of two cohorts. *Eur J Epidemiol* 2010;**25**:115–24.

22. Sanz C, Gautier J-F, Hanaire H. Physical exercise for the prevention and treatment of type 2 diabetes. *Diabetes Metab*; 2010. doi:10.1016/j.diabet.2010.06.001.

23. Rana JS, Li TY, Manson JE, Hu FB. Adiposity compared with physical inactivity and risk of type 2 diabetes in women. *Diabetes Care* 2007;**30**:53–8.

24. Sacks FM, Bray GA, Carey VJ, Smith SR, Ryan DH, Anton SD, McManus K, Champagne CM, Bishop LM, Laranjo N, Leboff MS, Rood JC, de Jonge L, Greenway FL, Loria CM, Obarzanek E, Williamson DA. Comparison of weight-loss diets with different compositions of fat, protein, and carbohydrates. *N Eng J Med* 2009;**360**:859–73.

25. Brehm BJ, Seeley RJ, Daniels SR, D'Alessio DA. A randomized trial comparing a very low carbohydrate diet and a calorie-restricted low fat diet on body weight and cardiovascular risk factors in healthy women. *J Clin Endocrinol Metab* 2003;**88**:1617–23.

26. Rolls BJ. Plenary Lecture 1: Dietary strategies for the prevention and treatment of obesity. *Proc Nutr Soc* 2010;**69**:70–9.

27. Brehm BJ, D'Alessio DA. Weight loss and metabolic benefits with diets of varying fat and carbohydrate content: separating the wheat from the chaff. *Nat Clin Pract Endocrinol Metab* 2008;**4**:140–6.

28. Barclay AW, Petocz P, McMillan-Price J, Flood VM, Prvan T, Mitchell P, Brand-Miller JC. Glycemic index, glycemic load, and chronic disease risk—a meta-analysis of observational studies. *Am J Clin Nutr* 2008;**87**:627–37.

29. Stanhope KL, Havel PJ. Fructose consumption: potential mechanisms for its effects to increase visceral adiposity and induce dyslipidemia and insulin resistance. *Curr Opin Lipidol* 2008;**19**:16–24.

30. Paddon-Jones D, Westman E, Mattes RD, Wolfe RR, Astrup A, Westerterp-Plantenga M. Protein, weight management, and satiety. *Am J Clin Nutr* 2008;**87**:1558S–61S.

31. Morenga LT, Williams S, Brown R, Mann J. Effect of a relatively high-protein, high-fiber diet on body composition and metabolic risk factors in overweight women. *Eur J Clin Nutr*; 2010. Sep 15. (Epub).

32. Hession M, Rolland C, Kulkarni U, Wise A, Broom J. Systematic review of randomized controlled trials of low-carbohydrate vs low-fat/low-calorie diets in the management of obesity and its comorbidities. *Obes Rev* 2009;**10**:36–50.

33. Fung TT, van Dam RM, Hankinson SE, Stampfer M, Willett WC, Hu FB. Low-carbohydrate diets and all-cause and cause-specific mortality: two cohort studies. *Ann Intern Med* 2010;**153**:289–98.

34. Brinkworth GD, Buckley JD, Noakes M, Clifton PM. Renal function following long-term weight loss in individuals with abdominal obesity on a very-low-carbohydrate diet vs high-carbohydrate diet. *J Am Diet Assoc* 2010;**110**:633–8.

35. Knight EL, Stampfer MJ, Hankinson SE, Spiegelman D, Curhan GC. The impact of protein intake on renal function decline in women with normal renal function or mild renal insufficiency. *Ann Intern Med* 2003;**138**:460–7.

36. Tuttle KR, Anderberg RJ, Cooney SK, Meek RL. Oxidative stress mediates protein kinase C activation and advanced glycation end product formation in a mesangial cell model of diabetes and high protein diet. *Am J Nephrol* 2009;**29**:171–80.

37. Cicerale S, Conlan XA, Sinclair AJ, Keast RS. Chemistry and health of olive oil phenolics. *Crit Rev Food Sci Nutr* 2009;**49**:218–36.

38. Trichopoulou A. Mediterranean diet: the past and the present. *Nutr Metab Cardiovasc Dis* 2001;**11**(Supp1. 4):1–4.

39. Martínez-González MA, de la Fuente-Arrillaga C, Nunez-Cordoba JM, Basterra-Gortari FJ, Beunza JJ, Vazquez Z, Benito S, Tortosa A, Bes-Rastrollo M. Adherence to Mediterranean diet and risk of developing diabetes: prospective cohort study. *BMJ* 2008;**336**:1348–51.

40. Nettleton JA, Steffen LM, Ni H, Liu K, Jacobs Jr DR. Dietary patterns and risk of incident type 2 diabetes in the Multi-Ethnic Study of Atherosclerosis (MESA). *Diabetes Care* 2008;**31**:1777–82.

41. Esposito K, Maiorino MI, Ceriello A, Giugliano D. Prevention and control of type 2 diabetes by Mediterranean diet: a systematic review. *Diabetes Res Clin Pract* 2010;**89**:97–102.

42. Walker KZ, O'Dea K. Is a low fat diet the optimal way to cut energy intake over the long-term in overweight people? *Nutr Metab Cardiovasc Dis* 2001;**11**:244–8.

43. Romaguera D, Norat T, Vergnaud AC, Mouw T, May AM, Agudo A, Buckland G, Slimani N, Rinaldi S,

Couto E, Clavel-Chapelon F, Boutron-Ruault MC, Cottet V, Rohrmann S, Teucher B, Bergmann M, Boeing H, Tjønneland A, Halkjaer J, Jakobsen MU, Dahm CC, Travier N, Rodriguez L, Sanchez MJ, Amiano P, Barricarte A, Huerta JM, Luan J, Wareham N, Key TJ, Spencer EA, Orfanos P, Naska A, Trichopoulou A, Palli D, Agnoli C, Mattiello A, Tumino R, Vineis P, Bueno-de-Mesquita HB, Büchner FL, Manjer J, Wirfält E, Johansson I, Hellstrom V, Lund E, Braaten T, Engeset D, Odysseos A, Riboli E, Peeters PH. Mediterranean dietary patterns and prospective weight change in participants of the EPIC-PANACEA project. Am J Clin Nutr 2010;92:912–21.

44. Buckland G, Bach A, Serra-Majem L. Obesity and the Mediterranean diet: A systematic review of observational and intervention studies. Obes Rev 2008;9:582–93.

45. McManus K, Antinoro L, Sacks F. A randomized controlled trial of a moderate-fat, low-energy diet compared with a low fat, low-energy diet for weight loss in overweight adults. Int J Obes Relat Metab Disord 2001;25:1503–11.

46. Shai I, Schwarzfuchs D, Henkin Y, Shahar DR, Witkow S, Greenberg I, Golan R, Fraser D, Bolotin A, Vardi H, Tangi-Rozental O, Zuk-Ramot R, Sarusi B, Brickner D, Schwartz Z, Sheiner E, Marko R, Katorza E, Thiery J, Fiedler GM, Blüher M, Stumvoll M, Stampfer MJ, Dietary Intervention Randomized Controlled Trial (DIRECT) Group. Weight loss with a low-carbohydrate, Mediterranean, or low-fat diet. N Engl J Med 2008;359:229–41.

47. Willcox CD, Bradley BJ, Todoriki H, Suzuki M. The Okinawan diet: health implications of a low-calorie, nutrient dense, antioxidant-rich dietary pattern low in glycemic load. J Am Coll Nutr 2009;28:500S–16S.

48. Jakicic JM, Clark K, Coleman E, Donnelly JE, Foreyt J, Melanson E, Volek J, Volpe SL, American College of Sports Medicine. American College of Sports Medicine position stand. Appropriate intervention strategies for weight loss and prevention of weight regain for adults. Med Sci Sports Exerc 2001;33:2145–56.

49. Horowitz JF. Exercise-induced alterations in muscle lipid metabolism improve insulin sensitivity. Exerc Sport Sci Rev 2007;35:192–6.

50. Svetkey LP, Stevens VJ, Brantley PJ, Appel LJ, Hollis JF, Loria CM, Vollmer WM, Gullion CM, Funk K, Smith P, Samuel-Hodge C, Myers V, Lien LF, Laferriere D, Kennedy B, Jerome GJ, Heinith F, Harsha DW, Evans P, Erlinger TP, Dalcin AT, Coughlin J, Charleston J, Champagne CM, Bauck A, Ard JD, Aicher K, Weight Loss Maintenance Collaborative Research Group. Comparison of strategies for sustaining weight loss: the weight loss maintenance randomized controlled trial. JAMA 2008;299:1139–48.

51. Calle MC, Fernandez ML. Effects of resistance training on the inflammatory response. Nutr Res Pract 2010;4:259–69.

52. Hamilton MT, Hamilton DG, Zderic TW. Role of low energy expenditure and sitting in obesity, metabolic syndrome, type 2 diabetes, and cardiovascular disease. Diabetes 2007;56:2655–67.

53. Healy GN, Dunstan DW, Salmon J, Shaw JE, Zimmet PZ, Owen N. Television time and continuous metabolic risk in physically active adults. Med Sci Sports Exerc 2008;40:639–45.

54. DeSouza CA, Shapiro LF, Clevenger CM, Dinenno FA, Monahan KD, Tanaka H, Seals DR. Regular aerobic exercise prevents and restores age-related declines in endothelium-dependent vasodilation in healthy men. Circulation 2000;102:1351–7.

55. Tjønna AE, Lee SJ, Rognmo Ø, Stølen TO, Bye A, Haram PM, Loennechen JP, Al-Share QY, Skogvoll E, Slørdahl SA, Kemi OJ, Najjar SM, Wisløff U. Aerobic interval training versus continuous moderate exercise as a treatment for the metabolic syndrome: a pilot study. Circulation 2008;118:346–54.

56. O'Donovan G, Kearney EM, Nevill AM, Woolf-May K, Bird SR. The effects of 24 weeks of moderate- or high-intensity exercise on insulin resistance. Eur J Appl Physiol 2005;95:522–8.

57. Haskell WL, Lee IM, Pate RR, Powell KE, Blair SN, Franklin BA, Macera CA, Heath GW, Thompson PD, Bauman A. Physical activity and public health: updated recommendation for adults from the American College of Sports Medicine and the American Heart Association. Med Sci Sports Exerc 2007;39:1423–34.

58. Hume C, Dunstan D, Salmon J, Healy G, Andrianopoulos N, Owen N. Are barriers to physical activity similar for adults with and without abnormal glucose metabolism? Diabetes Educ 2010;36:495–502.

59. Phillips SM. Resistance exercise: good for more than just Grandma and Grandpa's muscles. Appl Physiol Nutr Metab 2007;32:1198–205.

60. Sigal RJ, Kenny GP, Wasserman DH, Castaneda-Sceppa C. Physical activity/exercise and type 2 diabetes. Diabetes Care 2004;27:1023–5.

61. Miles MP. How do we solve the puzzle of unintended consequences of inflammation? Systematically. J Appl Physiol 2008;105:1023–5.

62. Shaw KA, Gennat HC, O'Rourke P, Del Mar C. Exercise for overweight or obesity. Cochrane Database Syst Rev 2009;3:1–97.

TYPES OF DIABETES AND ITS CORRELATION WITH OTHER DISEASES

The Role of Insulin Resistance in the Cardiorenal Syndrome

Jaya P. Buddineni*, Adam Whaley-Connell*,**,
James R. Sowers*,†,**

*Department of Internal Medicine, †Department of Medical Pharmacology & Physiology, University of Missouri School of Medicine **Harry S. Truman VA Medical Center, Columbia, MO, USA

INTRODUCTION

The metabolic syndrome is a cluster of metabolic abnormalities including diabetes that are risk factors for the development of cardiovascular disease (CVD) and chronic kidney disease (CKD). In the early 90s, the metabolic syndrome became an area of active investigative interest that ultimately led to a better understanding of the relationship between the presence of insulin resistance, CVD, and recently CKD, e.g., cardiorenal disease. There are various diagnostic criteria that have been developed such as National Cholesterol Education Program Adult Treatment Panel III (ATP III), European Group for Study of Insulin Resistance, American Association of Clinical Endocrinologists and the International

Nutritional and Therapeutic Interventions for Diabetes and Metabolic Syndrome
DOI: 10.1016/B978-0-12-385083-6.00011-5

137

Diabetes Federation. However, the common inclusion criteria between the various groups consistently rely on the presence of abdominal obesity and insulin resistance or overt diabetes mellitus. The central difference in defining the criteria of metabolic syndrome by the various organizations is noted in describing insulin resistance measurements, glycemic and blood pressure thresholds, measurements of abdominal obesity and/or the presence of microalbuminuria, defined as albumin excretion of 30–300 mg/day.[1,2]

Besides the well-established relationship between overt diabetes and the cardiorenal syndrome, there has been considerable focus on the association between insulin resistance and CKD in the past decade. Along with chronic hyperglycemia and hypertension, insulin resistance and obesity have emerged as key players in CKD development.[3] CKD is defined as the presence of a glomerular filtration rate (GFR) < 60 ml/min/1.73 m^2 with or without the presence of kidney damage, or in those with a GFR > 60 the presence of structural or functional abnormalities on biopsy, imaging, or blood or urine markers, albuminuria (e.g., proteinuria). Microalbuminuria is also an important component of the cardiorenal syndrome.[4]

EPIDEMIOLOGIC EVIDENCE

There is sufficient evidence from studies of patients with the metabolic syndrome and/or the cardiorenal syndrome to support a causal association between the presence of insulin resistance, obesity, and the presence of CKD. One such investigation, the Atherosclerosis Risk in Communities (ARIC) study noted an increased risk of developing CKD in non-diabetic subjects with the metabolic syndrome over a 9-year follow up, independent of baseline confounding factors and the development of diabetes and hypertension.[5] Subjects who fulfilled the NCEP/ATP III criteria for the metabolic syndrome at baseline had a 43% increased risk of developing CKD than those without it. Compared with subjects with no components of the syndrome, those with one, two, three, four or five components of it had an odds ratio (OR) for CKD of 1.13, 1.53, 1.75, 1.84, and 2.45, respectively.[5] Another study in overt type 1 diabetic subjects classified as having normal urinary albumin excretion (UAE), microalbuminuria, macroalbuminuria, or end-stage renal disease (ESRD); the prevalence of the metabolic syndrome rose significantly from 28% to 44%, 62%, and 68%, respectively. When considering a population without the presence of diabetes on inclusion, data from the Framingham heart study support that after adjustments, the presence of insulin resistance was significantly associated with development of CKD during 7-year follow-up.[6] Moreover, subjects at baseline had almost four times the risk of developing diabetic kidney disease in the presence of insulin resistance alone.[7] Data from the National Health and Nutrition Examination Survey (NHANES III) study further support the presence of insulin resistance is associated with both the presence of CKD and microalbuminuria after adjustment. Collectively, a trend has emerged wherein there is an increasing odds for CKD and microalbuminuria with increasing components of the metabolic (cardiorenal) syndrome irrespective of whether there is overt diabetes or not.[8]

Central to the discussion on whether insulin resistance or overt diabetes is associated with development of CKD, the presence of insulin resistance/hyperinsulinemia has been documented in a non-diabetic population at early, as well as advanced, stages of renal dysfunction.[9] This notion of an association between insulin resistance and CKD has been supported by NHANES data that suggest a strong association between the presence of insulin resistance and prevalent CKD in non-diabetic subjects after adjustment for age, gender, ethnicity, physical activity, blood pressure, total cholesterol and tobacco use.[10]

PATHOPHYSIOLOGIC LINKS BETWEEN INSULIN RESISTANCE, OBESITY, AND THE CARDIORENAL SYNDROME

The association between obesity and the development of insulin resistance, the cardiorenal syndrome, and diminishing kidney function appears to be multifactorial, including genetic and environmental factors. There have been reports of specific gene mutations in pathways that regulate lipolysis, insulin production, adipose tissue distribution, and appetite that seem to play a role in the development endothelial dysfunction as a precursor to development of CVD and CKD.[11,12] Environmental factors such as diet and exercise patterns also contribute to obesity, fat disposition and reductions in insulin sensitivity also seem to play a role in the development of the endothelial dysfunction.[13] The relationship between overweight/obesity and progressive renal dysfunction begins in early childhood and is related to increasing consumption of high-fructose corn syrup and insufficient physical activity.[1–3]

It is well established that adipose tissue acts as a complex autocrine/paracrine organ releasing multiple bioactive compounds that regulate glucose and lipid metabolism in the body. Mounting evidence supports a role for visceral adipose tissue in governing blood pressure regulation as well as glomerular filtration.[14] Numerous endocrine abnormalities have been suggested that explain the association between obesity, insulin resistance, and albuminuria of which the most significant ones are inappropriate activation of sympathetic nervous system (SNS), renin-angiotensin-aldosterone system (RAAS), activation of the sympathetic nervous system, and blunting actions of protective cytokines such as adiponectin.[15–17] Excessive visceral adipose tissue in obese individuals is a well-known source for pro-inflammatory adipokines such as tumor necrosis factor-α, interleukin-1, interleukin-6, leptin, and resistin which induce insulin resistance.[18] The resulting hyperinsulinemic state has been shown to induce structural glomerular changes which include glomerulosclerosis and thickening of glomerular basement membrane in animal models.[19]

MICROALBUMINURIA IN THE CARDIORENAL SYNDROME

Whether a risk predictor or outcome, the presence of microalbuminuria has been an area of contention in understanding the role of insulin resistance and proteinuria in the cardiorenal syndrome. The World Health Organization has previously included microalbuminuria in their definition of the metabolic syndrome. Despite growing preclinical evidence to support a microalbuminuria in the constellation of metabolic risk predictors, only a few epidemiologic studies have included microalbuminuria in non-diabetic subjects in evaluating CVD and/or CKD risk.[8,20–23] However, it is widely thought that microalbuminuria is a marker of generalized endothelial dysfunction and an independent, modifiable predictor of CVD as well as CVD-associated mortality.[24,25] Clinically, appropriate management targeting reductions in microalbuminuria can lead to reductions in CVD and CKD risk.[3]

INSULIN RESISTANCE IN THE CARDIORENAL SYNDROME

Persistent elevations of insulin levels can impair renal hemodynamics, causing, a rise in GFR in experimental studies[26] and in hypertensive individuals.[27] Hyperinsulinemia also leads to vascular sodium retention and salt sensitivity, thus contributing to increased glomerular pressure, hyperfiltration, and UAE in diabetic individuals.[28] The role of insulin resistance and hyperinsulinemia in activation of vascular sympathetic and vasoconstriction activity via release of increased catecholamines has been well documented.[2-29] In the insulin-resistant state, the normal production of nitric oxide (NO) mediated by insulin and its homologous peptide insulin-like growth factor-1 (IGF-1) through stimulation of phosphatidylinositol 3-kinase signaling pathways is impaired. This leads to decreased concentrations of NO and myosin light chain activation and adds to derangement of Na^+-K^+ exchange resulting in increased intracellular calcium concentration and increased calcium sensitivity in vascular smooth muscle cells.[29] All these changes potentially contribute not only to the development of vasoconstriction and hypertension, but also lead to glomerular hypertension and increased UAE.

In addition to the above enumerated adverse effects, hyperinsulinemia can also lead to vascular cell proliferation, mesangial expansion and increased extracellular matrix deposition.[30] These actions may be mediated directly by insulin and/or various other growth factors such as IGF-1, transforming growth factor-β (TGF-β), endothelin-1 (ET-1). IGF-1 and other insulin-dependent growth factors are potent smooth muscle mitogens that contribute to the formation of atherosclerotic lesions by paracrine, autocrine, or endocrine mechanisms.[31] IGF-1 has vascular effects similar to insulin and induces mesangial cell growth and glomerular expansion.[32] Insulin induces production of TGF-β by mesangial and proximal tubular cells [33] which in turn lead to extracellular matrix expansion and fibrosis.[34] Recent data suggest that ET-1 has been shown to be increased in response to hyperinsulinemia both *in vivo* and *in vitro*.[35,36] ET-1 is known to be a potent vasoconstrictor increasing vascular tone thus leading to glomerular hypertension. Moreover, ET-1 also has mesangial proliferative effects, which are mediated by protein kinase C signaling pathways.[37]

Finally, disequilibrium in the endogenous fibrinolytic system has been reported in conditions of insulin resistance and obesity that promote atherosclerosis.[38] Excess production of plasminogen activator inhibitor 1 (PAI-1) and coagulation factors such as factor VII have been noted in hyperinsulinemia, thus causing a hypercoaguable state and later leading to increased UAE in diabetic subjects.[39] There is sufficient preclinical data to support a role for TGF-β, angiotensin II, thrombin, and TNF-α in promoting the synthesis of PAI-1, which in turn inhibits plasmin formation and matrix metalloproteinase (MMP) activation, thus leading to fibrinolysis and extracellular membrane degradation resulting in fibrosis.[40]

OXIDATIVE STRESS AND ENDOPLASMIC STRESS IN THE CARDIORENAL SYNDROME

As iterated in the previous section, insulin resistance and the compensatory hyperinsulinemia contribute to alterations in numerous pathways that lead to vascular and renal remodeling. In the context of abnormal thrombolysis, hyperinsulinemia is also associated with excess reactive oxygen species formation and oxidant stress and low-grade inflammation leading to the development of endothelial dysfunction. Persistent hyperinsulinemia and hyperglycemia have been noted to produce reactive oxygen species by directing excessive glucose through anaerobic glycolysis, glucosamine production, glucose auto-oxidation pathways.[41] Endogenous antioxidant pathways such as superoxide dismutase and glutathione peroxidase are eventually used up leading to compensatory hyperinsulinemia-mediated renal effects. Endoplasmic reticulum stress is increasingly recognized as a molecular link between obesity deterioration of insulin action and development of the cardiorenal syndrome.[42] Dysregulation of insulin signaling via c-Jun N-terminal kinase-mediated phosphorylation of the insulin receptors was noted in endoplasmic reticulum stress conditions in rodent models of obesity.[42]

INAPPROPRIATE ACTIVATION OF THE RAAS

The role of RAAS in the pathogenesis of CKD is well studied in the context of diabetes. However, therapeutic use of pharmacological agents that inhibit the RAAS has equally been demonstrated to be integral in the management of CKD in the obese, insulin-resistant individual.[43] In obese individuals, activation of SNS and RAAS along with physical compression of kidneys lead to increased renal tubular sodium reabsorption, volume expansion, and hypertension.[44] Despite this level of salt retention and hyperfiltration, the RAAS is activated. The deleterious actions of angiotensin II on the kidneys include increased glomerular pressure, induction of intra-renal inflammatory cytokines and growth factors, apoptosis that lead to maladaptive mechanisms that contribute to development of albuminuria.[45] Angiotensin II is also shown to stimulate proliferation of mesangial cells, glomerular endothelial cells, and fibroblasts.[46] The interaction of angiotensin II with AT_1 receptors results in production of ROS by upregulating NADPH oxidase activity and intrarenal fibrosis, through production of growth factors such as TGF-β and connective tissue growth factor.[47] Smad signaling pathway and the Rho/Rho kinase system have been implicated in the angiotensin II-mediated impaired extracellular matrix remodelling.[47]

In the context of insulin resistance, our understanding of the role of aldosterone in the mechanisms of proteinuria and progression of CKD has been evolving in recent years. It has been reported that excess aldosterone levels promote the development of impaired insulin metabolic signaling which, in turn, contribute to hypertension leading to cardiovascular and renal structural and functional abnormalities.[48] Recent studies suggest that the increased non-genomic mineralocorticoid receptor signaling in response to the elevated levels of aldosterone and corticosteroids lead to the development of insulin resistance and albuminuria.[49]

CONCLUSIONS AND PERSPECTIVES

Diabetes is a well-recognized risk factor for development of CVD and CKD (Table 11.1). However, the role of insulin resistance is emerging as an equally important contributor to the cardiorenal risk and for progressive renal dysfunction in those with obesity. There is mounting evidence of strong association between these factors as components of insulin resistance and CKD. Various pathophysiologic mechanisms such as insulin resistance and compensatory hyperinsulinemia, visceral fat-induced adipokines, oxidative stress, inappropriate activation of the RAAS and SNS lead to glomerular hypertension, vascular proliferation, deposition of extracellular matrix causing impaired renal hemodynamics (Figure 11.1). The role of microalbuminuria and overt macro-albuminuria as a risk predictor is clear in the context of cardiorenal disease and progression of renal disease.

TABLE 11.1 Common Risk Factors for the Cardiorenal Syndrome

Visceral obesity
Insulin resistance/hyperinsulinemia
Hypertension
Dyslipidemia (high LDL and low HDL)
Salt sensitivity
Microalbuminuria
SNS overactivation
Inappropriate activation of RAAS
Inflammation—increased C-reactive protein
Oxidant stress—increased reactive oxygen species
Altered thrombolysis—increased PAI-1

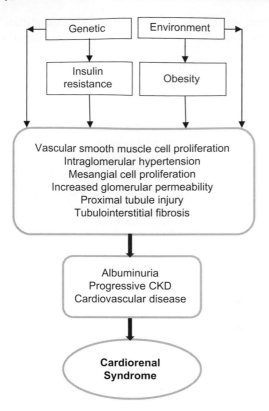

FIGURE 11.1 Multifactorial pathophysiologic mechanisms leading to cardiorenal syndrome.

In spite of the recognition of obesity as a critical pandemic, the impact on cardiorenal disease and the cardiorenal syndrome has yet to be fully elucidated. Further work should be focused in understanding and establishing the impact insulin resistance has on eliciting early kidney injury. However, non-pharmacological measures such as physical activity, weight reduction along with pharmacological interventions such as angiotensin-converting enzyme inhibitors, angiotensin receptor blockers, statins, insulin-sensitizing agents such as metformin, thiazolidinediones can be used in preventing the development of the cardiorenal metabolic syndrome as well as progression of CKD and CVD.

References

1. Sowers JR, Whaley-Connell A, Hayden MR. The role of overweight and obesity in the cardiorenal syndrome. *Cardiorenal Med* 2011;**1**:5–12.
2. Manrique C, Lastra G, Whaley-Connell A, Sowers JR. Hypertension and the cardiometabolic syndrome. *J Clin Hypertens (Greenwich)* Aug 2005;**7**(8):471–6.
3. Whaley Connell A, Pulakat L, DeMarco VG, Hayden MR, Habibi J, Hnerikson EJ, Sowers JR. Overnutrition and the cardiorenal syndrome: Use of a rodent model to examine mechanisms. *Cardiorenal Med* 2011;**1**:23–304.
4. Levey AS, Coresh J, Balk E, et al. National Kidney Foundation practice guidelines for chronic kidney disease: evaluation, classification, and stratification. *Ann Intern Med* Jul 15 2003;**139**(2):137–47.
5. Kurella M, Lo JC, Chertow GM. Metabolic syndrome and the risk for chronic kidney disease among nondiabetic adults. *J Am Soc Nephrol* Jul 2005;**16**(7):2134–40.
6. Fox CS, Larson MG, Leip EP, Meigs JB, Wilson PW, Levy D. Glycemic status and development of kidney disease: the Framingham Heart Study. *Diabetes Care* Oct 2005;**28**(10):2436–40.
7. Thorn LM, Forsblom C, Fagerudd J, et al. Metabolic syndrome in type 1 diabetes: association with diabetic nephropathy and glycemic control (the FinnDiane study). *Diabetes Care* Aug 2005;**28**(8):2019–24.
8. Chen J, Muntner P, Hamm LL, et al. The metabolic syndrome and chronic kidney disease in U.S. adults. *Ann Intern Med* Feb 3 2004;**140**(3):167–74.
9. Fliser D, Pacini G, Engelleiter R, et al. Insulin resistance and hyperinsulinemia are already present in patients with incipient renal disease. *Kidney Int* May 1998;**53**(5):1343–7.
10. Chen J, Muntner P, Hamm LL, et al. Insulin resistance and risk of chronic kidney disease in nondiabetic US adults. *J Am Soc Nephrol* Feb 2003;**14**(2):469–77.
11. El-Atat F, Aneja A, McFarlane S, Sowers J. Obesity and hypertension. *Endocrinol Metab Clin North Am* Dec 2003;**32**(4):823–54.
12. Cheng LS, Davis RC, Raffel LJ, et al. Coincident linkage of fasting plasma insulin and blood pressure to chromosome 7q in hypertensive hispanic families. *Circulation* Sep 11 2001;**104**(11):1255–60.
13. Lastra G, Manrique C, McFarlane SI, Sowers JR. Cardiometabolic syndrome and chronic kidney disease. *Curr Diab Rep* Jun 2006;**6**(3):207–12.
14. Sironi AM, Gastaldelli A, Mari A, et al. Visceral fat in hypertension: influence on insulin resistance and beta-cell function. *Hypertension* Aug 2004;**44**(2):127–33.
15. Rahmouni K, Correia ML, Haynes WG, Mark AL. Obesity-associated hypertension: new insights into mechanisms. *Hypertension* Jan 2005;**45**(1):9–14.

16. Qi Y, Takahashi N, Hileman SM, et al. Adiponectin acts in the brain to decrease body weight. *Nat Med* May 2004;**10**(5):524−9.

17. Massiera F, Bloch-Faure M, Ceiler D, et al. Adipose angiotensinogen is involved in adipose tissue growth and blood pressure regulation. *FASEB J* Dec 2001;**15**(14):2727−9.

18. Wisse BE. The inflammatory syndrome: the role of adipose tissue cytokines in metabolic disorders linked to obesity. *J Am Soc Nephrol* Nov 2004;**15**(11):2792−800.

19. Cusumano AM, Bodkin NL, Hansen BC, et al. Glomerular hypertrophy is associated with hyper-insulinemia and precedes overt diabetes in aging rhesus monkeys. *Am J Kidney Dis* Nov 2002;**40**(5):1075−85.

20. Mykkanen L, Zaccaro DJ, Wagenknecht LE, Robbins DC, Gabriel M, Haffner SM. Micro-albuminuria is associated with insulin resistance in nondiabetic subjects: the insulin resistance atherosclerosis study. *Diabetes* May 1998;**47**(5):793−800.

21. Hoehner CM, Greenlund KJ, Rith-Najarian S, Casper ML, McClellan WM. Association of the insulin resistance syndrome and microalbuminuria among nondiabetic native Americans. The Inter-Tribal Heart Project. *J Am Soc Nephrol* Jun 2002;**13**(6):1626−34.

22. Palaniappan L, Carnethon M, Fortmann SP. Association between microalbuminuria and the metabolic syndrome: NHANES III. *Am J Hypertens* Nov 2003;**16**(11 Pt 1):952−8.

23. Fujikawa R, Okubo M, Egusa G, Kohno N. Insulin resistance precedes the appearance of albuminuria in non-diabetic subjects: 6 years follow up study. *Diabetes Res Clin Pract* Aug 2001;**53**(2):99−106.

24. Mangrum A, Bakris GL. Predictors of renal and cardiovascular mortality in patients with non-insulin-dependent diabetes: a brief overview of micro-albuminuria and insulin resistance. *J Diabetes Complications* Nov-Dec 1997;**11**(6):352−7.

25. Abuaisha B, Kumar S, Malik R, Boulton AJ. Relationship of elevated urinary albumin excretion to components of the metabolic syndrome in non-insulin-dependent diabetes mellitus. *Diabetes Res Clin Pract* Feb 1998;**39**(2):93−9.

26. Cohen AJ, McCarthy DM, Stoff JS. Direct hemodynamic effect of insulin in the isolated perfused kidney. *Am J Physiol* Oct 1989;**257**(4 Pt 2):F580−5.

27. Dengel DR, Goldberg AP, Mayuga RS, Kairis GM, Weir MR. Insulin resistance, elevated glomerular filtration fraction, and renal injury. *Hypertension* Jul 1996;**28**(1):127−32.

28. Catalano C, Muscelli E, Quinones Galvan A, et al. Effect of insulin on systemic and renal handling of albumin in nondiabetic and NIDDM subjects. *Diabetes* May 1997;**46**(5):868−75.

29. McFarlane SI, Banerji M, Sowers JR. Insulin resistance and cardiovascular disease. *J Clin Endocrinol Metab* Feb 2001;**86**(2):713−8.

30. Young BA, Johnson RJ, Alpers CE, et al. Cellular events in the evolution of experimental diabetic nephropathy. *Kidney Int* Mar 1995;**47**(3):935−44.

31. Ferns GA, Motani AS, Anggard EE. The insulin-like growth factors: their putative role in atherogenesis. *Artery* 1991;**18**(4):197−225.

32. Conti FG, Striker LJ, Lesniak MA, MacKay K, Roth J, Striker GE. Studies on binding and mitogenic effect of insulin and insulin-like growth factor I in glomerular mesangial cells. *Endocrinology* Jun 1988;**122**(6):2788−95.

33. Anderson PW, Zhang XY, Tian J, et al. Insulin and angiotensin II are additive in stimulating TGF-beta 1 and matrix mRNAs in mesangial cells. *Kidney Int* Sep 1996;**50**(3):745−53.

34. Wang S, Denichilo M, Brubaker C, Hirschberg R. Connective tissue growth factor in tubulointerstitial injury of diabetic nephropathy. *Kidney Int* Jul 2001;**60**(1):96−105.

35. Ferri C, Pittoni V, Piccoli A, et al. Insulin stimulates endothelin-1 secretion from human endothelial cells and modulates its circulating levels in vivo. *J Clin Endocrinol Metab* Mar 1995;**80**(3):829−35.

36. Ferri C, Bellini C, Desideri G, De Mattia G, Santucci A. Endogenous insulin modulates circulating endothelin-1 concentrations in humans. *Diabetes Care* May 1996;**19**(5):504−6.

37. Simonson MS, Herman WH. Protein kinase C and protein tyrosine kinase activity contribute to mitogenic signaling by endothelin-1. Cross-talk between G protein-coupled receptors and pp60c-src. *J Biol Chem* May 5 1993;**268**(13):9347−57.

38. Juhan-Vague I, Alessi MC. PAI-1, obesity, insulin resistance and risk of cardiovascular events. *Thromb Haemost* Jul 1997;**78**(1):656−60.

39. Hirano T, Kashiwazaki K, Moritomo Y, Nagano S, Adachi M. Albuminuria is directly associated with increased plasma PAI-1 and factor VII levels in NIDDM patients. *Diabetes Res Clin Pract* Apr 1997;**36**(1):11−8.

40. Rerolle JP, Hertig A, Nguyen G, Sraer JD, Rondeau EP. Plasminogen activator inhibitor type 1 is a potential target in renal fibrogenesis. *Kidney Int* Nov 2000;**58**(5):1841−50.

41. Robertson RP, Harmon J, Tran PO, Tanaka Y, Takahashi H. Glucose toxicity in beta-cells: type 2 diabetes, good radicals gone bad, and the glutathione connection. *Diabetes* Mar 2003;**52**(3):581−7.

42. Ozcan U, Cao Q, Yilmaz E, et al. Endoplasmic reticulum stress links obesity, insulin action, and type 2 diabetes. *Science* Oct 15 2004;**306**(5695):457−61.

II. TYPES OF DIABETES AND ITS CORRELATION WITH OTHER DISEASES

43. Bomback AS, Toto R. Dual blockade of the renin-angiotensin-aldosterone system: beyond the ACE inhibitor and angiotensin-II receptor blocker combination. *Am J Hypertens* Oct 2009;**22**(10):1032—40.

44. Hall JE, Henegar JR, Dwyer TM, et al. Is obesity a major cause of chronic kidney disease? *Adv Ren Replace Ther* Jan 2004;**11**(1):41—54.

45. Ruster C, Wolf G. Renin-angiotensin-aldosterone system and progression of renal disease. *J Am Soc Nephrol* Nov 2006;**17**(11):2985—91.

46. Wolf G, Neilson EG. Angiotensin II induces cellular hypertrophy in cultured murine proximal tubular cells. *Am J Physiol* Nov 1990;**259**(5 Pt 2):F768—77.

47. Rodriguez-Vita J, Sanchez-Lopez E, Esteban V, Ruperez M, Egido J, Ruiz-Ortega M. Angiotensin II activates the Smad pathway in vascular smooth muscle cells by a transforming growth factor-beta-independent mechanism. *Circulation* May 17 2005;**111**(19):2509—17.

48. Whaley-Connell A, Johnson MS, Sowers JR. Aldosterone: role in the cardiometabolic syndrome and resistant hypertension. *Prog Cardiovasc Dis* Mar-Apr 2010;**52**(5):401—9.

49. Sowers JR, Whaley-Connell A, Epstein M. Narrative review: the emerging clinical implications of the role of aldosterone in the metabolic syndrome and resistant hypertension. *Ann Intern Med* Jun 2 2009;**150**(11):776—83.

12

An Overview of Diabetic Nephropathy

Kei Fukami*, Sho-ichi Yamagishi†

*Division of Nephrology, Department of Medicine, †Department of Pathophysiology and Therapeutics of Diabetic Vascular Complications, Kurume University School of Medicine, Fukuoka, Japan

OUTLINE

INTRODUCTION

Diabetes mellitus has been an increasing global health problem, and currently over 246 million people worldwide are affected by this disease. According to the report of the World Health Organization, it is expected that the number of people with diabetes will rise to 370 million worldwide by 2030.[1]

Among various disorders, diabetic nephropathy is the most common cause of end-stage renal disease, which could account for disability and high mortality rates in patients with diabetes. It has been considered that about 25–40% of patients with type 1 or type 2 diabetes develop nephropathy within 20–25 years of the onset of disease.[2] Large clinical trials such as United Kingdom Prospective Diabetes Study (UKPDS) and Diabetes Control and Complications Trial (DCCT) revealed that strict control of blood glucose or blood pressure significantly reduced the development and progression of diabetic nephropathy in both type 1 and type 2 diabetes.[3,4] However, current therapeutic options are far from satisfactory. The effects of intensive therapy on diabetic nephropathy are insufficient, and the number of diabetic patients with end-stage renal failure continues to increase in industrialized countries.

Several metabolic and hemodynamic pathways are implicated in diabetic nephropathy.

Nutritional and Therapeutic Interventions for Diabetes and Metabolic Syndrome
DOI: 10.1016/B978-0-12-385083-6.00012-7

Among them, there is widespread agreement that the renin-angiotensin system (RAS) plays a pivotal role in the pathogenesis of diabetic nephropathy. Large clinical trials have demonstrated substantial benefit of the blockade of this system for end-organ protection.[5–7] Indeed, interruption of the RAS with angiotensin-converting enzyme inhibitors (ACEIs) or angiotensin II type 1 receptor blockers (ARBs) has been shown to prevent the development and progression of renal disease in diabetic patients with hypertension.[5–7] On the basis of the findings, the American Diabetes Association (ADA) currently recommends ACEIs or ARBs as first-line therapy for hypertensive type 2 diabetic patients with micro- or macroalbuminuria. Further, it has been shown that irbesartan, an ARB, significantly prevents the progression of overt diabetic nephropathy in type 2 diabetic patients, compared with calcium channel blocker, amlodipine with an equipotent blood pressure lowering property.[8] These observations suggest that the inhibition of the RAS itself could be a therapeutic target for diabetic nephropathy. The RAS not only stimulates the expression of several inflammatory and fibrogenic factors such as monocyte chemoattractant protein-1 (MCP-1) and transforming growth factor-β (TGF-β) in the kidney, but also induces oxidative stress and activation of advanced glycation end products (AGEs)-receptor, mediating diabetic nephropathy.[9,10] Therefore, in this paper, we review the molecular mechanisms of diabetic nephropathy and discuss the therapeutic intervention for this devastating condition.

CLINICAL FEATURES OF DIABETIC NEPHROPATHY

The earliest clinical evidence for incipient diabetic nephropathy is the development of the persistent microalbuminuria (urinary albumin excretion rate, 20–200 µg/min), which is Albustix-negative. The natural history of diabetic nephropathy differs between type 1 and type 2 patients.[11] If left untreated, approximately 80% of type 1 diabetic patients will develop overt albuminuria (UAER > 200 µg/min) over a 15-year period. Of these patients, 50% will develop end-stage renal disease (ESRD) over the ensuing 10 years. In type 2 diabetes, if no treatment is initiated, up to 20–40% of patients will progress to overt albuminuria and 20% of those with overt albuminuria will develop ESRD over the next 20 years. Forty to fifty percent of patients with type 2 diabetes who have microalbuminuria are reported to finally die due to cardiovascular disease (CVD).[12]

The development of diabetic nephropathy is characterized by glomerular hyperfiltration, hypertrophy of glomerular and tubuloepithelial components, and thickening of glomerular basement membranes, followed by an expansion of extracellular matrix (ECM) in mesangial areas and an increased albumin excretion rate. Diabetic nephropathy ultimately progresses to glomerular sclerosis and tubulointerstitial fibrosis associated with renal dysfunction.[13] In type 1 diabetes, the prevalence of hyperfiltration has been reported approximately in 40–60% of the subjects.[14,15] The predominant causative factor of hyperfiltration in type 1 diabetes is considered to be "uncontrolled hyperglycemia" because intensive insulin therapy has been shown to normalize hyperfiltration in these patients.[16] However, the prevalence of hyperfiltration ranges from 35% to 45% in recently diagnosed type 2 diabetic subjects.[17,18] In older type 2 diabetic patients, hyperfiltration might be masked by age-related decline of glomerular filtration rate (GFR), while it could be exaggerated by the presence of obesity.[19] Cappuccio et al. have reported that obesity is associated with activation of the RAS and increased proximal tubular sodium reabsorption,[19,20] which could partly be involved in hyperfiltration in type 2 diabetes.

INVOLVEMENT OF METABOLIC FACTORS IN DIABETIC NEPHROPATHY

Chronic hyperglycemia is a major initiator of vascular complications of diabetes. Although various hyperglycemia-elicited metabolic derangements such as increased formation of AGEs, protein kinase C (PKC) activation, enhanced production of reactive oxygen species (ROS) have been proposed to contribute to the characteristic histopathological changes associated with diabetic nephropathy.[21–23] Recent clinical studies have substantiated the concept of "metabolic memory" in the pathogenesis of vascular complications of diabetes.[24] The DCCT-Epidemiology of Diabetes Interventions and Complications (DCCT-EDIC) Research, has revealed that the reduction in the risk of progressive retinopathy and nephropathy resulting from intensive therapy in patients with type 1 diabetes persists for at least several years after the DCCT trial, despite increasing hyperglycemia.[25,26] Intensive therapy during the DCCT resulted in decreased progression of intima-media thickness and subsequently reduction in the risk of non-fatal myocardial infarction, stroke, or death from CVD by 57%, 11 years after the completion of the trial.[27,28] Further, a recent follow-up study of UKPDS, called UKPDS80, also has shown that benefits of an intensive therapy in patients with type 2 diabetes are sustained after the cessation of the trial.[29] In this study, despite an early loss of glycemic differences between originally intensive and conventional therapy, a continued reduction in microvascular risk and emergent risk reductions for myocardial infarction and death from any cause were observed during 10 years of post-trial follow-up.[29] These findings

demonstrate that so-called "metabolic memory" may cause chronic abnormalities in diabetic vessels and kidney that are not easily reversed, even by subsequent, relatively good control of blood glucose, thus suggesting a long-term beneficial influence of early metabolic control (legacy effect) on the risk of diabetic retinopathy, nephropathy, CVD and death in both type 1 and type 2 diabetic patients. Among the various biochemical pathways implicated in vascular complications in diabetes, the biochemical nature of AGEs and their mode of action are most compatible with the concept of "metabolic memory".[28,30,31]

AGEs are generated as a result of a series of sequential biochemical reactions, including non-enzymatic glycation of free amino groups on protein, lipoproteins, and nucleic acids by reducing sugars, but some of which are poorly defined.[32] The formation and accumulation of AGEs progress at physiological aging, diabetes, or chronic renal failure conditions.[33] There is a growing body of evidence that AGEs play a central role in the pathogenesis of diabetic micro- and macrovascular complications.[34–36]

Diabetic nephropathy is characterized by glomerular and tubular basement membrane thickening, ECM expansion, microvascular damage, and fibrotic changes in the tubulointerstitium.[13,37] These renal structures accumulate AGEs[38] such as N-ε-carboxymethyllysine (CML) and pentosidine in the kidney which causes progressive alteration in renal structure and the loss of renal function in patients and rodents *via* various mechanisms, including their cross-linking properties of matrix proteins and activation of the downstream signaling pathways.[9,10,39–41] AGE formation on ECM proteins alters both matrix–matrix and cell–matrix interactions leading to diabetic glomerulosclerosis. Second, AGEs not only induce apoptotic cell death, but also stimulate vascular endothelial growth factor (VEGF) and MCP-1 production in cultured mesangial cells.[42]

Mesangial cells occupy a central anatomical position in the glomerulus, playing a crucial role in maintaining structure and function of glomerular capillary tufts.[43] They actually provide structural support for capillary loops and modulate glomerular filtration by its activity on the smooth muscles.[43–45] Thus, AGE-induced mesangial cell apoptosis and dysfunction may contribute in part to glomerular hyperfiltration, an early renal dysfunction in diabetes. Further, increased MCP-1 expression associated with monocyte infiltration in mesangium has been observed in the early phase of diabetic nephropathy.[46] Urinary MCP-1/creatinine ratios in type 2 diabetic patients with microalbuminuria were much higher than those in normal controls, and intensive insulin treatment significantly attenuated the urinary MCP-1 levels.[47] AGE accumulation in the glomerulus may be implicated in the initiation of diabetic nephropathy by promoting the secretion of MCP-1 by mesangial cells. Third, AGEs stimulate insulin-like growth factor-I, -II, platelet-derived growth factor, and TGF-β in mesangial cells, which in turn mediate production of type IV collagen, laminin, and fibronectin.[40,41,48] AGEs induce TGF-β overexpression in both podocytes and proximal tubular cells.[42,49,50] Ziyadeh et al. reported that long-term treatment of type 2 diabetic model mice with blocking antibodies raised against TGF-β suppressed excess matrix gene expression, glomerulosclerosis, and prevented the development of renal insufficiency.[51] These observations suggest that the AGE-induced TGF-β expression plays an important role in the pathogenesis of glomerulosclerosis and tubulointerstitial fibrosis in advanced diabetic nephropathy.

In early studies by Nicholls et al., renal AGE accumulation in diabetic mice was attenuated by either pancreatic islet transplantation or treatment with aminoguanidine (AG), an inhibitor of AGE formation.[52] A number of studies have demonstrated that AG decreases plasma and renal levels of AGEs and ameliorates functional and histopathological derangements in experimental diabetic nephropathy.[53,54] Double-blinded, placebo-controlled, randomized clinical trials of aminoguanidine (Pimagedine®), a prototype therapeutic agent for the prevention of AGE formation (ACTION; A Clinical Trial In Overt Nephropathy), were designed to evaluate the safety and efficacy of aminoguanidine in retarding the rate of progression of renal disease in patients with overt diabetic nephropathy. Pimagedine® therapy reduced the 24-h total urinary proteinuria and prevented the decrease in GFR and the progression of diabetic retinopathy in patients with type 1 diabetes.[55] Although the effects of Pimagedine® on serum creatinine doubling were found not to be significant, this study was noteworthy in providing the first clinical proof of the concept that inhibiting AGE formation can result in a clinically important attenuation of diabetic nephropathy.

ALT-946 (N-(2-acetamidoethyl) hydrozinecarboximidamide hydrochloride) is a newly developed, selective inhibitor of AGE formation devoid of nitric oxide synthase inhibition activity.[56] Forbes et al. have found that ALT-946 treatment reduces renal AGE accumulation and subsequently decreases albuminuria in streptozotocin (STZ)-induced diabetic rats.[57]

Vitamin B complexes such as pyridoxamine and thiamine have been found to inhibit the formation of AGEs.[48] Pyridoxamine was originally described as a post-Amadori inhibitor of AGE formation (so-called Amadorins). It inhibits AGE formation at three different levels by blocking oxidative degradation of the Amadori products, scavenging of toxic carbonyl products of glucose and lipid degradation, and trapping of ROS.[48] Administration of pyridoxal phosphate, an active form of vitamin B6, significantly inhibited albuminuria, glomerular hypertrophy, mesangial expansion, and interstitial fibrosis in association with the reduced expression of receptor for AGEs (RAGE) in the kidney.[48,58] Pyridoxamine and aminoguanidine had similar effects, supporting a mechanism of action involving AGE inhibition.[58] A multinational, double-blind study involving a total of 84 patients with either type 1 or type 2 diabetes and either mild-to-moderate or moderate-to-severe diabetic nephropathy revealed that the rate of rise in serum creatinine was decreased in 87% of patients receiving pyridoxamine compared to those receiving placebo. Furthermore, pyridoxamine prevented the rate of decline in creatinine clearance in diabetic subjects. Benfotiamine is a lipid-soluble thiamine derivative that reduces AGE accumulation in diabetes.[59] Recent studies have demonstrated that benfotiamine is able to block major biochemical pathways implicated in the pathogenesis of diabetic complications, including the accumulation of AGEs.[60] Further, in the STZ-induced diabetic model, Thornalley *et al.* have reported that benfotiamine therapy increases transketolase expression in renal glomeruli, increases the conversion of triosephosphates to ribose-5-phosphate, and subsequently inhibits the development of microalbuminuria.[61] Since hyperglycemia-induced generation of triosephosphates elicits mitochondrial oxidative stress production and stimulates the formation of AGEs such as methylglyoxal, benfotiamine may prevent the progression of diabetic nephropathy *via* the increased conversion of triosephosphates to ribose-5-phosphate.[23]

OPB-9195 ([±]-2-isopropylidenehydrazone-4-oxo-thiazolidin-5-ylacetanilide), a synthetic thiazolidine derivative and novel inhibitor of AGEs, prevented the progression of diabetic nephropathy by lowering serum concentrations of AGEs and their deposition of glomeruli in Otsuka-Long-Evans-Tokushima-Fatty rats, a model of type II diabetes with obesity.[62] OPB-9195 was also found to retard the progression of diabetic nephropathy by blocking type IV collagen production and suppressing overproduction of two growth factors, TGF-β and VEGF.[57]

RAGE has a central role in mediating the biological effects of AGEs. There is accumulating evidence that the AGE—RAGE interaction is involved in the development and progression of diabetic nephropathy.[63] Indeed, the engagement of RAGE by its ligands such as AGEs induces inflammatory cell infiltration and stimulates expression of adhesion molecules and cytokines in the diabetic kidney.[64,65] Since RAGE expression is enhanced in human diabetic glomeruli and tubules, and its level is correlated with AGE accumulation,[66] it is conceivable that the sustained activation of the AGE—RAGE axis elicits inflammatory and fibrogenic reactions in the kidney through oxidative stress generation and nuclear factor-kappa B (NF-κB) activation, thereby contributing to tubuloglomerular injury and sclerosis in diabetic nephropathy.

RAGE-overexpressing diabetic mice have been found to show progressive glomerulosclerosis with renal dysfunction, compared with diabetic littermates lacking the RAGE transgene.[67] Levels of AGEs and RAGE were elevated in the diabetic kidney, and blockade of the AGE—RAGE interaction decreased podocyte VEGF expression and albuminuria, which were associated with decreased numbers of inflammatory cells and reduced TGF-β expression in the glomerulus.[49] Furthermore, diabetic homozygous RAGE null mice failed to develop mesangial matrix expansion or thickening of the glomerular basement membrane.[49] Deletion of RAGE is also reported to prevent diabetic nephropathy in the OVE26 type 1 mouse, a model of progressive glomerulosclerosis and decline of renal function.[68] Taken together, these findings suggest that the activation of the AGE—RAGE system contributes to expression of VEGF and enhanced attraction/activation of inflammatory cells in the diabetic glomerulus, thereby setting the stage for mesangial activation and TGF-β production; processes which converge to cause albuminuria and glomerulosclerosis (Figure 12.1).

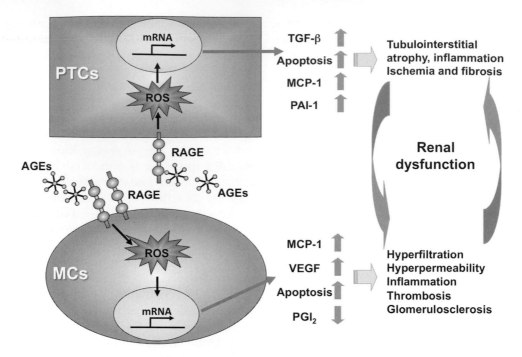

FIGURE 12.1 Molecular mechanisms of AGE−RAGE−ROS-induced renal injury in diabetic nephropathy. PTCs; proximal tubular cells, MCs; mesangial cells, ROS; reactive oxygen species, RAGE; receptor for advanced glycation end products, AGEs; advanced glycation end products, TGF-β; transforming growth factor-β, MCP-1; monocyte chemoattractant protein-1, PAI-1; plasminogen activator inhibitor-1, VEGF; vascular endothelial growth factor, PGI₂; prostaglandin I₂.

ROLE OF RAS IN DIABETIC NEPHROPATHY

The RAS has a critical role in the development and progression of diabetic nephropathy.[69] The inappropriate activation of this system induces hypertension, fluid retention, inflammation, and atherogenic responses that could lead to renal and cardiovascular damages in diabetes. In patients with diabetic nephropathy, although serum levels of renin or angiotensin II (Ang II) are low, the intrarenal RAS level is dramatically increased, thus suggesting the involvement of the intrarenal RAS activation in diabetic nephropathy. Micropuncture studies revealed a variety of intrarenal hemodynamic derangements in the kidney of diabetic rats, including increased intraglomerular pressure, increased single nephron

GFR and preferential afferent *vs* efferent arteriolar vasodilatation, all of which could lead to hyperfiltration, followed by renal dysfunction in diabetic nephropathy.[70] The increased intraglomerular pressure was reduced by the treatment with ACEIs,[70] which was associated with the alleviation of renal damage in experimental diabetic nephropathy. Therefore, Ang II-induced vasoconstriction of glomerular efferent artery, followed by the increase in the intraglomerular pressure, may play a role in hyperfiltration in early stage of diabetic nephropathy.

Although the renoprotective effects of RAS inhibitor are largely ascribed to its blood pressure-lowering properties in humans, a recent clinical study suggests a pleiotropic effect of the RAS inhibitor, beyond its blood pressure-lowering effects, on diabetic nephropathy.

Taguma *et al.* have shown that in ACEIs, captopril administered at a dose that does not lower blood pressure significantly improves nephrotic syndrome in type 1 diabetic patients.[71] Further, Lewis *et al.* reported in the collaborative study that 3 years of captopril treatment was associated with a reduction in the end point including doubling of serum creatinine, progression of ESRD or death, independently of its effects on blood pressure.[5] Treatment with captopril also reduced the risk of cardiovascular mortality in type 1 diabetic patients.[5]

There are a couple of large trials to show the clinical utility of ARBs for the treatment of hypertensive type 2 diabetic patients with microalbuminuria (IRMA-II)[72] or overt nephropathy (RENAAL, IDNT).[73,74] However, a number of diabetic patients treated with ARBs did show only partial anti-proteinuric response, and this heralded a progressive loss of renal function in most cases[5,72–74] Thus, a multidrug approach may likely be the better strategy. However, the ONTARGET (Ongoing Telmisartan Alone and in combination with Ramipril Global Endpoint Trial) study, which randomly assigned 25,620 patients with high-risk group, established cardiovascular disease, including 6,982 diabetic patients to telmisartan, ramipril, or a combination therapy, has shown that the excess of adverse renal outcomes on combination therapy was driven by the more frequent need for acute hemodialysis to treat transient renal dysfunction.[75] Therefore, one should be careful to use dual blockade therapy in patients with high cardiovascular risk and/or diabetes.

Combination therapy using RAS inhibitor and calcium channel blocker, have been studied in multicenter randomized trials, such as BENEDICT (Bergamo Nephrologic Diabetes Complications Trial).[76] This study aimed to explore whether ACEI alone or in combination with a non-dihydropyridinic calcium channel blocker reduced the albumin excretion rate and slowed GFR decline compared with placebo plus conventional antihypertensive therapy in patients with type 2 diabetic nephropathy, hypertension, and normo- or microalbuminuria. However, the beneficial effect of ACEIs was not enhanced by combined non-dihydropyridine calcium channel blocker therapy.[77]

RAS inhibitors such as ACEIs and ARBs could cause an increase in prorenin level and plasma renin activity (PRA). When renin binds to the renin receptor, its enzymatic activity to convert angiotensinogen to angiotensin I is dramatically increased. Moreover, the interaction of renin with the receptor directly activates the downstream signals and stimulates TGF-β production in the kidney leading to glomerular sclerosis and fibrosis in diabetic nephropathy.[78,79] Blockade of prorenin binding to the receptor by a decoy peptide has been shown to prevent renal damage in STZ-induced diabetic rats.[80] Since the plasma level of prorenin is increased in patients with diabetic nephropathy, it is probable that the compensated increase in prorenin level and PRA may reduce the expected benefits of RAS inhibitors in diabetic nephropathy. Therefore, the addition of a direct renin inhibitor such as aliskiren to RAS inhibitors may represent a promising approach for the treatment of diabetic nephropathy. Indeed, combination therapy with aliskiren and irbesartan was more effective for reducing urinary albumin excretion rate in type 2 diabetic patients compared with each monotherapy.[81] In the Aliskiren in the eValuation of prOteinuria In Diabetes (AVOID) trial, treatment with 300 mg of aliskiren daily, as compared with placebo, reduced the urinary albumin-to-creatinine ratio by 20% in hypertensive type 2 diabetic patients who were already treated with an ARB, losartan.[82] In this study, only a small difference in blood pressure was seen between the two groups. Therefore, aliskiren might have renoprotective effects that are independent of blood pressure-lowering properties in patients with hypertension, type 2 diabetes and nephropathy.

Recent experiments have focused on the interaction of the RAS and other metabolic pathways thought to be critical to the development of diabetic nephropathy. A number of studies have shown that the RAS and PKC-β are closely interrelated with each other in the diabetic kidney. Diabetic glomerular hyperfiltration is likely to be the consequence of hyperglycemia-induced decreases in afferent arteriolar resistance, which could lead to glomerular hypertension.[83,84] Some of the vasoconstrictive actions of Ang II are mediated by PKC activity.[85] Diacylglycerol-PKC pathway may enhance the action of Ang II in the glomeruli, thus being involved in hyperfiltration in early diabetic nephropathy. PKC-β is also activated by Ang II in the proximal nephrons, while ACEIs reduce diabetes-associated

increase in PKC-β activity in the glomeruli, which was in parallel with the suppression of albuminuria.[86,87] There are several reports to suggest an interaction between the RAS and AGEs in diabetic nephropathy as well (Figure 12.2). ACEIs reduce the accumulation of renal and serum AGEs, probably *via* its antioxidative properties.[88] Long-term treatment with an ARB may exert salutary effects on AGEs level in the rat remnant kidney model, probably due to improved renal function.[89] Candesartan, an ARB, reduces AGE accumulation and subsequent albuminuria by down-regulating the NADPH oxidase p47phox component and inducible nitric oxide synthase expression and by attenuating RAGE expression in type 2

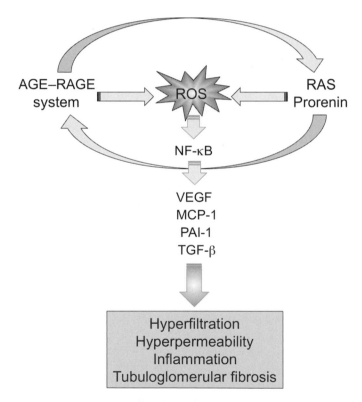

FIGURE 12.2 Crosstalk between the AGE–RAGE axis and RAS in diabetic nephropathy. AGEs; advanced glycation end products, RAGE; receptor for advanced glycation end products, RAS; renin angiotensin system, ROS; reactive oxygen species, NF-κB; nuclear factor-kappa B, VEGF; vascular endothelial growth factor, MCP-1; monocyte chemoattractant protein-1, PAI-1; plasminogen activator inhibitor-1, TGF-β; transforming growth factor-β.

diabetic KK/Ta mouse kidneys.[90] In humans, administration of ramipril has been recently shown to result in a mild decline of fluorescent non-CML-AGEs and malondialdehyde concentrations in non-diabetic nephropathy patients.[91] In type 2 diabetic subjects, a low dose of valsartan treatment also decreases serum AGE levels in a blood pressure-independent manner.[92] In addition, we have previously found that the AGE–RAGE-mediated ROS generation activates TGF-β-Smad signaling and subsequently induces mesangial cell hypertrophy and fibronectin synthesis by autocrine production of Ang II.[9] AGEs induce mitogenesis and collagen production in renal interstitial fibroblasts *via* the Ang II-CTGF pathway.[93] Further, olmesartan medoxomil, an ARB, protects against glomerulosclerosis and renal tubular injury in AGE-injected rats, thus supporting the concept that AGEs could induce renal damage in diabetes *via* the activation of RAS.[94] Our recent study shows that AGEs induce apoptosis and inflammatory, thrombogenic, and fibrogenic reactions in proximal tubular cells, all of which are blocked by irbesartan.[95,96] Taken together, these findings may provide an important mechanistic link between metabolic factors and the RAS, which could promote the development and progression of diabetic nephropathy.

CONCLUSION

In this review, we summarized the molecular mechanisms of diabetic nephropathy and provided potential therapeutic targets that could prevent this devastating disorder. Multifactorial intensified intervention should be needed for halting diabetic nephropathy.

References

1. Wild S, Roglic G, Green A, Sicree R, King H. Global prevalence of diabetes: estimates for the year 2000 and projections for 2030. *Diabetes Care* 2004;**27**:1047–53.
2. Remuzzi G, Schieppati A, Ruggenenti P. Clinical practice. Nephropathy in patients with type 2 diabetes. *N Engl J Med* 2002;**346**:1145–51.
3. Intensive blood-glucose control with sulphonylureas or insulin compared with conventional treatment and risk of complications in patients with type 2 diabetes (UKPDS 33). UK Prospective Diabetes Study (UKPDS) Group. *Lancet* 1998;**352**:837–53.
4. The effect of intensive treatment of diabetes on the development and progression of long-term complications in insulin-dependent diabetes mellitus. The Diabetes Control and Complications Trial Research Group. *N Engl J Med* 1993;**329**:977–86.
5. Lewis EJ, Hunsicker LG, Bain RP, Rohde RD. The effect of angiotensin-converting-enzyme inhibition on diabetic nephropathy. The Collaborative Study Group. *N Engl J Med* 1993;**329**:1456–62.
6. Ravid M, Savin H, Jutrin I, Bental T, Katz B, Lishner M. Long-term stabilizing effect of angiotensin-converting enzyme inhibition on plasma creatinine and on proteinuria in normotensive type II diabetic patients. *Ann Intern Med* 1993;**118**:577–81.
7. Sica DA, Bakris GL. Type 2 diabetes: RENAAL and IDNT—the emergence of new treatment options. *J Clin Hypertens (Greenwich)* 2002;**4**:52–7.
8. Pohl MA, Blumenthal S, Cordonnier DJ, De Alvaro F, Deferrari G, Eisner G, Esmatjes E, Gilbert RE, Hunsicker LG, de Faria JB, Mangili R, Moore J, Reisin E, Ritz E, Schernthaner G, Spitalewitz S, Tindall H, Rodby RA, Lewis EJ. Independent and additive impact of blood pressure control and angiotensin II receptor blockade on renal outcomes in the irbesartan diabetic nephropathy trial: clinical implications and limitations. *J Am Soc Nephrol* 2005;**16**:3027–37.
9. Fukami K, Ueda S, Yamagishi S, Kato S, Inagaki Y, Takeuchi M, Motomiya Y, Bucala R, Iida S, Tamaki K, Imaizumi T, Cooper ME, Okuda S. AGEs activate mesangial TGF-beta-Smad signaling via an angiotensin II type I receptor interaction. *Kidney Int* 2004;**66**:2137–47.
10. Fukami K, Yamagishi S, Ueda S, Okuda S. Role of AGEs in diabetic nephropathy. *Curr Pharm Des* 2008;**14**:946–52.
11. Ismal N, Cornell S. In: Ritz E, Rychlik I, editors. *Nephropathy in type 2 diabetes*. New York: Oxford University Press; 1999. p. 12–24.
12. Eurich DT, Majumdar SR, Tsuyuki RT, Johnson JA. Reduced mortality associated with the use of ACE inhibitors in patients with type 2 diabetes. *Diabetes Care* 2004;**27**:1330–4.
13. Sharma K, Ziyadeh FN. Hyperglycemia and diabetic kidney disease. The case for transforming growth factor-beta as a key mediator. *Diabetes* 1995;**44**:1139–46.

14. Mogensen CE, Christensen CK. Predicting diabetic nephropathy in insulin-dependent patients. *N Engl J Med* 1984;**311**:89—93.

15. Dahlquist G, Stattin EL, Rudberg S. Urinary albumin excretion rate and glomerular filtration rate in the prediction of diabetic nephropathy; a long-term follow-up study of childhood onset type-1 diabetic patients. *Nephrol Dial Transplant* 2001;**16**:1382—6.

16. Wiseman MJ, Saunders AJ, Keen H, Viberti G. Effect of blood glucose control on increased glomerular filtration rate and kidney size in insulin-dependent diabetes. *N Engl J Med* 1985;**312**:617—21.

17. Chaiken RL, Eckert-Norton M, Bard M, Banerji MA, Palmisano J, Sachimechi I, Lebovitz HE. Hyperfiltration in African-American patients with type 2 diabetes. Cross-sectional and longitudinal data. *Diabetes Care* 1998;**21**:2129—34.

18. Silveiro SP, Friedman R, de Azevedo MJ, Canani LH, Gross JL. Five-year prospective study of glomerular filtration rate and albumin excretion rate in normofiltering and hyperfiltering normoalbuminuric NIDDM patients. *Diabetes Care* 1996;**19**:171—4.

19. Chagnac A, Herman M, Zingerman B, Erman A, Rozen-Zvi B, Hirsh J, Gafter U. Obesity-induced glomerular hyperfiltration: its involvement in the pathogenesis of tubular sodium reabsorption. *Nephrol Dial Transplant* 2008;**23**:3946—52.

20. Cappuccio FP, Strazzullo P, Siani A, Trevisan M. Increased proximal sodium reabsorption is associated with increased cardiovascular risk in men. *J Hypertens* 1996;**14**:909—14.

21. Bohlender JM, Franke S, Stein G, Wolf G. Advanced glycation end products and the kidney. *Am J Physiol Renal Physiol* 2005;**289**:F645—59.

22. Kelly DJ, Zhang Y, Hepper C, Gow RM, Jaworski K, Kemp BE, Wilkinson-Berka JL, Gilbert RE. Protein kinase C beta inhibition attenuates the progression of experimental diabetic nephropathy in the presence of continued hypertension. *Diabetes* 2003;**52**:512—8.

23. Nishikawa T, Edelstein D, Du XL, Yamagishi S, Matsumura T, Kaneda Y, Yorek MA, Beebe D, Oates PJ, Hammes HP, Giardino I, Brownlee M. Normalizing mitochondrial superoxide production blocks three pathways of hyperglycaemic damage. *Nature* 2000;**404**:787—90.

24. Tonna S, El-Osta A, Cooper ME, Tikellis C. Metabolic memory and diabetic nephropathy: potential role for epigenetic mechanisms. *Nat Rev Nephrol* 2010;**6**:332—41.

25. Retinopathy and nephropathy in patients with type 1 diabetes four years after a trial of intensive therapy. The Diabetes Control and Complications Trial/Epidemiology of Diabetes Interventions and Complications Research Group. *N Engl J Med* 2000;**342**:381—9.

26. Group, W. T. f. t. D.C. a. C.T.E. o. D.I. a. C.R. Sustained effect of intensive treatment of type 1 diabetes mellitus on development and progression of diabetic nephropathy: the Epidemiology of Diabetes Interventions and Complications (EDIC) study. *JAMA* 2003;**290**:2159—67.

27. Nathan DM, Lachin J, Cleary P, Orchard T, Brillon DJ, Backlund JY, O'Leary DH, Genuth S, Trial, D. C. a. C. and Group, E. o. D.I. a. C.R. Intensive diabetes therapy and carotid intima-media thickness in type 1 diabetes mellitus. *N Engl J Med* 2003;**348**:2294—303.

28. Nathan DM, Cleary PA, Backlund JY, Genuth SM, Lachin JM, Orchard TJ, Raskin P, Zinman B, Group, D. C. a. C.T.E. o. D.I. a. C.D.E.S.R. Intensive diabetes treatment and cardiovascular disease in patients with type 1 diabetes. *N Engl J Med* 2005;**353**:2643—53.

29. Holman RR, Paul SK, Bethel MA, Matthews DR, Neil HA. 10-year follow-up of intensive glucose control in type 2 diabetes. *N Engl J Med* 2008;**359**: 1577—89.

30. Monnier VM, Bautista O, Kenny D, Sell DR, Fogarty J, Dahms W, Cleary PA, Lachin J, Genuth S. Skin collagen glycation, glycoxidation, and crosslinking are lower in subjects with long-term intensive versus conventional therapy of type 1 diabetes: relevance of glycated collagen products versus HbA1c as markers of diabetic complications. DCCT Skin Collagen Ancillary Study Group. Diabetes Control and Complications Trial. *Diabetes* 1999;**48**:870—80.

31. Genuth S, Sun W, Cleary P, Sell DR, Dahms W, Malone J, Sivitz W, Monnier VM, Group, D.S.C.A. S. Glycation and carboxymethyllysine levels in skin collagen predict the risk of future 10-year progression of diabetic retinopathy and nephropathy in the diabetes control and complications trial and epidemiology of diabetes interventions and complications participants with type 1 diabetes. *Diabetes* 2005;**54**:3103—11.

32. Brownlee M. Lilly Lecture 1993. Glycation and diabetic complications. *Diabetes* 1994;**43**:836—41.

33. Förster A, Kühne Y, Henle T. Studies on absorption and elimination of dietary maillard reaction products. *Ann N Y Acad Sci* 2005;**1043**:474—81.

34. Makita Z, Radoff S, Rayfield EJ, Yang Z, Skolnik E, Delaney V, Friedman EA, Cerami A, Vlassara H. Advanced glycosylation end products in patients with diabetic nephropathy. *N Engl J Med* 1991;**325**:836—42.

35. Vlassara H. Recent progress in advanced glycation end products and diabetic complications. *Diabetes* 1997; **46**(Suppl. 2):S19—25.

36. Yamagishi S, Yonekura H, Yamamoto Y, Katsuno K, Sato F, Mita I, Ooka H, Satozawa N, Kawakami T, Nomura M, Yamamoto H. Advanced glycation end products-driven angiogenesis in vitro. Induction of the

growth and tube formation of human microvascular endothelial cells through autocrine vascular endothelial growth factor. *J Biol Chem* 1997;**272**:8723−30.

37. Gilbert RE, Cooper ME. The tubulointerstitium in progressive diabetic kidney disease: more than an aftermath of glomerular injury? *Kidney Int* 1999;**56**:1627−37.

38. Gugliucci A, Bendayan M. Reaction of advanced glycation endproducts with renal tissue from normal and streptozotocin-induced diabetic rats: an ultrastructural study using colloidal gold cytochemistry. *J Histochem Cytochem* 1995;**43**:591−600.

39. Yamagishi S, Inagaki Y, Okamoto T, Amano S, Koga K, Takeuchi M, Makita Z. Advanced glycation end product-induced apoptosis and overexpression of vascular endothelial growth factor and monocyte chemoattractant protein-1 in human-cultured mesangial cells. *J Biol Chem* 2002;**277**:20309−15.

40. Cooper ME. Interaction of metabolic and haemodynamic factors in mediating experimental diabetic nephropathy. *Diabetologia* 2001;**44**:1957−72.

41. Fukami K, Cooper ME, Forbes JM. Agents in development for the treatment of diabetic nephropathy. *Expert Opin Investig Drugs* 2005;**14**:279−94.

42. Yamagishi S, Inagaki Y, Okamoto T, Amano S, Koga K, Takeuchi M. Advanced glycation end products inhibit de novo protein synthesis and induce TGF-beta overexpression in proximal tubular cells. *Kidney Int* 2003;**63**:464−73.

43. Dworkin LD, Ichikawa I, Brenner BM. Hormonal modulation of glomerular function. *Am J Physiol* 1983;**244**:F95−104.

44. Kreisberg JI, Venkatachalam M, Troyer D. Contractile properties of cultured glomerular mesangial cells. *Am J Physiol* 1985;**249**:F457−63.

45. Schlondorff D. The glomerular mesangial cell: an expanding role for a specialized pericyte. *FASEB J* 1987;**1**:272−81.

46. Banba N, Nakamura T, Matsumura M, Kuroda H, Hattori Y, Kasai K. Possible relationship of monocyte chemoattractant protein-1 with diabetic nephropathy. *Kidney Int* 2000;**58**:684−90.

47. Ye SD, Zheng M, Zhao LL, Qian Y, Yao XM, Ren A, Li SM, Jing CY. Intensive insulin therapy decreases urinary MCP-1 and ICAM-1 excretions in incipient diabetic nephropathy. *Eur J Clin Invest* 2009;**39**:980−5.

48. Yamagishi S, Fukami K, Ueda S, Okuda S. Molecular mechanisms of diabetic nephropathy and its therapeutic intervention. *Curr Drug Targets* 2007;**8**:952−9.

49. Wendt TM, Tanji N, Guo J, Kislinger TR, Qu W, Lu Y, Bucciarelli LG, Rong LL, Moser B, Markowitz GS, Stein G, Bierhaus A, Liliensiek B, Arnold B, Nawroth PP, Stern DM, D'Agati VD, Schmidt AM.

RAGE drives the development of glomerulosclerosis and implicates podocyte activation in the pathogenesis of diabetic nephropathy. *Am J Pathol* 2003;**162**:1123−37.

50. Oldfield MD, Bach LA, Forbes JM, Nikolic-Paterson D, McRobert A, Thallas V, Atkins RC, Osicka T, Jerums G, Cooper ME. Advanced glycation end products cause epithelial-myofibroblast transdifferentiation via the receptor for advanced glycation end products (RAGE). *J Clin Invest* 2001;**108**:1853−63.

51. Ziyadeh FN, Hoffman BB, Han DC, Iglesias-De La Cruz MC, Hong SW, Isono M, Chen S, McGowan TA, Sharma K. Long-term prevention of renal insufficiency, excess matrix gene expression, and glomerular mesangial matrix expansion by treatment with monoclonal antitransforming growth factor-beta antibody in db/db diabetic mice. *Proc Natl Acad Sci USA* 2000;**97**:8015−20.

52. Nicholls K, Mandel TE. Advanced glycosylation endproducts in experimental murine diabetic nephropathy: effect of islet isografting and of aminoguanidine. *Lab Invest* 1989;**60**:486−91.

53. Raj DS, Choudhury D, Welbourne TC, Levi M. Advanced glycation end products: a nephrologist's perspective. *Am J Kidney Dis* 2000;**35**:365−80.

54. Kelly DJ, Gilbert RE, Cox AJ, Soulis T, Jerums G, Cooper ME. Aminoguanidine ameliorates overexpression of prosclerotic growth factors and collagen deposition in experimental diabetic nephropathy. *J Am Soc Nephrol* 2001;**12**:2098−107.

55. Bolton WK, Cattran DC, Williams ME, Adler SG, Appel GB, Cartwright K, Foiles PG, Freedman BI, Raskin P, Ratner RE, Spinowitz BS, Whittier FC, Wuerth JP, Group, A.I. I. Randomized trial of an inhibitor of formation of advanced glycation end products in diabetic nephropathy. *Am J Nephrol* 2004;**24**:32−40.

56. Wilkinson-Berka JL, Kelly DJ, Koerner SM, Jaworski K, Davis B, Thallas V, Cooper ME. ALT-946 and aminoguanidine, inhibitors of advanced glycation, improve severe nephropathy in the diabetic transgenic (mREN-2)27 rat. *Diabetes* 2002;**51**:3283−9.

57. Forbes JM, Soulis T, Thallas V, Panagiotopoulos S, Long DM, Vasan S, Wagle D, Jerums G, Cooper ME. Renoprotective effects of a novel inhibitor of advanced glycation. *Diabetologia* 2001;**44**:108−14.

58. Degenhardt TP, Alderson NL, Arrington DD, Beattie RJ, Basgen JM, Steffes MW, Thorpe SR, Baynes JW. Pyridoxamine inhibits early renal disease and dyslipidemia in the streptozotocin-diabetic rat. *Kidney Int* 2002;**61**:939−50.

59. Cameron NE, Gibson TM, Nangle MR, Cotter MA. Inhibitors of advanced glycation end product formation and neurovascular dysfunction in experimental diabetes. *Ann N Y Acad Sci* 2005;**1043**:784−92.

II. TYPES OF DIABETES AND ITS CORRELATION WITH OTHER DISEASES

60. Hammes HP, Du X, Edelstein D, Taguchi T, Matsumura T, Ju Q, Lin J, Bierhaus A, Nawroth P, Hannak D, Neumaier M, Bergfeld R, Giardino I, Brownlee M. Benfotiamine blocks three major pathways of hyperglycemic damage and prevents experimental diabetic retinopathy. *Nat Med* 2003;9:294–9.

61. Babaei-Jadidi R, Karachalias N, Ahmed N, Battah S, Thornalley PJ. Prevention of incipient diabetic nephropathy by high-dose thiamine and benfotiamine. *Diabetes* 2003;52:2110–20.

62. Tsuchida K, Makita Z, Yamagishi S, Atsumi T, Miyoshi H, Obara S, Ishida M, Ishikawa S, Yasumura K, Koike T. Suppression of transforming growth factor beta and vascular endothelial growth factor in diabetic nephropathy in rats by a novel advanced glycation end product inhibitor, OPB-9195. *Diabetologia* 1999;42:579–88.

63. Bierhaus A, Humpert PM, Morcos M, Wendt T, Chavakis T, Arnold B, Stern DM, Nawroth PP. Understanding RAGE, the receptor for advanced glycation end products. *J Mol Med* 2005;83:876–86.

64. Basta G, Lazzerini G, Massaro M, Simoncini T, Tanganelli P, Fu C, Kislinger T, Stern DM, Schmidt AM, De Caterina R. Advanced glycation end products activate endothelium through signal-transduction receptor RAGE: a mechanism for amplification of inflammatory responses. *Circulation* 2002;105:816–22.

65. Hofmann MA, Drury S, Fu C, Qu W, Taguchi A, Lu Y, Avila C, Kambham N, Bierhaus A, Nawroth P, Neurath MF, Slattery T, Beach D, McClary J, Nagashima M, Morser J, Stern D, Schmidt AM. RAGE mediates a novel proinflammatory axis: a central cell surface receptor for S100/calgranulin polypeptides. *Cell* 1999;97:889–901.

66. Soulis T, Thallas V, Youssef S, Gilbert RE, McWilliam BG, Murray-McIntosh RP, Cooper ME. Advanced glycation end products and their receptors co-localise in rat organs susceptible to diabetic microvascular injury. *Diabetologia* 1997;40:619–28.

67. Yamamoto Y, Kato I, Doi T, Yonekura H, Ohashi S, Takeuchi M, Watanabe T, Yamagishi S, Sakurai S, Takasawa S, Okamoto H, Yamamoto H. Development and prevention of advanced diabetic nephropathy in RAGE-overexpressing mice. *J Clin Invest* 2001;108:261–8.

68. Reiniger N, Lau K, McCalla D, Eby B, Cheng B, Lu Y, Qu W, Quadri N, Ananthakrishnan R, Furmansky M, Rosario R, Song F, Rai V, Weinberg A, Friedman R, Ramasamy R, D'Agati V, Schmidt AM. Deletion of the receptor for advanced glycation end products reduces glomerulosclerosis and preserves renal function in the diabetic OVE26 mouse. *Diabetes* 2010;59:2043–54.

69. Ruggenenti P, Cravedi P, Remuzzi G, Medscape. The RAAS in the pathogenesis and treatment of diabetic nephropathy. *Nat Rev Nephrol* 2010;6:319–30.

70. Zatz R, Dunn BR, Meyer TW, Anderson S, Rennke HG, Brenner BM. Prevention of diabetic glomerulopathy by pharmacological amelioration of glomerular capillary hypertension. *J Clin Invest* 1986;77:1925–30.

71. Taguma Y, Kitamoto Y, Futaki G, Ueda H, Monma H, Ishizaki M, Takahashi H, Sekino H, Sasaki Y. Effect of captopril on heavy proteinuria in azotemic diabetics. *N Engl J Med* 1985;313:1617–20.

72. Parving HH, Lehnert H, Bröchner-Mortensen J, Gomis R, Andersen S, Arner P, Group, I. i. P. w. T.D. a. M.S. The effect of irbesartan on the development of diabetic nephropathy in patients with type 2 diabetes. *N Engl J Med* 2001;345:870–8.

73. Lewis EJ, Hunsicker LG, Clarke WR, Berl T, Pohl MA, Lewis JB, Ritz E, Atkins RC, Rohde R, Raz I, Group C S. Renoprotective effect of the angiotensin-receptor antagonist irbesartan in patients with nephropathy due to type 2 diabetes. *N Engl J Med* 2001;345:851–60.

74. Brenner BM, Cooper ME, de Zeeuw D, Keane WF, Mitch WE, Parving HH, Remuzzi G, Snapinn SM, Zhang Z, Shahinfar S, Investigators, R. S. Effects of losartan on renal and cardiovascular outcomes in patients with type 2 diabetes and nephropathy. *N Engl J Med* 2001;345:861–9.

75. Mann JF, Schmieder RE, McQueen M, Dyal L, Schumacher H, Pogue J, Wang X, Maggioni A, Budaj A, Chaithiraphan S, Dickstein K, Keltai M, Metsärinne K, Oto A, Parkhomenko A, Piegas LS, Svendsen TL, Teo KK, Yusuf S, investigators, O. Renal outcomes with telmisartan, ramipril, or both, in people at high vascular risk (the ONTARGET study): a multicentre, randomised, double-blind, controlled trial. *Lancet* 2008;372:547–53.

76. Ruggenenti P, Fassi A, Ilieva AP, Bruno S, Iliev IP, Brusegan V, Rubis N, Gherardi G, Arnoldi F, Ganeva M, Ene-Iordache B, Gaspari F, Perna A, Bossi A, Trevisan R, Dodesini AR, Remuzzi G, Investigators, B.N.D.C.T. B. Preventing microalbuminuria in type 2 diabetes. *N Engl J Med* 2004;351:1941–51.

77. Remuzzi G, Macia M, Ruggenenti P. Prevention and treatment of diabetic renal disease in type 2 diabetes: the BENEDICT study. *J Am Soc Nephrol* 2006;17:S90–7.

78. Nguyen G, Delarue F, Burcklé C, Bouzhir L, Giller T, Sraer JD. Pivotal role of the renin/prorenin receptor in angiotensin II production and cellular responses to renin. *J Clin Invest* 2002;109:1417–27.

79. Nguyen G, Delarue F, Berrou J, Rondeau E, Sraer JD. Specific receptor binding of renin on human mesangial cells in culture increases plasminogen activator inhibitor-1 antigen. *Kidney Int* 1996;50:1897–903.

80. Ichihara A, Hayashi M, Kaneshiro Y, Suzuki F, Nakagawa T, Tada Y, Koura Y, Nishiyama A, Okada H, Uddin MN, Nabi AH, Ishida Y, Inagami T, Saruta T.

Inhibition of diabetic nephropathy by a decoy peptide corresponding to the "handle" region for non-proteolytic activation of prorenin. *J Clin Invest* 2004;**114**:1128—35.

81. Estacio RO. Renin-angiotensin-aldosterone system blockade in diabetes: role of direct renin inhibitors. *Postgrad Med* 2009;**121**:33—44.

82. Parving HH, Persson F, Lewis JB, Lewis EJ, Hollenberg NK, Investigators, A. S. Aliskiren combined with losartan in type 2 diabetes and nephropathy. *N Engl J Med* 2008;**358**:2433—46.

83. O'Donnell MP, Kasiske BL, Keane WF. Glomerular hemodynamic and structural alterations in experimental diabetes mellitus. *FASEB J* 1988;**2**:2339—47.

84. Ruan X, Arendshorst WJ. Role of protein kinase C in angiotensin II-induced renal vasoconstriction in genetically hypertensive rats. *Am J Physiol* 1996;**270**:F945—52.

85. Williams B, Schrier RW. Glucose-induced protein kinase C activity regulates arachidonic acid release and eicosanoid production by cultured glomerular mesangial cells. *J Clin Invest* 1993;**92**:2889—96.

86. Boesch DM, Garvin JL. Age-dependent activation of PKC isoforms by angiotensin II in the proximal nephron. *Am J Physiol Regul Integr Comp Physiol* 2001;**281**:R861—7.

87. Osicka TM, Yu Y, Lee V, Panagiotopoulos S, Kemp BE, Jerums G. Aminoguanidine and ramipril prevent diabetes-induced increases in protein kinase C activity in glomeruli, retina and mesenteric artery. *Clin Sci (Lond)* 2001;**100**:249—57.

88. Forbes JM, Cooper ME, Thallas V, Burns WC, Thomas MC, Brammar GC, Lee F, Grant SL, Burrell LM, Burrell LA, Jerums G, Osicka TM. Reduction of the accumulation of advanced glycation end products by ACE inhibition in experimental diabetic nephropathy. *Diabetes* 2002;**51**:3274—82.

89. Sebeková K, Schinzel R, Münch G, Krivosíková Z, Dzúrik R, Heidland A. Advanced glycation end-product

levels in subtotally nephrectomized rats: beneficial effects of angiotensin II receptor 1 antagonist losartan. *Miner Electrolyte Metab* 1999;**25**:380—3.

90. Fan Q, Liao J, Kobayashi M, Yamashita M, Gu L, Gohda T, Suzuki Y, Wang LN, Horikoshi S, Tomino Y. Candesartan reduced advanced glycation end-products accumulation and diminished nitro-oxidative stress in type 2 diabetic KK/Ta mice. *Nephrol Dial Transplant* 2004;**19**:3012—20.

91. Sebeková K, Gazdíková K, Syrová D, Blazícek P, Schinzel R, Heidland A, Spustová V, Dzúrik R. Effects of ramipril in nondiabetic nephropathy: improved parameters of oxidatives stress and potential modulation of advanced glycation end products. *J Hum Hypertens* 2003;**17**:265—70.

92. Saisho Y, Komiya N, Hirose H. Effect of valsartan, an angiotensin II receptor blocker, on markers of oxidation and glycation in Japanese type 2 diabetic subjects: blood pressure-independent effect of valsartan. *Diabetes Res Clin Pract* 2006;**74**:201—3.

93. Lee CI, Guh JY, Chen HC, Hung WC, Yang YL, Chuang LY. Advanced glycation end-product-induced mitogenesis and collagen production are dependent on angiotensin II and connective tissue growth factor in NRK-49F cells. *J Cell Biochem* 2005;**95**:281—92.

94. Yamagishi S, Takeuchi M, Inoue H. Olmesartan medoxomil, a newly developed angiotensin II type 1 receptor antagonist, protects against renal damage in advanced glycation end product (age)-injected rats. *Drugs Exp Clin Res* 2005;**31**:45—51.

95. Matsui T, Yamagishi S, Ueda S, Fukami K, Okuda S. Irbesartan inhibits albumin-elicited proximal tubular cell apoptosis and injury in vitro. *Protein Pept Lett* 2010;**17**:74—7.

96. Matsui T, Yamagishi S, Takeuchi M, Ueda S, Fukami K, Okuda S. Irbesartan inhibits advanced glycation end product (AGE)-induced proximal tubular cell injury in vitro by suppressing receptor for AGEs (RAGE) expression. *Pharmacol Res* 2010;**61**:34—9.

An Overview of Diabetes and Ocular Health

Shintaro Nakao[*,†], *Yasuaki Hata*[*]

[*]Section of Ophthalmology, Department of Medicine, Fukuoka Dental College, Fukuoka,
Japan [†]Department of Ophthalmology, Graduate School of Medical Sciences,
Kyushu University, Fukuoka, Japan

INTRODUCTION

Diabetes, a metabolism disorder, is a lifestyle disease that has been dramatically on the rise.

Dietary patterns are shifting from plant-based to animal-based proteins and fats with urbanization of the developing countries. One of the major concerns that our society faces today in

Nutritional and Therapeutic Interventions for Diabetes and Metabolic Syndrome
DOI: 10.1016/B978-0-12-385083-6.00013-9

not only developed countries, but also in developing ones is the various chronic complications associated with the disease[1] such as cardiovasculopathy, nephropathy, neuropathy, and retinopathy (Figure 13.1). Among the various ocular diabetic complications, including ocular neuropathy, uveitis, and cataract, diabetic retinopathy has been recognized as the most significant damage that results in impaired vision and eventual vision loss. Recent advanced surgeries and treatments allow diabetic patients who long suffered from devastating complications to have a better quality of life; however, diabetic retinopathy still remains as one of the leading causes of blindness. A possible contributing factor is the prolonged duration of diabetes from improved glycemic control. While poorly managed glycemic control had led to deaths in many diabetic cases in the past, patients with improved glycemic control tend to live longer with the disease. Studies have suggested that serious complications, especially microvascular, are most likely to occur

in those who have had diabetes for many years. Other complicated systemic diseases such as hyperlipidemia are also contributing factors. The latest experimental and clinical studies have revealed the pathophysiological mechanisms of ocular diabetic complications. The basic mechanism of ocular diabetic complications is microvasculopathy by persistent hyperglycemia. In this chapter, we would like to introduce epidemiology, pathophysiological mechanisms, and recent advances in the management of diabetic ocular complications, mainly diabetic retinopathy.

EPIDEMIOLOGY/RISK FACTORS

In many countries, diabetic retinopathy is the most frequent cause of preventable blindness in working ages.[2] In the US, an estimated 50% of people with type 2 diabetes and 86% with type 1 diabetes have diabetic retinopathy.[3] Various population-based studies in the other countries showed similar prevalence of diabetic retinopathy.[4] However, in developed countries, the prevalence is decreasing due to improvement in the control of systemic risk factors, whereas in developing countries, the incidence of diabetes is growing at an alarming rate due to the lifestyle change.[5,6]

The Wisconsin Epidemiologic Study of Diabetic Retinopathy in 1984 indicated that the severity of retinopathy was related to longer-duration, high levels of glycosylated hemoglobin (HbA1c), presence of proteinuria, higher diastolic BP, and male gender after diabetes for 10 years.[7] Recent study in the US confirmed that the steepest increase in retinopathy prevalence occurs among individuals with certain HbA1c level ($\geq 5.5\%$) and fasting plasma glucose (FPG) ($\geq 5.8\,\mathrm{mmol/l}$).[8] A Japanese study (Hisayama study) also suggested that measuring HbA1c or fasting plasma glucose is useful for predicting diabetic retinopathy.[9]

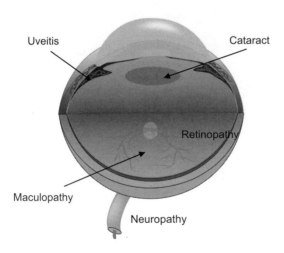

FIGURE 13.1 **Ocular complications of diabetes.** Ocular diabetic complications include keratitis, cataract, uveitis, retinopathy, maculopathy and ocular neuropathy. Diabetic retinopathy and maculopathy are the most important ocular complications because they lead to vision loss. (*See the color plate section at the back of the book.*)

Table 13.1 shows several important risk factors for diabetic retinopathy. Findings from population-based studies suggest that the prevalence and severity of diabetic retinopathy are higher in African Americans, Hispanics, and south Asians than in Caucasians, and are not fully accounted for by differences in the distribution of retinopathy risk factors. Population-based incidence study in type 1 diabetes suggests that a reduction of hyperglycemia and hypertension may result in a beneficial decrease in the progression to proliferative retinopathy.[10] In males, increased alcohol consumption was related to increased severity of retinopathy.[11] Previous epidemiological studies have shown that diabetic retinopathy is associated with many other systemic and lifestyle factors including nephropathy, obesity,[12] hematological markers of anemia,[13] hypothyroidism,[14] inflammation, and endothelial dysfunction.[15] Several epidemiological studies suggest that diabetic retinopathy could be a predictive marker for systemic vascular disorders including stroke, atherosclerosis, and coronary heart diseases.[16-18]

TABLE 13.1 Risk Factors of Diabetic Retinopathy

☐ Hyperglycemia
☐ Hypertension
☐ Dyslipidemia
☐ Diabetes duration
☐ Ethnic origin
   (African Americans, Hispanic, South Asian)
☐ Pregnancy
☐ Puberty
☐ Cataract surgery
☐ Presence of proteinuria
☐ Smoking
☐ Alcohol

This table shows important risk factors of diabetic retinopathy. Hyperglycemia and hypertension are the most important. One percent decrease in HbA1c and 10 mmHg decrease in systolic blood pressure can decrease the risk of retinopathy by 40% and 35%, respectively. The duration of diabetes is also a major risk factor. The 25-year cumulative rates of progression to diabetic retinopathy and macular edema are 83% and 29%, respectively.

PATHOPHYSIOLOGY

Basic Mechanism: Microvascular Damage

The role of the eye is to serve as a light receptor. Because blood vessels can disturb the transparency, the minimum network of blood vessels is developed to meet the demand of the blood supply required. So the eye is fragile with regard to hypoxia, and the vessels and surrounding cells are easily influenced by hypoxia.[19] Furthermore, the oxygen demand of the eye is known to be higher than the other central neuronal systems (e.g., brain) because the dark adaptation needs much oxygen.[20,21] Retinal microvascular damage could be observed in earlier stages of diabetes than damage to other organs. However, the eye has to get the most oxygen and nutrition from blood circulation. This means that retinal vascular damage affects the retinal functions. The diabetes-related vascular damage always initiates from capillaries, but not veins or arteries. However, the reasons why the initial sites of the diabetes-related vascular damage are always the capillaries are unknown.[22] Diabetic microvascular damage is mainly characterized by microthrombosis, hyperpermeability, and angiogenesis (Figure 13.2). Because these mechanisms are not independent, and they affect each other in the progression of diabetic retinopathy, the clinical findings are not simple.

Microthrombosis

Why does microvascular thrombosis occur in the diabetic retina? After the thrombosis occurs in retinal capillaries, thrombosis of the macrovascular level can form a retinal non-perfusion area. Thrombosis could be induced under these conditions: changes in vascular wall structure, changes in blood components, and changes in blood flow. Because of abnormal coagulation, fibrinolysis and blood flow in diabetic patients,

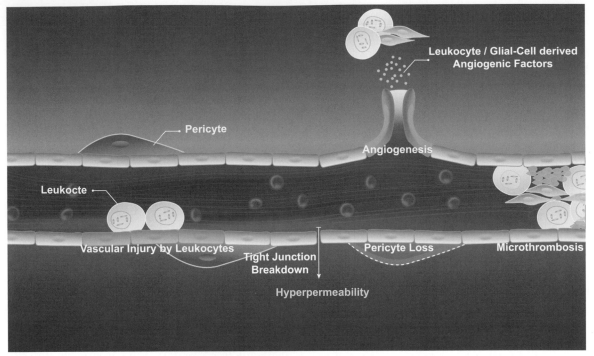

FIGURE 13.2   Vascular damage in diabetic retinopathy. The basic mechanism of diabetic retinopathy is hyperglycemia-induced vascular damage. Various cellular components also play important roles in the pathogenesis.

clots are easily formed and the dissolution is difficult in diabetes.[23,24] Abnormality of bloodstream and components as well as vascular endothelium and pericytes in diabetes also promote clot formation[25-27] (Figure 13.2). In the early stages of microvascular thrombosis, platelets, fibrin, and leukocytes play important roles for clot formation.[24,25,28] Furthermore, adhered leukocytes and platelets are known to damage retinal endothelium (Figure 13.2).[29,30] Activated glial cells and the proliferation would make the obstruction irreversible (Figure 13.2), leading to retinal hypoxia by the wider nonperfusion area (Table 13.2).

Hyperpermeability

Retinal vessel hyperpermeability induces dot/blot hemorrhage, retinal edema (leakage of plasma protein), and hard exudate (deposition of lipoprotein) (Table 13.2). Endothelial cells in retinal blood vessels have tight junctions which are known to compose the blood—retinal barrier. This barrier protects the neural retina from the leakage of toxic components from blood circulation. It is difficult for intravenous injection of drugs to reach the neuronal retina due to this barrier. The tight junction in the retina is regulated by not only the special character of retinal endothelium but also by various surrounding cells, especially neuronal cells or glial cells[31] (Figure 13.2). In diabetic retinopathy, the breakdown of the blood—retinal barrier leads to the hyperpermeability, resulting in vascular leakage.[32] Moreover, an experimental diabetic retina shows that some endothelial cytoplasms are thin and have fenestration. These fenestrations that are

TABLE 13.2 Pathogenesis, Clinical Features and Cellular Reaction of Diabetic Retinopathy

Pathogenesis	Stage	Clinical features	Cellular reaction
Hyperpermeabilty	Non-proliferative diabetic retinopathy (NPDR)	Retinal hemorrhage/Hard exudate	Endothelial cell fenestration/Pericyte loss
Microthrombosis	Moderate NPDR	Soft exudate/Intraretinal microvascular abonormalities	Thrombosis by leukocytes & platelets
Angiogenesis	Proliferative diabetic retinopathy (PDR)	Retinal angiogenesis/Vitreous hemorrhage	Endothelial cell proliferation/Angiogenic factors by glial cells & leukocytes
Fibrosis	PDR	Proliferative membrane/Tractional retinal detachment	Glial cell proliferation/Hyalocytes activation

seen in both capillaries and venules are closed by a thin diaphragm. Transendothelial channels are also observed in the endothelial cytoplasm. The tight junctions between endothelial cells are rarely altered. The junctions are open with short adherent regions in which the junctional membranes show increased electron density. These morphological changes account for the characteristic breakdown of the blood–retinal barrier in the diabetic retina.[33] Furthermore, pericyte loss and glial cell proliferation are often observed in diabetic eyes (Table 13.2). Because pericytes also regulate the blood–retinal barrier, pericyte loss contributes to the hyperpermeability.[34] Glial cells or leukocyte-derived vascular endothelial growth factor-A (VEGF-A) are known to be the main players in diabetes-induced hyperpermeability in retina[35,36] (Figure 13.2). It is known that neutrophil or platelet adhesion to endothelial cells induces hyperpermeability of retina vessels[37,38] (Figure 13.2). These observations indicate that the interactions between retinal endothelial cells and the surrounding cells play important roles for the pathogenesis of diabetic retinopathy. However, once retinal blood vessels are damaged, the blood vessel function can not be recovered with any current therapy.

Angiogenesis

Abnormal angiogenesis in diabetes is most clinically apparent in proliferative diabetic retinopathy (Table 13.2). The following vitreous hemorrhage and tractional retinal detachment cause severe visual loss. Because a blood vessel is a tube for carrying red blood cells, leukocytes, and platelets, the body induces angiogenesis in order to compensate for the lack of these cells. Red blood cells, leukocytes, and platelets play certain roles in hypoxia, inflammation, and tissue damage, respectively. So hypoxia, inflammation, or tissue damage causes angiogenesis. As described above, capillary occlusions are characteristic features of early diabetic retinopathy. Hypoxia by the retinal ischemia upregulates VEGF-A expression and the VEGF-A induces angiogenesis. Activated leukocytes, especially macrophages, are well-known to induce angiogenesis by secretion of various angiogenic factors[39,40] (Figure 13.2). Because platelets are also known to support angiogenesis, platelets contribute to retinal angiogenesis in diabetes.[25,38,41] Proliferative diabetic retinopathy is characterized by proliferation of fibrovascular tissue formed by the extension of retinal angiogenesis into the vitreous cavity. Matrix metalloproteinase-2 (MMP-2) can contribute to the pathogenesis by degradation of inner limiting membrane.[42] Upregulations in numerous other cytokines, chemokines, adhesion molecules, vasoactive hormones, and immune cells in the vitreous cavity of diabetic retinopathy have been reported[43,44] (Table 13.3). Angiogenic factors including VEGF-A in vitreous must contribute to the invasion of retinal angiogenesis into vitreous.

Inflammation

Several mechanisms have been proposed to modulate the pathogenesis of diabetic retinopathy. Main pathways include advanced glycation endo-products (AGE), oxidative stress, protein kinase C activation, inflammation, Rho-associated, coiled−coil−containing protein kinase (ROCK), and growth factors. Diabetic retinopathy is also known to be inflammation. Diabetic retinopathy was initially termed "diabetic retinitis", although this usage fell out of favor in the 1970s.[45] Chronic inflammation is characterized by increased vascular permeability, edema, inflammatory cell infiltration, cytokine and chemokine expression, tissue destruction, and neovascularization, and diabetic retinopathy shows most of these features. Activated macrophages and granulocytes can cause microvascular occlusions and cell damage by the release of cytotoxic products[30] (Figure 13.2). Furthermore, retinal leukostasis by intercellular adhesion molecule-1 (ICAM-1), mainly neutrophils

adhesion, causes retinal vascular damage.[29,37] Vascular adhesion protein-1 (VAP-1) is an endothelial adhesion molecule that possesses semicarbazide-sensitive amine oxidase (SSAO) activity and is involved in leukocyte recruitment. Recent study reveals the critical contribution of VAP-1 to leukocyte transmigration, with little impact on firm leukocyte adhesion in the retinas of diabetic animals. VAP-1 inhibition might be beneficial in the treatment of diabetic retinopathy.[46] Nonsteroidal anti-inflammatory drugs also might prevent vascular damage of the early diabetic retinopathy.[47] An animal experimental study shows that neither tumor necrosis factor-α (TNF-α) nor inflammation is required for early blood−retinal barrier (BRB) breakdown in diabetic retinopathy (DR); however, TNF-α is critical for the later complications including BRB breakdown, retinal leukostasis, and apoptosis associated with diabetic retinopathy.[48]

VEGF

VEGF is a highly specific mitogen for vascular endothelial cells. The expression of VEGF is upregulated in response to hypoxia, by activated oncogenes, and by a variety of cytokines. VEGF induces endothelial cell proliferation, promotes cell migration, and inhibits apoptosis. *In vivo* VEGF induces angiogenesis as well as permeabilization of blood vessels, and plays a central role in the regulation of vasculogenesis.[49] In the eye, VEGF is also known to play a central role in ocular angiogenesis including diabetic retinopathy. VEGF expression could be observed in glial cells as well as in leukocytes in the diabetic retina[35] (Figure 13.2). VEGF levels in ocular tissues from patients with diabetes are greater than in non-diabetic subjects[43] (Table 13.3). Numerous preclinical studies point to a central role for VEGF in the pathogenesis of both diabetic macular edema and proliferative diabetic retinopathy.[50] VEGF is also known to play an important role in the breakdown of the blood−retinal barrier.[36] Recent accumulating clinical evidences

TABLE 13.3 Increased Cytokines and Growth Factors in Vitreous/Retina of Diabetic Retinopathy

Increased cytokines in vitreous/retina
VEGF-A
MCP-1
IL-6
IL-8
SDF-1
TNF-α
Erythropoietin
TGF-β2

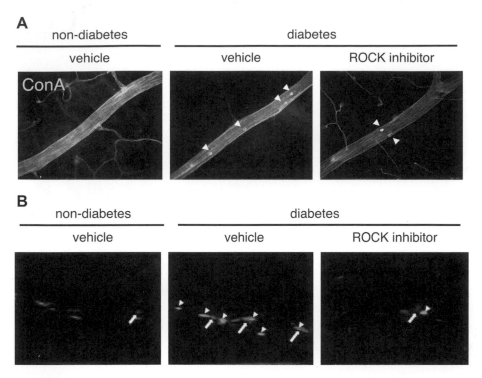

FIGURE 13.3   ROCK as a target for diabetic retinopathy. A: More leukocyte adhesion is observed in diabetic retina compared with normal retina. ROCK inhibitor fasudil blocks the leukocyte adhesion on retinal vessels. White arrowheads indicate firmly adhering leukocytes. B: Dead or injured endothelial cells [red, propidium iodide (PI)] and endothelial nuclei (blue, DAPI). Injured retinal endothelium (white arrowhead) with adherent leukocytes (white arrow) is increased in diabetic retina which is blocked by ROCK inhibitor. (*See the color plate section at the back of the book.*)

also indicate that VEGF plays a critical role in pathogenesis of both diabetic macular edema and neovascularization in proliferative diabetic retinopathy.

ROCK

Rho-associated, coiled—coil—containing protein kinases (ROCKs) play key roles in a variety of physiologic functions, including cytoskeletal rearrangement, contractility of smooth muscle, adhesion, proliferation, and migration.[51] Some studies have shown that Rho and its target protein ROCK are implicated in the important role for diabetes. It is reported that ROCK could be increased in endothelial cells by high glucose.[52] *In vivo* studies revealed that ROCK

could be involved in the pathogenesis of renal and aortic complications during diabetic states.[53,54] Recent study showed that the Rho/ROCK pathway is activated in retinal microvessels during diabetes and promotes leukocyte adhesion to the retinal endothelium by increasing ICAM-1 and integrins[55] (Figure 13.3A). Furthermore, a specific ROCK inhibitor, fasudil, could inhibit VEGF-A-induced angiogenesis, indicating that ROCK is also important for angiogenesis.[56] In the late stages of diabetic retinopathy, proliferative membranes could form and the contraction could cause retinal detachment. ROCK inhibition suppresses critical contraction of proliferative membrane, suggesting that ROCK inhibitor might be useful for the management of later stages of diabetic

FIGURE 13.4 **Hyalocytes in diabetic retinopathy.** A: Histologic characteristics of hyalocytes. Under an electron microscope, hyalocytes assumed many forms and possessed lysosome-like granules, mitochondria, and micropinocytotic vesicles, presenting the characteristics of a macrophage lineage. B; Vitreous fluids from patients with proliferative diabetic retinopathy can induce gel contraction by hyalocytes. This contraction can be inhibited by TGF-β blocking as well as ROCK inhibitor.

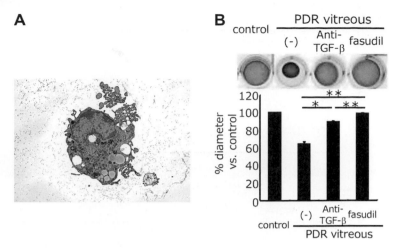

retinopathy[57,58] (Figure 13.4). Statin that could suppress ROCK activity must treat diabetic retinopathy.[59] These findings suggest that ROCK is a candidate for the molecular targeting of diabetic retinopathy.[60]

Hyalocytes

Hyalocytes have been described as occurring in the peripheral or cortical region of the vitreous close to the inner surface of the retina.[61] Although hyalocytes were discovered more than 100 years ago, the molecular and cellular biological characteristics of hyalocytes have yet to be fully elucidated. Hyalocytes are resident macrophages and originate from the blood monocytes[62,63] (Figure 13.4A). Hyalocytes have rare mitotic activity under physiological conditions.[64] However, under pathological conditions hyalocytes play important roles in the pathogenesis of proliferative vitreoretinal diseases including proliferative diabetic retinopathy and they are a candidate for cellular targeting therapy[57,58,65] (Figure 13.4B). Various studies using clinical samples showed upregulation of TNF-α in diabetic patients[66] (Table 13.3). TNF-α promoted proliferation, migration, and gel contraction by hyalocyte, suggesting that TNF-α-activated hyalocytes contribute to the

late stage of diabetic retinopathy.[67] Moreover, because hyalocytes could secrete VEGF-A, hyalocytes might affect retinal vascular hyperpermeability and angiogenesis.[68]

CLINICAL ASSESSMENT

Retinopathy

Diabetic retinopathy is the most common cause of blindness in working people in various countries. As described above, diabetic retinopathy is a consequence of microvascular changes (Figure 13.1). Non-proliferative diabetic retinopathy is characterized by microaneurysms, hemorrhages, venous beading, capillary loss, and intraretinal microvascular abnormalities[69] (Figure 13.5A). Proliferative diabetic retinopathy develops secondary to capillary thrombosis which upregulates VEGF and inflammatory cytokines. It is defined by angiogenesis from the retina or optic nerve on the posterior surface of the vitreous or the iris. Angiogenic vessels are easy to rupture, causing vitreous hemorrhage. In the advanced stage, these angiogenic vessels form fibrovascular membranes that induce traction on the retina, leading to tractional retinal detachment[69] (Figure 13.5B).

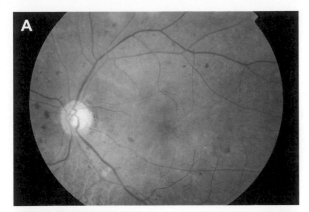

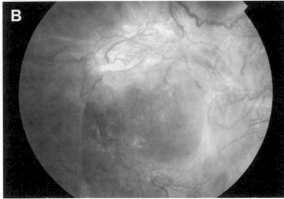

FIGURE 13.5 Clinical features of diabetic retinopathy. A: Non-proliferative diabetic retinopathy. Cardinal signs are retinal microaneurysms, hemorrhages and hard exudates. B: Proliferative diabetic retinopathy is characterized by angiogenesis and fibrovascular membranes. (*See the color plate section at the back of the book.*)

The main symptom of diabetic retinopathy is reduced vision, but this occurs mostly when the stage is advanced and sometimes irreversible. Early changes in diabetic retinopathy are generally asymptomatic and treatment is needed before patients are aware of visual acuity loss.[69]

After pupil dilatation, the fundus can be observed by direct and indirect ophthalmoscopy. It is often difficult to detect the retinal ischemia by the fundus observation. Fluorescein angiography (FAG) is a useful tool to recognize retinal ischemic lesion, abnormalities of retinal vessels and neovascularization (Figure 13.6A–C).

Maculopathy

The macula is located in the center of the retina, the light-sensitive tissue at the back of the eye (Figure 13.1). Diabetic maculopathy occurs when retinopathy affects the macula and central visual acuity is threatened. Patients with type 2 diabetes have a higher prevalence of maculopathy than those with type 1 diabetes. The maculopathy can be classified into macular edema and macular ischemia. Macular ischemia is characterized by capillary loss in the macular area and is currently untreatable. Macular edema is cause by hyperpermeability of retinal vessels and/or decreased efflux of fluid across the retinal pigment epithelium which can be induced by outer/inner blood–retinal barrier dysfunction. These cause retinal swelling by the accumulation of intraretinal fluid which results in central vision loss. Diabetic macular edema is focal and diffuse. Leaky microaneurysms cause circinate hard exudates which can also induce visual loss.[69] FAG identifies leaky vascular abnormalities responsible for fluid accumulation (Figure 13.6C). Optical coherence tomography (OCT) is also a useful examination for diagnosis of diabetic macular edema. OCT allows the recognition of tractional edema by visualizing the relationships between retina and posterior hyaloid (Figure 13.6D, E).

Neuropathy

Diabetic neuropathies are neuropathic disorders that are associated with diabetes mellitus. Neuropathies are characterized by a progressive loss of nerve fibers that can be assessed non-invasively by several tests of nerve function including the pupils of the eyes, making them less responsive to changes in light (Figure 13.1). Diabetes may have led to the loss of function of

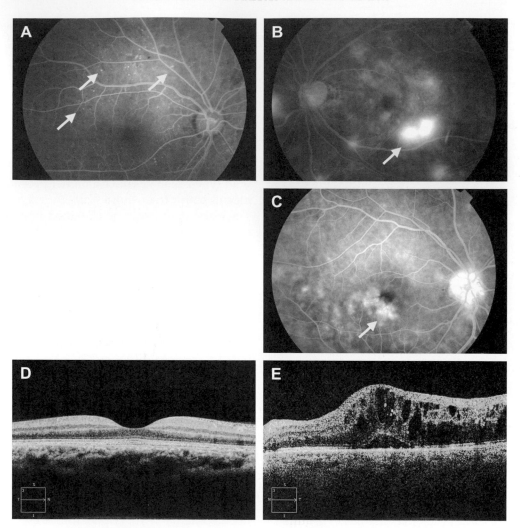

FIGURE 13.6 Imaging of diabetic retinopathy. A–C: Fluorescein retinal angiography (FA). A: FA images of non-proliferative diabetic retinopathy which is characterized by microaneurysms (arrows). B: FA images of non-proliferative diabetic retinopathy. Fluorescein leakage is angiogenesis (arrows). C: Pooling of fluorescein dye by macular edema (arrows). D, E: Optical coherence tomography (OCT). OCT images of normal retina (D) and diabetic macular edema (E). (*See the color plate section at the back of the book.*)

a nerve that controls a single muscle (e.g., oculo-motor nervecan). For example, focal neuropathy causes problems with eye movement that results in double vision.

Diabetic retinopathy is microvascular damage; however, the retina is a vascularized neural tissue but not a network of blood vessels.[70]

Histopathological study showed the loss of neurons in diabetic retinopathy.[71] Various investigations have also demonstrated that the loss of neuroretinal function occurs before the onset of vascular damage in humans with electroretinography, dark adaptation, contrast sensitivity, and color vision test.[70] These observations suggest that diabetic retinopathy is part of neuropathy in retina.

Uveitis

It has been reported that 6% of the patients with anterior uveitis had diabetes mellitus (Figure 13.1). This is significantly higher than the prevalence of 1.4% in the normal population. Furthermore, the onset of diabetes mellitus preceded the onset of anterior uveitis in most cases.[72]

Cataract

Cataracts are lens opacities that cause 50% of blindness in developing countries[73] (Figure 13.1). Diabetes raises the risk for senile cataract by about 40%. Cataract is a common complication of diabetes. Indeed it has been estimated that up to 15% of cataract surgery is performed on diabetics.

THERAPY

Glycemic Control

Improved glycemic control (HbA1c 7%) can reduce but not abolish the risk of diabetic retinopathy.[74] The Diabetes Control and Complications Trial (DCCT) showed that intensive treatment reduced the risk of development and progression of diabetic maculopathy compared with usual management in both type 1 and type 2 diabetes.[75] UK Prospective Diabetes Study (UKPDS) presented that tight control of blood glucose can show 17% reduction in the risk of progression of retinopathy, a 29% reduction in the need for laser treatment, and a 16% reduction in the risk of legal blindness compared with usual management.[76] Although there could be a small risk of worsening of retinopathy by the onset of therapy, the long-term benefits outweigh this risk.[77] One percent reduction of HbA1c decreases risk of retinopathy by 30–40% and the effect appears to be long-lasting (metabolic memory).[78]

Blood Pressure Control

Hypertension might exacerbate diabetic retinopathy through increased blood flow and mechanical damage of retinal endothelial cells, stimulating expression of VEGF and VEGF receptor-2.[79] Epidemiological studies support that hypertension is a major risk factor for diabetic retinopathy. The UKPDS study showed that the progression of diabetic retinopathy was reduced by 35% in the tight control group compared with the less tight group. The risk of moderate vision loss and the need for laser treatment could be rescued by 47% and 35%, respectively. Some blood pressure-lowering drugs including renin angiotensin inhibitors could show a benefit for diabetic retina beyond their blood pressure-lowering effects.[80]

Lipid-Lowering Therapy

Dyslipidemia could play an important role in the pathogenesis of diabetic retinopathy.[81] Elevation of serum lipid levels is a risk factor for retinal hard exudates and diabetic retinal edema leading to visual loss.[82,83] Retinal hard exudates form as a result of increased vascular permeability that causes the leakage of fluid and lipids and is often accompanied by retinal thickness. Retinal lipid deposition might cause loss of retinal function. The DCCT study showed that severity of diabetic retinopathy was associated with increasing triglycerides and inversely associated with high-density lipoprotein (HDL) cholesterol.[84] Fibrates and statins are lipid-lowering drugs which are widely used for dyslipidemia. Peroxisome proliferator activated receptor-α (PPARα) agonist fenofibrate suppresses endothelial proliferation and inhibits VEGF expression resulting in angiogenesis inhibition. A study showed that fewer patients who received feno-fibrate needed laser treatment than in the placebo group.[85] Statin produces anti-inflammatory and vasoprotective results in diabetic retina.[86]

Steroid

Locally administered (topical, sub-tenon, intravitreal) corticosteroid has been used to treat diabetic macular edema and diabetes-related inflammatory conditions. However, the mechanism of the action is not fully understood. A possible mechanism is to inhibit VEGF expression via nuclear factor kappaB (NFκB) regulation.[68,87] Previous studies have suggested that peribulbar steroid, with or without focal photocoagulation, is unlikely to be of substantial benefit in cases of diabetic macular edema with good visual acuity[88] (Figure 13.7A, B). However, peribulbar steroid injections are associated with an increased incidence of intraocular pressure (IOP) elevation and an increased risk of cataract development compared with laser or posterior peribulbar injections.[89] Intraocular (intravitreal) injection of steroid has been reported to reduce the progression and even induce regression of diabetic retinopathy.[90] Intravitreal injection of steroid is also reported to be beneficial for improving visual acuity in patients with clinically significant diffuse diabetic macular edema.[91] Recent study showed that intravitreal steroid injection is effective in improving visual acuity in patients with refractory diabetic macular edema in the short term, but the benefits do not seem to persist in the long term.[92] Intraocular steroids are also associated with increased risk of cataract and intraocular pressure elevation. These side effects often limit the treatment for patients because it is difficult to predict which patients will show a rise in intraocular pressure or which will have cataract. Furthermore, injection-related side effects include retinal detachment, vitreous

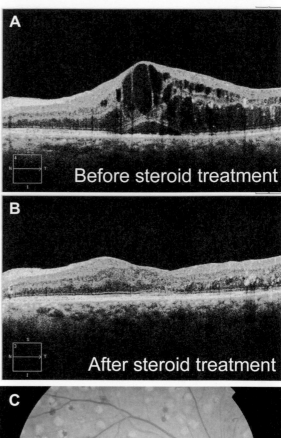

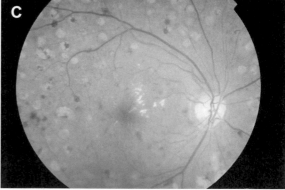

FIGURE 13.7 Therapy for diabetic retinopathy. A: Steroid therapy for diabetic macular edema. B: OCT images before and after steroid (triamcinolone acetonide) treatment. Steroid treatment resolves diabetic macular edema. OCT is a useful tool to estimate the efficiency of steroid for diabetic macular edema. B: Laser photocoagulation. Laser photocoagulation reduces retinal oxygen demand. This treatment causes regression of retinal neovascularization and reduces central macular thickening. (*See the color plate section at the back of the book.*)

hemorrhage, bacterial endophthalmitis, and sterile endophthalmitis.[93]

VEGF Inhibitors

Bevacizumab (Avastin) is a humanized mouse antibody that blocks VEGF and was fFDA-approved as a treatment for metastatic colorectal cancer in 2004. Bevacizumab is not formulated for use within the eye but was reported as being used off-label as an intravitreal injection to treat diabetic macular edema in 2006.[94] A monoclonal fragment, ranibizumab (Lucentis), is derived from bevacizumab and specifically formulated for eye treatment. Because ranibizumab (48 kDa) is much smaller than bevacizumab (149 kDa), ranibizumab could penetrate the retina faster than bevacizumab. Accumulating clinical studies indicate that anti-VEGF drugs including pegaptanib (Macugen), bevacizumab (Avastin), and ranibizumab (Lucentis) are potentially useful and they improve outcomes for treating diabetic retinopathy.[50] In a recent large randomized trial of intravitreal ranibizumab, patients treated with ranibizumab were more likely to gain at least 10 letters of visual acuity and less likely to lose 10 or more letters after 1 year of the treatment. However, patients received an average of eight ot nine injections in the first year.[95] Bevacizumab has also been reported to cause regression of retinal angiogenesis. A longer-term study with anti-VEGF drugs is needed to assess if the repeated injections affect visual acuity outcome. Recent histological study with bevacizumab treatment suggests the effect of VEGF inhibition on diabetic neovascular tissue. Bevacizumab could lead to endothelial apoptosis with vascular regression and induce normalization of premature vessels by increasing pericyte coverage and reducing endothelial fenestration.[96] A few reports suggest an increased risk of tractional retinal detachment with the treatment of VEGF inhibitor.[97,98] Some experimental studies showed that VEGF is essential for the maintenance of the choriocapillaris or for survival on muller cells and photoreceptors.[99–101] These data also alert us to the effect of VEGF inhibition for eye homeostasis.

Laser Photocoagulation

Laser photocoagulation is a well-established treatment for diabetic retinopathy (Figure 13.7C). The main aim of photocoagulation is to reduce retinal oxygen demand which is a regulator for angiogenesis. This treatment causes regression of retinal neovascularization and reduces central macular thickening and thus prevents visual loss from proliferative diabetic retinopathy and diabetic maculopathy. The Early Treatment of Diabetic Retinopathy Study (ETDRS) indicated laser photocoagulation could reduce the risk of moderate visual loss by 50%.[102] However, in some patients this treatment can not prevent loss of vision.

Vitrectomy

Vitrectomy has been the mainstay surgical treatment for proliferative diabetic retinopathy including persistent vitreous hemorrhage and tractional retinal detachment. Its aim is to improve vision by removing hemorrhage in or behind the vitreous or proliferative membranes, reattaching detached retina and reducing the factors for angiogenesis by complete pan-retinal laser photocoagulation. Furthermore, vitrectomy can remove various cytokines and growth factors from the vitreous cavity. The Diabetic Retinopathy Vitrectomy Study (DRVS) showed that type 1 diabetes patients with severe vitreous hemorrhage achieve visual outcome if earlier vitrectomy was undertaken.[103,104] Vitrectomy has also been suggested as a treatment for diabetic macular edema regardless of vitreo-macular traction. Studies showed further benefits of vitrectomy combined with peeling of the internal limiting membrane in the treatment of diabetic macular edema for early regression of the edema.[105]

CONCLUSIONS

Despite recent advances in the understating of the pathogenesis of diabetic retinopathy and in the development of new therapies including VEGF inhibitor, diabetic retinopathy is still a developing, vision-threatening disease. Physicians and ophthalmologists should be aware not only of the apparent benefits but also of the potential risks of present and future therapies. Through understanding the various mechanisms in diabetic complications, we see that blood glucose control is the most important factor for the prevention of diabetic retinopathy.

References

1. Hossain P, Kawar B, El Nahas M. Obesity and diabetes in the developing world—a growing challenge. N Engl J Med 2007;356:213–5.
2. Cheung N, Mitchell P, Wong TY. Diabetic retinopathy. Lancet 2010;376:124–36.
3. Kempen JH, O'Colmain BJ, Leske MC, Haffner SM, Klein R, Moss SE, Taylor HR, Hamman RF. The prevalence of diabetic retinopathy among adults in the United States. Arch Ophthalmol 2004;122:552–63.
4. Wang FH, Liang YB, Zhang F, Wang JJ, Wei WB, Tao QS, Sun LP, Friedman DS, Wang NL, Wong TY. Prevalence of diabetic retinopathy in rural China: the Handan Eye Study. Ophthalmology 2009;116:461–7.
5. Klein R, Lee KE, Knudtson MD, Gangnon RE, Klein BE. Changes in visual impairment prevalence by period of diagnosis of diabetes: the Wisconsin Epidemiologic Study of Diabetic Retinopathy. Ophthalmology 2009;116:1937–42.
6. Chan JC, Malik V, Jia W, Kadowaki T, Yajnik CS, Yoon KH, Hu FB. Diabetes in Asia: epidemiology, risk factors, and pathophysiology. JAMA 2009;301:2129–40.
7. Klein R, Klein BE, Moss SE, Davis MD, DeMets DL. The Wisconsin epidemiologic study of diabetic retinopathy. II. Prevalence and risk of diabetic retinopathy when age at diagnosis is less than 30 years. Arch Ophthalmol 1984;102:520–6.
8. Cheng YJ, Gregg EW, Geiss LS, Imperatore G, Williams DE, Zhang X, Albright AL, Cowie CC, Klein R, Saaddine JB. Association of A1C and fasting plasma glucose levels with diabetic retinopathy prevalence in the U.S. population: Implications for
9. Miyazaki M, Kubo M, Kiyohara Y, Okubo K, Nakamura H, Fujisawa K, Hata Y, Tokunaga S, Iida M, Nose Y, Ishibashi T. Comparison of diagnostic methods for diabetes mellitus based on prevalence of retinopathy in a Japanese population: the Hisayama Study. Diabetologia 2004;47:1411–5.
10. Klein R, Klein BE, Moss SE, Cruickshanks KJ. The Wisconsin Epidemiologic Study of Diabetic Retinopathy: XVII. The 14-year incidence and progression of diabetic retinopathy and associated risk factors in type 1 diabetes. Ophthalmology 1998;105:1801–15.
11. Kohner EM, Aldington SJ, Stratton IM, Manley SE, Holman RR, Matthews DR, Turner RC. United Kingdom Prospective Diabetes Study, 30: diabetic retinopathy at diagnosis of non-insulin-dependent diabetes mellitus and associated risk factors. Arch Ophthalmol 1998;116:297–303.
12. Cheung N, Wong TY. Obesity and eye diseases. Surv Ophthalmol 2007;52:180–95.
13. Conway BN, Miller RG, Klein R, Orchard TJ. Prediction of proliferative diabetic retinopathy with hemoglobin level. Arch Ophthalmol 2009;127:1494–9.
14. Yang JK, Liu W, Shi J, Li YB. An association between subclinical hypothyroidism and sight-threatening diabetic retinopathy in type 2 diabetic patients. Diabetes Care 2010;33:1018–20.
15. Klein BE, Knudtson MD, Tsai MY, Klein R. The relation of markers of inflammation and endothelial dysfunction to the prevalence and progression of diabetic retinopathy: Wisconsin epidemiologic study of diabetic retinopathy. Arch Ophthalmol 2009;127:1175–82.
16. Cheung N, Rogers S, Couper DJ, Klein R, Sharrett AR, Wong TY. Is diabetic retinopathy an independent risk factor for ischemic stroke? Stroke 2007;38:398–401.
17. Cheung N, Wang JJ, Klein R, Couper DJ, Sharrett AR, Wong TY. Diabetic retinopathy and the risk of coronary heart disease: the Atherosclerosis Risk in Communities Study. Diabetes Care 2007;30:1742–6.
18. Cheung N, Wang JJ, Rogers SL, Brancati F, Klein R, Sharrett AR, Wong TY. Diabetic retinopathy and risk of heart failure. J Am Coll Cardiol 2008;51:1573–8.
19. Kern TS, Engerman RL. Capillary lesions develop in retina rather than cerebral cortex in diabetes and experimental galactosemia. Arch Ophthalmol 1996;114:306–10.
20. Arden GB, Wolf JE, Tsang Y. Does dark adaptation exacerbate diabetic retinopathy? Evidence and a linking hypothesis. Vision Res 1998;38:1723–9.
21. Arden GB. The absence of diabetic retinopathy in patients with retinitis pigmentosa: implications for

pathophysiology and possible treatment. *Br J Ophthalmol* 2001;**85**:366−70.

22. Duffy A, Liew A, O'Sullivan J, Avalos G, Samali A, O'Brien T. Distinct effects of high-glucose conditions on endothelial cells of macrovascular and microvascular origins. *Endothelium* 2006;**13**:9−16.

23. Carr ME. Diabetes mellitus: a hypercoagulable state. *J Diabetes Complications* 2001;**15**:44−54.

24. Ishibashi T, Inoue S, Tanaka K. Fibrinolytic activity of the retinae in streptozotocin-diabetic rats. *Invest Ophthalmol Vis Sci* 1985;**26**:125−7.

25. Ishibashi T, Tanaka K, Taniguchi Y. Platelet aggregation and coagulation in the pathogenesis of diabetic retinopathy in rats. *Diabetes* 1981;**30**:601−6.

26. Ashton N. Studies of the retinal capillaries in relation to diabetic and other retinopathies. *Br J Ophthalmol* 1963;**47**:521−38.

27. Mizutani M, Kern TS, Lorenzi M. Accelerated death of retinal microvascular cells in human and experimental diabetic retinopathy. *J Clin Invest* 1996;**97**: 2883−90.

28. Murata T, Ishibashi T, Inomata H. Immunohistochemical detection of extravasated fibrinogen (fibrin) in human diabetic retina. *Graefes Arch Clin Exp Ophthalmol* 1992;**230**:428−31.

29. Joussen AM, Murata T, Tsujikawa A, Kirchhof B, Bursell SE, Adamis AP. Leukocyte-mediated endothelial cell injury and death in the diabetic retina. *Am J Pathol* 2001;**158**:147−52.

30. Schroder S, Palinski W, Schmid-Schonbein GW. Activated monocytes and granulocytes, capillary nonperfusion, and neovascularization in diabetic retinopathy. *Am J Pathol* 1991;**139**:81−100.

31. Gardner TW, Lieth E, Khin SA, Barber AJ, Bonsall DJ, Lesher T, Rice K, Brennan Jr WA. Astrocytes increase barrier properties and ZO-1 expression in retinal vascular endothelial cells. *Invest Ophthalmol Vis Sci* 1997;**38**:2423−7.

32. Ishibashi T, Tanaka K, Taniguchi Y. Disruption of blood−retinal barrier in experimental diabetic rats: an electron microscopic study. *Exp Eye Res* 1980;**30**: 401−10.

33. Ishibashi T, Inomata H. Ultrastructure of retinal vessels in diabetic patients. *Br J Ophthalmol* 1993;**77**: 574−8.

34. Uemura A, Ogawa M, Hirashima M, Fujiwara T, Koyama S, Takagi H, Honda Y, Wiegand SJ, Yancopoulos GD, Nishikawa S. Recombinant angiopoietin-1 restores higher-order architecture of growing blood vessels in mice in the absence of mural cells. *J Clin Invest* 2002;**110**:1619−28.

35. Hata Y, Nakagawa K, Ishibashi T, Inomata H, Ueno H, Sueishi K. Hypoxia-induced expression of

vascular endothelial growth factor by retinal glial cells promotes in vitro angiogenesis. *Virchows Arch* 1995;**426**:479−86.

36. Murata T, Nakagawa K, Khalil A, Ishibashi T, Inomata H, Sueishi K. The relation between expression of vascular endothelial growth factor and breakdown of the blood−retinal barrier in diabetic rat retinas. *Lab Invest* 1996;**74**:819−25.

37. Miyamoto K, Khosrof S, Bursell SE, Rohan R, Murata T, Clermont AC, Aiello LP, Ogura Y, Adamis AP. Prevention of leukostasis and vascular leakage in streptozotocin-induced diabetic retinopathy via intercellular adhesion molecule-1 inhibition. *Proc Natl Acad Sci USA* 1999;**96**:10836−41.

38. Yamashiro K, Tsujikawa A, Ishida S, Usui T, Kaji Y, Honda Y, Ogura Y, Adamis AP. Platelets accumulate in the diabetic retinal vasculature following endothelial death and suppress blood−retinal barrier breakdown. *Am J Pathol* 2003;**163**:253−9.

39. Sunderkotter C, Steinbrink K, Goebeler M, Bhardwaj R, Sorg C. Macrophages and angiogenesis. *J Leukoc Biol* 1994;**55**:410−22.

40. Nakao S, Kuwano T, Tsutsumi-Miyahara C, Ueda S, Kimura YN, Hamano S, Sonoda KH, Saijo Y, Nukiwa T, Strieter RM, Ishibashi T, Kuwano M, Ono M. Infiltration of COX-2-expressing macrophages is a prerequisite for IL-1 beta-induced neovascularization and tumor growth. *J Clin Invest* 2005;**115**:2979−91.

41. Kisucka J, Butterfield CE, Duda DG, Eichenberger SC, Saffaripour S, Ware J, Ruggeri ZM, Jain RK, Folkman J, Wagner DD. Platelets and platelet adhesion support angiogenesis while preventing excessive hemorrhage. *Proc Natl Acad Sci USA* 2006;**103**:855−60.

42. Noda K, Ishida S, Inoue M, Obata K, Oguchi Y, Okada Y, Ikeda E. Production and activation of matrix metalloproteinase-2 in proliferative diabetic retinopathy. *Invest Ophthalmol Vis Sci* 2003;**44**: 2163−70.

43. Aiello LP, Avery RL, Arrigg PG, Keyt BA, Jampel HD, Shah ST, Pasquale LR, Thieme H, Iwamoto MA, Park JE, et al. Vascular endothelial growth factor in ocular fluid of patients with diabetic retinopathy and other retinal disorders. *N Engl J Med* 1994;**331**:1480−7.

44. Yoshimura T, Sonoda KH, Sugahara M, Mochizuki Y, Enaida H, Oshima Y, Ueno A, Hata Y, Yoshida H, Ishibashi T. Comprehensive analysis of inflammatory immune mediators in vitreoretinal diseases. *PLoS One* 2009;**4**:e8158.

45. Dana GW. Type of diabetes mellitus associated with diabetic retinitis. *AMA Arch Ophthalmol* 1953;**50**:123−4.

II. TYPES OF DIABETES AND ITS CORRELATION WITH OTHER DISEASES

46. Noda K, Nakao S, Zandi S, Engelstadter V, Mashima Y, Hafezi-Moghadam A. Vascular adhesion protein-1 regulates leukocyte transmigration rate in the retina during diabetes. *Exp Eye Res* 2009;**89**:774—81.

47. Joussen AM, Poulaki V, Mitsiades N, Kirchhof B, Koizumi K, Dohmen S, Adamis AP. Nonsteroidal anti-inflammatory drugs prevent early diabetic retinopathy via TNF-alpha suppression. *Faseb J* 2002;**16**:438—40.

48. Huang H, Gandhi JK, Zhong X, Wei Y, Gong J, Duh EJ, Vinores SA. TNF{alpha} is required for late BRB breakdown in diabetic retinopathy and its inhibition prevents leukostasis and protects vessels and neurons from apoptosis. *Invest Ophthalmol Vis Sci* 2011.

49. Ferrara N, Gerber HP, LeCouter J. The biology of VEGF and its receptors. *Nat Med* 2003;**9**:669—76.

50. Nicholson BP, Schachat AP. A review of clinical trials of anti-VEGF agents for diabetic retinopathy. *Graefes Arch Clin Exp Ophthalmol* 2010;**248**:915—30.

51. Riento K, Ridley AJ. Rocks: multifunctional kinases in cell behaviour. *Nat Rev Mol Cell Biol* 2003;**4**: 446—56.

52. Iwasaki H, Okamoto R, Kato S, Konishi K, Mizutani H, Yamada N, Isaka N, Nakano T, Ito M. High glucose induces plasminogen activator inhibitor-1 expression through Rho/Rho-kinase-mediated NF-kappaB activation in bovine aortic endothelial cells. *Atherosclerosis* 2008;**196**:22—8.

53. Kolavennu V, Zeng L, Peng H, Wang Y, Danesh FR. Targeting of RhoA/ROCK signaling ameliorates progression of diabetic nephropathy independent of glucose control. *Diabetes* 2008;**57**:714—23.

54. Tang J, Kusaka I, Massey AR, Rollins S, Zhang JH. Increased RhoA translocation in aorta of diabetic rats. *Acta Pharmacol Sin* 2006;**27**:543—8.

55. Arita R, Hata Y, Nakao S, Kita T, Miura M, Kawahara S, Zandi S, Almulki L, Tayyari F, Shimokawa H, Hafezi-Moghadam A, Ishibashi T. Rho kinase inhibition by fasudil ameliorates diabetes-induced microvascular damage. *Diabetes* 2009;**58**:215—26.

56. Hata Y, Miura M, Nakao S, Kawahara S, Kita T, Ishibashi T. Antiangiogenic properties of fasudil, a potent Rho-Kinase inhibitor. *Jpn J Ophthalmol* 2008;**52**:16—23.

57. Kita T, Hata Y, Kano K, Miura M, Nakao S, Noda Y, Shimokawa H, Ishibashi T. Transforming growth factor-beta2 and connective tissue growth factor in proliferative vitreoretinal diseases: possible involvement of hyalocytes and therapeutic potential of Rho kinase inhibitor. *Diabetes* 2007;**56**:231—8.

58. Kita T, Hata Y, Arita R, Kawahara S, Miura M, Nakao S, Mochizuki Y, Enaida H, Goto Y, Shimokawa H, Hafezi-Moghadam A, Ishibashi T. Role of TGF-beta in proliferative vitreoretinal diseases and ROCK as a therapeutic target. *Proc Natl Acad Sci USA* 2008;**105**:17504—9.

59. Kawahara S, Hata Y, Kita T, Arita R, Miura M, Nakao S, Mochizuki Y, Enaida H, Kagimoto T, Goto Y, Hafezi-Moghadam A, Ishibashi T. Potent inhibition of cicatricial contraction in proliferative vitreoretinal diseases by statins. *Diabetes* 2008;**57**:2784—93.

60. Arita R, Hata Y, Ishibashi T. ROCK as a therapeutic target of diabetic retinopathy. *J Ophthalmol* 2010; **2010**:175163.

61. Hamburg A. Some investigations on the cells of the vitreous body. *Ophthalmologica* 1959;**138**:81—107.

62. Noda Y, Hata Y, Hisatomi T, Nakamura Y, Hirayama K, Miura M, Nakao S, Fujisawa K, Sakamoto T, Ishibashi T. Functional properties of hyalocytes under PDGF-rich conditions. *Invest Ophthalmol Vis Sci* 2004;**45**:2107—14.

63. Qiao H, Hisatomi T, Sonoda KH, Kura S, Sassa Y, Kinoshita S, Nakamura T, Sakamoto T, Ishibashi T. The characterisation of hyalocytes: the origin, phenotype, and turnover. *Br J Ophthalmol* 2005;**89**: 513—7.

64. Haddad A, Andre JC. Hyalocyte-like cells are more numerous in the posterior chamber than they are in the vitreous of the rabbit eye. *Exp Eye Res* 1998;**66**: 709—18.

65. Kita T, Hata Y, Miura M, Kawahara S, Nakao S, Ishibashi T. Functional characteristics of connective tissue growth factor on vitreoretinal cells. *Diabetes* 2007;**56**:1421—8.

66. Armstrong D, Augustin AJ, Spengler R, Al-Jada A, Nickola T, Grus F, Koch F. Detection of vascular endothelial growth factor and tumor necrosis factor alpha in epiretinal membranes of proliferative diabetic retinopathy, proliferative vitreoretinopathy and macular pucker. *Ophthalmologica* 1998;**212**: 410—4.

67. Hata Y, Nakao S, Kohno R, Oba K, Kita T, Miura M, Sassa Y, Schering A, Ishibashi T. Role of tumour necrosis factor-{alpha} (TNF{alpha}) in the functional properties of hyalocytes. *Br J Ophthalmol* 2011;**95**:261—5.

68. Hata Y, Sassa Y, Kita T, Miura M, Kano K, Kawahara S, Arita R, Nakao S, Shih JL, Ishibashi T. Vascular endothelial growth factor expression by hyalocytes and its regulation by glucocorticoid. *Br J Ophthalmol* 2008;**92**:1540—4.

69. Ockrim Z, Yorston D. Managing diabetic retinopathy. *BMJ* 2010;**341**:c5400.

70. Antonetti DA, Barber AJ, Bronson SK, Freeman WM, Gardner TW, Jefferson LS, Kester M, Kimball SR, Krady JK, LaNoue KF, Norbury CC, Quinn PG, Sandirasegarane L, Simpson IA. Diabetic retinopathy: seeing beyond glucose-induced microvascular disease. *Diabetes* 2006;**55**:2401—11.

71. Wolter JR. Diabetic retinopathy. *Am J Ophthalmol* 1961;**51**:1123—41.

72. Rothova A, Meenken C, Michels RP, Kijlstra A. Uveitis and diabetes mellitus. *Am J Ophthalmol* 1988;**106**:17—20.

73. Javitt JC, Wang F, West SK. Blindness due to cataract: epidemiology and prevention. *Annu Rev Public Health* 1996;**17**:159—77.

74. The effect of intensive treatment of diabetes on the development and progression of long-term complications in insulin-dependent diabetes mellitus. The Diabetes Control and Complications Trial Research Group. *N Engl J Med* 1993;**329**:977—86.

75. Progression of retinopathy with intensive versus conventional treatment in the Diabetes Control and Complications Trial. Diabetes Control and Complications Trial Research Group. *Ophthalmology* 1995;**102**:647—61.

76. Intensive blood-glucose control with sulphonylureas or insulin compared with conventional treatment and risk of complications in patients with type 2 diabetes (UKPDS 33). UK Prospective Diabetes Study (UKPDS) Group. *Lancet* 1998;**352**:837—53.

77. Early worsening of diabetic retinopathy in the Diabetes Control and Complications Trial. *Arch Ophthalmol* 1998;**116**:874—86.

78. Jax TW. Metabolic memory: a vascular perspective. *Cardiovasc Diabetol* 2010;**9**:51.

79. Suzuma I, Hata Y, Clermont A, Pokras F, Rook SL, Suzuma K, Feener EP, Aiello LP. Cyclic stretch and hypertension induce retinal expression of vascular endothelial growth factor and vascular endothelial growth factor receptor-2: potential mechanisms for exacerbation of diabetic retinopathy by hypertension. *Diabetes* 2001;**50**:444—54.

80. Nagai N, Izumi-Nagai K, Oike Y, Koto T, Satofuka S, Ozawa Y, Yamashiro K, Inoue M, Tsubota K, Umezawa K, Ishida S. Suppression of diabetes-induced retinal inflammation by blocking the angiotensin II type 1 receptor or its downstream nuclear factor-kappaB pathway. *Invest Ophthalmol Vis Sci* 2007;**48**:4342—50.

81. Silva PS, Cavallerano JD, Sun JK, Aiello LM, Aiello LP. Effect of systemic medications on onset and progression of diabetic retinopathy. *Nat Rev Endocrinol* 2010;**6**:494—508.

82. Chew EY, Klein ML, Ferris 3rd FL, Remaley NA, Murphy RP, Chantry K, Hoogwerf BJ, Miller D. Association of elevated serum lipid levels with retinal hard exudate in diabetic retinopathy. Early Treatment Diabetic Retinopathy Study (ETDRS) Report 22. *Arch Ophthalmol* 1996;**114**:1079—84.

83. Klein BE, Moss SE, Klein R, Surawicz TS. The Wisconsin Epidemiologic Study of Diabetic Retinopathy. XIII. Relationship of serum cholesterol to retinopathy and hard exudate. *Ophthalmology* 1991;**98**:1261—5.

84. Lyons TJ, Jenkins AJ, Zheng D, Lackland DT, McGee D, Garvey WT, Klein RL. Diabetic retinopathy and serum lipoprotein subclasses in the DCCT/EDIC cohort. *Invest Ophthalmol Vis Sci* 2004;**45**:910—8.

85. Keech AC, Mitchell P, Summanen PA, O'Day J, Davis TM, Moffitt MS, Taskinen MR, Simes RJ, Tse D, Williamson E, Merrifield A, Laatikainen LT, d'Emden MC, Crimet DC, O'Connell RL, Colman PG. Effect of fenofibrate on the need for laser treatment for diabetic retinopathy (FIELD study): a randomised controlled trial. *Lancet* 2007;**370**:1687—97.

86. Miyahara S, Kiryu J, Yamashiro K, Miyamoto K, Hirose F, Tamura H, Katsuta H, Nishijima K, Tsujikawa A, Honda Y. Simvastatin inhibits leukocyte accumulation and vascular permeability in the retinas of rats with streptozotocin-induced diabetes. *Am J Pathol* 2004;**164**:1697—706.

87. Nakao S, Hata Y, Miura M, Noda K, Kimura YN, Kawahara S, Kita T, Hisatomi T, Nakazawa T, Jin Y, Dana MR, Kuwano M, Ono M, Ishibashi T, Hafezi-Moghadam A. Dexamethasone inhibits interleukin-1beta-induced corneal neovascularization: role of nuclear factor-kappaB-activated stromal cells in inflammatory angiogenesis. *Am J Pathol* 2007;**171**:1058—65.

88. Chew E, Strauber S, Beck R, Aiello LP, Antoszyk A, Bressler N, Browning D, Danis R, Fan J, Flaxel C, Friedman S, Glassman A, Kollman C, Lazarus H. Randomized trial of peribulbar triamcinolone acetonide with and without focal photocoagulation for mild diabetic macular edema: a pilot study. *Ophthalmology* 2007;**114**:1190—6.

89. Chew EY, Glassman AR, Beck RW, Bressler NM, Fish GE, Ferris FL, Kinyoun JL. Ocular side effects associated with peribulbar injections of triamcinolone acetonide for diabetic macular edema. *Retina* 2011;**31**:284—9.

90. Bressler NM, Edwards AR, Beck RW, Flaxel CJ, Glassman AR, Ip MS, Kollman C, Kuppermann BD, Stone TW. Exploratory analysis of diabetic retinopathy progression through 3 years in a randomized clinical trial that compares intravitreal triamcinolone acetonide with focal/grid photocoagulation. *Arch Ophthalmol* 2009;**127**:1566—71.

91. Jonas JB, Kreissig I, Sofker A, Degenring RF. Intravitreal injection of triamcinolone for diffuse diabetic macular edema. *Arch Ophthalmol* 2003;**121**:57—61.

92. Yilmaz T, Weaver CD, Gallagher MJ, Cordero-Coma M, Cervantes-Castaneda RA, Klisovic D, Lavaque AJ, Larson RJ. Intravitreal triamcinolone acetonide injection for treatment of refractory diabetic macular edema: a systematic review. *Ophthalmology* 2009;**116**:902—11. quiz 912—3.

93. Roth DB, Chieh J, Spirn MJ, Green SN, Yarian DL, Chaudhry NA. Noninfectious endophthalmitis associated with intravitreal triamcinolone injection. *Arch Ophthalmol* 2003;**121**:1279—82.

94. Haritoglou C, Kook D, Neubauer A, Wolf A, Priglinger S, Strauss R, Gandorfer A, Ulbig M, Kampik A. Intravitreal bevacizumab (Avastin) therapy for persistent diffuse diabetic macular edema. *Retina* 2006;**26**:999—1005.

95. Elman MJ, Aiello LP, Beck RW, Bressler NM, Bressler SB, Edwards AR, Ferris 3rd FL, Friedman SM, Glassman AR, Miller KM, Scott IU, Stockdale CR, Sun JK. Randomized trial evaluating ranibizumab plus prompt or deferred laser or triamcinolone plus prompt laser for diabetic macular edema. *Ophthalmology* 2010;**117**:1064—77. e1035.

96. Kohno R, Hata Y, Mochizuki Y, Arita R, Kawahara S, Kita T, Miyazaki M, Hisatomi T, Ikeda Y, Aiello LP, Ishibashi T. Histopathology of neovascular tissue from eyes with proliferative diabetic retinopathy after intravitreal bevacizumab injection. *Am J Ophthalmol* 2010;**150**:223—9. e221.

97. Arevalo JF, Maia M, Flynn Jr HW, Saravia M, Avery RL, Wu L, Eid Farah M, Pieramici DJ, Berrocal MH, Sanchez JG. Tractional retinal detachment following intravitreal bevacizumab (Avastin) in patients with severe proliferative diabetic retinopathy. *Br J Ophthalmol* 2008;**92**:213—6.

98. Moradian S, Ahmadieh H, Malihi M, Soheilian M, Dehghan MH, Azarmina M. Intravitreal bevacizumab in active progressive proliferative diabetic retinopathy. *Graefes Arch Clin Exp Ophthalmol* 2008;**246**:1699—705.

99. Saint-Geniez M, Maharaj AS, Walshe TE, Tucker BA, Sekiyama E, Kurihara T, Darland DC, Young MJ, D'Amore PA. Endogenous VEGF is required for visual function: evidence for a survival role on muller cells and photoreceptors. *PLoS One* 2008;**3**:e3554.

100. Saint-Geniez M, Kurihara T, Sekiyama E, Maldonado AE, D'Amore PA. An essential role for RPE-derived soluble VEGF in the maintenance of the choriocapillaris. *Proc Natl Acad Sci USA* 2009;**106**:18751—6.

101. Murakami Y, Ikeda Y, Yonemitsu Y, Miyazaki M, Inoue M, Hasegawa M, Sueishi K, Ishibashi T. Inhibition of choroidal neovascularization via brief subretinal exposure to a newly developed lentiviral vector pseudotyped with Sendai viral envelope proteins. *Hum Gene Ther* 2010;**21**:199—209.

102. Treatment techniques and clinical guidelines for photocoagulation of diabetic macular edema. Early Treatment Diabetic Retinopathy Study Report Number 2. Early Treatment Diabetic Retinopathy Study Research Group. *Ophthalmology* 1987;**94**:761—74.

103. Two-year course of visual acuity in severe proliferative diabetic retinopathy with conventional management. Diabetic Retinopathy Vitrectomy Study (DRVS) report #1. *Ophthalmology* 1985;**92**:492—502.

104. Early vitrectomy for severe vitreous hemorrhage in diabetic retinopathy. Two-year results of a randomized trial. Diabetic Retinopathy Vitrectomy Study report 2. The Diabetic Retinopathy Vitrectomy Study Research Group. *Arch Ophthalmol* 1985;**103**:1644—52.

105. Gandorfer A, Messmer EM, Ulbig MW, Kampik A. Resolution of diabetic macular edema after surgical removal of the posterior hyaloid and the inner limiting membrane. *Retina* 2000;**20**:126—33.

An Overview of Diabetic Retinopathy

Stephen G. Schwartz*, Harry W. Flynn, Jr.[†]

*Bascom Palmer Eye Institute, University of Miami Miller School of Medicine, Naples, FL, USA
[†]Bascom Palmer Eye Institute, University of Miami Miller School of Medicine, Miami, FL, USA

INTRODUCTION

Despite improvements in the medical care of patients with diabetes mellitus, diabetic retinopathy remains an important worldwide cause of visual loss. This chapter briefly reviews the clinical features and evidence-based management of diabetic retinopathy, including investigational pharmacotherapies currently in clinical trials.

EPIDEMIOLOGY

In the US, diabetic retinopathy is a very common complication of diabetes mellitus as well as the leading cause of visual loss among adults aged 20–64 years.[1] The natural history of diabetic retinopathy is that of progressive disease.

The Wisconsin Epidemiologic Study of Diabetic Retinopathy (WESDR) reported that, among patients diagnosed with diabetes mellitus at age 30 years or older, the prevalence of diabetic retinopathy increased from 28.8% in persons with disease duration of less than 5 years to 77.8% in persons with disease duration of 15 or more years. Similarly, the rate of proliferative diabetic retinopathy (PDR) increased from 2% in persons with disease duration of less than 5 years to 15.5% in persons with disease duration of 15 or more years.[2] WESDR also reported that, among patients diagnosed with diabetes

Nutritional and Therapeutic Interventions for Diabetes and Metabolic Syndrome
DOI: 10.1016/B978-0-12-385083-6.00014-0

mellitus at age 30 years or older, the prevalence of diabetic macular edema (DME) increased from 3% in persons with disease duration of less than 5 years to 28% in persons with disease duration of 20 or more years.[3]

More recently, the National Health and Nutrition Examination Survey (NHANES) reported the estimated prevalence of diabetic retinopathy at 28.5% of US adult diabetics aged 40 years and older. The estimated prevalence of vision-threatening diabetic retinopathy was 4.4%. Diabetic retinopathy was more prevalent among males, among non-Hispanic black individuals, and in patients with longer durations of diabetes, higher systolic blood pressure, and higher hemoglobin A1c levels.[4]

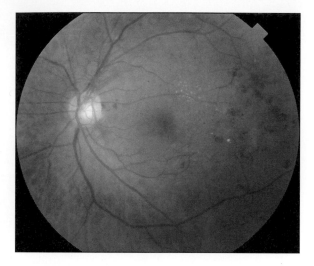

FIGURE 14.1 **Proliferative diabetic retinopathy.** Fundus photograph, left eye, demonstrating proliferative diabetic retinopathy with prominent neovascularization of the disc. (*See the color plate section at the back of the book.*)

CLASSIFICATION

Diabetic retinopathy is classified as either nonproliferative diabetic retinopathy (NPDR) or PDR. NPDR is characterized by the presence of retinal microaneurysms, intraretinal hemorrhages, intraretinal exudates, and other retinal vascular anomalies, including intraretinal microvascular abnormalities (IRMA) and venous beading.

PDR is characterized by the presence of neovascularization. Neovascularization may occur on the optic disc [neovascularization of the disc (NVD)] or elsewhere on the retina [neovascularization elsewhere (NVE)] (Figure 14.1). PDR may progress to vitreous hemorrhage and traction retinal detachment, with subsequent severe visual loss. Neovascularization may also occur on the iris [neovascularization of the iris (NVI)] which may progress to neovascular glaucoma (NVG).

RANDOMIZED CLINICAL TRIALS

The treatment of diabetic retinopathy is guided by the results of many large, prospective,

multicenter randomized clinical trials (RCTs). The Diabetes Control and Complication Trial (DCCT) reported that intensive control of systemic metabolic factors, including blood sugar, blood pressure, and serum lipids, is associated with a reduced incidence of diabetic retinopathy in patients with type 1 diabetes mellitus.[5] The United Kingdom Prospective Diabetic Study (UKPDS) reported similar outcomes in patients with type 2 diabetes mellitus.[6] Patients with diabetic retinopathy are generally advised to consult with their internist or endocrinologist to achieve tighter control of their metabolic factors.

The Diabetic Retinopathy Study (DRS) reported that panretinal photocoagulation (PRP) reduced the incidence of severe visual loss (defined as visual acuity worse than 5/200 at two consecutive visits) in patients with PDR.[7] In this trial, the DRS defined certain high-risk characteristics, including NVD greater than that visualized on a standard photograph, or any NVD or NVE in the presence of preretinal or vitreous hemorrhage. PRP is typically performed in a clinic setting using topical anesthesia and an argon-green laser or similar instrument (Figure 14.2).

The Early Treatment Diabetic Retinopathy Study (ETDRS) reported that focal/grid photocoagulation reduced the incidence of moderate visual loss (defined as doubling of the visual angle) in patients with clinically significant macular edema (CSME).[8] In this trial, CSME was defined as thickening of the retina at or within 500 μm of the center of the macula; hard exudates at or within 500 μm of the center of the macula, if associated with thickening of the adjacent retina; or a zone of retinal thickening one disc area or larger in size, any part of which is within one disc area of the center of the macula. Focal/grid photocoagulation is typically performed in a clinic setting using topical anesthesia and an argon-green laser or similar instrument (Figures 14.3–14.5).

The Diabetic Retinopathy Vitrectomy Study (DRVS) compared treatments of patients with

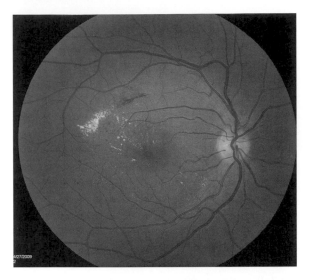

FIGURE 14.3 Diabetic macular edema. Fundus photograph, right eye, demonstrating diabetic macular edema with retinal thickening and hard exudates. (*See the color plate section at the back of the book.*)

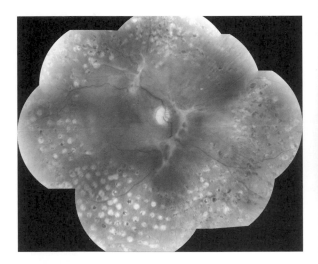

FIGURE 14.2 Panretinal photocoagulation. Montage fundus photograph, right eye, demonstrating regressed proliferative diabetic retinopathy following treatment with panretinal photocoagulation. (*See the color plate section at the back of the book.*)

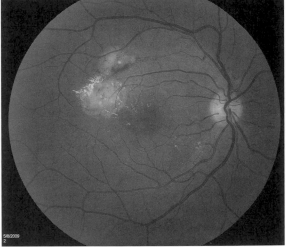

FIGURE 14.4 Focal photocoagulation. Fundus photograph, right eye, demonstrating the same patient as in Figure 14.3, immediately following focal photocoagulation of diabetic macular edema. (*See the color plate section at the back of the book.*)

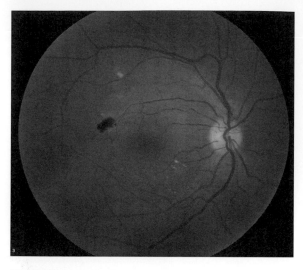

FIGURE 14.5 **Focal photocoagulation.** Fundus photograph, right eye, demonstrating the same patient as in Figures 14.3 and 14.4, approximately one year following focal photocoagulation of diabetic macular edema. (*See the color plate section at the back of the book.*)

severe vitreous hemorrhage. Patients were randomized to receive early (defined as within 1–6 months) pars plana vitrectomy (PPV) or deferred (defined as 1 year) PPV. The DRVS reported that early PPV was associated with a greater incidence of achieving 20/40 or better visual acuity.[9] The Diabetic Retinopathy Clinical Research (DRCR) Network reported that PPV may also be beneficial in patients with DME associated with vitreomacular traction.[10] PPV is typically performed in an operating room setting using local (retrobulbar) or occasionally general anesthesia.

The ETDRS subsequently reported that aspirin use was not associated with an increased rate of vitreous hemorrhage and was not associated with progression of diabetic retinopathy.[11] Therefore, aspirin is generally not contraindicated in patients with existing diabetic retinopathy.

The benefits of photocoagulation and PPV have been known for decades. Unfortunately, some patients continue to lose vision despite these interventions. This has led to the investigation of various pharmacotherapies to treat DME and PDR.[12] These include local (ocular) and systemic agents. Local agents are frequently delivered via office-based intravitreal injection. Although the visual benefits may be significant, there is a small risk of vision-threatening infection, or endophthalmitis, in about 0.05% of injections.[13]

Intravitreal triamcinolone acetonide (IVTA) is associated with short-term anatomic and visual improvement of DME. The DRCR Network completed a large, multicenter RCT comparing two doses (1 mg and 4 mg) of IVTA *vs* photocoagulation for DME. After 2 years of follow-up, treatment with photocoagulation was associated with generally more favorable visual outcomes than was treatment with IVTA.[14] In a subsequent study, the generally more favorable outcomes associated with photocoagulation persisted for 3 years of follow-up.[15] Intravitreal corticosteroids are associated with risks of cataract formation and intraocular pressure (IOP) elevation. IVTA is not currently approved by the US FDA for this indication.

A fluocinolone-eluting intravitreal implant (Iluvien, Alimera Sciences, Alpharetta, GA), which may be administered through a 25-gauge injection in a clinic setting, has been studied as a longer-term treatment for DME. In the FAMOUS (Pharmacokinetic and Efficiency Study of Fluocinolone Acetonide Inserts in Patients with DME) trial, the implant was reported to release fluocinolone for at least 1 year in patients with DME.[16] The FAME (Fluocinolone Acetonide in Diabetic Macular Edema) Study comprises two phase 3 RCTs, which reported that the fluocinolone implant was associated with generally more favorable anatomic and visual outcomes than was standard treatment, although the implant was associated with an increased risk of IOP elevation[17]. The fluocinolone implant is not currently approved by the US FDA.

Vascular endothelial growth factor (VEGF) antagonists have also been studied as pharmacotherapies for DME. Ranibizumab (Lucentis, Genentech, South San Francisco, CA) is FDA-approved in the treatment of exudative age-related macular degeneration and macular edema associated with retinal vein occlusion. It is also being studied as a treatment for DME. The READ-2 (Ranibizumab for Edema of the Macula in Diabetes) Study reported generally favorable outcomes in patients with DME for up to 2 years.[18]

The DRCR reported that combination therapy with ranibizumab and photocoagulation was more effective than photocoagulation alone for up to 1 year.[19] In spite of the strongly positive RCT data, ranibizumab is not currently approved by the US FDA for this indication.

Bevacizumab (Avastin, Genentech, South San Francisco, CA) is FDA-approved for the systemic treatment of various malignancies. Because of its ready availability and relatively low cost, it is commonly used as an off-label intravitreal treatment of various retinal diseases, including DME and PDR. The DRCR network conducted a phase 2 RCT and reported some evidence of efficacy.[20] The BOLT (Bevacizumab or Laser Therapy in the Management of DME) Study randomized patients with persistent DME to receive either bevacizumab or additional focal/grid photocoagulation and reported more favorable outcomes in the bevacizumab group.[21]

Bevacizumab is also used as an adjunctive therapy for PDR. A small RCT reported that preoperative bevacizumab improved surgical outcomes in patients undergoing PPV for severe PDR by reducing retinal and iris neovascularization.[22] Another small RCT reported that preoperative bevacizumab reduced the incidence of postoperative vitreous hemorrhage following PPV.[23]

Activation of protein kinase C (PKC) may play an important role in the pathogenesis of diabetic retinopathy. Ruboxistaurin, an orally administered selective antagonist of the PKC β isoforms, has been studied in multiple RCTs as a systemic therapy for diabetic retinopathy. The PKC-Diabetic Retinopathy Study (PKC-DRS) reported that ruboxistaurin reduced the incidence of moderate visual loss (doubling of the visual angle) in some patients with NPDR.[24] The PKC-DRS2 study reported that ruboxistaurin reduced sustained moderate visual loss (for 6 months) in some patients with NPDR.[25] The PKC-DME Study (PKC-DMES) reported evidence that ruboxistaurin delayed progression of DME, although the study's primary end point was not achieved.[26] Ruboxistaurin is not currently approved by the US FDA.

TREATMENT GUIDELINES

Patients with diabetes mellitus generally receive dilated eye examinations on a regular basis. Communication between the ophthalmologist and the internist or endocrinologist caring for the patient is encouraged.

Most patients with CSME, and some patients with milder DME, are considered for focal/grid photocoagulation. Patients with recurrent DME, and patients judged to be poor candidates for photocoagulation, may be considered for pharmacological therapies. In phakic patients, off-label intravitreal bevacizumab may be considered, because of its relatively low cost and its lack of association with cataract formation. IVTA may be considered in pseudophakic patients and in patients with severe DME unresponsive to other therapies.

Most patients with "high-risk" PDR, and some patients with milder PDR and severe NPDR, are considered for PRP. Patients with vitreous hemorrhage that precludes PRP may be observed for a period of time, or may be considered for off-label intravitreal bevacizumab. Although intravitreal bevacizumab may provide short-term regression of PDR in many patients, the effect is typically temporary and subsequent PRP is generally recommended. Patients with chronic vitreous hemorrhage unresponsive to observation and/or bevacizumab may be considered for PPV. Some patients with other structural abnormalities (including vitreomacular traction and traction retinal detachment) may also be considered for PPV.

Acknowledgments

Partially supported by NIH Center Grant P30-EY014801 and by an unrestricted grant from the University of Miami from Research to Prevent Blindness, New York, NY.

References

1. Fong DS, Aiello LP, Ferris, 3rd FL, Klein R. Diabetic retinopathy. *Diabetes Care* 2004;**27**:2540−53.
2. Klein R, Klein BE, Moss SE, Davis MD, DeMets DL. The Wisconsin epidemiologic study of diabetic retinopathy. III. Prevalence and risk of diabetic retinopathy when age at diagnosis is 30 or more years. *Arch Ophthalmol* 1984;**102**:527−32.
3. Klein R, Klein BE, Moss SE, Davis MD, DeMets DL. The Wisconsin epidemiologic study of diabetic retinopathy. IV. Diabetic macular edema. *Ophthalmology* 1984;**91**:1464−74.
4. Zhang X, Saaddine JB, Chou CF, Cotch MF, Cheng YJ, Geiss LS, Gregg EW, Albright AL, Klein BEK, Klein R. Prevalence of diabetic retinopathy in the United States, 2005−2008. *JAMA* 2010;**304**:649−56.
5. Diabetes Control and Complication Trial Research Group. The effect of intensive treatment of diabetes on the development and progression of long-term complications in insulin-dependent diabetes mellitus. *N Engl J Med* 1993;**329**:977−86.
6. UK Prospective Diabetes Study Group. Intensive blood-glucose control with sulphonylureas or insulin compared with conventional treatment and risk of complications in patients with type 2 diabetes. UKPDS 33. *Lancet* 1998;**352**:837−53.
7. The Diabetic Retinopathy Study Research Group. Photocoagulation treatment of proliferative diabetic retinopathy. Clinical application of Diabetic Retinopathy Study (DRS) findings, DRS Report Number 8. The Diabetic Retinopathy Study Research Group. *Ophthalmology* 1981;**88**:583−600.
8. Early Treatment Diabetic Retinopathy Study Research Group. Photocoagulation for diabetic macular edema. Early Treatment Diabetic Retinopathy Study report number 1. *Arch Ophthalmol* 1985;**103**:1796−806.
9. Diabetic Retinopathy Vitrectomy Study Research Group. Early vitrectomy for severe vitreous hemorrhage in diabetic retinopathy. Two-year results of a randomized trial. Diabetic Retinopathy Vitrectomy Study report 2. *Arch Ophthalmol* 1985;**103**:1644−52.
10. Diabetic Retinopathy Clinical Research Network Writing Committee, Haller JA, Qin H, Apte RS, Beck RR, Bressler NM, Browning DJ, Danis RP, Glassman AR, Googe JM, Kollman C, Lauer AK, Peters MA, Stockman ME. Vitrectomy outcomes in eyes with diabetic macular edema and vitreomacular traction. *Ophthalmology* 2010;**117**:1087−93.
11. Chew EY, Klein ML, Murphy RP, Remaley NA, Ferris 3rd FL. Effects of aspirin on vitreous/preretinal hemorrhage in patients with diabetes mellitus. Early Treatment Diabetic Retinopathy Study report no. 20. *Arch Ophthalmol* 1995;**113**:52−5.
12. Schwartz SG, Flynn Jr HW, Scott IU. Pharmacotherapy for diabetic retinopathy. *Expert Opinion on Pharmacotherapy* 2009;**10**:1123−31.
13. Schwartz SG, Flynn Jr HW, Scott IU. Endophthalmitis after intravitreal injections. *Expert Opinion on Pharmacotherapy* 2009;**10**:2119−26.
14. Diabetic Retinopathy Clinical Research Network. A randomized trial comparing intravitreal triamcinolone acetonide and focal/grid photocoagulation for diabetic macular edema. *Ophthalmology* 2008;**115**:1447−9.
15. Diabetic Retinopathy Clinical Research Network (DRCR.net), Beck RW, Edwards AR, Aiello LP, Bressler NM, Ferris F, Glassman AR, Hartnett E, Ip MS, Kim JE, and Kollman C. Three-year follow-up of a randomized trial comparing focal/grid photocoagulation and intravitreal triamcinolone for diabetic macular edema. *Arch Ophthalmol* 2009;**127**:245−51.
16. Campochiaro PA, Hafiz G, Shah SM, Bloom S, Brown DM, Busquets M, Ciulla T, Feiner L, Sabates N, Billman K, Kapik B, Green K, Kane F, FAMOUS Study Group. Sustained ocular delivery of fluocinolone acetonide by an intravitreal insert. *Ophthalmology* 2010;**117**:1393−9.
17. Campochiaro PA, Brown DM, Pearson A, Ciulla T, Boyer D, Holz FG, Tolentino M, Gupta A, Duarte L, Madreperla S, Gonder J, Kapik B, Billman K, Kane FE, FAME Study Group. Long-term benefit of sustained-delivery fluocinolone acetonide vitreous inserts for diabetic macular edema. *Ophthalmology* 2011;**188**:626−35.
18. Nguyen QD, Shah SM, Khwaja AA, Channa R, Hatef E, Do DV, Boyer D, Heier JS, Abraham P, Thach AB, Lit ES, Foster BS, Kruger E, Dugel P, Chang T, Das A, Ciulla TA, Pollack JS, Lim JI, Eliot D, Campochiaro PA,

READ-2 Study Group. Two-year outcomes of the ranibizumab for edema of the macula in diabetes (READ-2) study. *Ophthalmology* 2010;**117**:2146–51.

19. Diabetic Retinopathy Clinical Research Network, Elman MJ, Aiello LP, Beck RW, Bressler NM, Bressler SB, Edwards AR, Ferris 3rd FL, Friedman SM, Glassman AR, Miller KM, Scott IU, Stockdale CR, Sun JK. Randomized trial evaluating ranibizumab plus prompt or deferred laser or triamcinolone plus prompt laser for diabetic macular edema. *Ophthalmology* 2010;**117**:1064–77.

20. Diabetic Retinopathy Clinical Research Network, Scott IU, Edwards AR, Beck RW, Bressler NM, Chan CK, Elman MJ, Friedman SM, Greven CM, Maturi RK, Pieramici DJ, Shami M, Singerman LJ, Stockdale CR. A phase II randomized clinical trial of intravitreal bevacizumab for diabetic macular edema. *Ophthalmology* 2007;**114**:1860–7.

21. Michaelides M, Kaines A, Hamilton RD, Fraser-Bell S, Rajendram R, Quhill F, Boss CJ, Xing W, Egan C, Peto T, Bunce C, Leslie RD, Hykin PG. A prospective randomized trial of intravitreal bevacizumab or laser therapy in the management of diabetic macular edema (BOLT study) 12 month data: report 2. *Ophthalmology* 2010;**117**:1078–86.

22. di Lauro R, De Ruggiero P, di Lauro MT, Romano MR. Intravitreal bevacizumab for surgical treatment of severe proliferative diabetic retinopathy. *Graefes Arch Clin Exp Ophthalmol* 2010;**248**:785–91.

23. Ahmadieh H, Shoeibi N, Entezari M, Monshizadeh R. Intravitreal bevacizumab for prevention of early post-vitrectomy hemorrhage in diabetic patients: a randomized clinical trial. *Ophthalmology* 2009;**116**:1943–8.

24. PKC-DRS Study Group. The effect of ruboxistaurin on visual loss in patients with moderately severe to very severe nonproliferative diabetic retinopathy: initial results of the Protein Kinase C beta Inhibitor Diabetic Retinopathy Study (PKC-DRS) multicenter randomized clinical trial. *Diabetes* 2005;2188–97.

25. PKC-DRS2 Group, Aiello LP, Davis MD, Girach A, Kles KA, Milton RC, Sheetz MJ, Vignati L, Zhi XE. Effect of ruboxistaurin on visual loss in patients with diabetic retinopathy. *Ophthalmology* 2006;**113**:2221–30.

26. PKC-DMES Study Group. Effect of ruboxistaurin in patients with diabetic macular edema: thirty-month results of the randomized PKC-DMES clinical trial. *Arch Ophthalmol* 2007;**125**:318–24.

15

Role of Peripheral Neuropathy in the Development of Foot Ulceration and Impaired Wound Healing in Diabetes Mellitus

Francesco Tecilazich*, Thanh L. Dinh[†], Aristidis Veves*

*Joslin-Beth Israel Deaconess Foot Center and Microcirculation Laboratory, Harvard Medical School, Boston, MA, USA [†]Division of Podiatry, Beth Israel Deaconess Medical Center, Harvard Medical School, Boston, MA, USA

INTRODUCTION

The nervous system is the most dependent tissue on glucose and oxygen hematic supply.

Diabetic neuropathy is an insidious, frequently silent and undetected, chronic complication of diabetes mellitus (DM), characterized by the progressive loss of somatic and autonomic

Nutritional and Therapeutic Interventions for Diabetes and Metabolic Syndrome
DOI: 10.1016/B978-0-12-385083-6.00015-2

185

nerve fibers.[1] Diabetic neuropathy is a heterogeneous disorder that encompasses a wide range of abnormalities. DM, in fact, may virtually affect any part of the nervous system, and thus we can distinguish seven major types of diabetic neuropathies: distal symmetric polyneuropathy, autonomic neuropathy, nerve entrapment syndromes, proximal asymmetric mononeuropathy (or diabetic amyotrophy), truncal radiculopathy, cranial mononeuropathy, chronic inflammatory demyelinating polyradiculopathy. Statistical data of the International Diabetes Federation (IDF) and World Health Organization (WHO) show a pandemic picture of DM (250 million people and prevalence 4.4%, in 2000), with a projected near doubling in the next two decades, of people affected by the disease (prevalence 2.8%).[2] Following the increased prevalence of DM, it is reasonable to assume there will be a dramatic increase of all its complications, neuropathy included.

DIABETIC NEUROPATHY

Diabetic neuropathies can fundamentally be distinct in two subgroups depending on their natural course and relationship with duration and control of DM. The first, the gradually progressive group in which severity is related to duration of disease, and that includes sensory and autonomic neuropathies; and the second, the remissive group, whic includes mononeuropathies, radiculopathies, and the acute painful neuropathies. Diagnosis of diabetic neuropathy relies on neurological symptom score (NSS), nerve disability score (NDS) and on electromyography (EMG). Of note, the 10-g monofilament and the Achilles tendon reflex are good tools for predicting the development of foot ulcers, but are not sensitive in detecting early-stage neuropathy.[3]

Comparison of incidence and prevalence of neuropathy in type 1 (T1) and T2DM is very difficult because the two major studies [the Diabetes Control and Complication Trial (DCCT) for T1DM and the United Kingdom Prospective Diabetes Study (UKPDS) for T2DM] used different time intervals and methods for defining neuropathy. In fact, DCCT showed that 15–30% of patients with tightly controlled DM developed neuropathy (abnormal nerve conduction in at least two nerves) at 5 years, compared to 40–52% of control patients.[4] UKPDS instead showed 19% of patients with tightly controlled DM developed neuropathy (abnormal biothesiometer readings in both toes) at 6 years, and 21% of standard treated patients.[5] Taken together, these data suggest that tight control is more effective in reducing the onset of diabetic neuropathy in T1DM than in T2DM patients. With regards to impaired fasting glycemia, available data are controversial and therefore it is still not possible to determine whether it increases the risk of diabetic sensory or autonomic neuropathy.[6–8]

Classification

Peripheral Neuropathy

Diabetic Peripheral Neuropathy (DPN) is a distal symmetric polyneuropathy, is the most common form of neuropathy in the developed world,[9] and is the most frequent neurological complication of DM. It is usually referred to as diabetic neuropathy, in fact at least 50% of patients with DM have clinically manifest DPN. Besides DM, DPN can be caused by other metabolic diseases (such as amyloidosis, uremia, porphyria, and myxedema), vitamin deficiencies (vitamins B_1, B_6, and B_{12}), drugs and chemicals (alcohol, cytotoxic agents, chlorambucil, nitrofurantoin, isoniazid), neoplastic disorders (bronchial and gastric carcinoma, lymphoma), infective or inflammatory diseases (such as Guillain–Barré Syndrome and Lyme borreliosis) and genetic disorders (like Charcot–Marie–Tooth disease and hereditary sensory neuropathies). DPN can be either sensory or motor, even though patients generally present with symmetrical distal sensory-motor polyneuropathy, and may involve small or large fibers.[10] Of note, small and large fiber neuropathy are not separate entities, but belong to the spectrum of the same condition and frequently coexist. Peripheral sensory neuropathy manifests as pain, numbness, and reduced touch and vibration sensation, especially at the limbs, in a stocking distribution. It is considered to be a major contributor to foot amputations, increasing the risk of foot amputations by 1.7-fold alone and by 36-fold if there is a prior history of ulceration.[11] Motor neuropathy in the diabetic foot causes hypotrophia and hypotonia of the intrinsic muscles, the so-called "intrinsic minus foot", that leads to muscular imbalance. The toes assume a clawing aspect and the metatarsal heads flex plantarly. These biomechanical modifications cause prominences at the metatarsal head and digital level, representing areas of focal pressures. Coupled with sensory neuropathy, the increased pressures are susceptible to increased forces with subsequent ulceration.

SMALL FIBER NEUROPATHY

Small fiber neuropathy generally occurs early in the course of DM and is classified as an acute or a chronic painful neuropathy based on the persistence of pain (less or more than 6 months, respectively). Frequently there is absence of clinical and electrophysiological signs of nerve damage. Initially the clinic presentation is dominated by C-fiber type pain and allodynia, these are later substituted by hypoalgesia and impaired warm thermal perception, associated with defective autonomic function. This foot presents impaired blood flow and appears cold. Histologically, there is loss of nerve fiber staining with PGP 9.5 in the skin.

LARGE FIBER NEUROPATHY

Large fibers, contrarily to the small, are myelinated and rapidly conducting fibers, that originate in the toes and have the first synapse in the medulla oblongata. Large fibers subserve motor function, vibration perception, position sense, and cold thermal sensation, and because of their length, they tend to be affected first in DM. Symptoms generally are minimal, but electromyography abnormalities are readily detected. Generally the first objective evidence is the impairment in vibration perception, and other clinical signs are Aδ-type pain (dull sensation, eventually cramp-like), depressed tendon reflexes, *pes equinus* (due to shortening of the Achilles tendon) with hypotrophia of intrinsic muscles. This foot presents increased blood flow and appears warm.

Autonomic Neuropathy

Clinically, autonomic neuropathy may affect systems like the cardiovascular (causing orthostatic hypotension, silent myocardial infarction, sudden death, and resting tachycardia), metabolic (hypoglycemia unawareness and unresponsiveness), gastrointestinal (gastroparesis and diarrhea), genitourinary (bladder and erectile dysfunction) and the peripheral (gustatory sweating, papillary abnormalities, edema). In the lower extremity, autonomic neuropathy can cause arteriovenous shunting, resulting in a vasodilatation in the small arteries,[12] which does not diminish even with foot elevation. Clinically, the neuropathic foot will present as swollen (secondary to neuropathic edema), warm (as a result of the arteriovenous shunting), and dry (because of the decreased activity of the sweat glands).[13] When combined, these changes can result in a skin that is dramatically prone to fissuring, predisposing the patient foot to risk of infection.[14]

Nerve—Axon Reflex

Physiologically, C-nociceptive nerve fibers are activated under conditions of stress such as pain and trauma, and antidromically stimulate the adjacent C fibers to secrete numerous neuropeptides (substance P, neuropeptide Y, neurotensin, calcitonin gene-related peptide, and histamine) which exert vasodilatation and increase vessel permeability. This protective mechanism, also known as Lewis' triple flare response or the Nerve—Axon Reflex Vasodilation (NARV), is impaired in both diabetic patients with and without neuropathy,[15] but with the largest reduction in neuropathic feet. NARV depends on the existence of an intact neurogenic vascular response and is equal to one-third of the maximal vasodilatory capacity. Because of the nerve—axon reflex impairment, the diabetic neuropathic patients present a reduced hyperemic response in the infected or injured foot,[16] thus diabetic neuropathy renders the diabetic foot functionally ischemic. (Figure 15.1) This characteristic impairment at the foot level may be another possible mechanism that explains poor wound healing in DFU.

Pathophysiology

They key factor in the vascular concept of DPN seems to be decreased nerve blood flow, secondary to vasa nervorum endothelial dysfunction. The subsequent endoneural hypoxia

determines functional and morphological nerve changes.[17] The major pathogenetic mechanisms responsible for vasa nervorum endothelium impairment have been postulated to include polyol pathway abnormalities, non-enzymatic glycation, activation of protein kinase C (PKC) and oxidative stress as possible mediators.

Polyol Pathway Abnormalities

In the presence of hyperglycemia, glucose enters the polyol pathway that consists of two reactions. In the first, the enzyme aldose-reductase (AR) using NADPH as a cofactor, catalyzes the reduction of glucose to sorbitol (of note, NADPH will no longer be available for synthesizing nitric oxide and glutathione). Then, sorbitol dehydrogenase oxidizes sorbitol to fructose, with production of NADH from NAD+. The polyol pathway activation results therefore, on the one hand, in an increase of intracellular sorbitol (with subsequent osmotic stress), fructose (which is a 10-times more potent glycation agent than glucose), and reactive oxygen species, and on the other hand, in a decrease in

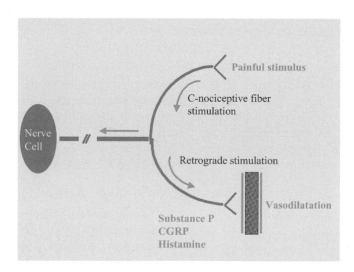

FIGURE 15.1 The nerve—axon reflex. Injury or inflammation stimulate the C-nociceptive fibers and cause retrograde stimulation of the adjacent fibers that release active vasodilators (such as histamine, SP and CGRP). This results finally in hyperemic reaction during stress.

nitric oxide and glutathione.[18] The role for AR in the pathogenesis of DPN has been extensively reviewed.[19] Recently, new evidence emerged on AR increased activity in hyperglycemia- and diabetes-induced oxidative-nitrosative stress[20] and downstream activation of MAPK (mitogen-activated protein kinase),[21] PARP (poly ADP-ribose polymerase)[20] and nuclear factor kappa-B (NF-κB).[21] Accumulation of the organic osmolyte sorbitol also determines depletion of other osmolytes, like myo-inositol and taurine.[22] This phenomenon causes impairment of the phosphoinositide metabolism, through activation of neural protein kinase C by diminished phosphoinositide derived diacylglycerols, and subsequent reduction in Na^+/K^+-ATPase activity.[23] Na^+-K^+ ATPase is involved in the maintenance of cellular integrity and functions of contractility, growth, and differentiation, and its impairment is responsible for the early reversible nerve conduction defect in experimental diabetes.[24]

Over 32 randomized controlled trials, involving almost 5,000 participants, in the last 30 years have tested AR inhibitors (ARI) in treating diabetic neuropathy. The results of ARI agents (like ranirestat, epalrestat, and many others) for DPN treatment remain inconclusive, in fact a meta-analysis involving 879 ARI treated and 909 control (placebo or no treatment) participants, showed no overall significant difference between the groups in the treatment of diabetic polyneuropathy.[25]

Non-Enzymatic Glycation

Non-enzymatic glycation of proteins exposed to an hyperglycemic environment determines the formation of the advanced glycosylated end products (AGEs). RAGE is the AGE receptor and is localized in the peripheral nerve, both on the endothelial and the Schwann cells.[26] Increased AGE levels contribute to the increased vascular permeability of diabetes, since blockade of RAGE reverses diabetes-mediated vascular hyperpermeability.[27] Meerwarldt et al.,

showed the existence of a correlation between increased AGE accumulation in the skin and clinical manifestations of diabetic neuropathy.[28]

Oxidative Stress

Oxidative stress contributes to the development of diabetic neuropathic complications, through an increased production of reactive oxygen species (ROS) and decreased endogenous capacity of neutralizing them (via scavengers such as superoxide dismutase).[29] Oxidative stress causes a series of changes in endothelial cell function and gene expression in diabetes. ROS are generated from the electron transport chains in mitochondria and by activated phagocytes. The mechanisms underlying the increased levels of ROS and the impaired activity of antioxidant factors in DM are multifold and not completely understood.[29] Increased ROS levels lead to increased peroxidation of lipid membranes, proteins and DNA with alteration of cellular function and structure. Of note, oxidative stress increases the levels of two vasogenic factors, endothelin-1 and angiotensin II, respectively, via increase of NF-κB and renin–angiotensin system upregulation. Endothelin-1 and angiotensin II are potent vasoconstrictors and possible contributors to the reduced peripheral nerve blood flow, which results in endoneurial hypoxia, an important and early pathogenetic factor in diabetic neuropathy in both patients and animal models.[30]

Protein Kinase C

PKC includes a superfamily of isoenzymes, key players in intercellular signal transduction for hormone and cytokines. Increased activation of PKC may be determined by hyperglycemia, and results in the phosphorylation of intracellular proteins. PKC seems to contribute to diabetic neuropathy by a neurovascular mechanism such as blood flow and conduction velocity, however its role in endothelial function remains controversial.[31–34] Ruboxistaurin (RBX) mesylate is a PKC inhibitor that specifically inhibits PKC-β overactivation and that has been shown to improve neural function in diabetic animals.[35] In a double-blinded randomized clinical trial, however, treatment with RBX in patients with DPN failed to achieve the primary end point of improving quantitative sensory testing for vibration detection threshold among all symptomatic patients. It is noteworthy that the study shows a significant improvement in the neuropathy total symptoms score-6 (NTSS-6) at 6 and at 12 months, in the group classified at baseline with clinically significant sensorial neuropathy (NTSS-6 > 6) and treated with RBX 64 mg, compared to placebo.[36]

DIABETIC FOOT ULCERS

Diabetic foot ulcers (DFU) are characterized by an inability to self-repair in a timely and orderly manner,[37] and occurs as a consequence of the interaction of several contributory factors. These contributory factors may be schematically divided into intrinsic (neuropathy, peripheral vascular disease, and diabetes severity) and extrinsic (wound infection, callus formation, and excessive pressure to the site).[38] There is a triad of factors that contribute ultimately to ulceration, and they are: presence of peripheral neuropathy, foot deformities, and acute (or chronic) repetitive trauma. In the diabetic foot, peripheral sensory neuropathy is responsible for the pain insensitivity, while autonomic sensory neuropathy causes impaired sweat gland function, resulting in dry, atrophic skin. Motor neuropathy commonly causes intrinsic muscle wasting with a characteristic foot with joint contractures and prominent bones to the metatarsal plantar region with limited fat padding.[39] All together the three components determine loss of sensation, changes in foot structure with consequent deformity, and skin changes. The diabetic foot is therefore more vulnerable to injury with poor defenses. Of note, it has been shown that loss of peripheral sensory and autonomic nerves along with diminished neuropeptide production precedes clinical symptoms of neuropathy.[40] Moreover, skin biopsies from patients with type 2 DM with active foot ulcers, with and without peripheral sensory neuropathy, presented severe denervation, irrespective of clinically identifiable sensory neuropathy.[41] Internal or external traumas are generally the next key factor and are generally related to the development of abnormally high foot pressures during walking. Internal traumas typically result from repetitive stresses from high-pressure areas, external traumas derive instead from the environment, such as an object in the shoe. (Figure 15.2).

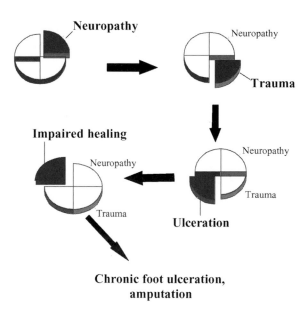

FIGURE 15.2 The pathway to foot ulceration. Sensory neuropathy, associated with pain insensitivity, is the first component. Internal or external traumas are the next key component. Impaired wound healing is the third component leading to the development of chronic ulceration. (From Pecoraro et al.[52])

WOUND HEALING

Wound healing requires sufficient circulation, proper nutrition, adequate immune status, and the avoidance of traumatic mechanical forces. Microscopically, it involves a well-orchestrated, complex series of biological and molecular events consisting of cell migration, cell proliferation, and deposition of extracellular matrix (ECM).[42] This cascade of wound healing can physiologically be divided into four different and overlapping phases: hemostasis, inflammation, proliferation, and remodeling. In DM, there are major abnormalities in all these four different phases and there is no linear progression through the phases of wound healing like the acute wounds.

Impaired wound healing has been implicated as a significant cause for poor healing in the DFU. Initially it was thought that failure to heal a diabetic ulcer was related to presence of infection and ischemia, and to the continuous walking on the injured foot, mainly because of the pain insensitivity. Two other major factors contribute to this impairment, the functional changes in microcirculation and in cellular activity, and the expression of various growth factors and cytokines physiologically involved in the healing process. Recent investigation has in fact revealed that impairments at the microvascular level as well as abnormal expression of growth factors and other cytokines are involved in tissue repair and wound healing. As a result, diabetic ulcers become stalled in the inflammatory phase and fail to progress to the proliferative phase, remaining in a chronic inflammatory state.[42]

The contributions of peripheral nerves and cutaneous neurobiology to wound healing have recently become evident. Vasomodulators secreted by the palindromic stimulation of the C-nociceptive fibers are important mediators of the angiogenesis process. In the presence of somatic neuropathy, the nerve–axon reflex-related secretion of these vasomodulators is profoundly impaired and this defect contributes to the insufficient formation of new vessels in the wound area and to the subsequent impaired wound healing. In the last decade, it has also been realized that numerous neuropeptides that are secreted by the small nerve fibers, both sensory and autonomic, play a key role during the inflammatory and proliferative phases via regulation of cytokine expression and/or function.[43] The neuropeptides commonly involved in wound healing are substance P (SP) and neuropeptide Y (NPY). SP is widely distributed in both the central nervous system (CNS) and peripheral nervous system (PNS).[44–46] SP is released from peripheral neurons in response to noxious stimuli and it promotes vasodilatation, leukocyte chemotaxis, and leukocyte–endothelial cell adhesion. In this way SP elicits the extravasation, migration and subsequent accumulation of leukocytes at sites of injury.[47] In patients with diabetes SP-positive nerve fibers[40] are shown to be reduced and it is evident that dysregulation in the SP pathway in diabetes can significantly impair the wound repairing process. Similarly to SP, NPY is also important for both the inflammatory and angiogenic phases of wound healing. NPY's angiogenic action consists in stimulating EC proliferation and migration leading to angiogenesis.[48] The levels of NPY in the skin are reduced in patients with diabetes.[49]

Currently, the cornerstones of the treatment of DFUs consist of adequate debridement, offloading of pressure, correction of ischemia, treatment of infection, and local wound care. However, even when optimal treatment is provided, not more than 50% of ulcers will be healed after 12–20 weeks (Figure 15.3).[50] Advanced wound care treatments (such as local growth factors, living skin equivalents and negative pressure wound therapy) should be reserved for wounds that fail to progress to healing in a linear fashion, and that are identified by comparing the wound area at different visits.

FIGURE 15.3 Mean percent ulcer area reduction during the first 4 weeks in a prospective study that followed up patients for a 12-week period. Patients who completely healed their ulcer during the 12-week period were defined as *healers,* and those who failed to heal as *nonhealers.* The area was calculated by multiplying length by width. During the first 4 weeks, *healers* had a mean percent ulcer area reduction of 82% (95% CI 70–94), significantly higher to that of the *nonhealers* (25% reduction, 95% CI 15–35, $p < 0.001$). The midpoint between percentage area reduction from baseline at 4 weeks in *healers vs nonhealers* at 12 weeks was 53%. Subjects with an ulcer area reduction above presented a 12-week healing rate of 58%, meanwhile those below the 4-week median had a healing rate of only 9% ($p < 0.01$). Patients who fail to reduce their ulcer area to half of initial size over a 4-week period should therefore be considered as unlikely to heal, and the use of advanced wound care products may be justifiable in this subgroup of patients. *Indicates $p < 0.01$. (From Sheehan *et al.* 50)

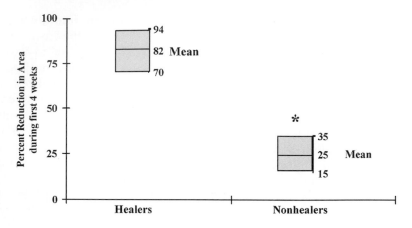

CONCLUSIONS

There is no question that the growth of DM in the industrialized world is reaching epidemic proportions. As the incidence of DM rises, secondary complications such as neuropathy and diabetic foot ulcerations will follow. Therefore, precocious nutritional and therapeutic interventions in DM may be the best means of preventing the onset of diabetic complications, among which DPN is one of the most devastating and represents the leading cause of foot amputation.[51]

References

1. Urbancic-Rovan V. Causes of diabetic foot lesions. *Lancet* 2005;**366**:1675–6.

2. Wild S, Roglic G, Green A, Sicree R, King H. Global prevalence of diabetes: estimates for the year 2000 and projections for 2030. *Diabetes Care* 2004;**27**:1047–53.

3. Vinik AINP, Milicevic Z, et al. Diabetic neuropathies: An overview of clinical aspects. In: LeRoith D TS, Olefsky JM, editors. *Diabetes Mellitus: A Fundamental and Clinical Text.* Philadelphia: Lippincot-Raven; 1996.

4. The effect of intensive diabetes therapy on the development and progression of neuropathy. The Diabetes Control and Complications Trial Research Group. *Ann Intern Med* 1995;**122**:561–8.

5. Intensive blood-glucose control with sulphonylureas or insulin compared with conventional treatment and risk of complications in patients with type 2 diabetes (UKPDS 33). UK Prospective Diabetes Study (UKPDS) Group. *Lancet* 1998;**352**:837–53.

6. Eriksson KF, Nilsson H, Lindgarde F, et al. Diabetes mellitus but not impaired glucose tolerance is associated with dysfunction in peripheral nerves. *Diabet Med* 1994;**11**:279–85.

7. Franklin GM, Kahn LB, Baxter J, Marshall JA, Hamman RF. Sensory neuropathy in non-insulin-dependent diabetes mellitus. The San Luis Valley Diabetes Study. *Am J Epidemiol* 1990;**131**:633—43.

8. Singh JP, Larson MG, O'Donnell CJ, et al. Association of hyperglycemia with reduced heart rate variability (The Framingham Heart Study). *Am J Cardiol* 2000;**86**: 309—12.

9. Dyck PJ, Kratz KM, Karnes JL, et al. The prevalence by staged severity of various types of diabetic neuropathy, retinopathy, and nephropathy in a population-based cohort: the Rochester Diabetic Neuropathy Study. *Neurology* 1993;**43**:817—24.

10. Bird SJ, Brown MJ. The clinical spectrum of diabetic neuropathy. *Semin Neurol* 1996;**16**:115—22.

11. Vinik AI, Park TS, Stansberry KB, Pittenger GL. Diabetic neuropathies. *Diabetologia* 2000;**43**:957—73.

12. Ward JD, Boulton AJ, Simms JM, Sandler DA, Knight G. Venous distension in the diabetic neuropathic foot (physical sign of arteriovenous shunting). *J R Soc Med* 1983;**76**:1011—4.

13. Boulton AJ, Scarpello JH, Ward JD. Venous oxygenation in the diabetic neuropathic foot: evidence of arteriovenous shunting? *Diabetologia* 1982;**22**:6—8.

14. Tegner R. The effect of skin temperature on vibratory sensitivity in polyneuropathy. *J Neurol Neurosurg Psychiatry* 1985;**48**:176—8.

15. Caselli A, Rich J, Hanane T, Uccioli L, Veves A. Role of C-nociceptive fibers in the nerve axon reflex-related vasodilation in diabetes. *Neurology* 2003;**60**:297—300.

16. Hernandez C, Burgos R, Canton A, Garcia-Arumi J, Segura RM, Simo R. Vitreous levels of vascular cell adhesion molecule and vascular endothelial growth factor in patients with proliferative diabetic retinopathy: a case-control study. *Diabetes Care* 2001;**24**:516—21.

17. Cameron NE, Eaton SE, Cotter MA, Tesfaye S. Vascular factors and metabolic interactions in the pathogenesis of diabetic neuropathy. *Diabetologia* 2001;**44**:1973—88.

18. Brownlee M. Biochemistry and molecular cell biology of diabetic complications. *Nature* 2001;**414**:813—20.

19. Oates PJ. Polyol pathway and diabetic peripheral neuropathy. *Int Rev Neurobiol* 2002;**50**:325—92.

20. Obrosova IG, Van Huysen C, Fathallah L, Cao XC, Greene DA, Stevens MJ. An aldose reductase inhibitor reverses early diabetes-induced changes in peripheral nerve function, metabolism, and antioxidative defense. *FASEB J* 2002;**16**:123—5.

21. Price SA, Agthong S, Middlemas AB, Tomlinson DR. Mitogen-activated protein kinase p38 mediates reduced nerve conduction velocity in experimental diabetic neuropathy: interactions with aldose reductase. *Diabetes* 2004;**53**:1851—6.

22. Stevens MJ, Lattimer SA, Kamijo M, Van Huysen C, Sima AA, Greene DA. Osmotically-induced nerve taurine depletion and the compatible osmolyte hypothesis in experimental diabetic neuropathy in the rat. *Diabetologia* 1993;**36**:608—14.

23. Winegrad AI. Banting lecture 1986. Does a common mechanism induce the diverse complications of diabetes? *Diabetes* 1987;**36**:396—406.

24. Greene DA, Chakrabarti S, Lattimer SA, Sima AA. Role of sorbitol accumulation and myo-inositol depletion in paranodal swelling of large myelinated nerve fibers in the insulin-deficient spontaneously diabetic bio-breeding rat. Reversal by insulin replacement, an aldose reductase inhibitor, and myo-inositol. *J Clin Invest* 1987;**79**:1479—85.

25. Chalk C, Benstead TJ, Moore F. Aldose reductase inhibitors for the treatment of diabetic polyneuropathy. *Cochrane Database Syst Rev*; 2007. CD004572.

26. Wada R, Yagihashi S. Role of advanced glycation end products and their receptors in development of diabetic neuropathy. *Ann N Y Acad Sci* 2005;**1043**: 598—604.

27. Makita Z, Radoff S, Rayfield EJ, et al. Advanced glycosylation end products in patients with diabetic nephropathy. *N Engl J Med* 1991;**325**:836—42.

28. Meerwaldt R, Links TP, Graaff R, et al. Increased accumulation of skin advanced glycation end-products precedes and correlates with clinical manifestation of diabetic neuropathy. *Diabetologia* 2005;**48**:1637—44.

29. Van Dam PS, Van Asbeck BS, Erkelens DW, Marx JJ, Gispen WH, Bravenboer B. The role of oxidative stress in neuropathy and other diabetic complications. *Diabetes Metab Rev* 1995;**11**:181—92.

30. Low PA, Lagerlund TD, McManis PG. Nerve blood flow and oxygen delivery in normal, diabetic, and ischemic neuropathy. *Int Rev Neurobiol* 1989;**31**: 355—438.

31. Ohara Y, Sayegh HS, Yamin JJ, Harrison DG. Regulation of endothelial constitutive nitric oxide synthase by protein kinase C. *Hypertension* 1995;**25**:415—20.

32. Beckman JA, Goldfine AB, Gordon MB, Garrett LA, Creager MA. Inhibition of protein kinase C beta prevents impaired endothelium-dependent vasodilation caused by hyperglycemia in humans. *Circ Res* 2002;**90**:107—11.

33. Beckman JA, Goldfine AB, Goldin A, Prsic A, Kim S, Creager MA. Inhibition of protein kinase C beta does not improve endothelial function in type 2 diabetes. *J Clin Endocrinol Metab* 2010;**95**:3783—7.

34. Mehta NN, Sheetz M, Price K, et al. Selective PKC beta inhibition with ruboxistaurin and endothelial function in type-2 diabetes mellitus. *Cardiovasc Drugs Ther* 2009;**23**:17—24.

35. Yamagishi S, Uehara K, Otsuki S, Yagihashi S. Differential influence of increased polyol pathway on protein kinase C expressions between endoneurial and epineurial tissues in diabetic mice. *J Neurochem* 2003;**87**: 497–507.
36. Vinik AI, Bril V, Kempler P, et al. Treatment of symptomatic diabetic peripheral neuropathy with the protein kinase C beta-inhibitor ruboxistaurin mesylate during a 1-year, randomized, placebo-controlled, double-blind clinical trial. *Clin Ther* 2005;**27**:1164–80.
37. Lazarus GS, Cooper DM, Knighton DR, et al. Definitions and guidelines for assessment of wounds and evaluation of healing. *Arch Dermatol* 1994;**130**: 489–93.
38. Shaw JE, Boulton AJ. The pathogenesis of diabetic foot problems: an overview. *Diabetes* 1997;**46**(Suppl. 2): S58–61.
39. Boulton A. Late sequelae of diabetic neuropathy. In: Boulton A, editor. *Diabetic Neuropathy.* Lancaster: Marius Press; 1997. p. 63–76.
40. Lindberger M, Schroder HD, Schultzberg M, et al. Nerve fibre studies in skin biopsies in peripheral neuropathies. I. Immunohistochemical analysis of neuropeptides in diabetes mellitus. *J Neurol Sci* 1989;**93**:289–96.
41. Galkowska H, Olszewski WL, Wojewodzka U, Rosinski G, Karnafel W. Neurogenic factors in the impaired healing of diabetic foot ulcers. *J Surg Res* 2006;**134**:252–8.
42. Falanga V. Wound healing and its impairment in the diabetic foot. *Lancet* 2005;**366**:1736–43.
43. Pradhan L, Nabzdyk C, Andersen ND, LoGerfo FW, Veves A. Inflammation and neuropeptides: the connection in diabetic wound healing. *Expert Rev Mol Med* 2009;**11**: e2.
44. Hokfelt T, Kellerth JO, Nilsson G, Pernow B. Substance p: localization in the central nervous system and in some primary sensory neurons. *Science* 1975;**190**:889–90.
45. Harrison S, Geppetti P. Substance p. *Int J Biochem Cell Biol* 2001;**33**:555–76.
46. Khawaja AM, Rogers DF. Tachykinins: receptor to effector. *Int J Biochem Cell Biol* 1996;**28**:721–38.
47. Pernow B. Substance P. *Pharmacol Rev* 1983;**35**:85–141.
48. Zukowska-Grojec Z, Karwatowska-Prokopczuk E, Rose W, et al. Neuropeptide Y: a novel angiogenic factor from the sympathetic nerves and endothelium. *Circ Res* 1998;**83**:187–95.
49. Wallengren J, Badendick K, Sundler F, Hakanson R, Zander E. Innervation of the skin of the forearm in diabetic patients: relation to nerve function. *Acta Derm Venereol* 1995;**75**:37–42.
50. Sheehan P, Jones P, Caselli A, Giurini JM, Veves A. Percent change in wound area of diabetic foot ulcers over a 4-week period is a robust predictor of complete healing in a 12-week prospective trial. *Diabetes Care* 2003;**26**:1879–82.
51. Effect of intensive therapy on the microvascular complications of type 1 diabetes mellitus. *JAMA* 2002;**287**:2563–9.
52. Pecoraro RE, Reiber GE, Burgess EM. Pathways to diabetic limb amputation. Basis for prevention. *Diabetes Care* 1990;**13**:513–21.

An Overview of Gestational Diabetes

Christopher Federico, Gabriella Pridjian

Department of Obstetrics & Gynecology, Tulane University School of Medicine,
New Orleans, LA, USA

INTRODUCTION

Gestational diabetes mellitus, described as a new onset of glucose intolerance first diagnosed during pregnancy,[1] now complicates up to 7% of all pregnancies.[2,3,4] For many years, and to a great extent still today, gestational diabetes has been a subject of great controversy. If left undiagnosed and untreated, gestational diabetes can have vast ill effects on both mother and baby, including excessive fetal growth, birth injuries, fetal hypoglycemia, cesarean delivery,[5] and long-term medical risks for mother and baby. This chapter will examine the pathophysiology, epidemiology, diagnosis, dietary and other treatment, and prognosis, and outcome of gestational diabetes.

PATHOPHYSIOLOGY

The primary mechanisms of action of the glucose intolerance seen in gestational diabetes

Nutritional and Therapeutic Interventions for Diabetes and Metabolic Syndrome
DOI: 10.1016/B978-0-12-385083-6.00016-4

are peripheral insulin resistance and decreased pancreatic insulin secretion.[6] Specifically, Buchanan *et al.* found that insulin sensitivity in normal pregnant women was reduced to about one-third of that of nonpregnant women of similar weight and age.[7] Insulin resistance worsens as the pregnancy progresses. In a longitudinal study of healthy pregnant women using the hyperinsulinemic-euglycemic clamp, Catalano *et al.* found a 56% decrease in insulin sensitivity in nonobese women by late pregnancy.[8] This insulin resistance is more profound in obese pregnant women and at advancing gestational ages.[9]

It is postulated that insulin resistance in pregnancy is related to post-receptor handling of glucose. Several aspects of pregnancy contribute to this altered handling of glucose including impaired tyrosine kinase activity,[10] which is normally responsible for the phosphorylation of cellular substrates; decreased expression of insulin receptor substrate-1,[11] a cytosolic protein that binds phosphorylated intracellular substrates and transmits signals downstream; and decreased expression of the GLUT4 glucose transport protein in adipose tissue,[12] which normally promotes glucose uptake.

Additionally seen in pregnancy is marked pancreatic β-cell hypertrophy and hyperplasia in order to compensate for decreased insulin sensitivity and increased insulin requirements.[13,14] In experimental diabetes in rat models, the endocrine pancreas, and in particular the insulin-producing β-cells have an impaired capacity to compensate during pregnancy.[15] Growth hormone, prolactin, and human placental lactogen, which are present in elevated levels in pregnant women, are important stimulators of β-cell growth and proliferation. Specific receptors for both prolactin and growth hormone are present in β-cells, and their expression is upregulated during pregnancy.[14] This impaired β-cell function and reduced β-cell adaptation results in insufficient insulin secretion to maintain euglycemia in all pregnancies.

EPIDEMIOLOGY

In recent years, there has been an increase in the prevalence of both obesity and type 2 diabetes. There is evidence for an increasing prevalence of gestational diabetes, especially in younger obese women in the US. Increasing rates of obesity in the younger population was only one explanation for the rise. Another factor for this increase is the improved survival of female infants whose birth weights were at the extremes of the normal range during the past few decades. As adults, the latter individuals have altered insulin action that may predispose them to develop gestational diabetes.

Several maternal factors have been associated with an increased risk for developing gestational diabetes. Age, race, and parity have all been shown to be associated with increasing rates of gestational diabetes.[16] A retrospective cohort study of over 111,000 pregnancies in Canada found positive relationships between gestational diabetes and mothers who were obese, had a history of a fetal demise or a history of a prior cesarean delivery.[17]

Prior gestational diabetes is a strong risk factor for recurrence. In general, the risk of recurrence of gestational diabetes is between 33 and 56%.[18,19] In a study of 78 women in California with gestational diabetes in an index pregnancy, 69% were found to have gestational diabetes in a subsequent pregnancy.[20] Additionally, a between-pregnancy interval of less than 24 months, a between-pregnancy weight gain of greater than 15 lb, a diagnosis of gestational diabetes at less than 24 weeks' gestation, and insulin therapy in the previous pregnancy were all found to be highly predictive of recurrence. Other risk factors for development of gestational diabetes have been published and are divided into relative strength of risk (Table 16.1).

TABLE 16.1 Risk Factors for Development of Gestational Diabetes

Risk factors for development of gestational diabetes	Some risk, but low	Medium	High
	Overweight	Obesity	Severe obesity
	Asian ethnicity (some subsets medium risk)	Polycystic ovarian syndrome	Prior gestational diabetes
	African American ethnicity	Parents with type 2 diabetes	Sibling with diabetes
	Low maternal birth weight	Prior macrosomic infant	Persistent glucosuria
	Prior stillborn	Maternal age > 35 years	
	Prior cesarean	Hispanic ethnicity	
	Polyhydramnios	Multiple gestation	
		Periodontal disease	

Table compiled from the following epidemiologic studies and generally categorized based upon published odds ratios:

Torloni M. R., Betran A. P. and Horta B. L. (2009) Prepregnancy BMI and the risk of gestational diabetes: a systematic review of the literature with meta-analysis. Obes. Rev. **10**, 194—203.

Chu S., Kim S. Y. and Lau J. (2009) Re: Prepregnancy BMI and the risk of gestational diabetes: a systematic review of the literature with meta-analysis. Obes. Rev. **10**, 489—490.

McGuire V., Rauh M. J. and Mueller B. A. (1996) The risk of diabetes in a subsequent pregnancy associated with prior history of gestational diabetes or a macrosomic infant. Paediatr. Perinat. Epidemiol. **10**, 64—72.

Cypryk K., Szymczak W. and Czupryniak L. (2008) Gestational diabetes — an analysis of risk factors. Endokrynol. Polska 59, 393—397.

Rauh-Hain J. A., Rana S. and Tamez, H. (2009) Risk for developing gestational diabetes in women with twin pregnancies. J. Maternal-Fetal Neonatal Med. **22**, 293—299.

Rao A. K., Daniels K. and El-Sayed Y. Y. (2006) Perinatal outcomes among Asian American and Pacific Islander women. Am. J. Obstet. Gynecol. **195**, 834—838.

Dooley S., Metzger, B. and Cho N. (1991) Gestational diabetes mellitus: influence of race on disease prevalence and perinatal outcome in the US population. Diabetes 20, 25—29.

Toulis K. A., Goulis D. G. and Kolibianakis E. M. (2009) Risk of gestational diabetes mellitus in women with polycystic ovarian syndrome: a systematic review and a meta-analysis. Fertility & Sterility **92**, 667—677.

Kim C., Liu T. and Valdez R. (2009) Does frank diabetes in first degree relatives of a pregnant woman affect the likelihood of her developing gestational diabetes mellitus or nongestational diabetes? Am. J. Obstet. Gynecol. **201**, 576.

Xiong X., Ellkind-Hirsch K. E. and Vastardis S. (2009) Periodontal disease is associated with gestational diabetes mellitus, a case-control study. J. Periodontol. **80**, 1742—1749.

Seghieri G., Anichini R. and de Bellis A. (2002) Relationship between gestational diabetes mellitus and low maternal birth weight. Diabetes Care **25**, 1761—1765.

SCREENING AND DIAGNOSIS

Significant controversy exists in the screening and diagnosis of gestational diabetes. Universal screening and risk-based screening are acceptable approaches.[21,22] The American Diabetes Association (ADA) does not recommend screening for women who meet all of the following criteria: (i) are less than 25 years of age; (ii) are normal body weight; (iii) have no first-degree relatives with diabetes; (iv) have no personal history of abnormal glucose metabolism; (v) have no personal history of poor obstetric outcome; (vi) are not members of a racial/ethnic group with a high prevalence of diabetes (Hispanic American, Native American, Asian American, African American, Pacific Islander).[2] This risk assessment is best performed at the first prenatal visit. Women with a high risk of gestational diabetes should be screened as soon as possible. Women are otherwise screened between 24 and 28 weeks of gestation.

A two-step method for screening and diagnosis is used in the US. In the first step a 50-g glucose load is administered without regard to fasting state, and a plasma glucose level is measured 1 h later. If the 1-h glucose challenge test is abnormal (Table 16.2), a diagnostic 3-h glucose tolerance test (3-h GTT) is then administered. In the 3-h GTT, a 100-g oral glucose load is administered after a 6–8-h fast and with at least three days of no carbohydrate restriction prior to the test and three postprandial glucose levels measured (Table 16.2). When the two-step approach is used, an abnormal glucose threshold value of 140 mg/dl 1 h after the 50-g glucose load identifies 80% of women with gestational diabetes; use of 130 mg/dl as an abnormal cut-off increases this yield to 90%.[23] Controversy also exists as to what constitutes a positive confirmation test. Two sets of values are generally accepted to make the diagnosis of gestational diabetes (Table 16.2).

Some authors argue for the validity of using a 75-g, 2-h glucose tolerance test for diagnosis of gestational diabetes. Advantages of this test include convenience, cost, fewer side effects, and better reproducibility of results. Critics of this testing method worry that some women may not be identified with the 75-g load. Still, the World Health Organization (WHO) recommends the 75-g GTT,[24] and this is the method used most commonly outside of the US. The use of hemoglobin A1c is not recommended at this time for the diagnosis of gestational diabetes either by the ADA or the WHO[2] unless overt diabetes is suspected at the first prenatal visit.

Until recently, clear evidence-based guidelines to diagnose gestational diabetes have been lacking. The Hyperglycemia and Adverse Pregnancy Outcomes (HAPO) study, published in 2008, answered the questions about the effects of even mild levels of hyperglycemia.[5,25] The study was established as an observational, multicenter, multinational, multiethnic/racial blinded study, which included 15 health centers from around

TABLE 16.2　Diagnostic Parameters for Diagnosis of Gestational Diabetes

	Screening	Diagnosis	Glucose load (g)	Fasting		1-h		2-h		3-h	
				mg/dl	mmol/l	mg/dl	mmol/l	mg/dl	mmol/l	mg/dl	mmol/l
Current US	1-h, 50-g glucose [abnormal ≥ 130 or 140 mg/dl (7.2 or 7.8 mmol/l)]	National Diabetes Data Group[a]	100	105	5.8	190	10.6	165	9.2	145	8.0
		Carpenter-Coustan[a]	100	95	5.3	180	10.0	155	8.6	140	7.8
Current outside US[b]		2-h GTT	75					140	7.8		
Proposed international diagnostic testing[c]		2-h GTT	75	92	5.1	180	10.0	153	8.5		

[a] Two or more values met or exceeded required to make diagnosis. Table created from data from National Diabetes Data Group (1979) Classification and diagnosis of diabetes mellitus and categories of glucose intolerance. Diabetes **28**, 1039–1057 and Carpenter M.R., Coustan D.R. (1982) Criteria for screening tests for gestational diabetes. Am. J. Obstet. Gynecol **144**, 768–773.
[b] Only the 2-h value needed for assessment.
[c] International Association of Diabetes and Pregnancy Study Group, consensus statement[26], 2010 based upon HAPO study results.[5]
In the US, a 3-h, 100-g GTT performed after an abnormal 50-g 1-h glucose screen. Outside the US, a one-step diagnostic test is performed, most commonly the 75-g, 2-h GTT. The proposed international diagnostic test would make diagnosis similar.

the world. The study was accomplished with high-quality standardized data collection on roughly 25,000 women of varied ethnic, racial and socio-demographic backgrounds. The 10-year study produced clear evidence of fetal risk even with mild glucose intolerance.[5] Birth weight > 90th percentile for gestational age, elevated umbilical cord-blood C-peptide level (a proxy for fetal insulin levels), cesarean delivery, and neonatal hypoglycemic episodes all increased in direct proportion to higher maternal glucose levels and were even seen at mildly elevated glucose levels, levels lower than those diagnostic of gestational diabetes (Table 16.3).

Given the results of the HAPO study, the International Association of Diabetes and Pregnancy Study Groups convened to assess the best method for the diagnosis of gestational diabetes and reached consensus which was recently published.[26] The recommended testing paradigm involves a 75-g, 2-h glucose tolerance test (Table 16.2) and required one abnormal value.

Furthermore, at the first prenatal visit for detecting undiagnosed preexisting diabetes, either a fasting plasma glucose of greater than or equal to 126 mg/dl (7.0 mmol/l), a standardized hemoglobin A1c greater than or equal to 6.5%, or a random glucose greater than or equal to 200 mg/dl (11.1 mmol.l) and subsequently

confirmed is diagnostic of overt diabetes in pregnancy.[26]

EFFECTS OF UNTREATED GESTATIONAL DIABETES

If left untreated gestational diabetes can have profound effects on the mother, fetus, and newborn. Mothers have an increased cesarean delivery rate often to avoid potential birth trauma that may result from fetal macrosomia.

Most of the effects on the fetus can be directly related to the hyperinsulinemic state seen in gestational diabetes. As was first postulated by Jorgen Pedersen in 1952, maternal hyperglycemia leads to fetal hyperglycemia and resultant fetal hyperinsulinemia[27] which leads to macrosomia. Hypoglycemia, hypocalcemia, hypomagnesemia, polycythemia, hyperviscosity, hyperbilirubinemia, hypertrophic cardiomyopathy, and poor feeding have all been described in newborns of diabetic mothers.

The effects from gestational diabetes may also be seen throughout childhood and adulthood and in future generations. Infants born to mothers with gestational diabetes have a higher risk for developing childhood obesity,

TABLE 16.3   Hyperglycemia and Pregnancy Outcome Study (HAPO), Adjusted Odds Ratios (and 95% Confidence Intervals)

Risk factor	Birth weight > 90th percentile	Primary cesarean	Cord C-peptide level > 90th percentile
Fasting plasma glucose > 1 SD (9 mg/dl, 0.4 mmol/l)	1.38 (1.32−1.44)	1.11 (1.06−1.15)	1.55 (1.47−1.64)
1-h plasma glucose > 1 SD (9 mg/dl, 1.7 mmol/l)	1.46 (1.39−1.53)	1.10 (1.06−1.15)	1.46 (1.38−1.54)
2-h plasma glucose > 1 SD (5 mg/dl, 1.3 mmol/l)	1.28 (1.32−1.44)	1.08 (1.03−1.26)	1.37 (1.30−1.44)

Numbers are odds ratio (95% confidence interval). Table created with information from: The HAPO Study Cooperative Research Group (2008) Hyperglycemia and adverse pregnancy outcome. *N. Engl. J. Med.* **358,** 1991−1992. Women with blood sugar levels in the gestational diabetes range were excluded from the study. All three primary outcomes were statistically significantly increased, $p < 0.05$.

gestational diabetes, type 2 diabetes, and metabolic syndrome.[28] We can even see these changes on a molecular level. In a study done in 1979 experimental mild diabetes in a pregnant rat induced gestational diabetes in the second generation and macrosomia and pancreatic β-cell hyperplasia in the third generation.[29] The authors postulated that this initial overstimulation of β-cells *in utero* led to eventual β-cell dysfunction later in life.[30]

A similar effect is seen in human offspring. A prospective study that focused on the offspring of women with gestational and pregestational (type 1 or type 2) diabetes, found that the prevalence of impaired glucose tolerance was about 19% in offspring at 10—16 years of age.[31] In general, impaired glucose tolerance in children is a rare event occurring in less than 5% of the population. Thus, *in utero* exposure to high glucose and insulin levels has a profound effect on future insulin activity. This was further proven in a study by Plagemann, where *in utero* insulin levels as assessed by amniocentesis proved to be strong predictors of impaired glucose tolerance in childhood.[32]

EFFECTIVENESS OF TREATMENT

The fact that treatment of gestational diabetes is effective in reducing associated complications was only shown recently. In 2005, Crowther and associates proved that treatment of gestational diabetes decreases serious perinatal morbidity and improves a woman's health-related quality of life.[33] These authors found that the rate of serious perinatal complications was significantly lower among the infants of the 490 women in the treatment group than among the infants of the 510 women in the routine-care group (1% *vs* 4%). The Fifth International Workshop-Conference on Gestational Diabetes concluded that intensive management of gestational diabetes was associated with a decrease in infant morbidity

and mortality.[28] Langer *et al.*, in a retrospective study, compared pregnancy outcomes between pregnant women with diabetes diagnosed after 37 weeks (not treated) with treated diabetic women and control non-diabetic pregnant women. They found a composite adverse outcome of 59% for untreated, 18% for treated and 11% for non-diabetic subjects, respectively.[34]

Along with any type of treatment for gestational diabetes is glucose monitoring for the pregnant woman to assess the effectiveness of therapy in lowering blood glucose.

GLUCOSE MONITORING

Treatment of gestational diabetes begins with self-monitoring of blood glucose levels. A woman not taking insulin monitors her capillary glucose four times per day (fasting and 1 or 2 h after each meal) while women on insulin or an oral hypoglycemic agent may need to monitor up to six times a day (before meals and 1—2 h after each meal). Most diabetes experts believe that post prandial hyperglycemia is important to control in order to prevent complications and ask their diabetics to monitor at either 1 or 2 h postprandial.[35]

Based on a series of clinical trials that found comparable rates of macrosomia to non-diabetic controls in women, the Fifth International Workshop-Conference on Gestational Diabetes Mellitus recommended the following plasma glucose goals: fasting 90—99 mg/dl (5.0—5.5 mmol/l), a postprandial 1 h of less than 140 mg/dl (7.8 mmol/l), and a postprandial 2-h value of less than 120—127 mg/dl (6.7—7.1 mmol/l).[28]

LIFESTYLE MODIFICATION—DIET AND EXERCISE

The initial treatment of gestational diabetes includes dietary restriction and, if not contraindicated, moderate amounts of exercise. Dietary intervention, often termed "medical nutritional therapy", is designed to minimize postprandial glucose levels. The pregnant diabetic diet recommended is comprised of 24–30 calories/kg of present pregnancy weight, divided into three meals and three snacks daily, and composed of fewer than 40% carbohydrates.[36]

Magee *et al.* designed a study to evaluate strict caloric restriction as a treatment for obese subjects with gestational diabetes. They compared a 2,400 kcal/day diet with a 1,200 kcal/day diet. While the two groups differed significantly in average glucose levels and fasting insulin levels, fasting glucose levels and postglucose challenge levels were not significantly different. However, ketonemia and ketonuria developed in the calorie-restricted group after 1 week, and the investigators concluded that the 1,200 kcal diet may have an impact on the well-being of the fetus and therefore was not recommended.[37]

For overweight women, modest carbohydrate restriction may be appropriate, but starvation ketosis is best avoided. Furthermore, a low glycemic index diet has been shown to lead to a reduction in postprandial glucose levels and to decrease the number of diabetic women requiring insulin without compromising fetal or obstetric outcomes.[38] In general, medical nutritional therapy should focus on healthy food choices, portion control, and cooking practices that women may carry with them for the rest of their lives.

There is a role for modest amounts of exercise in women with gestational diabetes. Planned physical activity of 30 min/day is recommended for all individuals capable of participating. Advising diabetic women to walk briskly or do arm exercises while seated in a chair for at least 10 min after each meal accomplishes this goal. Regular aerobic exercise with proper warm-up and cool-down has been shown to lower fasting and postprandial glucose concentrations in several small studies.[39,40]

INSULIN THERAPY

For women who fail to reach glycemic control with diet and exercise alone, pharmacologic treatment is then initiated. For years this treatment has been with injectable insulin but has been replaced in many US centers by glyburide (see below and Table 16.4).

Since gestational diabetes varies in severity, one insulin regimen is insufficient to guide treatment. The most commonly used insulins for gestational diabetes are very-short-acting insulins (lispro, aspart), regular insulin, Neutral Protamine Hagedorn (NPH), and glargine. While there has been recent concern regarding glargine use in pregnancy, several studies, including a recent meta-analysis, report safety in pregnancy.[41]

When both basal and meal-related insulin is needed, total daily insulin requirements are calculated based on body weight and gestational week. In the first trimester, the insulin requirement using actual body weight is 0.7 units/kg/day, in the second trimester it is 0.8 units/kg/day, and in the third trimester, 0.9–1.0 units/kg/day. In obese women, the dose will need to be adjusted upwards. For example, in an extremely obese woman, the initial doses of insulin may need to be increased to 1.5–2.0 units/kg to overcome the combined insulin resistance of pregnancy and obesity.[42] However, caution requires that women who are insulin naïve begin on the lower doses and be adjusted upwards as needed. While there are several insulin regimens that can be used, a three- or four-injection per day regimen seems the most effective. Commonly two-thirds of the total daily insulin dose (TDD) calculated is given as NPH (two-thirds before breakfast and one-third at bedtime) and the remaining one-third of the TDD is given as regular insulin

TABLE 16.4   Pharmacologic Therapy for Gestational Diabetes

	Glyburide	Metformin	Insulin
Mechanism of action	Stimulates pancreatic β-cell insulin release	Increases sensitivity to insulin; stimulates insulin-induced glucose uptake	Receptor-mediated glucose uptake; other actions
Onset of action	~1 h	~1 h	Varies
Peak	4 h	2–4 h	Varies
Dosing	2.5 mg in a.m. or every 12 h, increase weekly by 2.5 mg to a maximum of 10 mg every 12 h	500 mg in a.m. or every 12 h; maximum 1000 mg every 12 h	Varies
Route	Oral	Oral	Subcutaneous
Placental transport	Yes (but conflicting studies)	Yes	Minimal (only antibody bound fraction)
US FDA pregnancy category	C[a]	B	B[b]
Experience with use in pregnancy	Modest	Limited	Substantial
Failure to achieve euglycemia requiring insulin	20%	35%	

[a] Limited experience in the first trimester.
[b] Certain newer insulin analogs category C; FDA = US Food and Drug Administration.

further divided into two-thirds before breakfast and one-third before dinner. Alternatively, an easier regimen which mimics more the endogenous pancreatic production of insulin, begins with administration of one half of the calculated TDD as glargine at bedtime and the remaining half of the TDD divided into thirds and administered as lispro or aspart with each meal.

Some women with gestational diabetes will only have fasting or postprandial hyperglycemia. Fasting hyperglycemia is best treated with bedtime NPH or glargine. Postprandial hyperglycemia is best treated with lispro or aspart.

ORAL HYPOGLYCEMIC AGENTS

In recent years, there has been growing interest in oral hypoglycemic agents for glucose control in women with gestational diabetes. Sulfonylurea drugs enhance insulin secretion and peripheral tissue sensitivity to insulin.[43–46] Since the primary mechanism of hyperglycemia in gestational diabetes is pancreatic β-cell hyperplasia with poor insulin secretion and poor tissue response, it seems logical that sulfonylurea drugs may prove beneficial in this female population.

Glibenclamide (glyburide), a newer generation sulfonylurea, was not found in significant levels in cord blood of neonates at birth nor did it cross a human perfused placental cotelydon model.[47,48] Based on these observations, Langer et al. conducted a randomized control trial to study the potential of glyburide as a first-line therapy for gestational diabetes. They found that glyburide and insulin were equally effective in achieving good glycemic control, and perinatal outcomes were not significantly different between the two groups.[49] Additionally, the cord-serum insulin concentrations were similar in the two groups, and glyburide was not detected in the cord serum of any infant in the glyburide group.

In attempting to apply Langer's findings to a large-scale managed care practice, Jacobson *et al.* similarly found that glyburide was at least as effective as insulin in achieving glycemic control and similar birth weights in women with gestational diabetes.[50] In a secondary review of their earlier data, Langer *et al.* further showed that glyburide and insulin are equally efficacious for treatment of gestational diabetes at all severity levels of diabetes when fasting glucose was between 95 and 139 mg/dl. In their study population, they found that over 80% of women requiring pharmacologic intervention will achieve glycemic control with glyburide.[51] Many US centers now use glyburide as the first-line pharmaceutical treatment for gestational diabetes.

Metformin (Table 16.4) is another oral hypoglycemic agent used in some pregnant women. Metformin is a biguanide drug that has been shown to cross the placenta;[52] however, evidence regarding use of metformin during pregnancy has been favorable with little significant risk of fetal malformations or neonatal hypoglycemia.[48,53,54] Rowan *et al.* compared metformin alone to metformin plus insulin and insulin alone and found no increase in perinatal complications with the metformin group.[55] Additionally, women in the study found the metformin arm preferable to the insulin arm. A recent randomized trial comparing metformin with glyburide as single agents for gestational diabetes therapy found the failure rate higher with metformin, with more elective cesarean deliveries and small birth weights in the metformin group. Other maternal and neonatal outcomes were similar between the two groups.[56]

FETAL SURVEILLANCE

Antepartum fetal testing is recommend in women with preexisting diabetes.[57] Women with well-controlled gestational diabetes are presumably at lower risk for fetal death, particularly if there is no fasting hyperglycemia, but there is no consensus regarding antepartum testing in women with well-controlled gestational diabetes.[21] A cohort study of women with gestational diabetes who required only diet control found no fetal deaths in women monitored by only fetal movement counts from 28 to 40 weeks' gestation, and weekly non-stress tests thereafter.[58] Based on this study, it seems reasonable to offer kick count monitoring to well-controlled gestational diabetics not requiring insulin, given the low cost and high compliance of this intervention. Despite the lack of conclusive data, the American Congress of Obstetricians and Gynecologists (ACOG) recommends that women whose diabetes is not well controlled, who require insulin, or have other risk factors such as hypertension or adverse obstetric history should be managed the same as individuals with preexisting diabetes.[21]

TIMING AND MODE OF DELIVERY

There are no data supporting delivery of women with gestational diabetes before 38 weeks' gestation in the absence of objective evidence of maternal or fetal compromise. In fact, the ACOG recommends that when glucose control is good and no other complications supervene, there is no good evidence to support routine delivery before 40 weeks of gestation.[21] In a cohort study, a policy of induction of labor at 38–39 weeks of gestation for women with insulin-treated gestational diabetes was compared with the results in expectantly managed historic controls. There was no significant difference in macrosomia or cesarean delivery rates, but shoulder dystocia was experienced by 10% of the expectant management group beyond

40 weeks of gestation *vs* 1.4% in the group induced at 38—39 weeks of gestation.[59]

Cesarean delivery rates are higher in women with gestational diabetes compared with non-diabetic controls, and the difference is not entirely attributable to fetal macrosomia.[60] Caregivers may be more prone to perform cesarean deliveries in women with gestational diabetes because of concern regarding risk of shoulder dystocia. There are no data to support a policy of cesarean delivery based purely on the diagnosis of gestational diabetes. It may be reasonable, however, to recommend cesarean delivery without a trial of labor at some particular threshold of fetal weight; both 4,250 and 4,500 g have been used as a threshold.[21] The Fifth International Workshop-Congress on Gestational Diabetes Mellitus concludes that strategies to reduce the risk of birth injury in women with gestational diabetes include a liberal policy toward cesarean delivery when fetal overgrowth is suspected.[28]

FOLLOW-UP TESTING AND LONG-TERM IMPLICATIONS

Since some of the earliest studies describing glucose intolerance in pregnancy, it has long been noted that the development of diabetes during pregnancy places a woman at high risk of developing overt diabetes later in life.[61] Although most women with gestational diabetes will return to normal glucose tolerance after delivery, a significant number will continue to display impaired glucose tolerance postpartum. In order to help identify these women who will develop type 2 diabetes, both American Congress of Obstetricians and Gynecologists[21] and the American Diabetes Association[62] recommend postpartum glucose testing, specifically a 75-g oral glucose load at about 6—12 weeks postpartum in women with gestational diabetes who do not have diabetes immediately postpartum. Fasting blood glucose alone is insufficient to test for type 2 diabetes in this setting.[63,64]

Given the high risk of developing type 2 diabetes in the years following a pregnancy complicated by gestational diabetes, the Fifth International Workshop-Conference on Gestational Diabetes recommends further screening including an oral glucose challenge test 1 year following delivery and every 3 years thereafter.[28] In one study of a group of Latino women with gestational diabetes, nearly 80% of those women that still demonstrated impaired glucose tolerance postpartum developed overt diabetes within 5 years.[65] Early diagnosis and treatment of type 2 diabetes can mitigate complications.

SUMMARY

Gestational diabetes now complicates about 7% of all pregnancies and is caused by peripheral insulin resistance and decreased insulin production, despite pancreatic β-cell proliferation. Left untreated, gestational diabetes can cause such adverse effects as increased cesarean delivery, macrosomia, birth trauma, and neonatal hypoglycemia as well as long-term metabolic effects on the newborn; childhood obesity and diabetes later in life can also be seen in the child of a diabetic mother. Pregnancy can be viewed as a "stress test" for type 2 diabetes in that women who develop gestational diabetes are at high risk for development of overt diabetes later in life. The postpartum period may be the ideal time to educate women regarding their risk of overt diabetes and institute lifestyle changes such as weight loss and exercise that may change that risk.

References

1. American Diabetes Association. Diagnosis and classification of diabetes mellitus. *Diabetes Care* 2011;**34**:S62—9.
2. Ferrara A, Kahn HS, Quesenberry CP, Riley C, Hedderson MM. An increase in the incidence of gestational diabetes mellitus: Northern California, 1991-2000. *Obstet Gynecol* 2004;**103**:526—33.

3. Coustan DR, Carpenter MW. Detection and treatment of gestational diabetes. *Clin Obstet Gynecol* 1985;**28**:507–15.

4. Mestman JH. Outcome of diabetes screening in pregnancy and perinatal morbidity in infants of mothers with mild impairment in glucose tolerance. *Diabetes Care* 1980;**3**:447–52.

5. The HAPO Study Research Group. Hyperglycemia and adverse pregnancy outcomes. *N Engl J Med* 2008;**358**:1991–2002.

6. Buchanan TA, Metzger BE, Freinkel N. Accelerated starvation in late pregnancy: A comparison between obese women with and without gestational diabetes mellitus. *Am J Obstet Gynecol* 1990;**162**:1015–20.

7. Buchanan TA, Metzger BE, Frienkel N. Insulin sensitivity and B-cell responsiveness to glucose during late pregnancy in lean and moderately obese women with normal glucose tolerance or mild gestational diabetes. *Am J Obstet Gynecol* 1990;**162**:1008–14.

8. Catalano PM, Tyzbir ED, Roman NM, Amini SB, Sims EA. Longitudinal changes in insulin release and insulin resistance in non-obese pregnant women. *Am J Obstet Gynecol* 1991;**165**:1667–72.

9. Catalano PM. Longitudinal changes in glucose metabolism during pregnancy in obese women with normal glucose tolerance and gestational diabetes mellitus. *Am J Obstet Gynecol* 1999;**180**:903–16.

10. Shao J, Catalano PM, Yamashita H, Ruyter I, Smith S, Younggren J, Friedman JE. Impaired insulin receptor tyrosine kinase activity and overexpression of PC-1 in skeletal muscle from obese women with gestational diabetes. *Diabetes* 2000;**49**:603–10.

11. Friedman JE, Ishizuka T, Huston L. Impaired glucose transport and insulin receptor tyrosine kinase phosphorylation in skeletal muscle from obese women with gestational diabetes. *Diabetes* 1999;**48**:1807–14.

12. Okuno S, Akazawa S, Yasuhi I. Decreased expression of GLUT4 glucose transpoter protein in adipose tissue during pregnancy. *Homr Metab Res* 1995;**27**:231–4.

13. Van Assche F, Aerts L, De Prins F. A morphological study of the endocrine pancreas in human pregnancy. *Br J Obstet Gynaecol* 1978;**85**:818–20.

14. Sorenson RL, Brelje TC. Adaptation of islets of Langerhans to pregnancy: beta-cell growth, enhanced insulin secretion and the role of lactogenic hormones. *Horm Metab Res* 1997;**29**:301–7.

15. Van Assche FA, Aerts L, Gepts W. Morphological changes in the endocrine pancreas in pregnant rats with experimental diabetes. *J Endocrinol* 1979;**80**:175–9.

16. Coustan DR, Nelson C, Carpenter MW, Carr SR, Rotondo L, Widness JA. Maternal age and screening for gestational diabetes: a population-based study. *Obstet Gynecol* 1989;**73**:557–61.

17. Xiong X, Saunders LD, Wang FL, Demianczuk NN. Gestational diabetes mellitus: prevalence, risk factors, maternal and infant outcomes. *Int J Gynaecol Obstet* 2001;**75**:221–8.

18. Gaudier FL, Hauth JC, Poist M, Corbett D, Cliver SP. Recurrence of gestational diabetes mellitus. *Obstet Gynecol* 1992;**80**:755–8.

19. Philipson EH, Super DM. Gestational diabetes mellitus: does it recur in subsequent pregnancy? *Am J Obstet Gynecol* 1989;**160**:1324–31.

20. Major CA, deVeciana M, Weeks J, Morgan MA. Recurrence of gestational diabetes: who is at risk? *Am J Obstet Gynecol* 1998;**179**:1038–42.

21. American College of Obstetricians and Gynecologists. *Gestational Diabetes. ACOG Practice Bulletin 30.* Washington, DC: ACOG; 2001.

22. Hillier TA, Vesco KK, Pedula KL, Beil TL, Whitlock EP, Pettitt DJ. Screening for gestational diabetes mellitus: a systematic review for the U.S. Preventive Services Task Force. *Ann Intern Med* 2008;**20**:766–75.

23. O'Sullivan JB, Mahan CM, Charles D, Dandrow RV. Screening criteria for high-risk gestational diabetic women. *Am J Obstet Gynecol* 1973;**116**:895–900.

24. World Health Organization Expert Committee on Diabetes Mellitus. *Second report of the WHO Expert Committee on diabetes mellitus. Geneva, Technical Report Series 646.* WHO; 1980.

25. Metzger B, Coustan D, Dyer A, Hadden D, Hod M, Lowe L, Oats J, Persson B, Trimble E. New findings in gestational diabetes – the HAPO Study. *Diabetes Voice* 2009;**54**:S25–8.

26. International Association of Diabetes and Pregnancy Study Groups. Recommendations on the diagnosis and classification of hyperglycemia in pregnancy. *Diabetes Care* 2010;**33**:676–82.

27. Pedersen J. Diabetes and pregnancy. *Blood sugar of newborn infants*; 1952. Thesis 230.

28. Metzger BE, Buchanan TA, Coustan DR, de Leiva A, Dunger DB, Hadden DR, Hod M, Kitzmiller JL, Kjos SL, Oats JN, Pettitt DJ, Sacks DA, Zoupas C. Summary and recommendations of the Fifth International Workshop-Conference on Gestational Diabetes Mellitus. *Diabetes Care* 2007;**30**:S251–60.

29. Aerts L, Van Assche FA. Is gestational diabetes an acquired condition? *J Dev Physiol* 1979;**1**:219–25.

30. Boloker J, Gertz SJ, Simmons RA. Gestational diabetes leads to the development of diabetes in adulthood in the rat. *Diabetes* 2002;**51**:1499–506.

31. Silverman BL, Metzger BE, Cho NH, Loeb CA. Impaired glucose tolerance in adolescent offspring of diabetic mothers. Relationship to fetal hyperinsulinism. *Diabetes Care* 1995;**18**:611–7.

32. Plagemann A, Harder T, Kohlhoff R, Rohde W, Dorner G. Glucose tolerance and insulin secretion in children of mothers with pregestational IDDM or gestational diabetes. *Diabetologia* 1997;**40**:1094–100.

33. Crowther CA, Hiller JE, Moss JR, McPhee AJ, Jeffries WS, Robinson JS. Effect of treatment of gestational diabetes mellitus on pregnancy outcomes. *N Engl J Med* 2005;**352**:2477–86.

34. Langer O, Yogev Y, Most O, Xenakis MJ. Gestational diabetes: the consequences of not treating. *Am J Obstet Gynecol* 2005;**192**:989–97.

35. DeVeciana M, Major CA, Morgan MA. Postprandial versus preprandial blood glucose monitoring in women with gestational diabetes mellitus requiring insulin therapy. *N Engl J Med* 1995;**333**:1237–41.

36. Jovanovic L. Role of diet and insulin treatment of diabetes in pregnancy. *Clin Obstet Gyn* 2000;**43**:46–55.

37. Magee MS, Knopp RH, Benedetti TJ. Metabolic effects of 1,200-kcal diet in obese pregnant women with gestational diabetes. *Diabetes* 1990;**39**:234–40.

38. Chew I, Brand J, Thorburn A, Truswell A. Application of glycemic index to mixed meals. *Am J Clin Nutr* 1988;**47**:53–6.

39. Jovanovic-Peterson L, Durak EP, Peterson CM. Randomized trial of diet versus diet plus cardiovascular conditioning on glucose levels in gestational diabetes. *Am J Obstet Gynecol* 1989;**161**:415–9.

40. Garcia-Patterson A, Martin E, Ubeda J, Maria MA, de Leiva A, Corcoy R. Evaluation of light exercise in the treatment of gestational diabetes. *Diabetes Care* 2001;**24**:2006–7.

41. Pollex E, Moretti ME, Koren G, Feig DS. Safety of insulin glargine use in pregnancy: A systematic review and meta-analysis. *The Annals of Pharmacotherapy* 2011;**45**:1–8.

42. Jovanovic-Peterson L, Peterson CM. Nutritional management of the obese gestational diabetic woman. *J Am Coll Nutr* 1992;**11**:246–50.

43. Groop L, Luzi L, Melanger A, Groop PH, DeFronzo RA. Different effects of glyburide and glipizide on insulin and hepatic glucose production in normal and NIDDM subjects. *Diabetes* 1987;**36**:1320–8.

44. Groop LC, Barzilai N, Ratheiser K, Luzi L, Wahlin-Boll E, Melander A. Dose-dependent effects of glyburide on insulin secretion and glucose uptake in humans. *Diabetes Care* 1991;**14**:724–7.

45. Rossetti L, Giaaccari A, DeFronzo RA. Glucose toxicity. *Diabetes Care* 1990;**13**:610–30.

46. Simonson DC, Ferrannini E, Bevilacqua S, Smith D, Barret E, Carlson R. Mechanism of improvement in glucose metabolism after chronic glyburide therapy. *Diabetes Care* 1984;**33**:838–45.

47. Elliott BD, Langer O, Schenker S, Johnson RF. Insignificant transfer of glyburide occurs across the human placenta. *Am J Obstet Gynecol* 1991;**165**(4 Pt 1):807–12.

48. Elliott BD, Schenker S, Langer O. Comparative placental transport of oral hypoglycemic agents in humans: a model of human placental drug transfer. *Am J Obstet Gynecol* 1994;**171**:653–60.

49. Langer O, Conway DL, Berkus MD. A comparison of glyburide and insulin in women with gestational diabetes mellitus. *N Engl J Med* 2000;**343**:1134–8.

50. Jacobson GF, Ramos GA, Ching JY, Kirby RS, Ferrara A, Field DR. Comparison of glyburide and insulin for the management of gestational diabetes in a large managed care organization. *Am J Obstet Gynecol* 2005;**193**:118–24.

51. Langer O, Yogev Y, Xenakis EM, Rosenn B. Insulin and glyburide therapy: dosage, severity level of gestational diabetes, and pregnancy outcome. *Am J Obstet Gynecol* 2005;**192**:134–9.

52. Charles B, Norris R, Xiao X, Hague W. Population pharmacokinetics of metformin in late pregnancy. *Ther Drug Monit* 2006;**28**:67–72.

53. Sivan E, Feldman B, Dolitzki M. Glyburide crosses the placenta in vivo in pregnant rats. *Diabetologia* 1995;**38**:753–6.

54. Koren G. Glyburide and fetal safety: transplacental pharmacokinetic considerations. *Reprod Toxicol* 2001;**15**:227–9.

55. Rowan JA, Hague WM, Gao W, Battin MR, Moore MP, MiG Trial Investigators. Metformin versus insulin for the treatment of gestational diabetes. *N Engl J Med* 2008;**358**:2003–15.

56. Moore LE, Clokey D, Rappaport VJ, Curet LB. Metformin compared with glyburide in gestational diabetes: a randomized controlled trial. *Obstet Gynecol* 2010;**115**:55–9.

57. American College of Obstetricians and Gynecologists. *Antepartum fetal surveillance. ACOG Practice Bulletin 9.* Washington, DC: ACOG; 1999.

58. Landon MB, Gabbe SG. Antepartum fetal surveillance in gestational diabetes mellitus. *Diabetes* 1985;**34**(Suppl. 2):50–4.

59. Lurie S, Insler V, Hagay ZJ. Induction of labor at 38 to 39 weeks of gestation reduces the incidence of shoulder dystocia in gestational diabetic women Class A2. *Am J Perinatol* 1996;**13**:293–6.

60. Casey BM, Lucas MJ, McIntire DD, Leveno KJ. Pregnancy outcomes in women with gestational diabetes compared with the general obstetric population. *Obstet Gynecol* 1997;**90**:869–73.

61. O'Sullivan JB, Mahan CM. Criteria for the oral glucose tolerance test in pregnancy. *Diabetes* 1964;**13**:278–85.

II. TYPES OF DIABETES AND ITS CORRELATION WITH OTHER DISEASES

62. American Diabetes Association. Gestational diabetes mellitus. *Diabetes Care* 2004;**27**:S88—90.

63. Kitzmiller J, Dang-Kilduff L, Taslimi M. Gestational diabetes after delivery: short-term management and long-term risks. *Diabetes Care* 2007;**30**: S225—35.

64. Ferrara A, Peng T, Kim C. Trends in postpartum diabetes screening and subsequent diabetes and impaired fasting glucose among women with histories of gestational diabetes mellitus: A report from the TRIAD Study. *Diabetes Care* 2009;**32**:269—74.

65. Kjos SL, Peters RK, Xiang A, Henry OA, Montoro M, Buchanan TA. Predicting future diabetes in Latino women with gestational diabetes: utility of early postpartum glucose tolerance testing. *Diabetes* 1995;**44**:586—91.

MOLECULAR INSIGHTS OF DIABETES AND METABOLIC SYNDROME

Gene—Environment Interaction in the Pathogenesis of Type 2 Diabetes

Kian-Peng Goh

Division of Endocrinology, Khoo Teck Puat Hospital, Alexandra Health, Singapore

INTRODUCTION

The study of complex diseases like type 2 diabetes mellitus (T2DM) classically posits that the determinants of biological variation are the genes and the environment. Unlike monogenic disorders where the gene has a strong impact on disease susceptibility when the penetrance is high, polygenic disorders are thought to result from the wrong interaction between the genes and the environment. In these cases, the impact of the gene on disease susceptibility is usually small to moderate.

The resources required to adequately study gene—environment interaction include a comprehensive human gene data bank which contains all known genes and their variants, accurate epidemiological records, well-defined disease populations and the human genomic epidemiology network (HuGE).[1] T2DM as a disease entity fulfills most if not all of these criteria, hence studies on the effect of gene–environment on its pathogenesis has garnered increased interest in recent years.

However, the road to elucidating the nature and contribution of the genes and the environment in the etiology of T2DM has not been easy and is usually fraught with more questions than answers. While the advent of epigenetic studies has provided possible hypotheses that may connect some of the dots, currently they remain speculative at best. The aim of this review is to examine the advances made so far in the genetic, epigenetic and environmental factors of T2DM pathogenesis and attempt to provide a plausible link between them.

THE GENETIC COMPONENT

Evidence of Genetic Contribution

T2DM has long been recognized as having a genetic component. The most convincing evidence comes from twin studies which indicate a concordance rate in monozygotic twins of 20–76%.[2–5] However, most of these studies suffer from flaws common in twin studies except for the study from Finland which is based on their national twin registry and is free from major methodological errors. In that study, the authors reported proband-wise and pair-wise concordance rates of 34% and 20% among monozygotic twins and 16% and 9% in dizygotic twins, respectively.[4]

The limitations of twin studies are also well-known. They do not tell us the genes responsible, mode of transmission or disease mechanism and do not consider intra-uterine factors. In addition, they pose a challenge in diseases with a late or variable onset. Nevertheless, these findings are useful in demonstrating that although a strong genetic contribution to disease susceptibility exists for T2DM, environmental influence also forms a significant contribution.[6]

Candidate Genes for T2DM

T2DM risk genes can be categorized into gene variants affecting insulin secretion, insulin sensitivity, glucagon secretion, or adiposity.[7] The interest in indentifying these genes is two-fold. Firstly, the discovery of such genes will lead to an increased understanding of the disease etiology which may provide new targets for treatment. Secondly, it may contribute to improved disease prediction allowing us to implement effective preventive strategies and intervene early.[8,9]

The Thrifty Gene Hypothesis

In 1962, Neel hypothesized the existence of thrifty genes or a "thrifty genotype" defined as one "which is exceptionally efficient in the intake and/or utilization of food".[10] This concept was later expanded by Chakravarthy and Booth to include the concept of coupled cycling between feast and famine; physical activity and rest; and metabolic processes. According to their hypothesis, thrifty genes were activated during feasting and rest and silenced during famine and physical activity. The advantage of such a genotype lies in its ability to maximize fuel storage in the form of fat and minimize caloric wastage, which ultimately offers the best chance of survival in a harsh and hostile environment where food availability is uncertain. Conversely, hunting and food gathering would occur during periods of low food supply. If food procurement was successful, feasting would resume in order to replenish depleted fuel stores and the cycling continued (Figure 17.1).

Over time, this would lead to the gradual elimination of those with non-thrifty genotypes from the human gene pool as they would not be able to conserve fuel efficiently and hence die off. This led to the selection of thrifty genes which would improve the likelihood of survival after unsuccessful hunts and during famines, and have remained with us since then. However, an obvious downside to this genotype is the metabolic cost that occurs when such

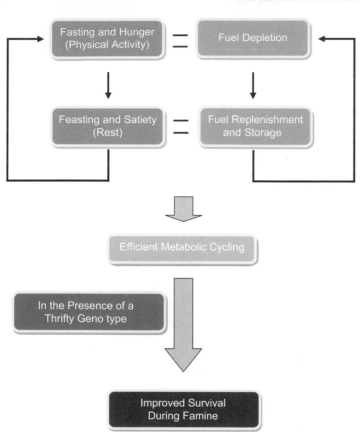

FIGURE 17.1 Normal feast-famine and physical activity-rest cycle and how the selection of thrifty genes and genotype leads to improved survival for the species during famine.

an environment no longer exists and food becomes plentiful. The cycling process is stalled and the excess fuel gets shunted into an unhealthy storage resulting in obesity and related metabolic diseases like T2DM (Figure 17.2). This phenomenon has been aptly described as a dissonance between "Stone Age" genes and "Space Age" circumstances.[11,12]

However, no thrifty genes or variants have been identified to date and only approximately 20–30% of the population is obese, although one would expect a proportion close to 100% since according to this hypothesis, everyone should have thrifty genes by now. Consequently, the debate on thrifty genes still rages on.[13,14]

Results of Genomewide Association Studies

The advent of genomewide association studies (GWAS) took the hunt for causative genes in complex diseases to the next level. In GWAS, single-nucleotide polymorphisms (SNPs) are tested for association with diseases and have revolutionized the way we hunt down genetic influences on complex traits. It is useful for detecting common risk alleles with a low effect size. So far, more than 500 GWAS covering 150 diseases with nearly 800 significant SNP-trait associations have been published.[15]

The landmark GWAS by the Wellcome Trust Case Control Consortium identified the following as possible candidate genes for T2DM: *PPARγ* (peroxisomal proliferative

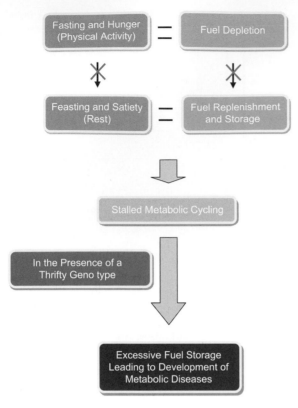

FIGURE 17.2 Stalling of the metabolic cycling and how the previous selection of thrifty genes and genotype leads to the development of metabolic diseases.

activated receptor gamma), *KCNJ11* (the inwardly-rectifying Kir6.2 component of the pancreatic β-cell KATP channel), *FTO* (fat-mass and obesity-associated), *CDKAL1* (CDK5 regulatory subunit associated protein 1-like 1), *HHEX* (homeobox, hematopoietically expressed), *IDE* (insulin degrading enzyme) and *TCF7L2* (transcription factor 7-like 2).[16]

To date, 38 SNPs associated with T2DM have been discovered, in addition to nearly two dozen associated with glycemic traits.[17] In one study, a genotype scoring system based on 18 known risk alleles was shown to be able to predict new cases of diabetes, but provided only a slightly better prediction of risk compared to knowledge of common risk factors

alone.[18] So the currently identified loci confer only a modest effect size in the variation of disease susceptibility and have yet to explain much of the genetic contribution believed to exist in T2DM.[19]

Some of these findings have increased our understanding of the fundamental biology of T2DM as well as implicated novel pathways. Interestingly, by increasing sample sizes and interrogating the genetic determinants of T2DM as a continuous glycemic trait rather than a dichotomous phenotype, most of the identified loci point to a primary defect in the β-cell.[17]

Collectively, these results imply three things. Firstly, although we have made substantial progress in identifying several gene variants associated with an increased risk of T2DM, a large portion of the genetic heritability remains unexplained. Hence, the burden of proof still lies upon us to demonstrate that thrifty genes or major T2DM risk genes exist. Secondly, the real value of genomic information may be in helping us understand the mechanism of disease, rather than providing clinically meaningful information.[20] Thirdly, although such genetic information may not be useful in the clinical prediction of T2DM, it may be useful in the younger age groups before the development of clinical risk factors.[17]

THE ENVIRONMENTAL COMPONENT

Physical Activity

Currently, there is substantial evidence to support the hypothesis that moderate to intensive physical activity is associated with the prevention of T2DM as well as a longer life expectancy.[21–23] Epidemiological data alone suggest that physically active individuals have a 30–50% lower risk of developing T2DM than sedentary persons.[24] Moreover, the risk of T2DM in physically inactive subjects is independent of obesity.[25]

The landmark Diabetes Prevention Program Study demonstrated the superiority of an intensive lifestyle exercise regimen over drug intervention in reducing the risk of diabetes in high-risk individuals. In this study, lifestyle intervention reduced the incidence by 58% and metformin by 31% as compared with placebo.[26] This result was also replicated in other population groups like the Da Qing Study in China and Finnish Diabetes Prevention Study in Finland, where similar effects of physical activity in reducing T2DM risk were demonstrated.[27,28] Taken together, these results firmly establish the importance of physical activity in decreasing the risk of T2DM.

Circadian Rhythm

The central circadian clock in mammals is located within the pacemaker neurons of the suprachiasmatic nucleus located in the anterior hypothalamus. Its function is to maintain proper phase alignment of the peripheral clocks in almost all other cells. There is mounting evidence that circadian clocks regulated by clock genes participate in glucose homeostasis, lipogenesis, and oxidative metabolism and the disruption of these genes is associated with an increased risk of metabolic diseases.[29]

A complex network involving the transcriptional activators circadian locomotor output cycles kaput (Clock), brain and muscle-Arnt-like 1 (Bmal1), and their targets genes Period (Per) and Cryptochrome (Cry) exists to coordinate the different metabolic responses within peripheral tissues according to the wake–sleep cycle. For example, 50% of the known nuclear receptors in white and brown adipose tissue, liver, and skeletal muscle in mice exhibit rhythmic expression.[30]

In terms of lifestyle factors, a high-fat diet leads to a disruption in clock gene expression and a phase delay in their downstream effectors.[31] Decreased sleep duration is also associated with an increased body mass index and

the risk of developing diabetes mellitus.[32–34] Even the reversal of the day–night cycle seen in night shift workers has been shown to be related to the metabolic syndrome.[35]

These findings are consistent with those from studies on clock gene mutants. Homozygous C57BL/6 J Clock mutant mice are obese and hyperphagic, have a greatly attenuated diurnal feeding rhythm and develop metabolic complications including hyperglycemia, hyperlipidemia and hyperleptinemia.[36]

While these results are far from conclusive, they do provide sufficient evidence to warrant further investigations into the relationship between the disruption of the circadian rhythm and the risk of metabolic diseases.

Gut Microbiota

The human gut microbiota is colonized at birth by maternal bacteria as well as the surrounding environment. It is composed of over 1,000 bacterial species resembling a multicellular organ which has evolved together with its host and provides it with the metabolic functions that it did not evolve with. More than 95% of the total microbiota is represented by the three dominant species: Firmicutes, Bacteroidetes, and Actinobacteria.[37]

There has been a recent interest in the possible role the gut microbiota plays in the pathogenesis of certain diseases. In both human and mice models, comparisons of the distal gut microbiota in both the obese and their lean counterparts have shown that obesity is associated with changes in the relative abundance of the two dominant bacterial divisions, the Bacteroidetes and the Firmicutes. Obese individuals have a decreased proportion of Bacteroidetes compared to lean people and this proportion increases with weight loss and a low-calorie diet.[38] Interestingly, the obese microbiome also has an increased capacity to harvest energy from the diet.[39] Consequently, there is increased fermentation capacity of the microbiota resulting in increased short-chain fatty acid production which has been implicated in the development of obesity through *de novo* lipogenesis.[37]

In subjects with T2DM, the proportions of *Firmicutes* and *Clostridia* were significantly reduced whereas the *Betaproteobacteria* was positively correlated with plasma glucose. The ratio of *Bacteroidetes* to *Firmicutes* also correlated positively with plasma glucose, but not with BMIs.[40]

Although the host genetics may impact on the microbiota, its effect is likely to be small. Conversely, the environment is likely to carry a more significant impact. For example, the host diet is one of the most important factors influencing host bacterial diversity. This dietary effect may be due to the variation in the ability of different species to use certain substrates like carbohydrates and fats. There is also mounting evidence that points to the heritability of the microbiota via a non-genetic transmission like the maternal micriobiome, also known as the maternal effect. Throughout life, other factors including antibiotic use, illnesses, travel, exercise, and socialization such as relocation have also been implicated.[41]

Currently, whether the difference in the gut microbiota in diabetic and obese individuals is a cause or effect remains unclear. In addition, the exact mechanism with which the gut microbiota affects the risk of T2DM is unknown.

Endocrine Disrupters[42]

In recent years, there has been a growing interest in the possible harm of endocrine-disrupting chemicals (EDCs) to our health. EDCs are defined as exogenous agents that interfere with the synthesis, secretion, transport, metabolism, binding action, or elimination of natural blood-borne hormones that are present in the body and are responsible for homeostasis, reproduction and developmental process.

EDCs are believed to interact with the genes and/or epigenome of key genes to alter the propensity for disease development later in life,

thus affecting not only the exposed individual but also subsequent generations.[43] Although the transgenerational epigenetic effects of environmental exposures are seen in animal models, epigenetic inheritance in humans remains to be convincingly elucidated.[44]

Epidemiological studies have found an association between high levels of dioxin and dioxin-like compounds with an increased risk for diabetes. The mechanism is postulated to be due to the antagonism of PPARγ functions through the activation of the aryl hydrocarbon receptor. Decreased PPARγ activity may lead to diabetes and continuous exposure to these compounds may reduce the expression and production of the glucose transporter protein GLUT4, thereby causing progressive insulin resistance.[45]

The widespread use of bisphenol A (BPA), an estrogenic compound, implies a great potential for exposure of the fetus and the young especially during early childhood development. Indeed, BPA has been found to cross the human placenta and has been measured in both maternal and fetal blood. Acute treatment with BPA through its estrogenic-like effect has been shown to cause temporary hyperinsulinemia, while longer-term exposure can lead to insulin resistance.[46] Low doses have also been found to inhibit the release of adiponectin, a hormone that improves insulin sensitivity.[47] In recognition of its potential for harm, Canada and the European Union have banned BPA in baby bottles.

Finally, advanced-glycation end products (AGEs), produced during high-temperature cooking, increase oxidative stress through the generation of reactive oxygen species. Oxidative stress has been implicated in the pathogenesis of T2DM through its effects on peripheral tissues and the pancreatic β-cell. In animal models, a high-AGE diet has been found to be associated with the development of T2DM and obesity.[48]

In summary, the evidence so far points to T2DM as a complex disease with genetic susceptibility being a prerequisite for its development, but requiring a significant environmental contribution for its clinical expression.

EPIGENETICS

As alluded to earlier, currently identified genetic variants explain only a small proportion of the heritability of T2DM leaving a large proportion of heritability unaccounted for. This unexplained heritability may be due to two possible reasons: (i) gene–environment interactions; and (ii) more complex pathways involving multiple genes and exposures.[49]

Epigenetics can be defined as the study of heritable changes in gene expression not attributable to changes in DNA sequence. Hence, it relates to the inheritance of genetic information on the basis of gene expression, in contrast to genetics which relates to gene sequence.[50] It can be seen as an intermediate event through which gene and environmental effects are mediated. Implicit to the understanding of epigenetics is its reactive and not proactive nature. What this means is that a change will only occur in response to an imposing event. On a molecular basis, epigenetics represent the structural adaptation of chromosomal regions to register, signal, or perpetuate altered activity states.[51] An epigenetic trait, then, is a stably heritable phenotype resulting from changes in a chromosome without alterations in the DNA sequence.[52]

At least four forms of epigenetic mechanisms have been described: (i) DNA methylation; (ii) small non-coding RNA-based silencing; (iii) polycomb-trithorax gene regulation; and (iv) post-translational modification of histone proteins by acetylation, methylation, phosphorylation, ubiquitinylation, glycosylation, sumoylation, and ADP ribosylation. Collectively, these marks form a combinatorial code, known as the histone code, that serves to determine whether the underlying DNA sequence is recognized in its active or inactive state.[53]

Once the genetic expression pattern has been set up, these epigenetic mechanisms ensure that they are stably inherited during cell division.[44,54,55]

Evidence from Population Studies[56]

Diamond provided further insight into the role of epigenetics in T2DM by comparing the prevalence rates of different population groups with their historical background in an attempt to prove a case for natural selection. The Nauruan Polynesian Islanders, whose ancestors depended on agriculture and fishing for food, experienced rampant starvation during World War 2 when a significant proportion of the population died. During the post-independence economic boom after the war, food became abundant again and the traditional lifestyle of fishing and farming gave way to a sedentary lifestyle. Within five decades, the prevalence of T2DM increased dramatically from 0% to 41%. This was difficult to account for from a genetic origin alone.

Similarly, the ancestors of the Arizona Pima Indians led a vigorous hunter–gatherer lifestyle. During the late 19th century, European immigrants diverted away the headwaters of the rivers, which reduced their capacity for irrigation and led to crop failures and widespread starvation. Hence, like their counterparts the Nauruans, the Pima Indians suffered an extra bout of natural selection in addition to the change to a sedentary lifestyle compared to their ancestors. This may explain the dramatic increase in T2DM prevalence within a relatively short time.

In contrast, Europeans enjoy a low prevalence of T2DM compared to any non-European population matched for lifestyle. As the originators of the Western lifestyle, they were spared much earlier from the severe famines which afflicted their ancestors and disappeared between 1650 and 1900.

These population studies provide compelling and thought-provoking evidence for natural selection. Since no thrifty gene has been found so far, the focus has shifted to searching for a thrifty epigenotype instead.[57]

Evidence from Famine Studies

The other piece of evidence for an epigenetic contribution stems from famine studies which provide the basis for the hypothesis that maternal malnutrition in pregnancy increases the risk of the progeny developing metabolic and cardiovascular related diseases in later life.

The earliest epidemiological study linking poor fetal growth and subsequent development of T2DM was by Hales and colleagues who showed that the proportion of men with impaired glucose tolerance fell progressively from 26% among those who were 18 lb (8.16 kg) or less at one year to 13% among those who had weighed 27 lb (12.25 kg) or more. Corresponding figures for T2DM were 17% and 0%, respectively.[58]

The recent study on the Chinese Famine (1959–1961) showed an association between the risk of metabolic syndrome in later life and the severity of the famine exposure. Similar associations were observed for adults who were exposed to the famine during early childhood, but not those exposed during mid- or late childhood. However, subjects born in severely affected famine areas with Western dietary habits in adulthood or who were overweight in adulthood had a particularly high risk of metabolic syndrome in later life.[59] Studies on the Dutch Winter Famine (1944–1945) and the Leningrad Siege (1941–1944) showed similar results.[60–62]

Developmental Plasticity

The findings from population and famine studies have led to the concept of developmental plasticity defined as the ability of an organism to develop in various ways, depending on the particular environment.[63] Developmental plasticity is a subset of phenotypic plasticity defined as the capacity of a single genotype to result in different phenotypes tailored to the environment. The consequence is a multipurpose genome, which allows the same genetic information to yield multiple cell types, highly dissimilar life stages, and alternative developmental pathways based on the organism's own and its ancestral environment.[64] Closely linked to this is the understanding of the developmental origins of health and disease which suggests that a stimulus in early development contributes to changes in the phenotype that predisposes it to later disease.[65]

It is now believed that nutritional cues in a developing organism in allowing it to predict a nutritionally harsh future environment, can condition the fetus to shift into a thrift mode. These phenotypic changes, collectively known as predictive adaptive response, include insulin resistance and a reduction of energy consuming tissues like skeletal and cardiac muscles. This is advantageous and improves the likelihood of postnatal survival should the environmental conditions remain consistent and the lack continues. However, it becomes maladaptive should the subsequent nutritional environment become favorable again, leading to a mismatch between a thrifty phenotype and a favorable environment.[66]

Through epigenetics, the evolutionarily valuable trait of metabolic thrift is maintained and future generations get their own chance to re-interpret the genotype in accordance with the environmental conditions encountered during early life. These changes, by virtue of the fact that they do not involve the genetic sequence, allow a prompt adaptation back to a less thrifty phenotype should the environment become favorable again.[57] This phenomenon was seen in the Nauruans when the incidence rate of T2DM decreased from 17.1 to 7.4 cases per 1,000 person-years within 10 years.[67]

This adaptive reversibility was also observed in animal models, which demonstrated that the magnitude of the programmed phenotypic expression decreases with successive generations, yet allowing the population to survive long enough to adapt.[68] Hence, epigenetic marks and alterations have an important role in population survival, by providing an intermediate level of control. However, the downside to this adaptive plasticity is its negative effect on evolvability through the weakening of the effect of natural selection.

The risk of T2DM is therefore contributed by genetic susceptibility, developmental environment and the adult environment. The risk is highest when the individual carries T2DM risk genes, the developmental environment is harsh and the adult environment is favorable. The opposite scenario is associated with the lowest risk (Figure 17.3).

The link between disease development and the two environments may thus be largely explained by epigenetic mechanisms. In one data-mining study, epigenetic factors scored among the highest in the pathogenesis of T2DM with adipocytes as the potential tissue of origin and cytokines or cytokine-like genes implicated as well.[69] It is therefore likely that phenotypic variation in terms of the differences among individuals in their risk for T2DM and obesity arises from variations in

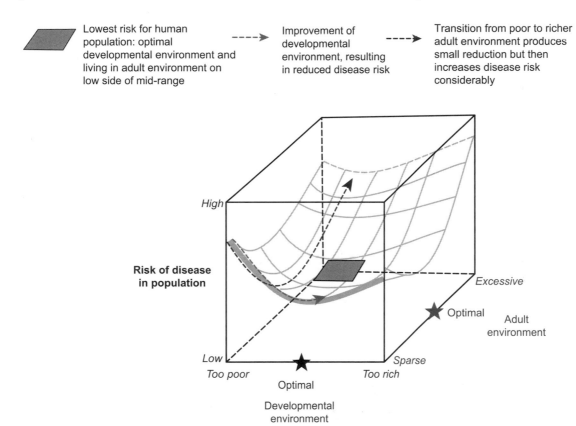

FIGURE 17.3 **Risk of disease development as a function of the adult and developmental environments**. *(Reprinted from Trends in Endocrinology and Metabolism, 21/4, Godfrey KM, Gluckman PD, Hanson MA. Developmental origins of metabolic disease: life course and intergenerational perspectives, 203. Copyright (2010), with permission from Elsevier.)*

programming events during critical stages of development.

Gene–Environment Interaction and Beyond

The paradigm in the understanding of T2DM development has shifted from a purely genetic or environmental origin to one in which there is a complex interdependent relationship between the genotype and the environment. This gene–environment interaction also spans across generations beginning with the ancestral environment to the maternal nutritional environment and finally to the adult environment. It is an interaction in which both genetic susceptibility and epigenetic mechanisms play a part, of which the latter may have a more dominant role. Hence, we should move beyond a gene–environment model to a gene/epigene–environment one as proposed by Bollati.[44] There is already early evidence of an epigene–environment interaction from a study which demonstrated

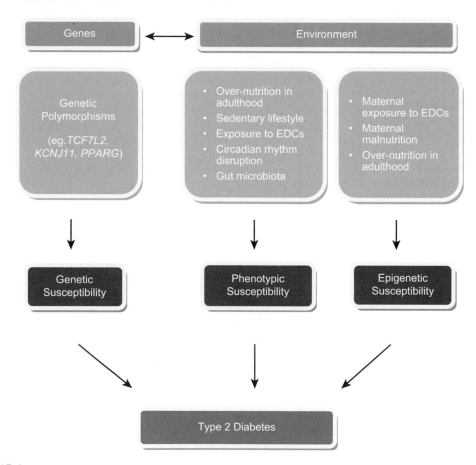

FIGURE 17.4 A model of gene-epigene-environment interaction which illustrates how genetic and environmental changes can result in the development of T2DM, either through an increase in genetic, phenotypic or epigenetic susceptibility.

a positive association between physical activity, a lifestyle—environmental factor, and global genomic DNA methylation, an epigenetic mark in humans.[70]

The presence of T2DM susceptibility gene variants predisposes an individual to the development of T2DM. Environmental factors can influence T2DM risk either through changes in the epigenome or as a purely phenotypic change. Epigenetic susceptibility may occur as a result of maternal exposure to EDCs or a mismatch between fetal programming from maternal malnutrition and subsequent over-nutrition in adulthood. Environmental factors that alter the phenotype without any genetic or epigenetic changes include exposure to EDCs, overnutrition in adulthood, circadian rhythm disruption and possibly, the gut microbiota. Finally, gene—environmental interaction can also occur when genetic susceptibility further lowers the threshold for the development of T2DM in the presence of phenotypic susceptibility. This model is summarized in Figure 17.4.

CONCLUSION

Both the genetic and environmental contribution to the development of T2DM have been well established. What is less elucidated is the interaction between them. Increasingly, the evidence is pointing to the interaction between the gene and the environment resulting in the proposed model of gene—environment interaction to explain much of the unexplained heritability of the disease. Unfortunately, this model is far from perfect and both epidemiological evidence and population studies suggest that epigenetic mechanisms are at least partly responsible. A proposed model, modified after Bollati's, takes into account the current genetic, epigenetic and environmental evidence in the development of T2DM.

As the technology to study epigenetic contribution to disease evolution advances, it is likely that this model will be further refined. Until that time, we should start to recognize that the seemingly separate threads of genetic, epigenetic, clinical, evolutionary, and epidemiological evidence are not independent of each other and should be pieced together in order to arrive at a more complete and integrated understanding of the etiology of T2DM.

References

1. Cumming AM. Lecture Notes: Complex Diseases (2007).
2. Medici F, Hawa M, Ianari A, Pyke DA, Leslie RD. Concordance rate for type II diabetes mellitus in monozygotic twins: actuarial analysis. *Diabetologia* 1999;**42**:146–50.
3. Poulsen P, Kyvik KO, Vaag A, Beck-Nielsen H. Heritability of type II (non-insulin-dependent) diabetes mellitus and abnormal glucose tolerance—a population-based twin study. *Diabetologia* 1999;**42**:139–45.
4. Kaprio J, Tuomilehto J, Koskenvuo M, Romanov K, Reunanen A, Eriksson J, Stengard J, Kesaniemi YA. Concordance for type 1 (insulin-dependent) and type 2 (non-insulin-dependent) diabetes mellitus in a population-based cohort of twins in Finland. *Diabetologia* 1992;**35**:1060–7.
5. Newman B, Selby JV, King MC, Slemenda C, Fabsitz R, Friedman GD. Concordance for type 2 (non-insulin-dependent) diabetes mellitus in male twins. *Diabetologia* 1987;**30**:763–8.
6. Hawkes CH. Twin studies in medicine—what do they tell us? *QJM* 1997;**90**:311–21.
7. Staiger H, Machicao F, Fritsche A, Haring HU. Pathomechanisms of type 2 diabetes genes. *Endocr Rev* 2009;**30**:557–85.
8. Frayling TM. A new era in finding type 2 diabetes genes—the unusual suspects. *Diabet Med* 2007;**24**: 696–701.
9. Florez JC, Jablonski KA, Bayley N, Pollin TI, de Bakker PI, Shuldiner AR, Knowler WC, Nathan DM, Altshuler D, Diabetes Prevention, Program Research Group. TCF7L2 polymorphisms and progression to diabetes in the Diabetes Prevention Program. *N Engl J Med* 2006;**355**:241–50.
10. Neel JV. Diabetes mellitus: a "thrifty" genotype rendered detrimental by "progress"? *Am J Hum Genet* 1962;**14**:353–62.
11. Chakravarthy MV, Booth FW. Eating, exercise, and "thrifty" genotypes: connecting the dots toward an

evolutionary understanding of modern chronic diseases. *J Appl Physiol* 2004;**96**:3–10.

12. Eaton SB, Konner M, Shostak M. Stone agers in the fast lane: chronic degenerative diseases in evolutionary perspective. *Am J Med* 1988;**84**:739–49.

13. Prentice AM, Hennig BJ, Fulford AJ. Evolutionary origins of the obesity epidemic: natural selection of thrifty genes or genetic drift following predation release? *Int J Obes (Lond)* 2008;**32**:1607–10.

14. Speakman JR. Thrifty genes for obesity, an attractive but flawed idea, and an alternative perspective: the 'drifty gene' hypothesis. *Int J Obes (Lond)* 2008;**32**:1611–7.

15. Manolio TA. Genomewide association studies and assessment of the risk of disease. *N Engl J Med* 2010;**363**:166–76.

16. Wellcome Trust Case Control Consortium. Genome-wide association study of 14,000 cases of seven common diseases and 3,000 shared controls. *Nature* 2007;**447**:661–78.

17. Billings LK, Florez JC. The genetics of type 2 diabetes: what have we learned from GWAS? *Ann N Y Acad Sci* 2010;**1212**:59–77.

18. Meigs JB, Shrader P, Sullivan LM, McAteer JB, Fox CS, Dupuis J, Manning AK, Florez JC, Wilson PW, D'Agostino Rb S, Cupples LA. Genotype score in addition to common risk factors for prediction of type 2 diabetes. *N Engl J Med* 2008;**359**:2208–19.

19. Maher B. Personal genomes: The case of the missing heritability. *Nature* 2008;**456**:18–21.

20. Evans JP, Meslin EM, Marteau TM, Caulfield T. Genomics. Deflating the genomic bubble. *Science* 2011;**331**:861–2.

21. Hu FB, Manson JE, Stampfer MJ, Colditz G, Liu S, Solomon CG, Willett WC. Diet, lifestyle, and the risk of type 2 diabetes mellitus in women. *N Engl J Med* 2001;**345**:790–7.

22. Jeon CY, Lokken RP, Hu FB, van Dam RM. Physical activity of moderate intensity and risk of type 2 diabetes: a systematic review. *Diabetes Care* 2007;**30**:744–52.

23. Jonker JT, De Laet C, Franco OH, Peeters A, Mackenbach J, Nusselder WJ. Physical activity and life expectancy with and without diabetes: life table analysis of the Framingham Heart Study. *Diabetes Care* 2006;**29**:38–43.

24. Bassuk SS, Manson JE. Epidemiological evidence for the role of physical activity in reducing risk of type 2 diabetes and cardiovascular disease. *J Appl Physiol* 2005;**99**:1193–204.

25. Rana JS, Li TY, Manson JE, Hu FB. Adiposity compared with physical inactivity and risk of type 2 diabetes in women. *Diabetes Care* 2007;**30**:53–8.

26. Knowler WC, Barrett-Connor E, Fowler SE, Hamman RF, Lachin JM, Walker EA, Nathan DM. Diabetes Prevention Program Research Group. Reduction in the incidence of type 2 diabetes with lifestyle intervention or metformin. *N Engl J Med* 2002;**346**:393–403.

27. Pan XR, Li GW, Hu YH, Wang JX, Yang WY, An ZX, Hu ZX, Lin J, Xiao JZ, Cao HB, Liu PA, Jiang XG, Jiang YY, Wang JP, Zheng H, Zhang H, Bennett PH, Howard BV. Effects of diet and exercise in preventing NIDDM in people with impaired glucose tolerance. The Da Qing IGT and Diabetes Study. *Diabetes Care* 1997;**20**:537–44.

28. Tuomilehto J, Lindstrom J, Eriksson JG, Valle TT, Hamalainen H, Ilanne-Parikka P, Keinanen-Kiukaanniemi S, Laakso M, Louheranta A, Rastas M, Salminen V, Uusitupa M. Finnish Diabetes Prevention Study Group. Prevention of type 2 diabetes mellitus by changes in lifestyle among subjects with impaired glucose tolerance. *N Engl J Med* 2001;**344**:1343–50.

29. Bass J, Takahashi JS. Circadian integration of metabolism and energetics. *Science* 2010;**330**:1349–54.

30. Yang X, Downes M, Yu RT, Bookout AL, He W, Straume M, Mangelsdorf DJ, Evans RM. Nuclear receptor expression links the circadian clock to metabolism. *Cell* 2006;**126**:801–10.

31. Barnea M, Madar Z, Froy O. High-fat diet delays and fasting advances the circadian expression of adiponectin signaling components in mouse liver. *Endocrinology* 2009;**150**:161–8.

32. Tuomilehto H, Peltonen M, Partinen M, Seppa J, Saaristo T, Korpi-Hyovalti E, Oksa H, Puolijoki H, Saltevo J, Vanhala M, Tuomilehto J. Sleep duration is associated with an increased risk for the prevalence of type 2 diabetes in middle-aged women—The FIN-D2D survey. *Sleep Med* 2008;**9**:221–7.

33. Hasler G, Buysse DJ, Klaghofer R, Gamma A, Ajdacic V, Eich D, Rossler W, Angst J. The association between short sleep duration and obesity in young adults: a 13-year prospective study. *Sleep* 2004;**27**:661–6.

34. Gottlieb DJ, Punjabi NM, Newman AB, Resnick HE, Redline S, Baldwin CM, Nieto FJ. Association of sleep time with diabetes mellitus and impaired glucose tolerance. *Arch Intern Med* 2005;**165**:863–7.

35. Karlsson B, Knutsson A, Lindahl B. Is there an association between shift work and having a metabolic syndrome? Results from a population based study of 27,485 people. *Occup Environ Med* 2001;**58**:747–52.

36. Turek FW, Joshu C, Kohsaka A, Lin E, Ivanova G, McDearmon E, Laposky A, Losee-Olson S, Easton A,

Jensen DR, Eckel RH, Takahashi JS, Bass J. Obesity and metabolic syndrome in circadian Clock mutant mice. *Science* 2005;**308**:1043–5.

37. Greiner T, Backhed F. Effects of the gut microbiota on obesity and glucose homeostasis. *Trends Endocrinol Metab* 2011;**22**:117–23.

38. Ley RE, Turnbaugh PJ, Klein S, Gordon JI. Microbial ecology: human gut microbes associated with obesity. *Nature* 2006;**444**:1022–3.

39. Turnbaugh PJ, Ley RE, Mahowald MA, Magrini V, Mardis ER, Gordon JI. An obesity-associated gut microbiome with increased capacity for energy harvest. *Nature* 2006;**444**:1027–31.

40. Larsen N, Vogensen FK, van den Berg FW, Nielsen DS, Andreasen AS, Pedersen BK, Al-Soud WA, Sorensen SJ, Hansen LH, Jakobsen M. Gut microbiota in human adults with type 2 diabetes differs from non-diabetic adults. *PLoS One* 2010;**5**: e9085.

41. Spor A, Koren O, Ley R. Unravelling the effects of the environment and host genotype on the gut microbiome. *Nat Rev Microbiol* 2011;**9**:279–90.

42. Diamanti-Kandarakis E, Bourguignon JP, Giudice LC, Hauser R, Prins GS, Soto AM, Zoeller RT, Gore AC. Endocrine-disrupting chemicals: an Endocrine Society scientific statement. *Endocr Rev* 2009;**30**: 293–342.

43. Skinner MK, Manikkam M, Guerrero-Bosagna C. Epigenetic transgenerational actions of environmental factors in disease etiology. *Trends Endocrinol Metab* 2010;**21**:214–22.

44. Bollati V, Baccarelli A. Environmental epigenetics. *Heredity* 2010;**105**:105–12.

45. Remillard RB, Bunce NJ. Linking dioxins to diabetes: epidemiology and biologic plausibility. *Environ Health Perspect* 2002;**110**:853–8.

46. Alonso-Magdalena P, Morimoto S, Ripoll C, Fuentes E, Nadal A. The estrogenic effect of bisphenol A disrupts pancreatic beta-cell function in vivo and induces insulin resistance. *Environ Health Perspect* 2006;**114**: 106–12.

47. Hugo ER, Brandebourg TD, Woo JG, Loftus J, Alexander JW, Ben-Jonathan N. Bisphenol A at environmentally relevant doses inhibits adiponectin release from human adipose tissue explants and adipocytes. *Environ Health Perspect* 2008;**116**:1642–7.

48. Sandu O, Song K, Cai W, Zheng F, Uribarri J, Vlassara H. Insulin resistance and type 2 diabetes in high-fat-fed mice are linked to high glycotoxin intake. *Diabetes* 2005;**54**:2314–9.

49. Thomas D. Gene-environment-wide association studies: emerging approaches. *Nat Rev Genet* 2010; **11**:259–72.

50. Sharp NC. The human genome and sport, including epigenetics, gene doping, and athleticogenomics. *Endocrinol Metab Clin North Am* 2010;**39**:201–15. xi.

51. Bird A. Perceptions of epigenetics. *Nature* 2007;**447**: 396–8.

52. Berger SL, Kouzarides T, Shiekhattar R, Shilatifard A. An operational definition of epigenetics. *Genes Dev* 2009;**23**:781–3.

53. Gottesfeld JM. Thematic minireview series: Epigenetics. *J Biol Chem* 2011. 10.1074/jbc.R111.243527.

54. Strachan T, Read AP. Human gene expression. In: *Human molecular genetics 3*. 3rd ed. NY: Garland; 2004. p. 294–5. 296.

55. van Vliet J, Oates NA, Whitelaw E. Epigenetic mechanisms in the context of complex diseases. *Cell Mol Life Sci* 2007;**64**:1531–8.

56. Diamond J. The double puzzle of diabetes. *Nature* 2003; **423**:599–602.

57. Stoger R. The thrifty epigenotype: an acquired and heritable predisposition for obesity and diabetes? *Bioessays* 2008;**30**:156–66.

58. Hales CN, Barker DJ, Clark PM, Cox LJ, Fall C, Osmond C, Winter PD. Fetal and infant growth and impaired glucose tolerance at age 64. *BMJ* 1991;**303**: 1019–22.

59. Li Y, Jaddoe VW, Qi L, He Y, Wang D, Lai J, Zhang J, Fu P, Yang X, Hu FB. Exposure to the Chinese famine in early life and the risk of metabolic syndrome in adulthood. *Diabetes Care* 2011;**34**:1014–8.

60. Roseboom T, de Rooij S, Painter R. The Dutch famine and its long-term consequences for adult health. *Early Hum Dev* 2006;**82**:485–91.

61. Sparen P, Vagero D, Shestov DB, Plavinskaja S, Parfenova N, Hoptiar V, Paturot D, Galanti MR. Long term mortality after severe starvation during the siege of Leningrad: prospective cohort study. *BMJ* 2004; **328**:11.

62. Stanner SA, Bulmer K, Andres C, Lantseva OE, Borodina V, Poteen VV, Yudkin JS. Does malnutrition in utero determine diabetes and coronary heart disease in adulthood? Results from the Leningrad siege study, a cross sectional study. *BMJ* 1997;**315**:1342–8.

63. Gluckman PD, Hanson MA, Cooper C, Thornburg KL. Effect of in utero and early-life conditions on adult health and disease. *N Engl J Med* 2008;**359**:61–73.

64. Johnson LJ, Tricker PJ. Epigenomic plasticity within populations: its evolutionary significance and potential. *Heredity* 2010;**105**:113–21.

65. Gluckman PD, Hanson MA. Living with the past: evolution, development, and patterns of disease. *Science* 2004;**305**:1733–6.

66. Godfrey KM, Gluckman PD, Hanson MA. Developmental origins of metabolic disease: life course and

intergenerational perspectives. *Trends Endocrinol Metab* 2010;**21**:199–205.

67. Dowse GK, Zimmet PZ, Finch CF, Collins VR. Decline in incidence of epidemic glucose intolerance in Nauruans: implications for the "thrifty genotype". *Am J Epidemiol* 1991;**133**:1093–104.

68. Benyshek DC, Johnston CS, Martin JF, Ross WD. Insulin sensitivity is normalized in the third generation (F3) offspring of developmentally programmed insulin resistant (F2) rats fed an energy-restricted diet. *Nutr Metab (Lond)* 2008;**5**:26.

69. Wren JD, Garner HR. Data-mining analysis suggests an epigenetic pathogenesis for type 2 diabetes. *J Biomed Biotechnol* 2005;**2005**:104–12.

70. Zhang FF, Cardarelli R, Carroll J, Zhang S, Fulda KG, Gonzalez K, Vishwanatha JK, Morabia A, Santella RM. Physical activity and global genomic DNA methylation in a cancer-free population. *Epigenetics* 2011;**6**:293–9.

18

Epigenetics in the Pathophysiology of Type 2 Diabetes

Charlotte Ling

Epigenetics and Diabetes, Lund University Diabetes Centre, Department of Clinical Sciences, Lund University, Malmö, Sweden

OUTLINE

INTRODUCTION

Type 2 diabetes is a polygenic multifactorial disease characterized by hyperglycaemia. The disease develops due to impaired insulin secretion from pancreatic β-cells and impaired insulin action in target tissues including skeletal muscle, adipose tissue, and the liver. It is well established that combinations of non-genetic and genetic risk factors influence the susceptibility for type 2 diabetes. While obesity, physical inactivity, and aging represent non-genetic risk factors for type 2 diabetes, genome-wide association studies have identified more than 40 polymorphisms associated with an increased risk for the disease.[1–9] The genome-wide association studies have been performed and replicated in cohorts of different ethnic backgrounds.[10–12] Common genetic variants do also affect insulin secretion and sensitivity as well as obesity and physical fitness, which may also affect the pathogenesis of type 2 diabetes.[7,13–19] Recent studies from our group and others do further show that epigenetic factors, including DNA methylation and histone modification, may affect the susceptibility for type 2 diabetes.[20] This chapter will summarize data from human and rodent studies, which demonstrate that epigenetic modifications influence the pathogenesis of type 2 diabetes.

AN OVERVIEW OF EPIGENETIC MECHANISMS

The epigenome includes DNA methylation and histone modifications. These chemical modifications of both the DNA sequence itself as well as of the proteins it is wrapped around, the histones, play a key role in controlling the function of the genome. Cells use these epigenetic modifications for parental imprinting, X-chromosome inactivation, to regulate cell differentiation, to control cell specific gene expression, and to silence junk DNA. In differentiated mammalian cells, DNA methylation mainly takes place on a cytosine residue in a CG dinucleotide.[21] Increased DNA methylation of promoter regions has been associated with transcriptional silencing.[22] This can be achieved through different mechanisms, i.e. methyl groups can prevent transcription factors from binding to promoters or methyl-binding proteins can bind to the methyl groups and further recruit co-repressors and histone deacetyltransferases (HDACs), which deacetylate the histones, resulting in a dense chromatin structure. Genomic DNA in eukaryotic cells is wrapped around histones to make up the densely packed chromatin. Furthermore, approximately 147 base pairs of DNA are wrapped around eight histone proteins to make up the nucleosome, which is the basic building block of the chromatin. Amino acids on N-terminal tails of the histones are subject to chemical modifications, i.e. methylation, acetylation, phosphorylation, sumoylation, and

ubiquitination, which are important in regulating the accessibility of DNA to the transcriptional machinery, replication, and recombination. Although these modifications may both increase and decrease the accessibility of the genomic DNA, it is proposed that multiple histone modifications act in combination and that the overall pattern of histone modifications at a specific locus influences whether a gene is active or not.[23] Nevertheless, histone acetylation of lysines is generally accepted to open up the chromatin structure and activate the genes.[24,25]

There are specific groups of enzymes which control the epigenetic modifications. DNA methyltransferases, including DNMT1, DNMT3a, and DNMT3b, regulate the methylation of DNA. While DNMT3a and DNMT3b are responsible for *de novo* methylation, DNMT1 maintains the DNA methylation pattern during cell replication. There are numerous groups of enzymes which control histone modifications. While histone acetyl transferases (HATs) acetylates, HDACs deacetylates the histones.[25,26] There are further histone methyl transferases and demethylases, which regulate methylation of lysine and arginine residues of histone tails.[27] Additional enzymes, not mentioned here, regulate other histone modifications.

Epigenetics has previously been defined as heritable changes in gene function that occur without a change in the nucleotide sequence and studies in both rodents and plants have shown that epigenetic variation can be inherited between generations.[28–32] A recent study has further shown that inherited epigenetic mechanisms may affect metabolic disease and pancreatic β-cell function due to a high-fat diet in fathers.[33]

EPIGENETIC MODIFICATIONS IN PATIENTS WITH TYPE 2 DIABETES

Although it is well established that epigenetic variation is associated with an increased risk for numerous disease, e.g., cancer, there is a limited number of studies demonstrating epigenetic changes in tissues from patients with type 2 diabetes. Nevertheless, pancreatic islets from patients with type 2 diabetes exhibit increased DNA methylation of the insulin promoter compared with non-diabetic donors.[34] Moreover, insulin promoter DNA methylation correlates negatively with insulin gene expression, proposing a role for DNA methylation in regulating the expression of the insulin gene. Data from Kuroda and co-workers support this hypothesis.[35] DNA methylation of the insulin promoter is lower in pancreatic β-cells compared with α-cells, supporting a role for DNA methylation in the cells' specific regulation of this gene.[34] HbA1c levels are measures of blood glucose levels over several months' time. In the study by Yang et al., HbA1c levels correlated positively with insulin promoter DNA methylation. Furthermore, treatment with hyperglycemia for 72 increases methylation of the insulin gene in clonal β-cells. These data show that glucose may influence the degree of DNA methylation and hence affect gene expression in pancreatic β-cells.

PGC1α is a transcriptional co-activator encoded by the *PPPARGC1A* gene and it is known to regulate oxidative function and ATP production in numerous cell types. Since ATP production and the ATP/ADP ratio play a key role in stimulating glucose-stimulated insulin secretion, we examined whether *PPPARGC1A* gene expression and DNA methylation are altered in pancreatic islets from patients with type 2 diabetes.[36] Indeed, while *PPPARGC1A* mRNA expression is decreased, *PPPARGC1A* promoter DNA methylation is increased in pancreatic islets from patients with type 2 diabetes compared with non-diabetic donors. Silencing *PPPARGC1A* in human pancreatic islets led to impaired glucose-stimulated insulin secretion. This study did also show that risk carriers of a *PPPARGC1A* genotype, the 482 gly/ser variant, is associated with decreased glucose-stimulated insulin secretion and decreased *PPPARGC1A* mRNA expression already in non-diabetic donors,[36] proposing that combinations of genetic and non-genetic factors play a role in the development of type 2 diabetes. Additional studies have shown that *PPPARGC1A* expression is decreased in skeletal muscle from patients with type 2 diabetes.[37,38] Moreover, a recent study showed that DNA methylation may also affect the *PPPARGC1A* gene in skeletal muscle of diabetic patients.[39] These studies show differential DNA methylation in tissues from patients with type 2 diabetes, which may affect gene expression and eventually insulin secretion and action.

AGING AND EPIGENETIC MODIFICATIONS

Increased age increases the risk for type 2 diabetes. Aging is also associated with impaired insulin secretion and action, possibly through mitochondrial dysfunction.[40] A study in young and elderly monozygotic twin pairs showed that while cells from young monozygotic twin pairs have a similar epigenetic pattern, both DNA methylation and histone modifications differed in cells from elderly monozygotic twin pairs.[41] This study proposes that the epigenome changes during life. If these changes take place in target tissues for type 2 diabetes, they may affect the susceptibility for the disease. Indeed, studies have found increased DNA methylation of candidate genes for type 2 diabetes in skeletal muscle of elderly compared with young twins.[42,43] It is well established that the expression of genes involved in oxidative phosphorylation, including *COX7A1* and *NDUFB6*, is reduced in skeletal muscle from patients with type 2 diabetes.[37] DNA methylation of the promoters of these genes was further increased in skeletal muscle of non-diabetic elderly compared with young twins.[42,43] In parallel, *COX7A1* and *NDUFB6* mRNA expression was decreased in muscle of the elderly twins and it was associated with insulin resistance *in vivo*. These studies demonstrate that age may affect DNA methylation of candidate genes for type 2 diabetes and hence affect gene expression and insulin sensitivity in skeletal muscle.

ENVIRONMENTAL FACTORS AND EPIGENETIC IMPACT ON TYPE 2 DIABETES

Obesity and physical inactivity are well established environmental risk factors for type 2 diabetes.[44,45] Epigenetic mechanisms have also been associated with obesity and diet in both rodent and human studies. Silencing of a histone methyltransferase, Jhdm2a, led to obesity in mice.[46] The agouti mouse is an additional rodent model where epigenetic modifications are associated with obesity.[47–49] A genome-wide DNA methylation study of 27,000 CpG sites in blood further proposed that epigenetic variation may play a role in obesity in humans.[50,51] Moreover, both a high-fat diet and weight loss are associated with epigenetic changes in skeletal muscle, adipose tissue, and blood from humans.[52–54] Some of these epigenetic differences are also associated with differential gene expression.

McGee and co-workers have studied the role of epigenetic mechanisms in skeletal muscle during exercise.[55–57] It is well established that exercise can increase the expression of glucose transporter 4 (GLUT4) in skeletal muscle[58] and this may lead to increased glucose uptake. Myocyte enhancer factor 2 (MEF2) is a transcription factor that binds to the GLUT4 promoter and regulates its expression. McGee *et al.* have shown that at rest MEF2 interacts with HDAC5 in the nucleus, resulting in deacetylation of histone tails at the GLUT4 promoter and a condensed inactive chromatin structure. After exercise, HDAC5 is phosphorylated by AMP-activated protein kinase and it hence dissociates

from MEF2 and leaves the nucleus. MEF2 does then interact with PGC1α and HATs at the GLUT4 gene, resulting in acetylation of histones at this gene and increased gene expression.

INTRAUTERINE ENVIRONMENT AND EPIGENETIC MODIFICATIONS

During embryonic development, epigenetic programming takes place, which affects cell differentiation. However, the epigenetic programming taking place *in utero* may also play a role later in life and affect the risk for metabolic disease.[59,60] Data from the Dutch Hunger Winter Families Study demonstrate epigenetic differences in blood from individuals who were prenatally exposed to famine in 1944—1945 compared with their unexposed same-sex siblings.[61–63] A low birth weight may represent a nutritionally restricted prenatal environment and a low birth weight is associated with impaired metabolism later in life.[52,64] Skeletal muscle from young healthy men born with a low birth weight does further show differential DNA methylation of *PPARGC1A* compared with age-matched men born with a normal birth weight.[52]

Animal studies have further shown that the prenatal environment plays an important role in programming the epigenome, which may affect the risk for diabetes later in life. One example is regulation of the *Pdx1* gene, which is a key transcription factor during the development of the pancreas *in utero*. Pdx1 does also regulate insulin gene expression in pancreatic β-cells postnatally. Park *et al.* found epigenetic changes of the *Pdx1* gene due to a restricted prenatal environment, which led to impaired insulin secretion and diabetes later in life.[65] A protein-restricted maternal diet alters the epigenetic control of the *Hnf4α* gene in pancreatic islets of the offspring.[66] Additional studies by Lillykrop *et al.* show the importance of the maternal diet for prenatal epigenetic programming and the impact on the metabolic profile later in life.[67-69]

GENETICS AND EPIGENETIC MODIFICATIONS

While epigenetic modifications affect the function of the genome, it is also possible that genetic variations, i.e. single nucleotide polymorphisms (SNPs), affect the epigenome. The impact of genetic variation on the epigenome may be either due to SNPs regulating epigenetic enzymes or SNPs introducing or deleting CpG sites and hence possible DNA methylation sites. Indeed, an SNP that introduces a CpG site in the *NDUFB6* gene is associated with both differential gene expression and DNA methylation in skeletal muscle.[42] Moreover, the effect on gene expression and DNA methylation was also influenced by aging. This study shows how genetic, epigenetic, and non-genetic factors all may interact to influence metabolism in humans.

SUMMARY

Epigenetic modifications in target tissues for type 2 diabetes are likely to play an important role in the development of the disease. Recent studies have identified epigenetic changes of candidate genes for type 2 diabetes in patients with the disease. Risk factors for type 2 diabetes do further change the epigenetic profile and hence gene expression, resulting in impaired insulin secretion and action. Nevertheless, additional genome-wide epigenetic analyses are needed to fully dissect the impact of epigenetic variation in the pathogenesis of type 2 diabetes.

References

1. McCarthy M, Genomics. Type 2 diabetes, and obesity. *The New England Journal of Medicine* 2010;**363**:2339—50.
2. Saxena R, Voight BF, Lyssenko V, Burtt NP, de Bakker PI, Chen H, Roix JJ, Kathiresan S, Hirschhorn JN, Daly MJ, Hughes TE, Groop L, Altshuler D, Almgren P, Florez JC, Meyer J, Ardlie K, Bengtsson Bostrom K, Isomaa B, Lettre G, Lindblad U, Lyon HN, Melander O, Newton-Cheh C, Nilsson P, Orho-Melander M, Rastam L, Speliotes EK, Taskinen MR, Tuomi T, Guiducci C, Berglund A, Carlson J, Gianniny L, Hackett R, Hall L, Holmkvist J, Laurila E, Sjogren M, Sterner M, Surti A, Svensson M, Svensson M, Tewhey R, Blumenstiel B, Parkin M, Defelice M, Barry R, Brodeur W, Camarata J, Chia N, Fava M, Gibbons J, Handsaker B, Healy C, Nguyen K, Gates C, Sougnez C, Gage D, Nizzari M, Gabriel SB, Chirn GW, Ma Q, Parikh H, Richardson D, Ricke D, Purcell S. Genome-wide association analysis identifies loci for type 2 diabetes and triglyceride levels. *Science* 2007;**316**:1331—6.
3. Scott LJ, Mohlke KL, Bonnycastle LL, Willer CJ, Li Y, Duren WL, Erdos MR, Stringham HM, Chines PS, Jackson AU, Prokunina-Olsson L, Ding CJ, Swift AJ, Narisu N, Hu T, Pruim R, Xiao R, Li XY, Conneely KN, Riebow NL, Sprau AG, Tong M, White PP, Hetrick KN, Barnhart MW, Bark CW, Goldstein JL, Watkins L, Xiang F, Saramies J, Buchanan TA, Watanabe RM, Valle TT, Kinnunen L, Abecasis GR, Pugh EW, Doheny KF, Bergman RN, Tuomilehto J, Collins FS, Boehnke M. A genome-wide association study of type 2 diabetes in Finns detects multiple susceptibility variants. *Science* 2007;**316**:1341—5.
4. Zeggini E, Weedon MN, Lindgren CM, Frayling TM, Elliott KS, Lango H, Timpson NJ, Perry JR, Rayner NW, Freathy RM, Barrett JC, Shields B, Morris AP, Ellard S, Groves CJ, Harries LW, Marchini JL, Owen KR, Knight B, Cardon LR, Walker M, Hitman GA, Morris AD, Doney AS, McCarthy MI, Hattersley AT. Replication of genome-wide association signals in UK samples reveals risk loci for type 2 diabetes. *Science* 2007;**316**:1336—41.
5. Zeggini E, Scott LJ, Saxena R, Voight BF, Marchini JL, Hu T, de Bakker PI, Abecasis GR, Almgren P, Andersen G, Ardlie K, Bostrom KB, Bergman RN, Bonnycastle LL, Borch-Johnsen K, Burtt NP, Chen H, Chines PS, Daly MJ, Deodhar P, Ding CJ, Doney AS, Duren WL, Elliott KS, Erdos MR, Frayling TM, Freathy RM, Gianniny L, Grallert H, Grarup N, Groves CJ, Guiducci C, Hansen T, Herder C, Hitman GA, Hughes TE, Isomaa B, Jackson AU, Jorgensen T, Kong A, Kubalanza K, Kuruvilla FG, Kuusisto J, Langenberg C, Lango H, Lauritzen T, Li Y, Lindgren CM, Lyssenko V, Marvelle AF, Meisinger C, Midthjell K, Mohlke KL, Morken MA, Morris AD, Narisu N, Nilsson P, Owen KR, Palmer CN, Payne F, Perry JR, Pettersen E, Platou C, Prokopenko I, Qi L, Qin L, Rayner NW, Rees M, Roix JJ, Sandbaek A,

Shields B, Sjogren M, Steinthorsdottir V, Stringham HM, Swift AJ, Thorleifsson G, Thorsteinsdottir U, Timpson NJ, Tuomi T, Tuomilehto J, Walker M, Watanabe RM, Weedon MN, Willer CJ, Illig T, Hveem K, Hu FB, Laakso M, Stefansson K, Pedersen O, Wareham NJ, Barroso I, Hattersley AT, Collins FS, Groop L, McCarthy MI, Boehnke M, Altshuler D. Meta-analysis of genome-wide association data and large-scale replication identifies additional susceptibility loci for type 2 diabetes. *Nat Genet* 2008;**40**:638—45.

6. Sladek R, Rocheleau G, Rung J, Dina C, Shen L, Serre D, Boutin P, Vincent D, Belisle A, Hadjadj S, Balkau B, Heude B, Charpentier G, Hudson TJ, Montpetit A, Pshezhetsky AV, Prentki M, Posner BI, Balding DJ, Meyre D, Polychronakos C, Froguel P. A genome-wide association study identifies novel risk loci for type 2 diabetes. *Nature* 2007;**445**:881—5.

7. Koeck T, Olsson AH, Nitert MD, Sharoyko VV, Ladenvall C, Kotova O, Reiling E, Ronn T, Parikh H, Taneera J, Eriksson JG, Metodiev MD, Larsson NG, Balhuizen A, Luthman H, Stancakova A, Kuusisto J, Laakso M, Poulsen P, Vaag A, Groop L, Lyssenko V, Mulder H, Ling C. A common variant in TFB1M is associated with reduced insulin secretion and increased future risk of type 2 diabetes. *Cell Metab* 2011;**13**:80—91.

8. Lyssenko V, Jonsson A, Almgren P, Pulizzi N, Isomaa B, Tuomi T, Berglund G, Altshuler D, Nilsson P, Groop L. Clinical risk factors, DNA variants, and the development of type 2 diabetes. *N Engl J Med* 2008;**359**:2220—32.

9. Lyssenko V, Nagorny CL, Erdos MR, Wierup N, Jonsson A, Spegel P, Bugliani M, Saxena R, Fex M, Pulizzi N, Isomaa B, Tuomi T, Nilsson P, Kuusisto J, Tuomilehto J, Boehnke M, Altshuler D, Sundler F, Eriksson JG, Jackson AU, Laakso M, Marchetti P, Watanabe RM, Mulder H, Groop L. Common variant in MTNR1B associated with increased risk of type 2 diabetes and impaired early insulin secretion. *Nat Genet* 2009;**41**:82—8.

10. Unoki H, Takahashi A, Kawaguchi T, Hara K, Horikoshi M, Andersen G, Ng DP, Holmkvist J, Borch-Johnsen K, Jorgensen T, Sandbaek A, Lauritzen T, Hansen T, Nurbaya S, Tsunoda T, Kubo M, Babazono T, Hirose H, Hayashi M, Iwamoto Y, Kashiwagi A, Kaku K, Kawamori R, Tai ES, Pedersen O, Kamatani N, Kadowaki T, Kikkawa R, Nakamura Y, Maeda S. SNPs in KCNQ1 are associated with susceptibility to type 2 diabetes in East Asian and European populations. *Nat Genet* 2008.

11. Ronn T, Wen J, Yang Z, Lu B, Du Y, Groop L, Hu R, Ling C. A common variant in MTNR1B, encoding melatonin receptor 1B, is associated with type 2 diabetes and fasting plasma glucose in Han Chinese individuals. *Diabetologia* 2009.

12. Wen J, Ronn T, Olsson A, Yang Z, Lu B, Du Y, Groop L, Ling C, Hu R. Investigation of type 2 diabetes risk alleles support CDKN2A/B, CDKAL1, and TCF7L2 as susceptibility genes in a Han Chinese cohort. *PLoS One* 2010;**5**. e9153.

13. Olsson AH, Ronn T, Ladenvall C, Parikh H, Isomaa B, Groop L, Ling C. Two common genetic variants near nuclear encoded OXPHOS genes are associated with insulin secretion in vivo. *Eur J Endocrinol* 2011.

14. Lyssenko V, Lupi R, Marchetti P, Del Guerra S, Orho-Melander M, Almgren P, Sjogren M, Ling C, Eriksson KF, Lethagen AL, Mancarella R, Berglund G, Tuomi T, Nilsson P, Del Prato S, Groop L. Mechanisms by which common variants in the TCF7L2 gene increase risk of type 2 diabetes. *J Clin Invest* 2007;**117**:2155—63.

15. Ling C, Poulsen P, Carlsson E, Ridderstrale M, Almgren P, Wojtaszewski J, Beck-Nielsen H, Groop L, Vaag A. Multiple environmental and genetic factors influence skeletal muscle PGC-1alpha and PGC-1beta gene expression in twins. *J Clin Invest* 2004;**114**:1518—26.

16. Ling C, Wegner L, Andersen G, Almgren P, Hansen T, Pedersen O, Groop L, Vaag A, Poulsen P. Impact of the peroxisome proliferator activated receptor-gamma coactivator-1beta (PGC-1beta) Ala203Pro polymorphism on in vivo metabolism, PGC-1beta expression and fibre type composition in human skeletal muscle. *Diabetologia* 2007;**50**:1615—20.

17. Ronn T, Poulsen P, Tuomi T, Isomaa B, Groop L, Vaag A, Ling C. Genetic variation in ATP5O is associated with skeletal muscle ATP50 mRNA expression and glucose uptake in young twins. *PLoS ONE* 2009;**4**. e4793.

18. Kacerovsky-Bielesz G, Chmelik M, Ling C, Pokan R, Szendroedi J, Farukuoye M, Kacerovsky M, Schmid AI, Gruber S, Wolzt M, Moser E, Pacini G, Smekal G, Groop L, Roden M. Short-term exercise training does not stimulate skeletal muscle ATP synthesis in relatives of humans with type 2 diabetes. *Diabetes* 2009.

19. Nilsson L, Olsson AH, Isomaa B, Groop L, Billig H, Ling C. A common variant near the PRL gene is associated with increased adiposity in males. *Mol Genet Metab* 2011;**102**:78—81.

20. Ling C, Groop L. Epigenetics: a molecular link between environmental factors and type 2 diabetes. *Diabetes* 2009;**58**:2718—25.

21. Lister R, Pelizzola M, Dowen RH, Hawkins RD, Hon G, Tonti-Filippini J, Nery JR, Lee L, Ye Z, Ngo QM, Edsall L, Antosiewicz-Bourget J, Stewart R, Ruotti V, Millar AH, Thomson JA, Ren B, Ecker JR. Human DNA methylomes at base resolution show widespread epigenomic differences. *Nature* 2009.

22. Weber M, Hellmann I, Stadler MB, Ramos L, Paabo S, Rebhan M, Schubeler D. Distribution, silencing potential and evolutionary impact of promoter DNA methylation in the human genome. *Nat Genet* 2007;**39**:457−66.

23. Wang Z, Zang C, Rosenfeld JA, Schones DE, Barski A, Cuddapah S, Cui K, Roh TY, Peng W, Zhang MQ, Zhao K. Combinatorial patterns of histone acetylations and methylations in the human genome. *Nat Genet* 2008;**40**:897−903.

24. Shahbazian MD, Grunstein M. Functions of site-specific histone acetylation and deacetylation. *Annu Rev Biochem* 2007;**76**:75−100.

25. Marmorstein R, Trievel RC. Histone modifying enzymes: structures, mechanisms, and specificities. *Biochim Biophys Acta* 2009;**1789**:58−68.

26. Wang Z, Zang C, Cui K, Schones DE, Barski A, Peng W, Zhao K. Genome-wide mapping of HATs and HDACs reveals distinct functions in active and inactive genes. *Cell* 2009;**138**:1019−31.

27. Teperino R, Schoonjans K, Auwerx J: Histone methyl transferases and demethylases; can they link metabolism and transcription? *Cell Metab* **12**:321−7.

28. Bird A. Perceptions of epigenetics. *Nature* 2007;**447**:396−8.

29. Skinner MK. Role of epigenetics in developmental biology and transgenerational inheritance. *Birth Defects Res C Embryo Today* **93**:51−5.

30. Cubas P, Vincent C, Coen E. An epigenetic mutation responsible for natural variation in floral symmetry. *Nature* 1999;**401**:157−61.

31. Chong S, Whitelaw E. Epigenetic germline inheritance. *Curr Opin Genet Dev* 2004;**14**:692−6.

32. Anway MD, Cupp AS, Uzumcu M, Skinner MK. Epigenetic transgenerational actions of endocrine disruptors and male fertility. *Science* 2005;**308**:1466−9.

33. Ng SF, Lin RC, Laybutt DR, Barres R, Owens JA, Morris MJ. Chronic high-fat diet in fathers programs beta-cell dysfunction in female rat offspring. *Nature* 2010;**467**:963−6.

34. Yang BT, Dayeh TA, Kirkpatrick CL, Taneera J, Kumar R, Groop L, Wollheim CB, Nitert MD, Ling C. Insulin promoter DNA methylation correlates negatively with insulin gene expression and positively with HbA(1c) levels in human pancreatic islets. *Diabetologia* 2010.

35. Kuroda A, Rauch TA, Todorov I, Ku HT, Al-Abdullah IH, Kandeel F, Mullen Y, Pfeifer GP, Ferreri K. Insulin gene expression is regulated by DNA methylation. *PLoS One* 2009;**4**. e6953.

36. Ling C, Del Guerra S, Lupi R, Ronn T, Granhall C, Luthman H, Masiello P, Marchetti P, Groop L, Del Prato S. Epigenetic regulation of PPARGC1A in human type 2 diabetic islets and effect on insulin secretion. *Diabetologia* 2008;**51**:615−22.

37. Mootha VK, Lindgren CM, Eriksson KF, Subramanian A, Sihag S, Lehar J, Puigserver P, Carlsson E, Ridderstrale M, Laurila E, Houstis N, Daly MJ, Patterson N, Mesirov JP, Golub TR, Tamayo P, Spiegelman B, Lander ES, Hirschhorn JN, Altshuler D, Groop LC. PGC-1alpha-responsive genes involved in oxidative phosphorylation are coordinately downregulated in human diabetes. *Nat Genet* 2003;**34**:267−73.

38. Patti ME, Butte AJ, Crunkhorn S, Cusi K, Berria R, Kashyap S, Miyazaki Y, Kohane I, Costello M, Saccone R, Landaker EJ, Goldfine AB, Mun E, DeFronzo R, Finlayson J, Kahn CR, Mandarino LJ. Coordinated reduction of genes of oxidative metabolism in humans with insulin resistance and diabetes: Potential role of PGC1 and NRF1. *Proc Natl Acad Sci USA* 2003;**100**:8466−71.

39. Barres R, Osler ME, Yan J, Rune A, Fritz T, Caidahl K, Krook A, Zierath JR. Non-CpG methylation of the PGC-1alpha promoter through DNMT3B controls mitochondrial density. *Cell Metab* 2009;**10**:189−98.

40. Petersen KF, Befroy D, Dufour S, Dziura J, Ariyan C, Rothman DL, DiPietro L, Cline GW, Shulman GI. Mitochondrial dysfunction in the elderly: possible role in insulin resistance. *Science* 2003;**300**:1140−2.

41. Fraga MF, Ballestar E, Paz MF, Ropero S, Setien F, Ballestar ML, Heine-Suner D, Cigudosa JC, Urioste M, Benitez J, Boix-Chornet M, Sanchez-Aguilera A, Ling C, Carlsson E, Poulsen P, Vaag A, Stephan Z, Spector TD, Wu YZ, Plass C, Esteller M. Epigenetic differences arise during the lifetime of monozygotic twins. *Proc Natl Acad Sci USA* 2005;**102**:10604−9.

42. Ling C, Poulsen P, Simonsson S, Ronn T, Holmkvist J, Almgren P, Hagert P, Nilsson E, Mabey AG, Nilsson P, Vaag A, Groop L. Genetic and epigenetic factors are associated with expression of respiratory chain component NDUFB6 in human skeletal muscle. *J Clin Invest* 2007;**117**:3427−35.

43. Ronn T, Poulsen P, Hansson O, Holmkvist J, Almgren P, Nilsson P, Tuomi T, Isomaa B, Groop L, Vaag A, Ling C. Age influences DNA methylation and gene expression of COX7A1 in human skeletal muscle. *Diabetologia* 2008;**51**:1159−68.

44. Lyssenko V, Almgren P, Anevski D, Perfekt R, Lahti K, Nissen M, Isomaa B, Forsen B, Homstrom N, Saloranta C, Taskinen MR, Groop L, Tuomi T. Predictors of and longitudinal changes in insulin sensitivity and secretion preceding onset of type 2 diabetes. *Diabetes* 2005;**54**:166−74.

45. Tuomilehto J, Lindstrom J, Eriksson JG, Valle TT, Hamalainen H, Ilanne-Parikka P, Keinanen-Kiukaanniemi S, Laakso M, Louheranta A, Rastas M, Salminen V, Uusitupa M. Prevention of type 2 diabetes mellitus by changes in lifestyle among subjects with

impaired glucose tolerance. *N Engl J Med* 2001;**344**:1343—50.

46. Tateishi K, Okada Y, Kallin EM, Zhang Y. Role of Jhdm2a in regulating metabolic gene expression and obesity resistance. *Nature* 2009;**458**:757—61.

47. Duhl DM, Vrieling H, Miller KA, Wolff GL, Barsh GS. Neomorphic agouti mutations in obese yellow mice. *Nat Genet* 1994;**8**:59—65.

48. Morgan HD, Sutherland HG, Martin DI, Whitelaw E. Epigenetic inheritance at the agouti locus in the mouse. *Nat Genet* 1999;**23**:314—8.

49. Wolff GL, Kodell RL, Moore SR, Cooney CA. Maternal epigenetics and methyl supplements affect agouti gene expression in Avy/a mice. *FASEB J* 1998;**12**:949—57.

50. Wang X, Zhu H, Snieder H, Su S, Munn D, Harshfield G, Maria BL, Dong Y, Treiber F, Gutin B, Shi H. Obesity related methylation changes in DNA of peripheral blood leukocytes. *BMC Med* 2011;**8**:87.

51. Franks PW, Ling C. Epigenetics and obesity: the devil is in the details. *BMC Med* 2010;**8**:88.

52. Brons C, Jacobsen S, Nilsson E, Ronn T, Jensen CB, Storgaard H, Poulsen P, Group L, Ling C, Astrup A, Vaag A. Deoxyribonucleic acid methylation and gene expression of PPARGC1A in human muscle is influenced by high-fat overfeeding in a birth-weight-dependent manner. *J Clin Endocrinol Metab* 2010;**95**:3048—56.

53. Bouchard L, Rabasa-Lhoret R, Faraj M, Lavoie ME, Mill J, Perusse L, Vohl MC. Differential epigenomic and transcriptomic responses in subcutaneous adipose tissue between low and high responders to caloric restriction. *Am J Clin Nutr* 2010;**91**:309—20.

54. Milagro FI, Campion J, Cordero P, Goyenechea E, Gomez-Uriz AM, Abete I, Zulet MA, Martinez JA. A dual epigenomic approach for the search of obesity biomarkers: DNA methylation in relation to diet-induced weight loss. *FASEB J* 2011.

55. McGee SL, Howlett KF, Starkie RL, Cameron-Smith D, Kemp BE, Hargreaves M. Exercise increases nuclear AMPK alpha2 in human skeletal muscle. *Diabetes* 2003;**52**:926—8.

56. McGee SL, Hargreaves M. Exercise and myocyte enhancer factor 2 regulation in human skeletal muscle. *Diabetes* 2004;**53**:1208—14.

57. McGee SL, van Denderen BJ, Howlett KF, Mollica J, Schertzer JD, Kemp BE, Hargreaves M. AMP-activated protein kinase regulates GLUT4 transcription by phosphorylating histone deacetylase 5. *Diabetes* 2008;**57**:860—7.

58. Neufer PD, Dohm GL. Exercise induces a transient increase in transcription of the GLUT-4 gene in skeletal muscle. *Am J Physiol* 1993;**265**:C1597—603.

59. Hales CN, Barker DJ, Clark PM, Cox LJ, Fall C, Osmond C, Winter PD. Fetal and infant growth and impaired glucose tolerance at age 64. *Bmj* 1991;**303**:1019—22.

60. Hales CN, Barker DJ. Type 2 (non-insulin-dependent) diabetes mellitus: the thrifty phenotype hypothesis. *Diabetologia* 1992;**35**:595—601.

61. Ravelli AC, van der Meulen JH, Michels RP, Osmond C, Barker DJ, Hales CN, Bleker OP. Glucose tolerance in adults after prenatal exposure to famine. *Lancet* 1998;**351**:173—7.

62. Heijmans BT, Tobi EW, Stein AD, Putter H, Blauw GJ, Susser ES, Slagboom PE, Lumey LH. Persistent epigenetic differences associated with prenatal exposure to famine in humans. *Proc Natl Acad Sci USA* 2008;**105**:17046—9.

63. Tobi EW, Lumey LH, Talens RP, Kremer D, Putter H, Stein AD, Slagboom PE, Heijmans BT. DNA methylation differences after exposure to prenatal famine are common and timing- and sex-specific. *Hum Mol Genet* 2009.

64. Jensen CB, Storgaard H, Madsbad S, Richter EA, Vaag AA. Altered skeletal muscle fiber composition and size precede whole-body insulin resistance in young men with low birth weight. *J Clin Endocrinol Metab* 2007;**92**:1530—4.

65. Park JH, Stoffers DA, Nicholls RD, Simmons RA. Development of type 2 diabetes following intrauterine growth retardation in rats is associated with progressive epigenetic silencing of Pdx1. *J Clin Invest* 2008;**118**:2316—24.

66. Sandovici IS NH, Dekker-Nitert M, Ackers-Johnson M, Jones RH, O'Neill LP, Marquez VE, Cairns WJ, Tadayyon M, Ling C, Constância M, Ozanne SE. *Dynamic epigenetic regulation by early-diet and aging of the type 2 diabetes susceptibility gene Hnf4a in pancreatic islets.* In: *Proc Natl Acad Sci USA In Press*; 2011.

67. Lillycrop KA, Phillips ES, Jackson AA, Hanson MA, Burdge GC. Dietary protein restriction of pregnant rats induces and folic acid supplementation prevents epigenetic modification of hepatic gene expression in the offspring. *J Nutr* 2005;**135**:1382—6.

68. Lillycrop KA, Phillips ES, Torrens C, Hanson MA, Jackson AA, Burdge GC. Feeding pregnant rats a protein-restricted diet persistently alters the methylation of specific cytosines in the hepatic PPAR alpha promoter of the offspring. *Br J Nutr* 2008;**100**:278—82.

69. Lillycrop KA, Slater-Jefferies JL, Hanson MA, Godfrey KM, Jackson AA, Burdge GC. Induction of altered epigenetic regulation of the hepatic glucocorticoid receptor in the offspring of rats fed a protein-restricted diet during pregnancy suggests that reduced DNA methyltransferase-1 expression is involved in impaired DNA methylation and changes in histone modifications. *Br J Nutr* 2007;**97**:1064—73.

Targeting the Metabolic Syndrome and Type 2 Diabetes by Preventing Inflammation

Amin Ardestani, Luan Shu, Kathrin Maedler

Centre for Biomolecular Interactions Bremen, University of Bremen, Germany

INTRODUCTION

β-cell apoptosis is a fundamental cause of T1DM and a hallmark of the reduced β-cell mass in T2DM.[1–3] In T1DM, β-cell destruction occurs through immune-mediated processes; mononuclear cell infiltration in the pancreatic islets and interaction between antigen-presenting cells and T-cells leads to high local concentrations of inflammatory cytokines, chemokines, and reactive oxygen species (ROS) which initiate a variety of signal cascades in β-cells that affect the expression of apoptotic genes and induce the β-cell destruction.[4,5]

T2DM is a multifactorial and multi-organ disease and pathways towards its progression are complex and a result of the interplay between environment and genes.

Nutritional and Therapeutic Interventions for Diabetes and Metabolic Syndrome
DOI: 10.1016/B978-0-12-385083-6.00019-X

233

Inflammation, glucotoxicity, lipotoxicity, and endoplasmic reticulum (ER) stress induce apoptotic signal transduction in the β-cell leading to impaired function and reduced β-cell mass in the advanced stage of disease.[6,7] Inflammatory cytokines are common mediators of pancreatic β-cell death in both types of diabetes. IL-1β was suggested many years ago as a key player in β-cell destruction mediated by the immune system. IL-1β is the most potent β-cell toxic cytokine and contributes to β-cell apoptosis by activation of multiple signal transduction pathways. TNF-α and interferon-gamma (IFN-γ) alone are weaker in this respect; however, in synergy with IL-1β, they potentiate its deleterious effect of IL-1β through induction of additional signaling pathways.[5,8]

Signaling pathways of IL-1β result in impaired insulin secretion and insulin action.[9] After the development of more sensitive analysis methods, subclinical inflammation has been identified as a major component of the metabolic diseases, and elevated cytokine levels were measured in obesity, insulin resistance, and type 2 diabetes mellitus (T2DM). Among other pro-inflammatory cytokines and chemokines, e.g., tumor necrosis factor-α (TNFα), IL-6, IL-8, MCP1, the cytokine interleukin-1β (IL-1β) has been associated with the metabolic syndrome such as atherosclerosis, chronic heart failure, and T2DM.

Earlier, IL-1β was already linked to autoimmune diseases such as rheumatoid arthritis, inflammatory bowel diseases, and type 1 diabetes (T1DM). IL-1β is a key regulator of the body's inflammatory response and is produced after infection, injury, and antigenic challenge. The macrophage is the primary source of IL-1, but also epidermal, epithelial, lymphoid, and vascular tissues synthesize IL-1. Macrophage-derived IL-1β production in insulin-sensitive organs leads to the progression of inflammation and induction of insulin resistance in obesity.

IL-1β LINKS OBESITY AND DIABETES

Chronic subclinical inflammation is present in obesity, insulin resistance, and T2DM. The diseases related to metabolic syndrome are characterized by abnormal cytokine production, including elevated circulating IL-1β, increased acute-phase proteins, e.g., C-reactive protein (CRP),[10] and activation of inflammatory signaling pathways.[11]

Proinflammatory cytokines can cause insulin resistance in adipose tissue, skeletal muscle, and liver by inhibiting insulin signal transduction. The sources of cytokines in insulin-resistant states are the insulin target tissues themselves, primarily fat and liver, but to a larger extent the activated tissue resident macrophages.[12]

Infiltration of macrophages in adipose tissue is tightly correlated with obesity in mice and humans.[13,14] Together with the detection of infiltrating macrophages in fat tissue, adipocytokines are produced in high amounts, i.e. leptin and resistin, while anti-inflammatory adiponectin is decreased. The adipokines in turn play a central role in the regulation of insulin resistance and β-cell function (Figure 19.1).[15,16]

IL-1β in Islets

While macrophage infiltration in adipose and brain tissue has been shown in many studies,[17] increased islet macrophage infiltration has only recently been observed in pancreatic sections from patients with T2DM,[18,19] and in T2DM animal models, such as the Goto-Kakizaki (GK) rat,[20] the high fat/high sucrose diet (HFD) and *db/db* mouse,[18] and the hyperglycemic Cohen diabetic rat.[21] The primary

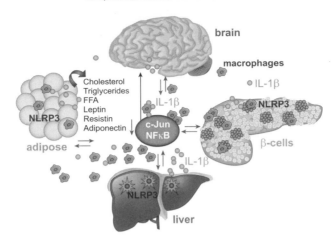

FIGURE 19.1 **The inflammatory axis in metabolic diseases and interplay between macrophage-derived IL-1β and its action in adipose, brain, pancreas, and liver (from[9,54]).** Macrophages migrate into insulin-sensitive organs and produce pro-inflammatory signals, which change the cell fate. In adipose, this leads to increased production of cholesterol, triglycerides, adipokines, and cytokines. Insulin sensitivity is impaired and glucose uptake disturbed. Mediated through intracellular signaling cascades, NFκB and c-Jun and the NALP3 inflammasome are activated and insulin resistance in the liver, fat, and brain and impaired insulin secretion in the β-cells develop. Reproduced with kind permission of Springer Science & Business Media. (*See the color plate section at the back of the book.*)

sources of IL-1β are blood monocytes, tissue macrophages, and dendritic cells. β-lymphocytes and natural killer (NK) cells also produce IL-1β.[22] The release of the leaderless cytokine, IL-1β, can not be initiated through the Golgi apparatus. Inactive pro-IL-1β precursor accumulates in the cytosol, and is processed by caspase-1 (also named interleukin converting enzyme, ICE) into the mature secreted IL-1β. The maturation occurs in a large multiprotein complex. Adenosine triphosphate (ATP) activates the $P2X_7$ receptor, which forms a pore in response to ligand stimulation and regulates cell permeability and cytokine release.[23]

Resident islet macrophages are fundamental in the development of autoimmune diabetes[24,25] and it is postulated that IL-1β secreted from such intra-islet macrophages results in β-cell destruction.[24] Recent studies show that the β-cells themselves are able to secrete IL-1β which is induced by double-stranded RNA, a mechanism by which viral infection may

mediate β-cell damage[26] by elevated glucose concentrations,[27–30] by leptin,[31] and by free fatty acids.[32]

In two animal models, *Psammomys obesus* and GK rat, pancreatic β-cells express IL-1β under hyperglycemic conditions.[27,33] In *Psammomys obesus*, normalizing hyperglycemia with phlorizin, an inhibitor of the renal tubular glucose re-uptake, inhibited intra-islet IL-1β expression.[27] In contrast, Jorns *et al.* found no IL-1β expression within the islets.[34] IL-1β production by islet cells was confirmed in several studies.[28,30,35,36] While glucose-induced IL-1β mRNA production was not found in human islets that had been preincubated in suspension for 3–5 days,[35] Boni-Schnetzler *et al.* show that glucose response in islets is negatively correlated with basal IL-1β expression levels.[28] These studies show that IL-β may mediate β-cell destruction also in T2DM (reviewed in[37]). IL-1β is also present in the β-cells in pancreatic sections from patients with T2DM.[27,28] It is tempting to suggest IL-1β as a target for the treatment of diabetes. However, whether changes in circulating cytokines are physiologically relevant in the face of locally produced inflammatory mediators remains unknown.

ACTIVATION OF THE NLRP3 INFLAMMASOME IN FAT, LIVER AND ISLETS RESULTS IN IL-1β PRODUCTION

IL-1β production is initiated by the activation of the NALP3 (nucleotide-binding domain, leucine-rich repeats containing family, pyrin domain-containing-3, also called NLRP3) inflammasome resulting in caspase-1 activation and subsequent maturation of IL-1β from proIL-1β. NLRs and Toll-like receptors (TLRs) are pattern recognition receptors through which innate immune cells such as macrophages detect pathogen-associated molecular patterns or danger-associated molecular patterns (DAMPs) derived from injured or damaged cells and, in response, release pro-inflammatory cytokines such as IL-1β.[38–40] The inflammasome is activated by bacterial toxins, endogenous stress signals (e.g., ATP, β-amyloid) through the formation of ROSs.[29,41]

Within pancreatic islets, elevated glucose[29] and islet amyloid polypeptide[42,43] are inducers of NLRP3 and IL-1β production in the pancreas. Glucose-induced IL-1β secretion involves caspase-8[27] and caspase-1 activation mediated by the NALP3 inflammasome. Glucose-induced IL-1β secretion is prevented in NALP3$^{-/-}$ mice, indicating that IL-1β is generated through glucose-induced ROS production and oxidative stress.[29] The thioredoxin (TRX)-interacting protein (TXNIP), which has been linked to insulin resistance,[44] functions as an activator of NALP3. In line with these data, another recent study shows that TXNIP is highly increased by elevated glucose in β-cells and that

TXNIP-deficient islets are protected against glucose toxicity.[45]

Human islet amyloid polypeptide induces activation of the NALP3 inflammasome and IL-1β within islets in bone-marrow-derived macrophages.[42] Oligomers of islet amyloid polypeptide (IAPP), a protein that forms amyloid deposits and replaces the area of β-cells in the pancreas during T2DM, triggers the NALP3 inflammasome and generates mature IL-1β, dependent on glucose metabolism, in islets, which strongly supports the role of IL-1β in the progression of T2DM.[46,47] IL-1β staining colocalizes to regions where amyloid was deposited. Macrophages in islets stained positive for IL-1β. In addition, a large area positive for IL-1β is localized in the islets outside of macrophages. Based on our observations in the human islet amyloid polypeptide transgenic rat,[48] there is evidence that IL-1β is expressed within the islets also in the β-cells after the induction of severe hyperglycemia (unpublished observation), indicating that β-cell IL-1β expression can be observed at high glucose levels when diabetes progresses. It remains to be elucidated whether toxicity of amylin oligomers on the β-cell involves IL-1β signals.

Despite the high expression of IL-1R1 in β-cells, expression of the NALP3 inflammasome components NALP3, ASC (apoptosis-associated speck-like protein containing a CARD), and caspase-1 show relatively low expression levels,[29] which may explain the modest release of IL-1β from islets.

Recently, high NALP3 expression has been found in fat and liver tissue in obesity,[40,49] linking inflammation-activation in the β-cell with insulin target tissue. In mice, NALP3 and IL-1β expression strongly correlates with adiposity. In patients with T2DM, NLRP3 and IL-1β mRNA expression is reduced and insulin sensitivity improved in response to calorie restriction. High-fat-diet-fed NALP3-KO mice have improved insulin signaling in fat and liver.[40] Wen *et al.* showed that NALP3-mediated IL-1β production is directly induced by the saturated fatty acid palmitate.[49] These recent studies show the association of obesity, inflammation in insulin target tissue and β-cells, and T2DM.

IL-1β and β-Cell Apoptosis: A Concert of Extrinsic and Intrinsic Pathways

Importantly, IL-1β induces its own and the expression of other cytokines, e.g., IL-2, -3, -6, and interferons.[50] In turn, cells that produce IL-1β also respond to IL-1β.[51] IL-1β initiates signal transduction by binding to IL-1R1 on the β-cell and once produced accelerates cell death.

IL-1R1 is highly expressed in the β-cell, more than 10-fold higher expression of IL-1RI mRNA was observed in isolated islets than in total pancreas, which is attributed to the expression in the β-cell. Furthermore, β-cell IL-1R1 expression levels are higher than in any other tissue,[32] which may explain the high sensitivity of the β-cell to IL-1. This leads to docking of the IL-1RAcP to the IL-1/IL-1R1 complex, which is followed by recruitment of the adaptor protein MyD88. Interleukin-1 receptor-associated kinase-4 (IRAK-4), Tollip and IRAK-1 are then bound, allowing IRAK-1 to activate TRAF6, which in turn triggers activation of transforming growth factor-β activating kinase-1 (TAK1). TAK1 is able to stimulate two main pathways; the IKK-NFκB pathway, and the mitogen-activated/stress-activated protein kinase (MAPK/SAPK) pathway.[52] In addition to TAK1, mitogen-activated protein kinase kinase kinase 1 (MEKK1) seems to participate in the activation of both NFκB and SAPK in β-cells.[53] Phosphorylation of IκB, a cytosolic inhibitor of NFκB, by inhibitory kappa B kinase (IKK) leads to inhibitory factor kappa B (IκB) degradation and nuclear factor kappa B (NFκB) translocation to the nucleus, thus regulating the transcription of many target genes, such as inducible nitric oxide synthase (iNOS) expression and NO production, a toxic reactive radical.[9,54] Consistently interfering with NFκB activation decreases IL-1β-induced β-cell death.[55,56] IL-1β signaling involves the MAPK/SAPK, c-Jun N-terminal kinase (JNK)/SAPK and protein kinase C delta pathways in the β-cell, which were described in detail before.[9,54]

IL-1β signals initiate apoptosis through two distinct pathways, the "extrinsic" (also called death receptor) and the "intrinsic" (also called mitochondrial) pathways.[57] In general, *the extrinsic pathway* is activated through death receptors, members of the tumor necrosis factor receptor (TNF-R) family that have an intracellular death domain (e.g., Fas, TNF-R1, DR4 and DR5). This activation through ligand/receptor binding results in the recruitment and cleavage of initiator caspase-8, which activates downstream effector caspases such as caspases-3, -6, and -7 and ultimately induces apoptosis.[57–59] The intrinsic pathway involves activation of the mitochondrial pathways; depolarization of the mitochondrial membrane leads to the release of cytochrome c which binds APAF-1 protein and procaspase 9 to form apaptosome complex which then activates initiator caspase-9 leading to the activation of downstream caspases.[57,60]

The extrinsic apoptotic pathway is causative for β-cell death in T1DM diabetes shown in *in vivo* mouse models and *in vitro*.[61–67] Pancreatic β-cells are sensitive to Fas ligand (FasL) or agonistic anti-Fas antibodies, and observations of FasL-expressing infiltrated-cytotoxic lymphocytes in T1DM implicated Fas-induced apoptosis as an important factor for β-cell destruction in T1DM.[62,66] IL-1β impairs insulin release via Fas induction enabling Fas-triggered apoptosis in rodent and human islets,[55,68–77] and shares similarities through the Fas pathway with glucose-induced apoptosis.[68]

The Fas receptor, activated through interactions between antigen-presenting β-cells and

T-cells as well as through local expression of inflammatory mediators, i.e. cytokines, chemokines, and other inflammatory compounds, binds to FasL which is constitutively expressed in the β-cell[68,72] and initiates β-cell apoptosis. IL-1β induces Fas expression on β-cells,[68,71,72,78–80] increasing their sensitivity to FasL and accelerating apoptosis via cleavage of downstream caspases.[81] Cytokine-induced Fas mRNA upregulation correlated directly with an increased surface expression of Fas and potentiates cytokine-induced apoptosis in islets.[82] In that regard, β-cells from FasL transgenic non-obese diabetic (NOD) mice are more susceptible to cytokine-induced apoptosis than wild-type β-cells whereas the administration of anti-FasL antibody at an early age to NOD mice prevented insulitis and diabetes.[83] Inflammatory insults specifically induce translocation of Fas to the β-cell surface[84] and interference with this cell surface Fas expression is a new strategy to improve β-cell survival in inflamed islets.

Intra-islet production of IL-1β mediates the inflammatory process in an autocrine/paracrine manner resulting in β-cell apoptosis.[85,86] Glucose-induced local production of IL-1β leads to Fas upregulation, caspase-8 and -3 activation, and β-cell apoptosis as a consequence of engagement by FasL, expressed on neighboring β-cells in the human islets.[86] Fas has also a physiological role on the β-cell and is needed for insulin secretion.[80] Fas-deficient mice[80] and also caspase-8-knockout[87] show impaired glucose tolerance. Also, a complete knockdown of pro-inflammatory IL-1 in the IL-1-KO mice results in impaired glucose tolerance, decreased β-cell mass, and decreased expression of β-cell transcription factors (e.g., PDX-1, Pax-4),[88] indicating that IL-1β has a dual role in the β-cell and activated pathways, e.g. FLIP, Fas, and NFκB might be needed for insulin secretion and survival.[80,87,88] Especially the dual role of

NFκB, which was long known to be responsible for IL-1β-induced β-cell destruction,[89] is shown through NFκB-induced activation of the anti-apoptotic gene A20, which protects against cell death,[90] promotes insulin secretion[91] and β-cell-specific NFκB depletion accelerates diabetes in the NOD mouse.[56] In contrast and despite their basally impaired glucose tolerance, IL-1β-KO mice are protected against the diabetogenic effects of the HFD as well as against glucotoxicity,[88] which supports the concept that IL-β mediates nutrient-induced β-cell dysfunction during the development of T2DM.

In NOD mice, IL-1R deficiency slows but does not prevent diabetes progression,[92] and caspase-1 (interleukin converting enzyme) deficiency has no effect on diabetes progression,[93] although both IL-1R subtype 1 and caspase-1 are highly expressed in islets from wild type NOD mice.[94] It is possible that pathways other than IL-1β signals are involved in diabetes in NOD mice since it was shown that IL-10 promotes diabetes in NOD mice independent of Fas, perforin, TNFR 1 and TNFR 2.[95] Also, only few, if any, Fas-expressing β-cells were found in islets of NOD mice close to the onset of hyperglycemia.[96] Such data suggest that one single pathway may not mediate β-cell apoptosis in diabetes.

This is supported by data showing that IL-1β-induced apoptosis occurs through activation of the *intrinsic pathway*, leading to mitochondrial-dependent caspase-9 cleavage, downstream caspase-3 activation, and cell death, in addition to the extrinsic pathway[97] (see Figure 19.2). The Bcl-2 family of proteins are critical regulators of the mitochondrial apoptotic pathway. Bcl-2 proteins are divided into two groups according to their function. The anti-apoptotic members, including Bcl-2, Bcl-xL, Bcl-w and Mcl-1, prevent mitochondrial outer membrane permeabilization (MOMP) and consequent release of cytochrome c.

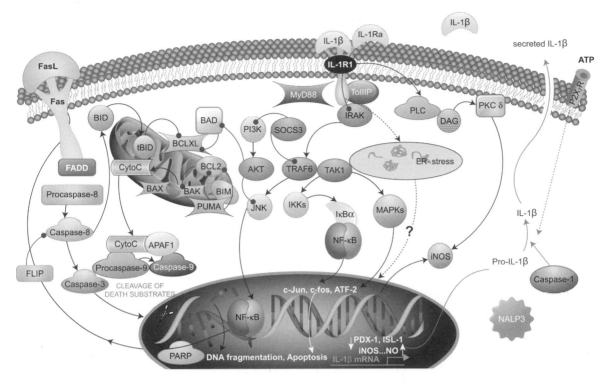

FIGURE 19.2 Cross-linking extrinsic and intrinsic pathways by IL-1β signaling in the β-cell. Details are described in the text. (*See the color plate section at the back of the book.*)

The pro-apoptotic Bcl-2 proteins are divided into the multi-domain effectors Bax, Bak and Bok (containing BH domains 1—3), or BH3-only proteins including Bid, Bad, Bik, Bim, Bmf, DP5, PUMA and Noxa (containing only the BH3 domain) which promote MOMP and are essential for apoptosis.[57,60] The BH3-only proteins act as either direct activators of pro-apoptotic Bax and Bak, or as de-repressors of anti-apoptotic Bcl-2 and Bcl-xL.[60,63] There are accumulating data showing that cytokine-induced cell death in β-cells involves the intrinsic pathway.[98—106] IL-1β together with TNF-α, and IFN-γ downregulate the expression of the Bcl-2 anti-apoptotic proteins in pancreatic islets[105,107] whereas overexpression of Bcl-2 or Mcl-1 protects against cytokine-induced β-cell death.[105,108,109] Bax as a pro-apoptotic

molecule is a critical element in the process of intrinsic cell death.[110] Bax translocates to the mitochondria which leads to cytochrome c release. Inhibition of Bax translocation by the potential Bax suppressor protein V5[98] or Bax deficiency[99] protects against cytokine-induced β-cell apoptosis. In line with these observations, Bcl-xL-deficient islets are critically sensitized to cytokines.[106] BH3-only proteins are essential for apoptosis initiation by IL-1β and other cytokines. Pro-inflammatory cytokines modulate BH3-only proteins through either transcriptional induction (e.g., Bim, PUMA and DP5) and/or post-translational modification (e.g., Bim, Bid, and Bad) prior to translocation to the mitochondria.[98,99,103,104,111] For example, IL-1β alone or in combination with TNF-α and IFN-γ increases Bim and Bid and decreases the inactive form of Bad (p-Bad) levels in Rinm5F cells and rat islets.[111] Specifically, Bad dephosphorylation and its dissociation form 14-3-3 inhibitory proteins, where it can translocate to the mitochondria and interact with anti-apoptotic proteins, is important for cytokine-induced β-cells.[98,111] The other BH3-only protein Bid is inactive in the cytosol in healthy cells and is predominantly regulated by cleavage by caspase-8. Following IL-1β treatment, Bid or tBid (truncated Bid) translocates to the mitochondria and interacts with Bax/Bak to promote cytochrome c release and apoptosis. Transcriptional upregulation of PUMA and BH3-only sensitizer DP5 play a key role for mitochondrial Bax translocation, cytochrome c release, caspase-3 cleavage resulting in β-cell apoptosis in IL-1β/IFN-γ-treated β-cells.[103,104] The BH3-only proteins mimetic, ABT-737, increases β-cell sensitivity to cytokines and accelerating apoptosis via cleavage of downstream caspases. Taken together, these studies show that pro-inflammatory cytokines, in particular IL-1β, modulate the expression of most of the Bcl-2-related proteins, indicating a complex regulation and a participation of these proteins in cytokine-induced β-cell apoptosis.

As a model, Scaffidi et al.[112] have introduced two cell types. In type I cells, death receptor (such as Fas) triggering leads to strong caspase-8 activation, which bypasses mitochondria, leading directly to activation of caspase-3 followed by apoptosis. In type II cells, death receptor-induced caspase-8 activation requires mitochondrial pathway-mediated amplification of the caspase cascade. Pancreatic β-cells are classified as type II cells.[99,113] It is now established that amplification of apoptosis signaling through caspase-8-mediated activation of the pro-apoptotic Bid leading to Bax/Bak-dependent activation of caspase-9 and effector caspases is essential for pancreatic β-cells.[99,113] Bid is required for FasL- and TNF-α-induced apoptosis of pancreatic islets and also

in lesser extent for cytokines cocktail including IL-1β. This shows that cytokine-induced death receptor activation through Fas upregulation amplify caspase cascade through mitochondrial pathway for efficient killing of β-cells. Understanding of the complex pathophysiological pathways how IL-1β or "cytokine toxicity" triggers β-cell apoptosis will shed new light on mechanisms of β-cell loss in diabetes and may therefore improve therapeutic intervention.

IL-1β AND β-CELL TRANSCRIPTIONAL REGULATION

Through a cascade of intracellular events, IL-1β causes β-cell dysfunction including decrease in glucose-stimulated insulin biosynthesis and secretion and β-cell apoptosis. IL-1β modulates β-cell transcription factors and gene expression profiles that initiate the process of β-cell failure. The transcription factor PDX1 (pancreatic duodenal homeobox-1, previously called IPF1, IDX1, STF1, or IUF1)[114] is as a key factor in pancreas development and function, with homozygous mutations resulting in pancreas agenesis associated with neonatal diabetes.[115,116] Heterozygosity for the null mutation, and hence reduced PDX1 expression levels affect insulin expression and secretion and predispose islets to apoptosis. PDX1 controls the expression of several genes which are vital for β-cell function such as insulin, Glut2 and glucokinase.[115] PDX1 also plays an essential role in the regulation of β-cell survival and susceptibility to apoptosis.[115,117,118] PDX1 deficiency contributes to impaired proliferation and enhanced apoptosis via transcriptional mechanisms in models of type 2 diabetes.[119] Overexpression of PDX1 restores β-cell mass and function, thereby preventing the onset of diabetes in IRS2 knockout mice showing the critical role of PDX1 in β-cell survival.[120] Also epigenetic changes of PDX1 gene expression can lead to the development of β-cell failure.[121]

PDX1 nuclear import and export signals (NLS/NES) suggest that this factor is subjected to regulation at the level of cellular localization[122,123] and that PDX1 nucleo-cytoplasmic shuttling regulates its function.[117,118,122,124] We have recently shown that the negative effect of IL-1β on β-cell function/survival is modulated by the shuttling of PDX1 to the cytoplasm, whereas IL-1β neutralizing by IL-1Ra results in enhancement of PDX1 nuclear translocation rescuing human islets *in vitro* and β-cells in diabetic mouse models from apoptosis and impaired function.[124] To establish whether IL-1β mediates β-cell death and impaired function via nuclear exclusion of PDX1. Overexpression of shuttling deficient-mutant PDX1-NES, which remains in the nucleus, reduced human islet apoptosis and improved islet function under IL-1β treatment. IL-1β-induced nuclear exclusion of PDX1 and its translocation to the cytoplasm was also JNK dependent and prevented by JNK inhibition further supporting JNK signaling as downstream of the IL-1 receptor.

Nucleocytoplasmic shuttling of PDX1 under diabetogenic conditions (IL-1β, chronically elevated glucose[124] or free fatty acids)[125] is a feature of diabetes. Our recent data[124] demonstrated that in all islets from patients with T2DM as well as in animal models, PDX1 protein was localized in the cytoplasm, whereas in the non-diabetic controls, PDX1 was in the nucleus. IL-1β antagonism by IL-1Ra overexpression or injections restored normoglycemia and β-cell function and survival in db/db and HFD-fed mice through redistribution of PDX1 into the nucleus. IL-1β-induced PDX1 cytoplasmic accumulation and its subsequent degradation may affect β-cell function in different levels. Cytosolic PDX1 may be inactive and regulation of gene expression is lost. As PDX1 regulates insulin and specific β-cell genes, altered localization may contribute to β-cell death and impaired

function and provides another explanation for the toxic effects of IL-1β on β-cells.

IL-1β AND GENETIC PREDISPOSITION

Genetic variation in the IL-1 gene family is associated with hyperglycemia and insulin resistance provides another proof for the involvement of IL-1β in the pathogenesis of diabetes.[126] Results from recent genome-wide association studies (GWAS) show that TCF7L2 (transcription factor 7-like 2, previously known as TCF-4) is a strong risk factor for type 2 diabetes.[127] This association of TCF7L2 variants with type 2 diabetes has been replicated in numerous study populations worldwide.[128] Since polymorphisms were found in the non-coding region of the gene, effects on the β-cell and whether there is a link between TCF7L2 and β-cell survival was previously unknown.

TCF7L2 is an important component of the WNT signaling cascade; the WNT/β-catenin signaling pathway is involved in many physiological and pathophysiological activities such as embryonic development, cell differentiation and tumorigenesis. WNT signal regulates lipid metabolism and glucose homeostasis as well, and regulates β-cell proliferation and function.[129] Mutations in LRP5 may lead to the development of diabetes and obesity.[130] The single nucleotide polymorphism locus in the Wnt5b gene confers susceptibility to type 2 diabetes in a Japanese population.[131] The Wnt antagonist sFRP inhibits β-cell proliferation and insulin secretion.[132]

TCF7L2 plays a role in glucose homeostasis through the regulation of pro-glucagon gene expression, which encodes incretin hormone GLP-1 (glucagon-like peptide-1) in intestinal cells.[133] TCF7L2 expression in the β-cells is correlated with β-cell function and survival. Reducing TCF7L2 gene expression by siRNA leads to increased β-cell apoptosis and impaired function.[134–137] A diabetic milieu, e.g., the cytokine mixture IL-1β and IFN-γ or high glucose, decreases TCF7L2 expression; conversely, overexpression of TCF7L2 protects islets from high glucose- and cytokine-induced apoptosis and impaired function,[136] suggesting that cytokine toxicity also interferes with TCF7L2 expression. One common pathway of IL-1β and the loss of TCF7L2 is the impaired activation of protein kinase B (AKT) and reduced phosphorylation of glycogen synthase kinase-3β (GSK3β) which indicates GSK3β regulation downstream of TCF7L2.[138] GSK3β is an enzyme that regulates glycogen synthesis in response to insulin.[139] When WNT signals are inactive, GSK3β interacts with β-catenin and phosphorylates it, leading to proteasome-mediated protein degradation. Loss of GSK3β phosphorylation leads to GSK3β activation, β-catenin degradation, and impaired β-cell proliferation and function.[140,141] GSK3β activity is necessary for full stimulation of the production of several pro-inflammatory cytokines,

such as IL-6, IL-1β, and TNF-α upon stimulation of Toll-like receptors in monocytes and peripheral blood mononuclear cells. Also, GSK3β reduces the production of the anti-inflammatory cytokine IL-10.[142] GSK3β regulates IL-1β-induced cytokine secretion by airway smooth muscle[143] and negatively regulates the levels of IL-1Ra produced by lipo-polysaccharide (LPS)-stimulated innate immune cells.[144]

Inhibitors of GSK3β reduce the production of pro-inflammatory cytokines and increase anti-inflammatory cytokine production. Inhibition of GSK3β activation results in stabilization of β-catenin which is then translocated to the nucleus and forms a transcriptor complex with TCF7L2 to activate target genes transcription.[145,146] Thus, small molecule inhibitors of GSK3β have potential therapeutic uses, including the treatment of neurodegenerative diseases, T2DM, as well as the associated chronic activation of inflammation.[146]

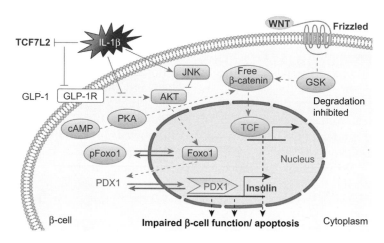

FIGURE 19.3   Genes and environment: IL-1β affects the transcription factors TCF7L2 and PDX1 and induces β-cell apoptosis and impaired function. IL-1β signals in the β-cell induce JNK and inhibit AKT activation, this enhances FoxO1 translocation after phosphorylation by JNK (c-Jun N-terminal kinase). TCF7L2 levels are reduced and inhibit GLP signaling. Decreases in the pool of free β-catenin (and inhibition of nuclear translocation) leads to reduced TCF7L2-mediated transcription. Decreased phosphorylation and activation of GSK-3β promotes proteosomal degradation, and degradation of TCF7L2 itself. Loss of TCF7L2 leads to a decrease in GLP-1R, AKT phosphorylation is reduced and increases the activity of FoxO1 and its translocation to the nucleus, while PDX1 is oppositely regulated and glucose-mediated insulin transcription is disturbed. Together, these effects all result in impaired insulin secretion and β-cell survival. (see the color plate section at the back of the book.)

We tested whether GSK3β inhibitors could reverse the deleterious effects of TCF7L2 depletion in isolated human islets.[138] Two specific GSK3β inhibitors 1-AKP (1-Azakenpaullone)[147] and SB216763[148] effectively restore GSK3β phosphorylation which was reduced by TCF7L2 knock-down, improve β-cell function in siTCF7L2-treated islets, restore β-cell proliferation, and decrease β-cell apoptosis.

GSK inhibitors directly stimulate β-cell proliferation, increase β-cell mass, mimic insulin action and would be therefore a potent therapy for diabetes.[149,150] Our recent study provides a possible treatment strategy of diabetes for patients carrying a TCF7L2 mutation (see Figure 19.3).[138]

One needs to carefully consider the multiplicity of substrates and complexity of regulation of GSK3β, which may result in unwanted side effects on various cells induced by dysregulated GSK3.[151]

THE DYSBALANCE OF IL-1β AND IL-1RA IN DIABETES[54]

Reminiscent to the essential role of glucose in mediating insulin secretion and proliferation at physiological concentrations but in inducing β-cell failure at chronically elevated concentration, a low concentration of IL-1β also stimulates insulin release and proliferation in rat and human islets (see Figure 19.4).[80,88,152−154] The beneficial IL-1β effects seem to be partly mediated by the increased secretion of the naturally occurring anti-inflammatory cytokine and antagonist of IL-1α and IL-1β, the interleukin-1 receptor antagonist. Similar to IL-1β, IL-1Ra binds to type 1 and 2 IL-1 receptors but lacks a second binding domain. Therefore, IL-1Ra does not recruit the IL-1 receptor accessory protein, the second component of the receptor complex.[155−157] While IL-1β is induced in islets and β-cells in T2DM, IL-1Ra is downregulated.[27,31]

Endogenous production and secretion of IL-1Ra limits inflammation and tissue damage.[22] *In vivo*, exogenous IL-1Ra counteracts low-dose streptozotocin-induced diabetes,[158] autoimmune diabetes,[159] and promotes graft survival[159−162] and islet survival after transplantation.[163] IL-1Ra is secreted from the β-cell and expressed in β-cell granules,[31] it protects cultured human islets from the deleterious effects of glucose[27] as well as IL-1β.[75,160,161,164,165] Inhibition of IL-1Ra with small interfering RNAs or long-term treatment with leptin lead to β-cell apoptosis and impaired function, which may provide a further link between obesity and diabetes.

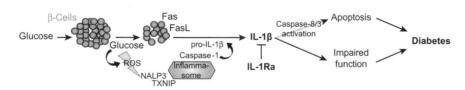

FIGURE 19.4 **Dual role of glucose on β-cell turnover (from[54]).** Stimulation of β-cells with glucose induces insulin secretion and β-cell proliferation. In contrast, chronic glucose exposure leads to upregulation of the Fas receptor and ligation with FasL to caspase activation, apoptosis, and impaired function, which contributes to β-cell failure in diabetes. Under such conditions, IL-1β is produced and secreted by the β-cell. This is mediated through ROS-induced induction of the NALP3 inflammasome, which activates caspase-1 and maturation of active IL-1β from pro-IL-1β. Pre-incubation of the islets with the naturally occurring IL-1 antagonist interleukin-1 receptor antagonist (IL-1Ra) inhibits glucose-induced apoptosis and improves β-cell function and could therefore be a valuable tool for diabetes therapy. Reproduced with kind permission of Springer Science + Business Media.

The definite secretion and regulation mechanisms of IL-1Ra are unknown. Like IL-1β, IL-1Ra may also be secreted by a leaderless pathway via activation of the P2X7 receptor.[166,167] In pancreatic islets from obese individuals P2X7 receptors are highly expressed and these receptors were almost undetectable in T2DM.[167] In accordance with the P2X7 receptor expression levels, increased IL-1Ra serum levels correlate with obesity and insulin resistance,[168-171] but IL-1Ra is decreased in T2DM.[172] Recent results from the Whitehall Study show that IL-1Ra levels increase before the onset of T2DM,[173] which are consistent with findings in HFD-fed mice. IL-1Ra levels were increased after 4 and 8 weeks of diet together with an increase in β-cell mass and body weight. Serum concentrations of IL-1Ra are influenced by adipose tissue, which is a major source of IL-1Ra.[174] After 16 weeks, when the HFD-fed mice display glucose intolerance and β-cell apoptosis, IL-1Ra levels are lower than in the normal diet-fed mice. Mice deficient for the P2X7 receptor, were unable to compensatorily increase β-cell mass in response to the HFD feeding and had no adaptive increase in IL-1Ra levels.[167]

The increased IL-1Ra could be an attempt of the body to counteract the deleterious effects of IL-1β and to preserve β-cell survival, insulin secretion and insulin sensitivity. It is hypothesized that IL-1Ra could have an additional metabolic effect which leads to insulin resistance. However, when we treated mice daily for 12 weeks with IL-1Ra we did not observe changes in insulin sensitivity at any time point.[175]

Whether serum IL-1Ra levels would explain the progression of diabetes in obese individuals and whether serum IL-1Ra affects IL-1Ra expression in the β-cell is not known. We hypothesize that a decreased β-cell IL-1Ra expression could trigger the progression from obesity to diabetes and high IL-1Ra expression could possibly protect the β-cell and enable it to adapt to conditions of higher insulin demand.[9,54]

BLOCKING IL-1β SIGNALS IN VIVO INHIBITS DIABETES PROGRESSION[54]

Recently, the hypothesis that blocking IL-1β is a successful strategy for the therapy of T2DM has been proven by several studies. Daily injection of IL-1Ra in mice fed a HFD improved glycemia, glucose-stimulated insulin secretion, and survival,[175] reduced hyperglycemia, and reversed the islet inflammatory phenotype in the GK rat.[176] Treatment with an IL-1β antibody also improved glycemic control in diet-induced obesity in mice.[177,178]

Importantly, results from a recent clinical study in patients with T2DM showed that IL-1Ra improved glycemic control and β-cell function.[179] After 13 weeks of treatment, C-peptide secretion was increased and inflammatory markers, e.g., IL-6 and C-reactive protein, were reduced in the IL-1Ra group. HbA1c was significantly lower in the IL-1Ra compared to the placebo group, which correlated with the body-surface area in the IL-1Ra group. The dose of 100 mg IL-1Ra was given daily to the patients without weight adjustment. Currently ongoing trials which include dose adjustment to the body weight may result in better glycemic control in the higher body surface area group. The effect of interleukin-1 antagonism on β-cell function is currently tested in patients with recent onset of T1DM.[180] Both, IL-1Ra as well as anti-IL-1β antibody XOMA 052 do not completely block IL-1β signalling. While IL-1Ra is a competitive antagonist to IL-1β, XOMA 052 has a novel mechanism of action that reduces IL-1β activity by 40–50-fold rather than completely blocking it.[178,181] Given the dual role of IL-1β on β-cell survival and insulin secretion, this may be an important characteristic of both drugs.

As shown by these recent studies, blocking IL-1β signaling may be a powerful new treatment for T2DM which does not rely on replacing insulin exogenously but acts at the level of the β-cell to improve β-cell survival and to improve endogenous insulin secretion and action. Moreover, blocking IL-1β may also improve insulin sensitivity. Further studies will be necessary to clarify the contradiction of IL-1Ra's modulation of insulin sensitivity and the impact of IL-β on β-cell survival in T2DM.

Acknowledgments

This work was supported by the European Research Council, the German Research Foundation (DFG, Emmy Noether Program) and the Juvenile Diabetes Research Foundation. The authors thank the members of the Islet Biology laboratory in Bremen for critical discussion.

References

1. Mandrup-Poulsen T. β-Cell apoptosis: stimuli and signaling. *Diabetes* 2001;**50**(Suppl. 1):S58–63.
2. Mathis D, Vence L, Benoist C. β-Cell death during progression to diabetes. *Nature* 2001;**414**:792–8.
3. Butler AE, Janson J, Bonner-Weir S, Ritzel R, Rizza RA, et al. Beta-cell deficit and increased beta-cell apoptosis in humans with type 2 diabetes. *Diabetes* 2003;**52**:102–10.
4. Mathis D, Vence L, Benoist C. Beta-cell death during progression to diabetes. *Nature* 2001;**414**:792–8.
5. Eizirik DL, Mandrup-Poulsen T. A choice of death—the signal-transduction of immune-mediated beta-cell apoptosis. *Diabetologia* 2001;**44**:2115–33.
6. Rhodes CJ. Type 2 diabetes—a matter of beta-cell life and death? *Science* 2005;**307**:380–4.
7. Donath MY, Ehses JA, Maedler K, Schumann DM, Ellingsgaard H, et al. Mechanisms of beta-cell death in type 2 diabetes. *Diabetes* 2005;**54**(Suppl. 2):S108–13.
8. Mandrup-Poulsen T, Bendtzen K, Dinarello CA, Nerup J. Human tumor necrosis factor potentiates human interleukin 1-mediated rat pancreatic beta-cell cytotoxicity. *J Immunol* 1987;**139**:4077–82.
9. Maedler K, Dharmadhikari G, Schumann DM, Storling J. Interleukin-1 beta targeted therapy for type 2 diabetes. *Expert Opin Biol Ther* 2009;**9**:1177–88.
10. Koenig W, Khuseyinova N, Baumert J, Thorand B, Loewel H, et al. Increased concentrations of C-reactive protein and IL-6 but not IL-18 are independently associated with incident coronary events in middle-aged men and women: results from the MONICA/KORA Augsburg case-cohort study, 1984–2002. *Arterioscler Thromb Vasc Biol* 2006;**26**:2745–51.
11. Wellen KE, Hotamisligil GS. Inflammation, stress, and diabetes. *J Clin Invest* 2005;**115**:1111–9.
12. de Luca C, Olefsky JM. Inflammation and insulin resistance. *FEBS Lett* 2008;**582**:97–105.
13. Weisberg SP, McCann D, Desai M, Rosenbaum M, Leibel RL, et al. Obesity is associated with macrophage accumulation in adipose tissue. *J Clin Invest* 2003;**112**:1796–808.
14. Xu H, Barnes GT, Yang Q, Tan G, Yang D, et al. Chronic inflammation in fat plays a crucial role in the development of obesity-related insulin resistance. *J Clin Invest* 2003;**112**:1821–30.
15. Koerner A, Kratzsch J, Kiess W. Adipocytokines: leptin—the classical, resistin—the controversial, adiponectin—the promising, and more to come. *Best Pract Res Clin Endocrinol Metab* 2005;**19**:525–46.
16. Tilg H, Moschen AR. Adipocytokines: mediators linking adipose tissue, inflammation and immunity. *Nat Rev Immunol* 2006;**6**:772–83.
17. Schenk S, Saberi M, Olefsky JM. Insulin sensitivity: modulation by nutrients and inflammation. *J Clin Invest* 2008;**118**:2992–3002.
18. Ehses JA, Perren A, Eppler E, Ribaux P, Pospisilik JA, et al. Increased number of islet-associated macrophages in type 2 diabetes. *Diabetes* 2007;**56**:2356–70.
19. Richardson SJ, Willcox A, Bone AJ, Foulis AK, Morgan NG. Islet-associated macrophages in type 2 diabetes. *Diabetologia* 2009;**52**:1686–8.
20. Homo-Delarche F, Calderari S, Irminger JC, Gangnerau MN, Coulaud J, et al. Islet inflammation and fibrosis in a spontaneous model of type 2 diabetes, the GK rat. *Diabetes* 2006;**55**:1625–33.
21. Weksler-Zangen S, Raz I, Lenzen S, Jorns A, Ehrenfeld S, et al. Impaired glucose-stimulated insulin secretion is coupled with exocrine pancreatic lesions in the Cohen diabetic rat. *Diabetes* 2008;**57**:279–87.
22. Dinarello CA. Immunological and inflammatory functions of the interleukin-1 family. *Annu Rev Immunol* 2009;**27**:519–50.
23. Narcisse L, Scemes E, Zhao Y, Lee SC, Brosnan CF. The cytokine IL-1beta transiently enhances P2X7 receptor expression and function in human astrocytes. *Glia* 2005;**49**:245–58.

24. Arnush M, Heitmeier MR, Scarim AL, Marino MH, Manning PT, et al. IL-1 produced and released endogenously within human islets inhibits beta cell function. *J Clin Invest* 1998 Aug 1;**102**(3):516–26. 26.

25. Lacy PE. The intraislet macrophage and type I diabetes. *Mt Sinai J Med* 1994;**61**:170–4.

26. Heitmeier MR, Arnush M, Scarim AL, Corbett JA. Pancreatic {beta}-cell damage mediated by β-cell production of IL-1: A novel mechanism for virus-induced diabetes. *J Biol Chem* 2001;**276**:11151–8.

27. Maedler K, Sergeev P, Ris F, Oberholzer J, Joller-Jemelka HI, et al. Glucose-induced beta-cell production of interleukin-1beta contributes to glucotoxicity in human pancreatic islets. *J Clin Invest* 2002; **110**:851–60.

28. Boni-Schnetzler M, Thorne J, Parnaud G, Marselli L, Ehses JA, et al. Increased interleukin (IL)-1beta messenger ribonucleic acid expression in beta -cells of individuals with type 2 diabetes and regulation of IL-1beta in human islets by glucose and autostimulation. *J Clin Endocrinol Metab* 2008;**93**:4065–74.

29. Zhou R, Tardivel A, Thorens B, Choi I, Tschopp J. Thioredoxin-interacting protein links oxidative stress to inflammasome activation. *Nat Immunol* 2010;**11**: 136–40.

30. Venieratos PD, Drossopoulou GI, Kapodistria KD, Tsilibary EC, Kitsiou PV. High glucose induces suppression of insulin signalling and apoptosis via upregulation of endogenous IL-1beta and suppressor of cytokine signalling-1 in mouse pancreatic beta cells. *Cell Signal* 2010;**22**:791–800.

31. Maedler K, Sergeev P, Ehses JA, Mathe Z, Bosco D, et al. Leptin modulates beta cell expression of IL-1 receptor antagonist and release of IL-1beta in human islets. *Proc Natl Acad Sci USA* 2004;**101**:8138–43.

32. Boni-Schnetzler M, Boller S, Debray S, Bouzakri K, Meier DT, et al. Free fatty acids induce a proinflammatory response in islets via the abundantly expressed interleukin-1 receptor I. *Endocrinology* 2009;**150**:5218–29.

33. Mine TMK, Okutsu T, Mitsui A, Kitahara Y. Gene expression profile in the pancreatic islets of Goto-Kakizaki (GK) rats with repeated postprandial hyperglycemia. *Diabetes* 2004;**53**(Suppl. 12):2475A.

34. Jorns A, Rath KJ, Bock O, Lenzen S. Beta cell death in hyperglycaemic Psammomys obesus is not cytokine-mediated. *Diabetologia* 2006;**49**:2704–12.

35. Welsh N, Cnop M, Kharroubi I, Bugliani M, Lupi R, et al. Is there a role for locally produced interleukin-1 in the deleterious effects of high glucose or the type 2 diabetes milieu to human pancreatic islets? *Diabetes* 2005;**54**:3238–44.

36. Fu AL, Zhou CY, Chen X. Thyroid hormone prevents cognitive deficit in a mouse model of Alzheimer's disease. *Neuropharmacology* 2010 Mar–Apr;**58**(4–5):722–9.

37. Donath MY, Ehses JA, Maedler K, Schumann DM, Ellingsgaard H, et al. Mechanisms of β-cell death in type 2 diabetes. *Diabetes* 2005;**54**(Suppl. 2):S108–13.

38. Martinon F, Gaide O, Petrilli V, Mayor A, Tschopp J. NALP inflammasomes: a central role in innate immunity. *Semin Immunopathol* 2007;**29**:213–29.

39. Martinon F, Mayor A, Tschopp J. The inflammasomes: guardians of the body. *Annu Rev Immunol* 2009; **27**:229–65.

40. Vandanmagsar B, Youm YH, Ravussin A, Galgani JE, Stadler K, et al. The NLRP3 inflammasome instigates obesity-induced inflammation and insulin resistance. *Nat Med* 2011;**17**:179–88.

41. Schroder K, Zhou R, Tschopp J. The NLRP3 inflammasome: a sensor for metabolic danger? *Science* 2010; **327**:296–300.

42. Masters SL, Dunne A, Subramanian SL, Hull RL, Tannahill GM, et al. Activation of the NLRP3 inflammasome by islet amyloid polypeptide provides a mechanism for enhanced IL-1beta in type 2 diabetes. *Nat Immunol* 2010;**11**:897–904.

43. Westwell-Roper C, Dai DL, Soukhatcheva G, Potter KJ, van Rooijen N, et al. IL-1 blockade attenuates islet amyloid polypeptide-induced proinflammatory cytokine release and pancreatic islet graft dysfunction. *J Immunol* 2011;**187**:2755–65.

44. Parikh H, Carlsson E, Chutkow WA, Johansson LE, Storgaard H, et al. TXNIP regulates peripheral glucose metabolism in humans. *PLoS Med* 2007; **4**:e158.

45. Chen J, Fontes G, Saxena G, Poitout V, Shalev A. Lack of TXNIP protects against mitochondria-mediated apoptosis, but not against fatty acid-induced, ER-stress-mediated beta cell death. *Diabetes* 2010 Feb;**59**(2):440–7.

46. Donath MY, Boni-Schnetzler M. IL-1beta activation as a response to metabolic disturbances. *Cell Metab* 2010;**12**:427–8.

47. Mandrup-Poulsen T. IAPP boosts islet macrophage IL-1 in type 2 diabetes. *Nat Immunol* 2010;**11**:881–3.

48. Butler AE, Jang J, Gurlo T, Carty MD, Soeller WC, et al. Diabetes due to a progressive defect in beta-cell mass in rats transgenic for human islet amyloid polypeptide (HIP Rat): a new model for type 2 diabetes. *Diabetes* 2004;**53**:1509–16.

49. Wen H, Gris D, Lei Y, Jha S, Zhang L, et al. Fatty acid-induced NLRP3-ASC inflammasome activation interferes with insulin signaling. *Nat Immunol* 2011; **12**:408–15.

50. Dinarello CA. Biology of interleukin 1. *FASEB J* 1988; **2**:108—15.

51. Warner SJ, Auger KR, Libby P. Human interleukin 1 induces interleukin 1 gene expression in human vascular smooth muscle cells. *J Exp Med* 1987;**165**: 1316—31.

52. Frobose H, Ronn SG, Heding PE, Mendoza H, Cohen P, et al. Suppressor of cytokine Signaling-3 inhibits interleukin-1 signaling by targeting the TRAF-6/TAK1 complex. *Mol Endocrinol* 2006;**20**: 1587—96.

53. Mokhtari D, Myers JW, Welsh N. The MAPK kinase kinase-1 is essential for stress-induced pancreatic islet cell death. *Endocrinology* 2008;**149**:3046—53.

54. Maedler K, Dharmadhikari G, Schumann DM, Storling J. Interleukin-targeted therapy for metabolic syndrome and type 2 diabetes. *Handb Exp Pharmacol* 2011;**257**—78.

55. Giannoukakis N, Mi Z, Rudert WA, Gambotto A, Trucco M, et al. Prevention of beta cell dysfunction and apoptosis activation in human islets by adenoviral gene transfer of the insulin-like growth factor I. *Gene Ther* 2000;**7**:2015—22.

56. Kim S, Millet I, Kim HS, Kim JY, Han MS, et al. NF-kappa B prevents beta cell death and autoimmune diabetes in NOD mice. *Proc Natl Acad Sci USA* 2007;**104**:1913—8.

57. Strasser A, O'Connor L, Dixit VM. Apoptosis signaling. *Annu Rev Biochem* 2000;**69**:217—45.

58. Adam-Klages S, Adam D, Janssen O, Kabelitz D. Death receptors and caspases: role in lymphocyte proliferation, cell death, and autoimmunity. *Immunol Res* 2005;**33**:149—66.

59. Krammer PH. CD95's deadly mission in the immune system. *Nature* 2000;**407**:789—95.

60. Lindsay J, Esposti MD, Gilmore AP. Bcl-2 proteins and mitochondria—Specificity in membrane targeting for death. *Biochim Biophys Acta* 2011;**1813**: 532—9.

61. Moriwaki M, Itoh N, Miyagawa J, Yamamoto K, Imagawa A, et al. Fas and Fas ligand expression in inflamed islets in pancreas sections of patients with recent-onset Type I diabetes mellitus. *Diabetologia* 1999;**42**:1332—40.

62. Chervonsky AV, Wang Y, Wong FS, Visintin I, Flavell RA, et al. The role of Fas in autoimmune diabetes. *Cell* 1997;**89**:17—24.

63. Allison J, Thomas HE, Catterall T, Kay TW, Strasser A. Transgenic expression of dominant-negative Fas-associated death domain protein in beta cells protects against Fas ligand-induced apoptosis and reduces spontaneous diabetes in nonobese diabetic mice. *J Immunol* 2005;**175**:293—301.

64. Yamada K, Takane-Gyotoku N, Yuan X, Ichikawa F, Inada C, et al. Mouse islet cell lysis mediated by interleukin-1-induced Fas. *Diabetologia* 1996;**39**: 1306—12.

65. Loweth AC, Williams GT, James RF, Scarpello JH, Morgan NG. Human islets of Langerhans express Fas ligand and undergo apoptosis in response to inter-leukin-1beta and Fas ligation. *Diabetes* 1998;**47**: 727—32.

66. Kay TW, Thomas HE, Harrison LC, Allison J. The beta cell in autoimmune diabetes: many mechanisms and pathways of loss. *Trends Endocrinol Metab* 2000;**11**: 11—5.

67. Ou D, Metzger DL, Wang X, Huang J, Pozzilli P, et al. TNF-related apoptosis-inducing ligand death pathway-mediated human beta-cell destruction. *Diabetologia* 2002;**45**:1678—88.

68. Maedler K, Spinas GA, Lehmann R, Sergeev P, Weber M, et al. Glucose induces beta-cell apoptosis via upregulation of the Fas-receptor in human islets. *Diabetes* 2001;**50**:1683—90.

69. Corbett JA, Sweetland MA, Wang JL, Lancaster Jr JR, McDaniel ML. Nitric oxide mediates cytokine-induced inhibition of insulin secretion by human islets of Langerhans. *Proc Natl Acad Sci USA* 1993;**90**:1731—5.

70. Giannoukakis N, Rudert WA, Ghivizzani SC, Gambotto A, Ricordi C, et al. Adenoviral gene transfer of the interleukin-1 receptor antagonist protein to human islets prevents IL-1beta-induced beta-cell impairment and activation of islet cell apoptosis in vitro. *Diabetes* 1999;**48**:1730—6.

71. Loweth AC, Watts K, McBain SC, Williams GT, Scarpello JH, et al. Dissociation between Fas expression and induction of apoptosis in human islets of Langerhans. *Diabetes Obes Metab* 2000;**2**:57—60.

72. Loweth AC, Williams GT, James RF, Scarpello JH, Morgan NG. Human islets of Langerhans express Fas ligand and undergo apoptosis in response to interleukin-1beta and Fas ligation. *Diabetes* 1998;**47**: 727—32.

73. Mandrup-Poulsen T, Bendtzen K, Nerup J, Dinarello CA, Svenson M, et al. Affinity-purified human interleukin I is cytotoxic to isolated islets of Langerhans. *Diabetologia* 1986;**29**:63—7.

74. Mandrup-Poulsen T, Bendtzen K, Nielsen JH, Bendixen G, Nerup J. Cytokines cause functional and structural damage to isolated islets of Langerhans. *Allergy* 1985;**40**:424—9.

75. Mandrup-Poulsen T, Zumsteg U, Reimers J, Pociot F, Morch L, et al. Involvement of interleukin 1 and interleukin 1 antagonist in pancreatic beta-cell destruction in insulin-dependent diabetes mellitus. *Cytokine* 1993;**5**:185—91.

III. MOLECULAR INSIGHTS OF DIABETES AND METABOLIC SYNDROME

76. Rabinovitch A, Sumoski W, Rajotte RV, Warnock GL. Cytotoxic effects of cytokines on human pancreatic islet cells in monolayer culture. *J Clin Endocrinol Metab* 1990;**71**:152–6.

77. Stassi G, De Maria R, Trucco G, Rudert W, Testi R, et al. Nitric oxide primes pancreatic beta cells for Fas-mediated destruction in insulin-dependent diabetes mellitus. *J Exp Med* 1997;**186**:1193–200.

78. Augstein P, Dunger A, Heinke P, Wachlin G, Berg S, et al. Prevention of autoimmune diabetes in NOD mice by troglitazone is associated with modulation of ICAM-1 expression on pancreatic islet cells and IFN-gamma expression in splenic T cells. *Biochem Biophys Res Commun* 2003;**304**:378–84.

79. Stassi G, Todaro M, Richiusa P, Giordano M, Mattina A, et al. Expression of apoptosis-inducing CD95 (Fas/Apo-1) on human beta-cells sorted by flow-cytometry and cultured in vitro. *Transplant Proc* 1995;**27**:3271–5.

80. Schumann DM, Maedler K, Franklin I, Konrad D, Storling J, et al. The Fas pathway is involved in pancreatic β cell secretory function. *Proc Natl Acad Sci USA* 2007;**104**:2861–6.

81. Donath MY, Storling J, Maedler K, Mandrup-Poulsen T. Inflammatory mediators and islet beta-cell failure: a link between type 1 and type 2 diabetes. *J Mol Med* 2003;**81**:455–70.

82. Zumsteg U, Frigerio S, Hollander GA. Nitric oxide production and Fas surface expression mediate two independent pathways of cytokine-induced murine beta-cell damage. *Diabetes* 2000;**49**:39–47.

83. Nakayama M, Nagata M, Yasuda H, Arisawa K, Kotani R, et al. Fas/Fas ligand interactions play an essential role in the initiation of murine autoimmune diabetes. *Diabetes* 2002;**51**:1391–7.

84. Augstein P, Dunger A, Salzsieder C, Heinke P, Kubernath R, et al. Cell surface trafficking of Fas in NIT-1 cells and dissection of surface and total Fas expression. *Biochem Biophys Res Commun* 2002;**290**:443–51.

85. Donath MY, Boni-Schnetzler M, Ellingsgaard H, Ehses JA. Islet inflammation impairs the pancreatic beta-cell in type 2 diabetes. *Physiology (Bethesda)* 2009;**24**:325–31.

86. Maedler K, Sergeev P, Ris F, Oberholzer J, Joller-Jemelka HI, et al. Glucose-induced beta cell production of IL-1beta contributes to glucotoxicity in human pancreatic islets. *J Clin Invest* 2002;**110**:851–60.

87. Liadis N, Salmena L, Kwan E, Tajmir P, Schroer SA, et al. Distinct in vivo roles of caspase-8 in beta-cells in physiological and diabetes models. *Diabetes* 2007;**56**:2302–11.

88. Maedler K, Schumann DM, Sauter N, Ellingsgaard H, Bosco D, et al. Low concentration of interleukin-1β induces FLICE-inhibitory protein-mediated β-cell proliferation in human pancreatic islets. *Diabetes* 2006;**55**:2713–22.

89. Flodstrom M, Welsh N, Eizirik DL. Cytokines activate the nuclear factor kappa B (NF-kappa B) and induce nitric oxide production in human pancreatic islets. *FEBS Lett* 1996;**385**:4–6.

90. Liuwantara D, Elliot M, Smith MW, Yam AO, Walters SN, et al. Nuclear factor-kappaB regulates beta-cell death: a critical role for A20 in beta-cell protection. *Diabetes* 2006;**55**:2491–501.

91. Hammar E, Parnaud G, Bosco D, Perriraz N, Maedler K, et al. Extracellular matrix protects pancreatic {beta}-cells against apoptosis: role of short- and long-term signaling pathways. *Diabetes* 2004;**53**:2034–41.

92. Thomas HE, Irawaty W, Darwiche R, Brodnicki TC, Santamaria P, et al. IL-1 receptor deficiency slows progression to diabetes in the NOD mouse. *Diabetes* 2004;**53**:113–21.

93. Schott WH, Haskell BD, Tse HM, Milton MJ, Piganelli JD, et al. Caspase-1 is not required for type 1 diabetes in the NOD mouse. *Diabetes* 2004;**53**:99–104.

94. Jafarian-Tehrani M, Amrani A, Homo-Delarche F, Marquette C, Dardenne M, et al. Localization and characterization of interleukin-1 receptors in the islets of Langerhans from control and nonobese diabetic mice. *Endocrinology* 1995;**136**:609–13.

95. Balasa B, La Cava A, Van Gunst K, Mocnik L, Balakrishna D, et al. A mechanism for IL-10-mediated diabetes in the nonobese diabetic (NOD) mouse: ICAM-1 deficiency blocks accelerated diabetes. *J Immunol* 2000;**165**:7330–7.

96. Thomas HE, Darwiche R, Corbett JA, Kay TW. Evidence that beta cell death in the nonobese diabetic mouse is Fas independent. *J Immunol* 1999;**163**:1562–9.

97. Papaccio G, Graziano A, Valiante S, D'Aquino R, Travali S, et al. Interleukin (IL)-1beta toxicity to islet beta cells: Efaroxan exerts a complete protection. *J Cell Physiol* 2005;**203**:94–102.

98. Grunnet LG, Aikin R, Tonnesen MF, Paraskevas S, Blaabjerg L, et al. Proinflammatory cytokines activate the intrinsic apoptotic pathway in beta-cells. *Diabetes* 2009;**58**:1807–15.

99. McKenzie MD, Carrington EM, Kaufmann T, Strasser A, Huang DC, et al. Proapoptotic BH3-only protein Bid is essential for death receptor-induced apoptosis of pancreatic beta-cells. *Diabetes* 2008;**57**:1284–92.

100. Saldeen J. Cytokines induce both necrosis and apoptosis via a common Bcl-2-inhibitable pathway in

rat insulin-producing cells. *Endocrinology* 2000;**141**: 2003—10.

101. Klein D, Ribeiro MM, Mendoza V, Jayaraman S, Kenyon NS, et al. Delivery of Bcl-XL or its BH4 domain by protein transduction inhibits apoptosis in human islets. *Biochem Biophys Res Commun* 2004;**323**:473—8.

102. Iwahashi H, Hanafusa T, Eguchi Y, Nakajima H, Miyagawa J, et al. Cytokine-induced apoptotic cell death in a mouse pancreatic beta-cell line: inhibition by Bcl-2. *Diabetologia* 1996;**39**:530—6.

103. Gurzov EN, Germano CM, Cunha DA, Ortis F, Vanderwinden JM, et al. p53 up-regulated modulator of apoptosis (PUMA) activation contributes to pancreatic beta-cell apoptosis induced by proinflammatory cytokines and endoplasmic reticulum stress. *J Biol Chem* 2010;**285**:19910—20.

104. Gurzov EN, Ortis F, Cunha DA, Gosset G, Li M, et al. Signaling by IL-1beta+IFN-gamma and ER stress converge on DP5/Hrk activation: a novel mechanism for pancreatic beta-cell apoptosis. *Cell Death Differ* 2009;**16**:1539—50.

105. Allagnat F, Cunha D, Moore F, Vanderwinden JM, Eizirik DL, et al. Mcl-1 downregulation by proinflammatory cytokines and palmitate is an early event contributing to beta-cell apoptosis. *Cell Death Differ* 2011;**18**:328—37.

106. Carrington EM, McKenzie MD, Jansen E, Myers M, Fynch S, et al. Islet beta-cells deficient in Bcl-xL develop but are abnormally sensitive to apoptotic stimuli. *Diabetes* 2009;**58**:2316—23.

107. Trincavelli ML, Marselli L, Falleni A, Gremigni V, Ragge E, et al. Upregulation of mitochondrial peripheral benzodiazepine receptor expression by cytokine-induced damage of human pancreatic islets. *J Cell Biochem* 2002;**84**:636—44.

108. Rabinovitch A, Suarez-Pinzon W, Strynadka K, Ju Q, Edelstein D, et al. Transfection of human pancreatic islets with an anti-apoptotic gene (bcl-2) protects beta-cells from cytokine-induced destruction. *Diabetes* 1999 Jun;**48**(6):1223—9.

109. Dupraz P, Rinsch C, Pralong WF, Rolland E, Zufferey R, et al. Lentivirus-mediated Bcl-2 expression in betaTC-tet cells improves resistance to hypoxia and cytokine-induced apoptosis while preserving in vitro and in vivo control of insulin secretion. *Gene Ther* 1999;**6**:1160—9.

110. Ghibelli L, Diederich M. Multistep and multitask Bax activation. *Mitochondrion* 2010;**10**:604—13.

111. Mehmeti I, Lenzen S, Lortz S. Modulation of Bcl-2-related protein expression in pancreatic beta cells by pro-inflammatory cytokines and its dependence on the antioxidative defense status. *Mol Cell Endocrinol* 2011;**332**:88—96.

112. Scaffidi C, Schmitz I, Zha J, Korsmeyer SJ, Krammer PH, et al. Differential modulation of apoptosis sensitivity in CD95 type I and type II cells. *J Biol Chem* 1999;**274**:22532—8.

113. Jost PJ, Grabow S, Gray D, McKenzie MD, Nachbur U, et al. XIAP discriminates between type I and type II FAS-induced apoptosis. *Nature* 2009;**460**: 1035—9.

114. Eizirik DL, Mandrup-Poulsen T. A choice of death—the signal-transduction of immune-mediated beta-cell apoptosis. *Diabetologia* 2001;**44**:2115—33.

115. McKinnon CM, Docherty K. Pancreatic duodenal homeobox-1, PDX-1, a major regulator of beta cell identity and function. *Diabetologia* 2001;**44**:1203—14.

116. Stoffers DA, Zinkin NT, Stanojevic V, Clarke WL, Habener JF. Pancreatic agenesis attributable to a single nucleotide deletion in the human IPF1 gene coding sequence. *Nat Genet* 1997;**15**:106—10.

117. Brissova M, Shiota M, Nicholson WE, Gannon M, Knobel SM, et al. Reduction in pancreatic transcription factor PDX-1 impairs glucose-stimulated insulin secretion. *J Biol Chem* 2002;**277**:11225—32.

118. Johnson JD, Ahmed NT, Luciani DS, Han Z, Tran H, et al. Increased islet apoptosis in Pdx1+/- mice. *J Clin Invest* 2003;**111**:1147—60.

119. Leibowitz G, Ferber S, Apelqvist A, Edlund H, Gross DJ, et al. IPF1/PDX1 deficiency and beta-cell dysfunction in Psammomys obesus, an animal With type 2 diabetes. *Diabetes* 2001;**50**:1799—806.

120. Kushner JA, Ye J, Schubert M, Burks DJ, Dow MA, et al. Pdx1 restores beta cell function in Irs2 knockout mice. *J Clin Invest* 2002;**109**:1193—201.

121. Pinney SE, Simmons RA. Epigenetic mechanisms in the development of type 2 diabetes. *Trends Endocrinol Metab* 2010;**21**:223—9.

122. Kawamori D, Kaneto H, Nakatani Y, Matsuoka TA, Matsuhisa M, et al. The forkhead transcription factor Foxo1 bridges the JNK pathway and the transcription factor PDX-1 through its intracellular translocation. *J Biol Chem* 2006;**281**:1091—9.

123. Moede T, Leibiger B, Pour HG, Berggren P, Leibiger IB. Identification of a nuclear localization signal, RRMKWKK, in the homeodomain transcription factor PDX-1. *FEBS Lett* 1999;**461**:229—34.

124. Ardestani A, Sauter NS, Paroni F, Dharmadhikari G, Cho JH, et al. Neutralizing IL-1β induces β -cell survival by maintaining PDX1 nuclear localization. *J Biol Chem* 2011.

125. Ryu GR, Yoo JM, Lee E, Ko SH, Ahn YB, et al. Decreased Expression and Induced Nucleocytoplasmic Translocation of Pancreatic and Duodenal Homeobox 1 in INS-1 Cells Exposed to High Glucose and Palmitate. *Diabetes Metab J* 2011;**35**:65—71.

126. Luotola K, Paakkonen R, Alanne M, Lanki T, Moilanen L, et al. Association of variation in the interleukin-1 gene family with diabetes and glucose homeostasis. *J Clin Endocrinol Metab* 2009;**94**:4575—83.

127. Grant SF, Thorleifsson G, Reynisdottir I, Benediktsson R, Manolescu A, et al. Variant of transcription factor 7-like 2 (TCF7L2) gene confers risk of type 2 diabetes. *Nat Genet* 2006;**38**:320—3.

128. Welters HJ, Kulkarni RN. Wnt signaling: relevance to beta-cell biology and diabetes. *Trends Endocrinol Metab* 2008;**19**:349—55.

129. Rulifson IC, Karnik SK, Heiser PW, ten Berge D, Chen H, et al. Wnt signaling regulates pancreatic beta cell proliferation. *Proc Natl Acad Sci USA* 2007;**104**:6247—52.

130. Guo YF, Xiong DH, Shen H, Zhao LJ, Xiao P, et al. Polymorphisms of the low-density lipoprotein receptor-related protein 5 (LRP5) gene are associated with obesity phenotypes in a large family-based association study. *J Med Genet* 2006;**43**:798—803.

131. Kanazawa A, Tsukada S, Sekine A, Tsunoda T, Takahashi A, et al. Association of the gene encoding wingless-type mammary tumor virus integration-site family member 5B (WNT5B) with type 2 diabetes. *Am J Hum Genet* 2004;**75**:832—43.

132. Schinner S, Ulgen F, Papewalis C, Schott M, Woelk A, et al. Regulation of insulin secretion, glucokinase gene transcription and beta cell proliferation by adipocyte-derived Wnt signalling molecules. *Diabetologia* 2008;**51**:147—54.

133. Yi F, Brubaker PL, Jin T. TCF-4 mediates cell type-specific regulation of proglucagon gene expression by beta-catenin and glycogen synthase kinase-3beta. *J Biol Chem* 2005;**280**:1457—64.

134. Loder MK, da Silva Xavier G, McDonald A, Rutter GA. TCF7L2 controls insulin gene expression and insulin secretion in mature pancreatic beta-cells. *Biochem Soc Trans* 2008;**36**:357—9.

135. da Silva Xavier G, Loder MK, McDonald A, Tarasov AI, Carzaniga R, et al. TCF7L2 regulates late events in insulin secretion from pancreatic islet β-cells. *Diabetes* 2009.

136. Shu L, Sauter NS, Schulthess FT, Matveyenko AV, Oberholzer J, et al. Transcription factor 7-like 2 regulates beta-cell survival and function in human pancreatic islets. *Diabetes* 2008;**57**:645—53.

137. Shu L, Matveyenko AV, Kerr-Conte J, Cho JH, McIntosh CH, et al. Decreased TCF7L2 protein levels in type 2 diabetes mellitus correlate with downregulation of GIP- and GLP-1 receptors and impaired beta-cell function. *Hum Mol Genet* 2009;**18**:2388—99.

138. Le Bacquer O, Shu L, Marchand M, Neve B, Paroni F, et al. TCF7L2 splice variants have distinct effects on {beta}-cell turnover and function. *Hum Mol Genet* 2011;**20**:1906—15.

139. Welsh GI, Wilson C, Proud CG. GSK3: a SHAGGY frog story. *Trends Cell Biol* 1996;**6**:274—9.

140. Mussmann R, Geese M, Harder F, Kegel S, Andag U, et al. Inhibition of GSK3 promotes replication and survival of pancreatic beta cells. *J Biol Chem* 2007;**282**:12030—7.

141. Liu Z, Tanabe K, Bernal-Mizrachi E, Permutt MA. Mice with beta cell overexpression of glycogen synthase kinase-3beta have reduced beta cell mass and proliferation. *Diabetologia* 2008;**51**:623—31.

142. Martin M, Rehani K, Jope RS, Michalek SM. Toll-like receptor-mediated cytokine production is differentially regulated by glycogen synthase kinase 3. *Nat Immunol* 2005;**6**:777—84.

143. Baarsma HA, Meurs H, Halayko AJ, Menzen MH, Schmidt M, et al. Glycogen synthase kinase-3 regulates cigarette smoke extract- and IL-1β-induced cytokine secretion by airway smooth muscle. *Am J Physiol Lung Cell Mol Physiol* **300**: L910—19.

144. Rehani K, Wang H, Garcia CA, Kinane DF, Martin M. Toll-like receptor-mediated production of IL-1Ra is negatively regulated by GSK3 via the MAPK ERK1/2. *J Immunol* 2009;**182**:547—53.

145. Wada A. GSK-3 inhibitors and insulin receptor signaling in health, disease, and therapeutics. *Front Biosci* 2009;**14**:1558—70.

146. Jope RS, Yuskaitis CJ, Beurel E. Glycogen synthase kinase-3 (GSK3): inflammation, diseases, and therapeutics. *Neurochem Res* 2007;**32**:577—95.

147. Kunick C, Lauenroth K, Leost M, Meijer L, Lemcke T. 1-Azakenpaullone is a selective inhibitor of glycogen synthase kinase-3 beta. *Bioorg Med Chem Lett* 2004;**14**:413—6.

148. Lochhead PA, Coghlan M, Rice SQ, Sutherland C. Inhibition of GSK-3 selectively reduces glucose-6-phosphatase and phosphatase and phosphoenolypyruvate carboxykinase gene expression. *Diabetes* 2001;**50**:937—46.

149. Stein J, Milewski WM, Hara M, Steiner DF, Dey A. GSK-3 inactivation or depletion promotes beta-cell replication via down regulation of the CDK inhibitor, p27 (Kip1). *Islets* 2011;**3**:21—34.

150. Liu Y, Tanabe K, Baronnier D, Patel S, Woodgett J, et al. Conditional ablation of Gsk-3beta in islet beta cells results in expanded mass and resistance to fat feeding-induced diabetes in mice. *Diabetologia* 2010;**53**:2600—10.

151. Jope RS, Johnson GV. The glamour and gloom of glycogen synthase kinase-3. *Trends Biochem Sci* 2004;**29**:95—102.

152. Spinas GA, Hansen BS, Linde S, Kastern W, Molvig J, et al. Interleukin 1 dose-dependently affects the biosynthesis of (pro)insulin in isolated rat islets of Langerhans. *Diabetologia* 1987;**30**:474—80.

153. Spinas GA, Mandrup-Poulsen T, Molvig J, Baek L, Bendtzen K, et al. Low concentrations of interleukin-1 stimulate and high concentrations inhibit insulin release from isolated rat islets of Langerhans. *Acta Endocrinol(Copenh)* 1986;**113**:551—8.

154. Spinas GA, Palmer JP, Mandrup-Poulsen T, Andersen H, Nielsen JH, et al. The bimodal effect of interleukin 1 on rat pancreatic beta-cells—stimulation followed by inhibition—depends upon dose, duration of exposure, and ambient glucose concentration. *Acta Endocrinol(Copenh)* 1988;**119**:307—11.

155. Dinarello CA. The role of the interleukin-1-receptor antagonist in blocking inflammation mediated by interleukin-1. *N Engl J Med* 2000;**343**:732—4.

156. Seckinger P, Lowenthal JW, Williamson K, Dayer JM, MacDonald HR. A urine inhibitor of interleukin 1 activity that blocks ligand binding. *J Immunol* 1987;**139**:1546—9.

157. Seckinger P, Williamson K, Balavoine JF, Mach B, Mazzei G, et al. A urine inhibitor of interleukin 1 activity affects both interleukin 1 alpha and 1 beta but not tumor necrosis factor alpha. *J Immunol* 1987;**139**:1541—5.

158. Sandberg JO, Andersson A, Eizirik DL, Sandler S. Interleukin-1 receptor antagonist prevents low dose streptozotocin induced diabetes in mice. *Bio chem-Biophys Res Commun* 1994;**202**:543—8.

159. Nicoletti F, Di Marco R, Barcellini W, Magro G, Schorlemmer HU, et al. Protection from experimental autoimmune diabetes in the non-obese diabetic mouse with soluble interleukin-1 receptor. *Eur J Immunol* 1994;**24**:1843—7.

160. Sandberg JO, Eizirik DL, Sandler S. IL-1 receptor antagonist inhibits recurrence of disease after syngeneic pancreatic islet transplantation to spontaneously diabetic non-obese diabetic (NOD) mice. *Clin Exp Immunol* 1997 May;**108**(2):314—7.

161. Stoffels K, Gysemans C, Waer M, Laureys J, Bouillon R, et al. Interleukin-1 receptor antagonist inhibits primary non-function and prolongs graft survival time of xenogeneic islets transplanted in sponaeously diabetic autoimmune NOD mice. *Diabetologia* 2002;**45**(Suppl. 2):424—4.

162. Tellez N, Montolio M, Estil-les E, Escoriza J, Soler J, et al. Adenoviral overproduction of interleukin-1 receptor antagonist increases beta cell replication and mass in syngeneically transplanted islets, and improves metabolic outcome. *Diabetologia* 2007;**50**:602—11.

163. Satoh M, Yasunami Y, Matsuoka N, Nakano M, Itoh T, et al. Successful islet transplantation to two recipients from a single donor by targeting proinflammatory cytokines in mice. *Transplantation* 2007;**83**:1085—92.

164. Sandberg JO, Eizirik DL, Sandler S, Tracey DE, Andersson A. Treatment with an interleukin-1 receptor antagonist protein prolongs mouse islet lograft survival. *Diabetes* 1993;**42**:1845—51.

165. Tellez N, Montolio M, Biarnes M, Castano E, Soler J, et al. Adenoviral overexpression of interleukin-1 receptor antagonist protein increases beta-cell replication in rat pancreatic islets. *Gene Ther* 2005;**12**:120—8.

166. Wilson HL, Francis SE, Dower SK, Crossman DC. Secretion of intracellular IL-1 receptor antagonist (type 1) is dependent on P2X7 receptor activation. *J Immunol* 2004;**173**:1202—8.

167. Glas R, Sauter NS, Schulthess FT, Shu L, Oberholzer J, et al. Purinergic P2X(7) receptors regulate secretion of interleukin-1 receptor antagonist and beta cell function and survival. *Diabetologia* 2009;**52**:1579—88.

168. Abbatecola AM, Ferrucci L, Grella R, Bandinelli S, Bonafe M, et al. Diverse effect of inflammatory markers on insulin resistance and insulin-resistance syndrome in the elderly. *J Am Geriatr Soc* 2004;**52**:399—404.

169. Meier CA, Bobbioni E, Gabay C, Assimacopoulos-Jeannet F, Golay A, et al. IL-1 receptor antagonist serum levels are increased in human obesity: a possible link to the resistance to leptin? *J Clin Endocrinol Metab* 2002;**87**:1184—8.

170. Ruotsalainen E, Salmenniemi U, Vauhkonen I, Pihlajamaki J, Punnonen K, et al. Changes in inflammatory cytokines are related to impaired glucose tolerance in offspring of type 2 diabetic subjects. *Diabetes Care* 2006;**29**:2714—20.

171. Salmenniemi U, Ruotsalainen E, Pihlajamaki J, Vauhkonen I, Kainulainen S, et al. Multiple abnormalities in glucose and energy metabolism and coordinated changes in levels of adiponectin, cytokines, and adhesion molecules in subjects with metabolic syndrome. *Circulation* 2004;**110**:3842—8.

172. Marculescu R, Endler G, Schillinger M, Iordanova N, Exner M, et al. Interleukin-1 receptor antagonist genotype is associated with coronary atherosclerosis in patients with type 2 diabetes. *Diabetes* 2002;**51**:3582—5.

173. Herder C, Brunner EJ, Rathmann W, Strassburger K, Tabak AG, et al. Elevated levels of the anti-inflammatory interleukin-1 receptor antagonist (IL-1Ra) precede the onset of type 2 diabetes (Whitehall II Study). *Diabetes Care* 2008.

174. Juge-Aubry CE, Somm E, Giusti V, Pernin A, Chicheportiche R, et al. Adipose tissue is a major source of interleukin-1 receptor antagonist: upregulation in obesity and inflammation. *Diabetes* 2003;**52**:1104—10.

175. Sauter NS, Schulthess FT, Galasso R, Castellani LW, Maedler K. The antiinflammatory cytokine interleukin-1 receptor antagonist protects from high-fat diet-induced hyperglycemia. *Endocrinology* 2008;**149**: 2208—18.

176. Ehses JA, Giroix M-H, Coulaud J, Akira S, Homo-Delarche F, et al. IL-1β-MyD88 signaling is central to islet chemokine secretion in response to metabolic stress: evidence from a spontaneous model of type 2 diabetes, the GK rat. *Diabetologia* 2008;**50** (Suppl. 1):S177.

177. Osborn O, Brownell SE, Sanchez-Alavez M, Salomon D, Gram H, et al. Treatment with an Interleukin 1 beta antibody improves glycemic control in diet-induced obesity. *Cytokine* 2008;**44**:141—8.

178. Owyang AM, Maedler K, Gross L, Yin J, Esposito L, et al. XOMA 052, an anti-IL-1β monoclonal antibody, improves glucose control and β-cell function in the diet-induced obesity mouse model. *Endocrinology* 2010.

179. Larsen CM, Faulenbach M, Vaag A, Volund A, Ehses JA, et al. Interleukin-1-receptor antagonist in type 2 diabetes mellitus. *N Engl J Med* 2007;**356**: 1517—26.

180. Pickersgill LM, Mandrup-Poulsen TR. The anti-interleukin-1 in type 1 diabetes action trial—background and rationale. *Diabetes Metab Res Rev* 2009;**25**:321—4.

181. Donath MY, Weder C, Brunner A, Keller C, Whitmore J, et al. XOMA 052, a potential disease modifying anti-IL-10 antibody shows sustained HbA1c reductions 3 months after single injection with no increases in safety parameters in subjects with T2DM. *Diabetes* 2008:58S1. A30.

Interleukin-18 in Metabolic Syndrome and Diabetes

Marius Trøseid*, Harald Arnesen[†],**, Ingebjørg Seljeflot[†],**

*Department of Infectious Diseases Oslo University Hospital, University of Oslo, Norway [†]Center for Clinical Heart Research, Department of Cardiology, Oslo University Hospital, University of Oslo, Norway **Faculty of Medicine, Oslo University Hospital, University of Oslo, Norway

INTRODUCTION

Diabetes mellitus and the metabolic syndrome are closely related multifactorial conditions. Metabolic syndrome is a strong predictor of type 2 diabetes, with an increased incidence rate of five- to seven-fold.[1,2] Both conditions increase the risk of future cardiovascular events, and the risk is increased in parallel with fasting glucose, from the normal range via impaired fasting glucose and metabolic syndrome to overt diabetes mellitus.[3] The risk of developing cardiovascular diease (CVD) is approximately doubled in subjects with the metabolic syndrome,[4] and tripled in subjects with type 2 diabetes.

There is increasing evidence that diabetes and the metabolic syndrome are associated with a chronic, low-grade inflammation. Indeed, some investigators have suggested that type 2 diabetes, metabolic syndrome, and atherosclerosis are multifactorial conditions which appear to have a common inflammatory basis.[5]

A growing body of evidence suggests that interleukin-18 (IL-18) is closely associated with both diabetes mellitus and the metabolic syndrome, and potentially related to the pathogenesis and complications of these conditions. The purpose of this review is to outline the role of IL-18 in diabetes and the metabolic syndrome, with particular emphasis on CVD risk and the effect of lifestyle interventions.

THE BIOLOGICAL EFFECT OF INTERLEUKIN-18 DEPENDS ON THE LOCAL CYTOKINE MILIEU

IL-18 is produced constitutively in many different cell types, including endothelial cells, smooth muscle cells, macrophages and antigen-presenting cells.[6–8] IL-18 is also produced in the adipocytes,[9] although non-adipocyte cells like macrophages have been identified as the main source of IL-18 in adipose tissue.[10]

IL-18 is subject to several regulatory steps. First, IL-18 is expressed as a precursor, pro-IL-18, which is inactive until cleaved by the enzyme caspase-1.[11] Also caspase-1 exists as an inactive precursor which requires the assembly of multi-unit complexes, known as inflammasomes, to be activated.[12,13]

IL-18, once secreted, is bound and inactivated by IL-18 binding protein, the synthesis of which is increased as a negative feedback mechanism in response to increased IL-18 production, ensuring protection from tissue damage due to uncontrolled proinflammatory activity.[14,15] IL-18 binds to its receptor, consisting of an α-chain which is responsible for extracellular binding of IL-18, and a β-chain which is responsible for intracellular signal transduction.[11,16,17] Notably, only the free fraction of IL-18 is able to activate the β-chain of the IL-18 receptor.[14,15]

IL-18 is a potent proinflammatory cytokine which enhances T-cell and natural killer cell maturation, as well as the production of cytokines, chemokines and cell adhesion molecules.[18,19] Importantly, in CD4 + T-cells IL-18 can stimulate both type 1 helper T (Th1) and Th2 responses depending on its cytokine milieu: IL-18 may stimulate a Th2 response in combination with IL-2, and may act synergistically with IL-12 to stimulate a Th1 response with production of interferon (IFN-γ),[11] a central feature in the atherosclerotic lesion (Figure 20.1).

Recently, increased levels of IL-12 have been reported in subjects with type 2 diabetes and in experimental hyperglycemia.[20,21] Hence, it could be proposed that IL-18 is more likely to trigger a Th1 response in the presence of a hyperglycemic proinflammatory milieu.[22] This might be relevant, since a Th1 response dominates among lymphocytes in the atherosclerotic plaque.[23,24]

INTERLEUKIN-18 IS CLOSELY ASSOCIATED WITH THE METABOLIC SYNDROME AND ITS COMPONENTS

The role of IL-18 in the metabolic syndrome has recently been reviewed by our group.[25] In several studies, elevated circulating levels of IL-18 have been associated with obesity,[26–29] insulin resistance,[30–32] hypertension,[33] and dyslipidemia.[27,28] Furthermore, IL-18 levels are elevated in subjects with the metabolic syndrome[34] and increase in parallel with an increasing number

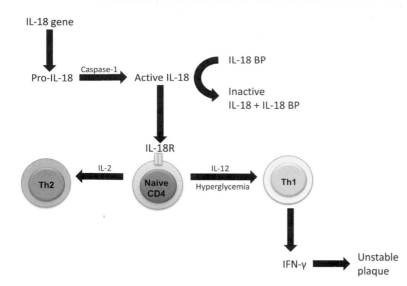

FIGURE 20.1 **IL-18 is subject to several regulatory steps**. The cytokine is expressed as a precursor, pro-IL-18, which is inactive until cleaved by caspase-1. Once secreted, IL-18 is bound and inactivated by IL-18 binding protein (IL-18 BP), and only the free fraction can stimulate a signal transduction via the β-chain of the IL-18 receptor (IL-18R). The biological effect is dependent on the cytokine milieu: IL-18 may stimulate a Th2 response in combination with IL-2, and may act synergistically with IL-12 to stimulate a Th1 response with production of IFN-γ, a central feature of the atherosclerotic lesion.

of components of the syndrome,[29,35] also after adjustment for insulin resistance, obesity, and inflammatory markers.[28]

Polymorphisms in the IL-18 gene have been shown to associate with circulating IL-18 levels.[36] Interestingly, a recent study showed that one such polymorphism located in the 3′untranslated region (3′UTR) was associated with increased serum levels of IL-18, impaired insulin sensitivity and increased risk of developing the metabolic syndrome.[37] All data taken together point to a strong association between IL-18 and the metabolic syndrome, and that IL-18 might be involved in the pathogenesis of the syndrome.

INTERLEUKIN-18 IS ASSOCIATED WITH THE INITIATION AND COMPLICATIONS OF DIABETES

Circulating levels of IL-18 have consistently been reported to be elevated in patients with type 2 diabetes mellitus in cross-sectional studies.[31,38,39] Also in type 1 diabetes, elevated levels of IL-18 have been reported, in particular in subjects with poor metabolic control.[40,41]

Interestingly, polymorphisms of the IL-12 and IL-18 genes have been associated with early onset of type 1 diabetes.[42] Furthermore, in healthy offspring of type 2 diabetic subjects, no suppression of IL-18 and other cytokines during experimental hyperinsulinemia was found, suggesting a role of low-grade inflammation in subjects at high risk of developing diabetes.[43]

Moreover, in two prospective study cohorts, elevated levels of IL-18 predicted and preceded the development of type 2 diabetes (Table 20.1).[44,45] However, fasting glucose or oral glucose tolerance tests were not taken into account in these studies. Hyperglycemia is a potential confounder, by enhancing the risk of future diabetes[3] as well as by increasing circulating levels of IL-18 in experimental settings.[46]

Regarding diabetic microvascular complications, IL-18 has been suggested to contribute to nephropathy in type 2 diabetes,[47] and IL-18 overexpression has been demonstrated in human tubular epithelial cells in nephropathy from patients with type 2 diabetes.[48] Notably, in a prospective study of type 2 diabetes, elevated IL-18 levels preceded the development of renal dysfunction measured by microalbuminuria.[49]

TABLE 20.1   Prospective Studies Evaluating the Effect of Elevated Circulating IL-18 Levels on Cardiovascular, Metabolic Syndrome, and Diabetes Related End Points

Study	Patients (n) and study population	Follow-up, years	End points	Outcome
Blankenberg et al.[54]	1,229 (known CAD)	4	Cardiovascular mortality	Increased risk of cardiovascular mortality
Hartford et al.[57]	1,261 (ACS)	8	Mortality	Increased all-cause and noncardiovascular mortality
Blankenberg et al.[58]	335 cases and 670 controls (healthy men)	5	CAD	Increased risk of CAD
Everett et al.[59]	253 cases and 253 controls (healthy women)	6	CVD	Increased risk of CVD
Koenig et al.[60]	382 cases and 1,980 controls (population based)	11	CAD	No increased risk of CAD
Espinola-Klein et al.[61]	1,263, stratified for MS (known CAD)	6	Cardiovascular mortality	Increased risk of cardiovascular mortality in MS strata
Trøseid et al.[22]	563, stratified for MS (elderly high-risk men)	3	CVD	Increased risk of CVD in MS strata
Thorand et al.[45]	527 cases and 1,698 controls (population based)	11	Type 2 diabetes	Increased risk of type 2 diabetes
Hivert et al.[44]	1,012 cases and 1,081 controls (women)	12	Type 2 diabetes	Increased risk of type 2 diabetes

ACS; acute coronary syndrome, CAD; coronary artery disease, CVD; cardiovascular disease, MS; metabolic syndrome.

However, another study reported that elevated IL-18 levels were associated with poor glycemic control but not with microvascular complications in young adults with type 1 diabetes.[40]

INTERLEUKIN-18 AND CARDIOVASCULAR DISEASE

Studies regarding associations between IL-18 and cardiovascular disease have been conflicting, in particular studies on stable atherosclerosis.

One study showed that elevated levels of IL-18 were associated with the presence of subclinical atherosclerosis evaluated with intima media thickness of the carotid artery, also after adjustment for traditional risk factors and inflammatory markers.[50] However, in two large population-based studies from the US and Australia, elevated levels of IL-18 were associated with carotid intima media thickness in univariate analyses, but not after adjustment for traditional risk factors.[29,51] In a recent study of a Finnish population, a polymorphism in the IL-18 gene was associated with substantially lower intima media thickness in men, but not women.[52]

Most studies in patients with diabetes or the metabolic syndrome have shown positive associations between elevated IL-18 levels and the presence of subclinical atherosclerosis. Hence, in a study of patients with type 2 diabetes, both carotid intima media thickness and brachial-ankle pulse wave velocity were significantly associated with serum levels of IL-18, although not in multivariate analyses.[53] Furthermore, we showed that arterial stiffness measured by brachial pulse wave propagation was associated with IL-18 levels and components of the metabolic syndrome, even in multivariate analyses, both cross-sectionally and during 3 years follow-up.[35]

Also data regarding IL-18 as a potential predictor of future cardiovascular events and mortality have so far been conflicting, although most studies show a positive association between elevated IL-18 levels and acute events (Table 20.1). In patients with known coronary artery disease, circulating IL-18 levels as well as polymorphisms in the IL-18 gene were associated with future cardiovascular mortality.[54,55] Interestingly, in patients with acute coronary syndromes, elevated IL-18 levels are related to the extent of coronary disease,[56] as well as future all-cause and noncardiovascular mortality.[57]

In two prospective studies, elevated IL-18 levels were associated with future cardiovascular disease in previously healthy men[58] and women.[59] However, another large population-based study with a follow-up of 11 years showed that increased levels of IL-6 and C-reactive protein (CRP), but not IL-18, were associated with future coronary events.[60]

To date, only two studies have prospectively evaluated IL-18 as a potential predictor of cardiovascular events in populations with the metabolic syndrome. In a large cohort consisting of men and women with known coronary artery disease, IL-18 was the only independent predictor of cardiovascular mortality in a subgroup with the metabolic syndrome, even after adjustment for CRP, IL-6, and fibrinogen.[61] In line with these results, we showed that IL-18 was a strong and independent predictor of cardiovascular events in elderly men with the metabolic syndrome, also after adjustment for CRP and IL-6, and with a synergistic effect of IL-18 and fasting glucose in the cardiovascular risk prediction.[22]

A point of discussion is whether circulating levels of total IL-18 are the most relevant measures of cardiovascular disease risk. IL-18 exists in free and protein-bound form, and only the free fraction of IL-18 is able to activate the β-chain of the IL-18 receptor, resulting in intracellular signal transduction.[14,15] Some data indicate that IL-18 binding protein might be protective of cardiovascular disease in the elderly, implicating that free rather than total IL-18 is involved in the atherosclerotic process.[14,62]

POTENTIAL MECHANISMS FOR THE ROLE OF INTERLEUKIN-18 IN DIABETES, METABOLIC SYNDROME AND ATHEROSCLEROSIS

Interleukin-18 in Atherosclerotic Lesions

IL-18 has been shown to be highly expressed in atherosclerotic plaques, mainly in plaque macrophages, and in particular in unstable plaques.[63] IL-18 is thought to exert its main pro-atherogenic effects by inducing IFN-γ production, which potentiates the inflammatory process and may lead to thinning or inhibition of the fibrous cap formation, resulting in vulnerable, rupture-prone plaques.[23,64] Furthermore, IL-18 seems to increase the expression of matrix metalloproteinases in vascular cells and macrophages, which might also contribute to plaque destabilization.[8,23]

Indeed, IL-18 might also directly cause plaque destabilization and cardiac dysfunction. In a model with ApoE-deficient mice, IL-18 overexpression enhanced the collagenolytic activity of smooth muscle cells, reduced intimal collagen content and fibrous cap thickness, leading to vulnerable plaque morphology.[65] Furthermore, in a mouse model with myocardial infarction, increased expression of cardiac IL-18 mRNA and a subsequent reduction of myocardial contractility were reported.[66] Interestingly, in a rat model with the metabolic syndrome, IL-18 overexpression aggravated insulin resistance, increased vascular inflammation, promoted remodeling by enhanced infiltration of macrophages, and increased medial thickness in the aortic wall.[67]

Interleukin-18 in Adipose Tissue

The classical perception of adipose tissue as a passive storage place of fatty acids has gradually been replaced by the notion of adipose tissue, and visceral fat in particular as an active endocrine organ. Visceral fat is now considered a central feature and potential cause of the metabolic syndrome,[68] in part mediated by release of a large number of metabolically active substances known as adipokines. Adipokines are involved in several biological processes, including inflammation, thrombosis, insulin sensitivity and energy balance.[69]

Human pre-adipocytes and adipocytes of all stages have been shown to constitutively express and secrete IL-18.[9,70] Of note, in obese individuals there is an increased expression of IL-18 in adipose tissue,[26] and a three-fold increased secretion from adipocytes compared with lean controls.[9] Interestingly, experimental hyperglycemia has been shown to increase the expression of IL-18 in adipocytes, an effect which was even more pronounced in the presence of intermittent hyperglycemia.[71] However, other studies have reported that non-adipocytes are the main sources of IL-18 in adipose tissue.[10]

Previous studies have reported macrophage infiltration in adipose tissue in obesity and insulin resistance.[72,73] A recent study showed that infiltration of T-lymphocytes preceded the infiltration of macrophages in adipose tissue in early stages of insulin resistance in obese mice.[74] Notably, in patients with type 2 diabetes, waist circumference correlated significantly with expression of IFN-γ in adipose tissue, suggesting a role of Th1 cells in insulin resistance.[74] Moreover, in another study of obese mice, there was a clear tendency towards Th1 polarization of lymphocytes in adipose tissue, which was associated with insulin resistance and could be reversed by immunotherapy.[75] IL-18 acts in synergy with IL-12 to stimulate Th1 polarization,[11] and levels of IL-12 have been reported to be increased in subjects with type 2 diabetes and by experimental hyperglycemia.[20,21] Hence, it could be speculated that IL-18 in combination with a hyperglycemic proinflammatory milieu might trigger Th1 activation and IFN-γ production,[22] both in adipose tissue and in the atherosclerotic plaque.

Interleukin-18 in Muscle Tissue

Several reports have suggested that adipose tissue might not be the main source of IL-18 in patients with obesity and the metabolic syndrome.[26,44,76,77] In one study, plasma levels of IL-18 were reduced by weight loss, whereas no effect was seen on adipose tissue expression of IL-18.[26] In another study, we showed that the reduction of IL-18 levels by exercise was significantly associated with improvement of the metabolic syndrome, but not with the reduction in visceral fat.[77]

There is increasing evidence that cytokines are involved in the regulation of skeletal muscle function, and tumor necrosis factor-α (TNF-α) has been associated with muscle catabolism and loss of muscle function.[78] IL-18 expression has been demonstrated in human skeletal muscles in a fiber specific way both in healthy individuals[79] and in patients with myopathy.[65]

Recently, it was shown experimentally that TNF-α infusion induced reduced glucose uptake and increased IL-18 expression in human skeletal muscle tissue, but not in adipose tissue, and the authors suggest that adipose tissue is unlikely to be a major source of IL-18.[76] Still, it remains to be demonstrated whether muscle tissue could be a major source of circulating IL-18 in subjects with and without diabetes and the metabolic syndrome.

Interleukin-18 Resistance

Paradoxically, genetically modified mice with IL-18 deficiency have been reported to develop hyperphagia, obesity, and insulin resistance, which might be reversed by recombinant IL-18 administration.[80] Furthermore, it was shown that patients with obesity and type 2 diabetes produce significantly less IFN-γ in peripheral blood mononuclear cells in response to IL-18 stimulation compared to lean controls, most likely due to reduced expression of the IL-18 receptor β-chain, and the authors have introduced a concept of IL-18 resistance as a potential explanation of elevated IL-18 levels in such patients.[81] This observation is supported by several studies that report defective leukocyte function and increased susceptibility to infections in patients with type 2 diabetes.[82–84] However, it remains to be determined whether this immunological phenomenon translates into a similar resistance to the metabolic effects of IL-18,[81] and which organs might be involved in such a process.

INTERLEUKIN-18 AND EFFECT OF LIFESTYLE INTERVENTIONS

Lifestyle interventions consisting of diet and exercise have been shown to improve several cardiovascular risk factors including the metabolic syndrome and to reduce the risk of developing type 2 diabetes.[85,86]

Weight loss mediated by calorie-restricted diet intervention was reported to decrease IL-18 levels in obese women.[87] Furthermore, combined interventions with diet and exercise have been shown to reduce IL-18 levels in both obese men[26] and women.[88] We have reported reduced serum levels of IL-18 by Mediterranean-like diet and omega-3 fatty acid supplementation in a population of elderly high-risk men.[89] In a *post hoc* analysis from the same trial, the reduction of IL-18 levels was associated with an increasing number of metabolic syndrome components that improved during 3 years of intervention.[35] Moreover, Mediterranean-like diet was shown to reduce levels of CRP, IL-6, and IL-18 in a middle-aged population with the metabolic syndrome.[90]

Aerobic exercise has been reported to reduce levels of CRP and IL-18 in subjects with type 2 diabetes,[91,92] and aerobic exercise, but not strength training, reduced circulating levels of CRP, IL-6, and IL-18 in older subjects.[93] However, both endurance training and strength training reduced plasma levels of IL-18 in a cohort of HIV-infected patients with lipodystrophy.[9,94] Furthermore, exercise performed on a rowing ergometer reduced adipose tissue expression of IL-18 in obese subjects.[95] Moreover, in a middle-aged cohort of men with the metabolic syndrome, we have reported reduced levels of IL-18 associated with improvement of metabolic syndrome components by a combined intervention consisting of aerobic exercise and strength training.[77]

CONCLUSIONS

Several lines of evidence support a pivotal role of IL-18 in the pathogenesis of diabetes mellitus and the metabolic syndrome. Importantly, IL-18 has been shown to be closely associated with the metabolic syndrome and its components,[28] to predict cardiovascular events and cardiovascular mortality in populations with the metabolic syndrome,[22,61] and to precede the development of diabetes.[44] Nonetheless, the exact role of IL-18 in these conditions needs to be clarified.

Although lifestyle interventions such as diet and exercise have been shown to reduce levels of IL-18 in populations with diabetes and the metabolic syndrome, it remains unclear whether such a reduction translates into reduced incidence of cardiovascular events. Furthermore, the contribution of adipose tissue, muscle tissue and other organs in regulating circulating levels of IL-18, as well as the potential role of IL-18 resistance, require further investigation.

Since IL-18 is subject to several regulatory steps including cleavage by caspase-1, inactivation by IL-18 binding protein, and signalling via the β-chain of the IL-18 receptor, it will be crucial to clarify to what extent circulating levels of total IL-18 relate to the biological actions of the cytokine. Finally, strategies for blocking IL-18 activity are currently investigated in various pathophysiological conditions such as sepsis and heart failure,[96,97] and could potentially represent future therapeutic tools for diabetes mellitus, the metabolic syndrome and the consequences of these conditions.

References

1. Eckel RH, Grundy SM, Zimmet PZ. The metabolic syndrome. *Lancet* 2005;**365**:1415–28.
2. Wilson PW, D'Agostino RB, Parise H, Sullivan L, Meigs JB. Metabolic syndrome as a precursor of cardiovascular disease and type 2 diabetes mellitus. *Circulation* 2005;**112**:3066–72.
3. Haffner SM, Stern MP, Hazuda HP, Mitchell BD, Patterson JK. Cardiovascular risk factors in confirmed prediabetic individuals. Does the clock for coronary heart disease start ticking before the onset of clinical diabetes? *JAMA* 1990;**263**:2893–8.
4. Grundy SM. Metabolic syndrome pandemic. *Arterioscler Thromb Vasc Biol* 2008;**28**:629–36.
5. Pradhan AD, Ridker PM. Do atherosclerosis and type 2 diabetes share a common inflammatory basis? *Eur Heart J* 2002;**23**:831–4.
6. Dinarello CA. The IL-1 family and inflammatory diseases. *Clin Exp Rheumatol* 2002;**20**:S1–13.
7. Dinarello CA. Interleukin-18 and the pathogenesis of inflammatory diseases. *Semin Nephrol* 2007;**27**:98–114.
8. Gerdes N, Sukhova GK, Libby P, Reynolds RS, Young JL, Schonbeck U. Expression of interleukin (IL)-18 and functional IL-18 receptor on human vascular endothelial cells, smooth muscle cells, and macrophages: implications for atherogenesis. *J Exp Med* 2002;**195**:245–57.
9. Skurk T, Kolb H, Muller-Scholze S, Rohrig K, Hauner H, Herder C. The proatherogenic cytokine interleukin-18 is secreted by human adipocytes. *Eur J Endocrinol* 2005;**152**:863–8.
10. Fain JN, Tichansky DS, Madan AK. Most of the interleukin 1 receptor antagonist, cathepsin S, macrophage migration inhibitory factor, nerve growth factor, and interleukin 18 release by explants of human adipose tissue is by the non-fat cells, not by the adipocytes. *Metabolism* 2006;**55**:1113–21.
11. Nakanishi K, Yoshimoto T, Tsutsui H, Okamura H. Interleukin-18 is a unique cytokine that stimulates both Th1 and Th2 responses depending on its cytokine milieu. *Cytokine Growth Factor Rev* 2001;**12**:53–72.
12. Shaw MH, Reimer T, Kim YG, Nunez G. NOD-like receptors (NLRs): bona fide intracellular microbial sensors. *Curr Opin Immunol* 2008;**20**:377–82.
13. Sirard JC, Vignal C, Dessein R, Chamaillard M. Nod-like receptors: cytosolic watchdogs for immunity against pathogens. *PLoS Pathog* 2007;**3**:e152.
14. Novick D, Kim SH, Fantuzzi G, Reznikov LL, Dinarello CA, Rubinstein M. Interleukin-18 binding protein: a novel modulator of the Th1 cytokine response. *Immunity* 1999;**10**:127–36.
15. Novick D, Schwartsburd B, Pinkus R, Suissa D, Belzer I, Sthoeger Z, Keane WF, Chvatchko Y, Kim SH, Fantuzzi G, Dinarello CA, Rubinstein M. A novel IL-18BP ELISA shows elevated serum IL-18BP in sepsis and extensive decrease of free IL-18. *Cytokine* 2001;**14**:334–42.
16. Kato Z, Jee J, Shikano H, Mishima M, Ohki I, Ohnishi H, Li A, Hashimoto K, Matsukuma E, Omoya K, Yamamoto Y, Yoneda T, Hara T, Kondo N, Shirakawa M. The structure and binding mode of interleukin-18. *Nat Struct Biol* 2003;**10**:966–71.
17. Torigoe K, Ushio S, Okura T, Kobayashi S, Taniai M, Kunikata T, Murakami T, Sanou O, Kojima H, Fujii M, Ohta T, Ikeda M, Ikegami H, Kurimoto M. Purification and characterization of the human interleukin-18 receptor. *J Biol Chem* 1997;**272**:25737–42.
18. Dinarello CA. Interleukin 1 and interleukin 18 as mediators of inflammation and the aging process. *Am J Clin Nutr* 2006;**83**:S447–55.
19. Gracie JA, Robertson SE, McInnes IB. Interleukin-18. *J Leukoc Biol* 2003;**73**:213–24.

20. Wegner M, Winiarska H, Bobkiewicz-Kozlowska T, Dworacka M. IL-12 serum levels in patients with type 2 diabetes treated with sulphonylureas. *Cytokine* 2008;**42**:312−6.

21. Wen Y, Gu J, Li SL, Reddy MA, Natarajan R, Nadler JL. Elevated glucose and diabetes promote interleukin-12 cytokine gene expression in mouse macrophages. *Endocrinology* 2006;**147**:2518−25.

22. Troseid M, Seljeflot I, Hjerkinn EM, Arnesen H. Interleukin-18 is a strong predictor of cardiovascular events in elderly men with the metabolic syndrome: synergistic effect of inflammation and hyperglycemia. *Diabetes Care* 2009;**32**:486−92.

23. Robertson AK, Hansson GK. T cells in atherogenesis: for better or for worse? *Arterioscler Thromb Vasc Biol* 2006;**26**:2421−32.

24. Hansson GK. Inflammation, atherosclerosis, and coronary artery disease. *N Engl J Med* 2005;**352**:1685−95.

25. Troseid M, Seljeflot I, Arnesen H. The role of interleukin-18 in the metabolic syndrome. *Cardiovasc Diabetol* 2010;**9**:11.

26. Bruun JM, Stallknecht B, Helge JW, Richelsen B. Interleukin-18 in plasma and adipose tissue: effects of obesity, insulin resistance, and weight loss. *Eur J Endocrinol* 2007;**157**:465−71.

27. Evans J, Collins M, Jennings C, van der Merwe L, Soderstrom I, Olsson T, Levitt NS, Lambert EV, Goedecke JH. The association of interleukin-18 genotype and serum levels with metabolic risk factors for cardiovascular disease. *Eur J Endocrinol* 2007;**157**: 633−40.

28. Hung J, McQuillan BM, Chapman CM, Thompson PL, Beilby JP. Elevated interleukin-18 levels are associated with the metabolic syndrome independent of obesity and insulin resistance. *Arterioscler Thromb Vasc Biol* 2005;**25**:1268−73.

29. Zirlik A, Abdullah SM, Gerdes N, MacFarlane L, Schonbeck U, Khera A, McGuire DK, Vega GL, Grundy S, Libby P, de Lemos JA. Interleukin-18, the metabolic syndrome, and subclinical atherosclerosis: results from the Dallas Heart Study. *Arterioscler Thromb Vasc Biol* 2007;**27**:2043−9.

30. Bosch M, Lopez-Bermejo A, Vendrell J, Musri M, Ricart W, Fernandez-Real JM. Circulating IL-18 concentration is associated with insulin sensitivity and glucose tolerance through increased fat-free mass. *Diabetologia* 2005;**48**:1841−3.

31. Fischer CP, Perstrup LB, Berntsen A, Eskildsen P, Pedersen BK. Elevated plasma interleukin-18 is a marker of insulin-resistance in type 2 diabetic and non-diabetic humans. *Clin Immunol* 2005;**117**:152−60.

32. Straczkowski M, Kowalska I, Nikolajuk A, Otziomek E, Adamska A, Karolczuk-Zarachowicz M, Gorska M. Increased serum interleukin-18 concentration is associated with hypoadiponectinemia in obesity, independently of insulin resistance. *Int J Obes (Lond)* 2007;**31**:221−5.

33. Rabkin SW. The role of interleukin 18 in the pathogenesis of hypertension-induced vascular disease. *Nat Clin Pract Cardiovasc Med* 2009;**6**:192−9.

34. Van Guilder GP, Hoetzer GL, Greiner JJ, Stauffer BL, Desouza CA. Influence of metabolic syndrome on biomarkers of oxidative stress and inflammation in obese adults. *Obesity (Silver Spring)* 2006;**14**:2127−31.

35. Troseid M, Seljeflot I, Weiss TW, Klemsdal TO, Hjerkinn EM, Arnesen H. Arterial stiffness is independently associated with interleukin-18 and components of the metabolic syndrome. *Atherosclerosis* 2010;**209**:337−9.

36. He M, Cornelis MC, Kraft P, van Dam RM, Sun Q, Laurie CC, Mirel DB, Chasman DI, Ridker PM, Hunter DJ, Hu FB, Qi L. Genome-wide association study identifies variants at the IL18-BCO2 locus associated with interleukin-18 levels. *Arterioscler Thromb Vasc Biol* 2010;**30**:885−90.

37. Presta I, Andreozzi F, Succurro E, Marini MA, Laratta E, Lauro R, Hribal ML, Perticone F, Sesti G. IL-18 gene polymorphism and metabolic syndrome. *Nutr Metab Cardiovasc Dis* 2009;**19**:e5−6.

38. Aso Y, Okumura K, Takebayashi K, Wakabayashi S, Inukai T. Relationships of plasma interleukin-18 concentrations to hyperhomocysteinemia and carotid intimal-media wall thickness in patients with type 2 diabetes. *Diabetes Care* 2003;**26**:2622−7.

39. Esposito K, Nappo F, Giugliano F, Di PC, Ciotola M, Barbieri M, Paolisso G, Giugliano D. Cytokine milieu tends toward inflammation in type 2 diabetes. *Diabetes Care* 2003;**26**:1647.

40. Altinova AE, Yetkin I, Akbay E, Bukan N, Arslan M. Serum IL-18 levels in patients with type 1 diabetes: relations to metabolic control and microvascular complications. *Cytokine* 2008;**42**:217−21.

41. Dong G, Liang L, Fu J, Zou C. Serum interleukin-18 levels are raised in diabetic ketoacidosis in Chinese children with type 1 diabetes mellitus. *Indian Pediatr* 2007;**44**:732−6.

42. Altinova AE, Engin D, Akbay E, Akturk M, Toruner F, Ersoy R, Yetkin I, Arslan M. Association of polymorphisms in the IL-18 and IL-12 genes with susceptibility to Type 1 diabetes in Turkish patients. *J Endocrinol Invest* 2010;**33**:451−4.

43. Ruotsalainen E, Stancakova A, Vauhkonen I, Salmenniemi U, Pihlajamaki J, Punnonen K, Laakso M. Changes in cytokine levels during acute hyperinsulinemia in offspring of type 2 diabetic subjects. *Atherosclerosis* 2010;**210**:536−41.

44. Hivert MF, Sun Q, Shrader P, Mantzoros CS, Meigs JB, Hu FB. Circulating IL-18 and the risk of type 2 diabetes in women. *Diabetologia* 2009;**52**:2101—8.
45. Thorand B, Kolb H, Baumert J, Koenig W, Chambless L, Meisinger C, Illig T, Martin S, Herder C. Elevated levels of interleukin-18 predict the development of type 2 diabetes: results from the MONICA/KORA Augsburg Study, 1984-2002. *Diabetes* 2005;**54**:2932—8.
46. Esposito K, Nappo F, Marfella R, Giugliano G, Giugliano F, Ciotola M, Quagliaro L, Ceriello A, Giugliano D. Inflammatory cytokine concentrations are acutely increased by hyperglycemia in humans: role of oxidative stress. *Circulation* 2002;**106**:2067—72.
47. Fujita T, Ogihara N, Kamura Y, Satomura A, Fuke Y, Shimizu C, Wada Y, Matsumoto K. Interleukin-18 contributes more closely to the progression of diabetic nephropathy than other diabetic complications. *Acta Diabetol* 2010, Feb 26 (Epub).
48. Miyauchi K, Takiyama Y, Honjyo J, Tateno M, Haneda M. Upregulated IL-18 expression in type 2 diabetic subjects with nephropathy: TGF-beta1 enhanced IL-18 expression in human renal proximal tubular epithelial cells. *Diabetes Res Clin Pract* 2009;**83**:190—9.
49. Araki S, Haneda M, Koya D, Sugimoto T, Isshiki K, Chin-Kanasaki M, Uzu T, Kashiwagi A. Predictive impact of elevated serum level of IL-18 for early renal dysfunction in type 2 diabetes: an observational follow-up study. *Diabetologia* 2007;**50**:867—73.
50. Yamagami H, Kitagawa K, Hoshi T, Furukado S, Hougaku H, Nagai Y, Hori M. Associations of serum IL-18 levels with carotid intima-media thickness. *Arterioscler Thromb Vasc Biol* 2005;**25**:1458—62.
51. Chapman CM, McQuillan BM, Beilby JP, Thompson PL, Hung J. Interleukin-18 levels are not associated with subclinical carotid atherosclerosis in a community population. The Perth Carotid Ultrasound Disease Assessment Study (CUDAS). *Atherosclerosis* 2006;**189**:414—9.
52. Hernesniemi JA, Heikkila A, Raitakari OT, Kahonen M, Juonala M, Hutri-Kahonen N, Marniemi J, Viikari J, Lehtimaki T. Interleukin-18 gene polymorphism and markers of subclinical atherosclerosis. The Cardiovascular Risk in Young Finns Study. *Ann Med* 2010;**42**:223—30.
53. Nakamura A, Shikata K, Hiramatsu M, Nakatou T, Kitamura T, Wada J, Itoshima T, Makino H. Serum interleukin-18 levels are associated with nephropathy and atherosclerosis in Japanese patients with type 2 diabetes. *Diabetes Care* 2005;**28**:2890—5.
54. Blankenberg S, Tiret L, Bickel C, Peetz D, Cambien F, Meyer J, Rupprecht HJ. Interleukin-18 is a strong predictor of cardiovascular death in stable and unstable angina. *Circulation* 2002;**106**:24—30.
55. Tiret L, Godefroy T, Lubos E, Nicaud V, Tregouet DA, Barbaux S, Schnabel R, Bickel C, Espinola-Klein C, Poirier O, Perret C, Munzel T, Rupprecht HJ, Lackner K, Cambien F, Blankenberg S. Genetic analysis of the interleukin-18 system highlights the role of the interleukin-18 gene in cardiovascular disease. *Circulation* 2005;**112**:643—50.
56. Chen MC, Chen CJ, Yang CH, Wu CJ, Fang CY, Hsieh YK, Chang HW. Interleukin-18: a strong predictor of the extent of coronary artery disease in patients with unstable angina. *Heart Vessels* 2007;**22**:371—5.
57. Hartford M, Wiklund O, Hulten LM, Persson A, Karlsson T, Herlitz J, Hulthe J, Caidahl K. Interleukin-18 as a predictor of future events in patients with acute coronary syndromes. *Arterioscler Thromb Vasc Biol* 2010;**30**:2039—46.
58. Blankenberg S, Luc G, Ducimetiere P, Arveiler D, Ferrieres J, Amouyel P, Evans A, Cambien F, Tiret L. Interleukin-18 and the risk of coronary heart disease in European men: the Prospective Epidemiological Study of Myocardial Infarction (PRIME). *Circulation* 2003;**108**:2453—9.
59. Everett BM, Bansal S, Rifai N, Buring JE, Ridker PM. Interleukin-18 and the risk of future cardiovascular disease among initially healthy women. *Atherosclerosis* 2009;**202**:282—8.
60. Koenig W, Khuseyinova N, Baumert J, Thorand B, Loewel H, Chambless L, Meisinger C, Schneider A, Martin S, Kolb H, Herder C. Increased concentrations of C-reactive protein and IL-6 but not IL-18 are independently associated with incident coronary events in middle-aged men and women: results from the MONICA/KORA Augsburg case-cohort study, 1984—2002. *Arterioscler Thromb Vasc Biol* 2006;**26**:2745—51.
61. Espinola-Klein C, Rupprecht HJ, Bickel C, Lackner K, Genth-Zotz S, Post F, Munzel T, Blankenberg S. Impact of inflammatory markers on cardiovascular mortality in patients with metabolic syndrome. *Eur J Cardiovasc Prev Rehabil* 2008;**15**:278—84.
62. Gangemi S, Basile G, Merendino RA, Minciullo PL, Novick D, Rubinstein M, Dinarello CA, Lo BC, Franceschi C, Basili S, D'Urbano E, Davi G, Nicita-Mauro V, Romano M. Increased circulating Interleukin-18 levels in centenarians with no signs of vascular disease: another paradox of longevity? *Exp Gerontol* 2003;**38**:669—72.
63. Mallat Z, Corbaz A, Scoazec A, Besnard S, Leseche G, Chvatchko Y, Tedgui A. Expression of interleukin-18 in human atherosclerotic plaques and relation to plaque instability. *Circulation* 2001;**104**:1598—603.

64. Leon ML, Zuckerman SH. Gamma interferon: a central mediator in atherosclerosis. *Inflamm Res* 2005;**54**: 395—411.

65. de Nooijer R, von der Thusen JH, Verkleij CJ, Kuiper J, Jukema JW, van der Wall EE, van Berkel JC, Biessen EA. Overexpression of IL-18 decreases intimal collagen content and promotes a vulnerable plaque phenotype in apolipoprotein-E-deficient mice. *Arterioscler Thromb Vasc Biol* 2004;**24**:2313—9.

66. Woldbaek PR, Tonnessen T, Henriksen UL, Florholmen G, Lunde PK, Lyberg T, Christensen G. Increased cardiac IL-18 mRNA, pro-IL-18 and plasma IL-18 after myocardial infarction in the mouse; a potential role in cardiac dysfunction. *Cardiovasc Res* 2003;**59**:122—31.

67. Tan HW, Liu X, Bi XP, Xing SS, Li L, Gong HP, Zhong M, Wang ZH, Zhang Y, Zhang W. IL-18 overexpression promotes vascular inflammation and remodeling in a rat model of metabolic syndrome. *Atherosclerosis* 2010;**208**:350—7.

68. Despres JP, Lemieux I, Bergeron J, Pibarot P, Mathieu P, Larose E, Rodes-Cabau J, Bertrand OF, Poirier P. Abdominal obesity and the metabolic syndrome: contribution to global cardiometabolic risk. *Arterioscler Thromb Vasc Biol* 2008;**28**:1039—49.

69. Lau DC, Dhillon B, Yan H, Szmitko PE, Verma S. Adipokines: molecular links between obesity and atheroslcerosis. *Am J Physiol Heart Circ Physiol* 2005; **288**:H2031—41.

70. Wood IS, Wang B, Jenkins JR, Trayhurn P. The pro-inflammatory cytokine IL-18 is expressed in human adipose tissue and strongly upregulated by TNFalpha in human adipocytes. *Biochem Biophys Res Commun* 2005;**337**:422—9.

71. Sun J, Xu Y, Dai Z, Sun Y. Intermittent high glucose stimulate MCP-l, IL-18, and PAI-1, but inhibit adiponectin expression and secretion in adipocytes dependent of ROS. *Cell Biochem Biophys* 2009;**55**:173—80.

72. Weisberg SP, McCann D, Desai M, Rosenbaum M, Leibel RL, Ferrante Jr AW. Obesity is associated with macrophage accumulation in adipose tissue. *J Clin Invest* 2003;**112**:1796—808.

73. Xu H, Barnes GT, Yang Q, Tan G, Yang D, Chou CJ, Sole J, Nichols A, Ross JS, Tartaglia LA, Chen H. Chronic inflammation in fat plays a crucial role in the development of obesity-related insulin resistance. *J Clin Invest* 2003;**112**:1821—30.

74. Kintscher U, Hartge M, Hess K, Foryst-Ludwig A, Clemenz M, Wabitsch M, Fischer-Posovszky P, Barth TF, Dragun D, Skurk T, Hauner H, Bluher M, Unger T, Wolf AM, Knippschild U, Hombach V, Marx N. T-lymphocyte infiltration in visceral adipose tissue: a primary event in adipose tissue inflammation and the development of obesity-mediated insulin resistance. *Arterioscler Thromb Vasc Biol* 2008;**28**: 1304—10.

75. Winer S, Chan Y, Paltser G, Truong D, Tsui H, Bahrami J, Dorfman R, Wang Y, Zielenski J, Mastronardi F, Maezawa Y, Drucker DJ, Engleman E, Winer D, Dosch HM. Normalization of obesity-associated insulin resistance through immunotherapy. *Nat Med* 2009;**15**:921—9.

76. Krogh-Madsen R, Plomgaard P, Moller K, Mittendorfer B, Pedersen BK. Influence of TNF-alpha and IL-6 infusions on insulin sensitivity and expression of IL-18 in humans. *Am J Physiol Endocrinol Metab* 2006;**291**:E108—14.

77. Troseid M, Lappegard KT, Mollnes TE, Arnesen H, Seljeflot I. The effect of exercise on serum levels of interleukin-18 and components of the metabolic syndrome. *Metab Syndr Relat Disord* 2009;**7**:579—84.

78. Li YP, Reid MB. Effect of tumor necrosis factor-alpha on skeletal muscle metabolism. *Curr Opin Rheumatol* 2001;**13**:483—7.

79. Plomgaard P, Penkowa M, Pedersen BK. Fiber type specific expression of TNF-alpha, IL-6 and IL-18 in human skeletal muscles. *Exerc Immunol Rev* 2005;**11**:53—63.

80. Netea MG, Joosten LA, Lewis E, Jensen DR, Voshol PJ, Kullberg BJ, Tack CJ, van KH, Kim SH, Stalenhoef AF, van de Loo FA, Verschueren I, Pulawa L, Akira S, Eckel RH, Dinarello CA, van den Berg W, van der Meer JW. Deficiency of interleukin-18 in mice leads to hyperphagia, obesity and insulin resistance. *Nat Med* 2006;**12**:650—6.

81. Zilverschoon GR, Tack CJ, Joosten LA, Kullberg BJ, van der Meer JW, Netea MG. Interleukin-18 resistance in patients with obesity and type 2 diabetes mellitus. *Int J Obes (Lond)* 2008;**32**:1407—14.

82. Delamaire M, Maugendre D, Moreno M, Le Goff MC, Allannic H, Genetet B. Impaired leucocyte functions in diabetic patients. *Diabet Med* 1997;**14**:29—34.

83. Gallacher SJ, Thomson G, Fraser WD, Fisher BM, Gemmell CG, MacCuish AC. Neutrophil bactericidal function in diabetes mellitus: evidence for association with blood glucose control. *Diabet Med* 1995; **12**:916—20.

84. Tsiavou A, Hatziagelaki E, Chaidaroglou A, Koniavitou K, Degiannis D, Raptis SA. Correlation between intracellular interferon-gamma (IFN-gamma) production by CD4+ and CD8+ lymphocytes and IFN-gamma gene polymorphism in patients with type 2 diabetes mellitus and latent autoimmune diabetes of adults (LADA). *Cytokine* 2005;**31**:135—41.

85. Anderssen SA, Carroll S, Urdal P, Holme I. Combined diet and exercise intervention reverses the metabolic syndrome in middle-aged males: results from the Oslo Diet and Exercise Study. *Scand J Med Sci Sports* 2007;**17**:687–95.

86. Tuomilehto J, Lindstrom J, Eriksson JG, Valle TT, Hamalainen H, Ilanne-Parikka P, Keinanen-Kiukaanniemi S, Laakso M, Louheranta A, Rastas M, Salminen V, Uusitupa M. Prevention of type 2 diabetes mellitus by changes in lifestyle among subjects with impaired glucose tolerance. *N Engl J Med* 2001;**344**: 1343–50.

87. Esposito K, Pontillo A, Ciotola M, Di Palo C, Grella E, Nicoletti G, Giugliano D. Weight loss reduces interleukin-18 levels in obese women. *J Clin Endocrinol Metab* 2002;**87**:3864–6.

88. Esposito K, Pontillo A, Di Palo C, Giugliano G, Masella M, Marfella R, Giugliano D. Effect of weight loss and lifestyle changes on vascular inflammatory markers in obese women: a randomized trial. *JAMA* 2003;**289**:1799–804.

89. Troseid M, Arnesen H, Hjerkinn EM, Seljeflot I. Serum levels of interleukin-18 are reduced by diet and n-3 fatty acid intervention in elderly high-risk men. *Metabolism* 2009;**58**:1543–9.

90. Esposito K, Marfella R, Ciotola M, Di Palo C, Giugliano F, Giugliano G, D'Armiento M, D'Andrea F, Giugliano D. Effect of a Mediterranean-style diet on endothelial dysfunction and markers of vascular inflammation in the metabolic syndrome: a randomized trial. *JAMA* 2004;**292**:1440–6.

91. Kadoglou NP, Iliadis F, Angelopoulou N, Perrea D, Ampatzidis G, Liapis CD, Alevizos M. The anti-inflammatory effects of exercise training in patients with type 2 diabetes mellitus. *Eur J Cardiovasc Prev Rehabil* 2007;**14**:837–43.

92. Kadoglou NP, Iliadis F, Sailer N, Athanasiadou Z, Vitta I, Kapelouzou A, Karayannacos PE, Liapis CD, Alevizos M, Angelopoulou N, Vrabas IS. Exercise training ameliorates the effects of rosiglitazone on traditional and novel cardiovascular risk factors in patients with type 2 diabetes mellitus. *Metabolism* 2010;**59**:599–607.

93. Kohut ML, McCann DA, Russell DW, Konopka DN, Cunnick JE, Franke WD, Castillo MC, Reighard AE, Vanderah E. Aerobic exercise, but not flexibility/resistance exercise, reduces serum IL-18, CRP, and IL-6 independent of beta-blockers, BMI, and psychosocial factors in older adults. *Brain Behav Immun* 2006;**20**:201–9.

94. Lindegaard B, Hansen T, Hvid T, van HG, Plomgaard P, Ditlevsen S, Gerstoft J, Pedersen BK. The effect of strength and endurance training on insulin sensitivity and fat distribution in human immunodeficiency virus-infected patients with lipodystrophy. *J Clin Endocrinol Metab* 2008;**93**:3860–9.

95. Leick L, Lindegaard B, Stensvold D, Plomgaard P, Saltin B, Pilegaard H. Adipose tissue interleukin-18 mRNA and plasma interleukin-18: effect of obesity and exercise. *Obesity (Silver Spring)* 2007; **15**:356–63.

96. Wang M, Markel TA, Meldrum DR. Interleukin 18 in the heart. *Shock* 2008;**30**:3–10.

97. Wang M, Tan J, Wang Y, Meldrum KK, Dinarello CA, Meldrum DR. IL-18 binding protein-expressing mesenchymal stem cells improve myocardial protection after ischemia or infarction. *Proc Natl Acad Sci USA* 2009;**106**:17499–504.

PATHOPHYSIOLOGY

CHAPTER

21

Sleep, Hypertension, and Diabetes

Michelle A. Miller, Francesco P. Cappuccio

University of Warwick, Warwick Medical School, Coventry, UK

BACKGROUND AND INTRODUCTION

There is now a wealth of evidence to support the epidemiological link between quantity of sleep (short and long duration of sleep) and quality of sleep (like difficulties in falling asleep or of maintaining sleep) and cardiovascular risk factors, namely hypertension and type 2 diabetes. Hypertension is an important cause of stroke and other cardiovascular diseases (CVDs). In the UK, 34% of men and 30% of women have been or are being treated for hypertension (as defined as a blood pressure of 140/90 mmHg or higher). However, many with high blood pressure are not being treated. It has been estimated recently that the prevalence of hypertension will soar to 1.56 billion

Nutritional and Therapeutic Interventions for Diabetes and Metabolic Syndrome
DOI: 10.1016/B978-0-12-385083-6.00021-8

267

by the year 2025.[1] The number of adults with diabetes in the world is estimated to be 170 million in 2000 and the prevalence is rising. It is estimated that just under 1.9 million people in the UK have been diagnosed with diabetes (4% of men and 3% of women) and that a large number of cases remain undiagnosed. Type 2 diabetes accounted for less than 3% of all cases of new-onset diabetes in children and adolescents 15 years ago but today accounts for up to 45% of new-onset adolescent cases.[2] An increased cardiovascular risk is seen in those individuals who have a cluster of risk factors as in the case of those individuals with metabolic syndrome (MetS).

SLEEP AND HYPERTENSION

Sleep-disordered breathing (SDB) refers to a spectrum of breathing disorders that occur during sleep and include snoring, the obesity-hypoventilation syndrome, and obstructive sleep apnoea (OSA). These sleep disturbances can result in abnormal ventilation, intermittent hypoxemia, and arousals from sleep. SDB has been linked to elevated blood pressure and risk of hypertension in several epidemiological observational studies.[3–7]

Cross-sectional analysis from the Sleep Heart Health Study on a sample of > 6,000 US adults showed a significant higher prevalence of hypertension among individuals with usual sleep duration above or below the median of 7–8 h per night.[8] Moreover, in a recent longitudinal analysis of the first National Health And Nutrition Examination Survey (NHANES-I), short sleep duration (< 5 h per night) was associated with a 60% higher risk of incident hypertension in middle-aged (32–59 years) American adults without apparent sleep disorders during a mean follow-up of 8–10 years.[9] The outcome was, however, based on self-reported diagnosis of hypertension, and no gender-specific analyses were included. Furthermore, in this study

no association was found in individuals > 60 years of age. More recent findings from the CARDIA study show that reduced sleep duration, measured by wrist actigraphy, predicts higher blood pressure levels and adverse changes in blood pressure over 5 years among 578 African Americans and whites aged 33–45 years at baseline.[10]

We recently examined both the cross-sectional and prospective associations of sleep duration with prevalent and incident hypertension in the Whitehall II Study, a prospective cohort of 10,308 white-collar British civil servants aged 35–55 years at baseline (phase 1: 1985–1988).[11] We conducted gender-specific analyses, as previous studies have indicated that reduced durations of sleep might be associated with more detrimental effects on cardiovascular outcomes among women.

In the cross-sectional analyses of over 5,000 individuals, short duration of sleep (< 5 h per night) was associated with higher risk of hypertension compared with the group sleeping 7 h but only among women (OR: 1.72; 1.07–2.75). In prospective analyses (mean follow-up: 5 years), the cumulative incidence of hypertension was 20.0% ($n = 740$) among 3,691 normotensive individuals. In women, short duration of sleep was associated with a higher risk of hypertension but the associations were attenuated after accounting for cardiovascular risk factors and psychiatric co-morbidities. The study indicated for the first time that sleep deprivation may produce detrimental cardiovascular effects among women. Similar results have since been confirmed in a cross-sectional analysis of the Heinz Nixdorf Recall Study in Germany.[12] They showed a significant association between reduced sleep duration (≤ 5 h per night) and hypertension only among women (OR: 1.24; 1.04–1.46).

We also examined the cross-sectional gender-specific association of sleep duration with hypertension in the Western New York Health Study, a large, well-characterized population-based sample of over 3,000 white men (43.5%) and women from the US.[13] In this study we decided *a priori* to perform subgroup analyses by menopausal status among women to further investigate potential mechanisms for the observed gender-specific effect of reduced sleep duration on the risk of hypertension. In multivariate analyses, < 6 h of sleep per night was associated with a significant increased risk of hypertension compared to sleeping ≥ 6 h per night but only among women (OR: 1.66; 1.09−2.53). Furthermore, the effect was stronger among pre-menopausal women (3.25; 1.37−7.76) than among post-menopausal women (1.49; 0.92−2.41).[14]

SLEEP AND PULMONARY ARTERIAL HYPERTENSION (PAH)

PAH refers to abnormally high blood pressure in the arteries of the lungs. It is defined as an elevation of mean pulmonary artery pressure to 20 mmHg at rest and 30 mmHg during exercise. Normally, the right side of the heart pumps blood through the lungs so that it can become re-oxygenated. If narrowing of the arteries within the lungs occurs, the blood flow is impeded and there is a resultant build-up of pressure. To overcome this pressure the heart needs to work harder and the right side of the heart may become enlarged. If insufficient blood flows to the lungs, right-sided heart failure may develop. In 1998, the World Health Organization (WHO) recognized SDB as a secondary cause of PAH.

MECHANISMS

There are a number of potential pathophysiological mechanisms that might underlie the association between sleep deprivation and hypertension, including overactivity of the sympathetic nervous system or the renin−angiotensin−aldosterone system. Mechanisms involving pro-inflammatory responses, endothelial dysfunction, and renal impairment may also be important. It is possible, however, that sleep habits may represent a marker of health status and quality of life rather than a causal factor for hypertension.

Sleep and Blood Pressure

During normal sleep there is a decrease in blood pressure, which is referred to as "nocturnal dipping". It is thought to arise as a result of a decrease in sympathetic activation. The magnitude of dipping is normally around 10−20% and those individuals who have less than 10% night-time dipping are referred to as "non-dippers". A lack of or diminished night-time dip is independently associated with an increase in CVD (see [15]). There are a number of diseases that have been associated with non-dipping, one of which is OSA.

Obstructive Sleep Apnoea

OSA is a condition characterized by the complete or partial collapse of the pharyngeal airway during sleep. Recurrent episodes of airway obstructions result in hypoxia and hypercapnia increasing sympathetic neural tone, which in turn causes vasoconstriction and marked increases in blood pressure. Patients with OSA exhibit increased resting heart rate, decreased time duration between two consecutive R waves of the electrocardiogram (RR interval) variability, and increased blood pressure variability.[16] Moreover, the evidence to suggest that there is a causal relationship between OSA syndrome and hypertension is growing and over 50% of the individuals with OSA have hypertension.[17] The blood pressure response to OSA may be important in understanding the absence of nocturnal blood pressure fall in "non-dippers".[18] Effective treatment of OSA may attenuate neurohumoral and metabolic abnormalities, improve diurnal blood pressure control and conceivably reduce cardiovascular risk. The 7th Report of the Joint National Committee (JNC) on Prevention, Detection, Evaluation and Treatment of High Blood Pressure has recommended not only that OSA be considered in all resistant hypertensive patients, but that all hypertensive patients with a BMI in excess of 27kg/m^2 should be examined for the presence of sleeping disorders.[17]

The current gold standard for the treatment of moderate to severe OSA is nasal continuous positive airway pressure (CPAP), which acts as a pneumatic splint to prevent the collapse of the pharyngeal airway. It is a long-term treatment and it is associated with an improvement in daytime and nocturnal blood pressure control, especially in patients with severe sleep apnoea,[19] and may reduce low-grade inflammatory activation, normally detected in patients with OSA. A number of randomized controlled trials have been conducted to look at the effectiveness of CPAP in individuals with different degrees of severity of OSA. The findings from many of these studies have been examined in four recent meta-analyses.[20–23] The findings from each of these meta-analyses have been examined in a recent review.[15] The studies seem to suggest that there is a modest reduction in blood pressure with CPAP use. Compliance to treatment is important and most trials indicate that usage of CPAP is around 4–5 hours per night but that the greatest fall in blood pressures are observed in the more compliant individuals. Treatment duration may also be a key factor but most of the trials were for 3 months or less. Many patients have OSA that has been undiagnosed for long periods of time before treatment and 3 months may be insufficient to reverse some long-term effects.

Traditionally it was believed that PAH in patients with sleep apnoea syndrome (SAS)/ OAS could be ascribed to associated chronic obstructive pulmonary disease (COPD). In 2000, Bady et al. retrospectively analyzed individuals with SAS but without COPD to evaluate the possible occurrence of PAH as a complication of OAS. They found that in patients with SAS the prevalence of PAH varied from 10 to 79% and stepwise multiple regression analysis showed that mean pulmonary artery pressure (PAPm) was positively correlated with BMI and negatively with arterial oxygen tension (PaO_2). This suggests that PAH may be related to the severity of concurrent obesity and its respiratory mechanical consequences.[24]

Gender

Studies have suggested that short sleep duration may be associated with hypertension in women but not in men.[12–14] The exact mechanisms underlying these gender-specific associations are unclear but may involve hormonal influences or psychosocial factors especially during periods marking shifts in the reproductive stages of women, such as menopause. Moreover, methodological issues such as differential self-reporting of sleep habits between men and women may also play a role. However, the possibility that reduced sleep duration may represent a risk marker rather than a causal risk factor for diseases cannot be excluded at present.

Inflammation

Inflammatory markers are related to sleep and blood pressure[25] and changes in inflammatory mediators including hs-CRP, fibrinogen, and plasminogen activator inhibitor, which are important in the development of hypertension and CVD, have also been observed in OSA patients.[16] Data from many studies including randomized controlled trials indicates that treatment with CPAP may reduce inflammation in such individuals.[26–28] In some RCTs, however, there were no observed differences in the measured markers of inflammation.[29,30]

Clock Genes

Sleep is a complex phenotype and an individual's sleep pattern may be under the control of many genes and their interaction with the environment. Whilst the results from twin studies suggest that the heritability of sleep may be around 44%,[31] to date an underlying genetic basis for only a few sleep disorders has been established.[32] Many biological processes exhibit a circadian rhythm; in mammals this rhythm is governed by a central circadian clock or circadian oscillator which is located in the hypothalamic suprachiasmatic nucleus (SCN). This in turn controls the millions of peripheral clocks throughout the body. The circadian oscillator is composed of many genes and proteins which interact together and have both positive and negative feedback loops.[33] Research in this area is ongoing but a number of genes, including the Period genes, have been identified as being important in sleep–wake regulation. Among others, the CLOCK and BMAL1 elements promote the expression of the Period (PER1, 2 and 3) and Crytochrome (Cry1 & 2) genes.

In a recent study Okamura et al have demonstrated the importance of the clock for the maintenance of health. They have used genetically modified mice as a tool to investigate the consequences of abolishing the circadian clock. In their study they demonstrated that mice which become arrhythmic as a result of deleting the Cry1 and Cry2 clock genes also suffer from salt-sensitive hypertension. The wild type mice as expected showed 24-hour variability in their mean arterial pressure (MAP) but whilst Cry-null mice had MAP within the normal range there was no diurnal variability. When the mice were exposed to a 3% salt-loaded diet there was an increase in MAP in the Cry-null but not wild type mice. Furthermore, they observed that in these mice, a novel 3β-hydroxyl-steroid dehydrogenase (3β-Hsd) gene under clock control is severely overexpressed specifically in aldosterone-producing cells in the adrenal cortex. This

led to hyperaldosteronism and ultimately to salt-sensitive hypertension. It was observed that the pathophysiology of the Cry-null mice was similar to that of idiopathic hyperaldosteronism. The human homologue of this aldosterone-producing, cell-specific enzyme was also characterized and represents a new possibility in the pathogenesis of hypertension.[34]

Melatonin

Melatonin plays an important part in maintaining the body's circadian rhythm. It is produced by the pineal gland when it is dark and the production falls on light exposure. The pineal gland stores melatonin during the day then releases it towards night and this induces sleepiness. This release is triggered naturally by lowering of light levels; however, if individuals are not exposed to low light at night this event does not occur and may contribute to the sleeping difficulties observed in individuals who are subject to night-time light pollution. Melatonin also exerts effect on peripheral circadian clocks and has been shown to affect NO synthase pathways. Emerging fields in melatonin research also suggest that it may be important in weight control.[35] These studies once more highlight the importance of sleep in regulating metabolism and potential disease development.

Further evidence suggests that the increase in obesity and metabolic disorders may be associated with the increase of exposure to light at night (LAN) and shift work. In a recent study in mice, the relationship between night-time light exposure and obesity was examined. The investigators found that despite equivalent caloric intake and total activity, mice which were exposed to either bright or dim LAN have significantly increased body mass and reduced glucose tolerance compared with mice in a standard (LD) light/dark cycle. It was noted however that the timing of food intake in the bright or dim LAN-exposed mice differed from that of the mice in the standard L/D cycle. These results suggest that even low levels of light at night may disrupt feeding cycles and lead to weight gain which may have important implications for human beings who are exposed to light at night.[36]

During the past 20 years a number of clinical trials have been performed to examine the therapeutic utility of melatonin. These have been reviewed by Sánchez-Barceló *et al*. In particular, the use of melatonin in the treatment of cardiovascular disease and diabetes has been examined. The authors conclude that melatonin may be a useful adjuvant therapy for the treatment of, amongst others, arterial hypertension and diabetes and, whilst in a few cases it was reported that melatonin may aggravate some conditions, the vast majority of studies document the very low toxicity of melatonin over a wide range of doses[37].

SLEEP AND TYPE 2 DIABETES

In short-term, acute, laboratory and cross-sectional observational studies disturbed or reduced sleep is associated with glucose intolerance, insulin resistance, reduced acute insulin response to glucose and a reduction in the disposition index,[38] thus predisposing to type 2 diabetes. The causality of the association and the generalizability of the results to longer-term effects of sustained sleep disturbances have been studied in our recent systematic review and meta-analysis of prospective population-based studies. This provides the global evidence in support of the presence of a relationship between sleep disturbances (in quantity and quality) and the development of type 2 diabetes, providing a quantitative estimate of the risk.[39] The study shows an unambiguous and consistent pattern of increased risk of developing type 2 diabetes on either end of the distribution of sleep duration, as well as for qualitative disturbances of sleep patterns. Pooled analyses indicate that the risk of developing type 2 diabetes varies between 28% in people who report habitual sleep of less than 5–6 h per night and 84% in those with difficulties in maintaining their sleep. For short duration of sleep ($\leq$5–6h per night) the RR was 1.28; 95% CI 1.03–1.60; P = 0.024; for long duration of sleep (>8–9h per night) 1.48 (1.13–1.96; P = 0.005). Similar increased risk was also observed for difficulty in initiating sleep 1.57 (1.25–1.97; P < 0.0001) and for difficulty in maintaining sleep 1.84 (1.39–2.43; P < 0.0001). This large analysis of over 100,000 participants and over 3,000 incident cases of type 2 diabetes adds support to the idea that sleep quantity and quality are causally related to the development of type 2 diabetes. The effects were, by and large, comparable in men and women, did not depend on the type of assessment of exposure and outcome nor on the variation in the definitions of short or long sleep. A large number of potential confounders, particularly age and body mass index, were considered in the primary analyses. The effect tended to increase with the duration of follow-up.

These results are of interest as the association is relatively consistent in different populations and they indicate an effect size of potential public health relevance. There are limitations. First, the quality of the data can not go beyond the quality of the individual studies included.[40] Second, a meta-analysis of observational data is open to fallacies in that it can not directly control for confounding. Third, the results can only be representative of the studies that have been included although the statistical analysis did not suggest that there was any evidence of publication bias. These results are therefore important in guiding the assessment of current evidence and the definition of future research strategies and public health policy decisions.

MECHANISMS

There are a number of potential mechanisms relating sleep problems to the development of type 2 diabetes including changes in appetite, caloric intake and energy expenditure,[38,41] and impaired glycemic control.[42] Sleep debt, arising either through behavioral sleep restriction or the presence of OSA, may be associated with a decrease in glucose tolerance, a higher evening cortisol level, and an increased sympathetic activity, leading to increased weight, which in turn may be associated with an increased risk of sleep disorders.[42] Moreover, it has been suggested that there may be a bi-directional association between diabetes mellitus and OSA.[43]

Changes in Appetite

Studies indicate that short or disturbed sleep may lead to an increase in appetite. Under conditions where there is no concurrent increase in energy expenditure, this would increase the risk of weight gain if food intake increased. A prolonged and substantial increase in weight may lead to the development of obesity, which is a major risk factor for the development of insulin resistance and type 2 diabetes. Feeding and appetite regulation occurs in the arcuate nucleus of the hypothalamus. Neurons in this nucleus are regulated by input from a variety of locations in the periphery, including adiposity-signals (leptin), gut-derived signals (ghrelin and peptide YY (PYY)), and nutrient-derived signals (free fatty acids).[44] Leptin produced from adipocytes has a negative effect on appetite whereas ghrelin, secreted by gastric cells, stimulates appetite. PYY, secreted by intestinal cells, also inhibits feeding.[44]

A number of laboratory studies have examined the effects of sleep restriction on one or more hormones involved in appetite regulation. Spiegel *et al.* looked at the effect of sleep restriction on appetite control. They found that 6 nights of 4-h bedtimes followed by 6 nights of 12-h bedtimes was associated with a mean decrease of 19% in leptin levels during the period of sleep restriction.[45] The caloric intake and physical activity were maintained at the same level in the sleep restriction and 12-h sleep periods and no change in weight was observed.[45]

Changes in the ratio of ghrelin-to-leptin have also been observed following periods of sleep restriction and were shown to be correlated to changes in hunger ratings suggesting that the individuals concerned may have increased their food intake had they been given free access to food.[46]

Impaired Glycemic Control

Studies using positron emission tomography (PET)[47] suggest that the increase in blood glucose levels in individuals subjected to total sleep deprivation is a result of decreased brain glucose utilization. Sleep restriction (6 days) has also been associated with an extended duration of elevated night-time growth hormone (GH) concentrations[48] and with an increase in evening cortisol levels.[49] Following sleep restriction, elevated evening cortisol concentrations may the following morning result in reduced insulin sensitivity, leading to an additional increase in blood glucose.[50]

Sympathetic Nervous Activity

Increased sympathetic nervous activity could result in a reduction of insulin secretion from pancreatic β-cells. Laboratory studies of sleep have demonstrated that cardiac sympathovagal balance, derived from estimations of heart rate variability, are elevated following sleep restriction and this may reflect an increased sympathetic tone.[45,49]

Sleep Disturbances and Obstructive Sleep Apnoea

Data from the Sleep Heart Health Study demonstrates that diabetic subjects exhibit a higher frequency of obstructive and central respiratory events than non-diabetic subjects, which is not entirely explained by the associated increased prevalence of obesity in these individuals.[51] Furthermore, increasing evidence suggests that the association may be bi-directional and that OSA may independently contribute to the incidence of type 2 diabetes, thus making it very difficult to establish the causal pathway.[52] In a sample of 69,852 women participating in the longitudinal Nurses' Health Study, the relative risk of developing diabetes in snorers over 10 years was compared to that of non-snorers. The relative risk for snorers was 2.03 (95% CI 1.71−2.40).[53]

Studies have also related OSA to changes in glucose metabolism. Longitudinal studies have shown that a major indictor of OSA, that is snoring, is associated with altered glucose metabolism. A limitation of such studies is that polysomnography, the accepted gold standard for the diagnosis of OSA, has not been used.[53,54] Support for a causal link between OSA and glucose metabolism is obtained from studies that have demonstrated that CPAP treatment for OSA has beneficial effects on glucose metabolism.[55,56] Whilst the exact mechanism by which OSA leads to the development of type 2 diabetes is unknown, it is suggested that hypoxia and sleep fragmentation may be important and candidate pathways may include effects on the sympathetic system, the hypothalamic−pituitary−adrenal (HPA) axis and on inflammation. Further evidence is accumulating to support a bi-directional, feed-forward model in which there is a pernicious association between OSA, sleepiness, inflammation, and insulin resistance. Furthermore, all of these effects would promote atherosclerosis and cardiovascular disease and may thus be of public health importance.[52]

Sleep, both quantity and quality, should be regarded as a behavioral risk factor for the development of type 2 diabetes, heavily determined by the environment and possibly amenable to modification through both education and counseling as well as through favorable modifications of physical and working environments to allow sufficient sleep and avoid habitual and sustained sleep deprivation and disruption.

Melatonin

As per obesity, emerging evidence suggests that disruption of the light−dark cycle and melatonin levels in individuals may have important consequences on metabolism and may contribute to the development of metabolic syndrome, type 2 diabetes and insulin resistance.[35]

SLEEP, PREGNANCY-INDUCED HYPERTENSION, PRE-ECLAMPSIA, AND GESTATIONAL DIABETES

The physiological and hormonal changes that occur in pregnancy increase the risk of developing SDB. It has been estimated that 10−27% of pregnant women may suffer from habitual snoring[57] and there is growing evidence to suggest that snoring and sleep apnoea during pregnancy are associated with an increased risk of gestational hypertension and pre-eclampsia. Furthermore, there is evidence to suggest that SDB and short sleep duration in pregnant women is associated with the risk of gestational diabetes. However, whilst poor sleep quantity and quality are associated with adverse maternal and fetal outcomes, there is little direct evidence, which makes it difficult to assign causality. Notwithstanding, it has been proposed that potential mechanisms for these associations might include activation of the sympathetic nervous system, oxidation, inflammation, and adipokines along with mechanisms leading to the development of insulin resistance. [58]

PREVENTION AND PUBLIC HEALTH IMPORTANCE

Evidence is accumulating to support the hypothesis that OSA has a causal role in systemic hypertension independent of known confounding factors such as BMI and gender. It is apparent that effective treatment for OSA with CPAP can lower systemic blood pressure in patients with severe OSA. A reduction in blood pressure is likely to be associated with a decrease in cerebrovascular and cardiovascular risk. Furthermore, since OSA is a risk factor for pulmonary artery hypertension, effective treatment possibly with CPAP may also decrease this condition.

The Guidelines for the Primary Prevention of Stroke: A Guideline for Healthcare Professionals from the American Heart Association/American Stroke Association have recently been published.[59] The guidelines provide an overview of the evidence on established and emerging risk factors for stroke to provide evidence-based recommendations for the reduction of risk of a first stroke. As expected, non-modifiable risk factors such as age, sex, and ethnicity were identified along with well-modifiable risk factors such as hypertension and exposure to cigarette smoke and diabetes. In addition, previously less well-documented or potentially modifiable risk factors were also identified and these included the metabolic syndrome, excessive alcohol consumption, inflammation, and sleep-disordered breathing.

The evidence linking short sleep and poor sleep quality with changes in glucose and insulin metabolism and development of type 2 diabetes is now apparent and it is crucial that the public is made aware of the potential health risks associated with sleep curtailment.

CONCLUSIONS

The prevalence of hypertension and type 2 diabetes within the population is high and is growing. Given that it has become apparent in the last decade that there is a strong epidemiological link between sleep disturbances (quality and quantity) and these risk factors for cardiovascular disease, it is imperative that the potential population and public health implications are assessed. Research needs to be conducted to understand fully the mechanism by which sleep can lead to these disease states and intervention studies are required to determine if sleep extension or sleep improvement can have beneficial effects.

References

1. Kearney PM, Whelton M, Reynolds K, Muntner P, Whelton PK, He J. Global burden of hypertension: analysis of worldwide data. *Lancet* 2005;**365**(9455): 217–23.
2. WHO Chronic diseases and health promotion: Part Two. The urgent need for action, http://www.who.int/chp/chronic_disease_report/part2_ch1/en/index13.html (accessed 11.02.11).
3. Duran J, Esnaola S, Rubio R, Iztueta A. Obstructive sleep apnea-hypopnea and related clinical features in a population-based sample of subjects aged 30 to 70 yr. *Am J Respir Crit Care Med* 2001;**163**(3 Pt 1):685–9.
4. Haas DC, Foster GL, Nieto FJ, Redline S, Resnick HE, Robbins JA, Young T, Pickering TG. Age-dependent associations between sleep-disordered breathing and hypertension: importance of discriminating between systolic/diastolic hypertension and isolated systolic hypertension in the Sleep Heart Health Study. *Circulation* 2005;**111**(5):614–21.
5. Nieto FJ, Young TB, Lind BK, Shahar E, Samet JM, Redline S, D'Agostino RB, Newman AB, Lebowitz MD, Pickering TG. Association of sleep-disordered breathing, sleep apnea, and hypertension in a large community-based study. Sleep Heart Health Study. *JAMA* 2000;**283**(14):1829–36.
6. Peppard PE, Young T, Palta M, Skatrud J. Prospective study of the association between sleep-disordered breathing and hypertension. *N Engl J Med* 2000;**342**(19): 1378–84.
7. Young T, Peppard P, Palta M, Hla KM, Finn L, Morgan B, Skatrud J. Population-based study of sleep-disordered breathing as a risk factor for hypertension. *Archives of Internal Medicine* 1997;**157**(15):1746–52.
8. Gottlieb DJ, Redline S, Nieto FJ, Baldwin CM, Newman AB, Resnick HE, Punjabi NM. Association of usual sleep duration with hypertension: the Sleep Heart Health Study. *Sleep* 2006;**29**(8):1009–14.

9. Gangwisch JE, Heymsfield SB, Boden-Albala B, Buijs RM, Kreier F, Pickering TG, Rundle AG, Zammit GK, Malaspina D. Short sleep duration as a risk factor for hypertension: analyses of the first National Health and Nutrition Examination Survey. *Hypertension* 2006;**47**(5):833–9.

10. Knutson KL, Spiegel K, Penev P, Van Cauter E. The metabolic consequences of sleep deprivation. *Sleep Med Rev* 2007;**11**(3):163–78.

11. Cappuccio FP, Stranges S, Kandala N-B, Miller MA, Taggart FM, Kumari M, Ferrie JE, Shipley MJ, Brunner EJ, Marmot G. Gender-specific associations of short sleep duration with prevalent and incident hypertension. The Whitehall II Study. *Hypertension* 2007;**50**(4):694–701.

12. Stang A, Moebus S, Mohlenkamp S, Erbel R. Gender-specific associations of short sleep duration with prevalent hypertension. *Hypertension* 2008; **51**(3):e15–6.

13. Stranges S, Dorn JM, Shipley MJ, Kandala NB, Trevisan M, Miller MA, Donahue RP, Hovey KM, Ferrie JE, Marmot MG, Cappuccio FP. Correlates of short and long sleep duration: a cross-cultural comparison between the United Kingdom and the United States: the Whitehall II Study and the Western New York Health Study. *Am J Epidemiol* 2008;**168**(12): 1353–64.

14. Stranges S, Dorn JM, Cappuccio FP, Donahue RP, Rafalson LB, Hovey KM, Freudenheim JL, Kandala NB, Miller MA, Trevisan M. A population-based study of reduced sleep duration and hypertension: the strongest association may be in premenopausal women. *J Hypertens* 2010;**28**:896–902.

15. Calhoun DA, Harding SM. Sleep and hypertension. *Chest. Aug* 2010;**138**(2):434–43.

16. Kasasbeh E, Chi DS, Krishnaswamy G. Inflammatory aspects of sleep apnea and their cardiovascular consequences. *South Med J* 2006;**99**(1):58–67.

17. Chobanian AV, Bakris GL, Black HR, Cushman WC, Green LA, Izzo Jr JL, Jones DW, Materson BJ, Oparil S, Wright Jr JT, Roccella EJ. Seventh report of the Joint National Committee on Prevention, Detection, Evaluation, and Treatment of High Blood Pressure. *Hypertension* 2003;**42**(6):1206–52.

18. Wolf J, Hering D, Narkiewicz K. Non-dipping pattern of hypertension and obstructive sleep apnea syndrome. *Hypertens Res* 2010;**33**(9):867–71.

19. Pepperell JC, Ramdassingh-Dow S, Crosthwaite N, Mullins R, Jenkinson C, Stradling JR, Davies RJ. Ambulatory blood pressure after therapeutic and subtherapeutic nasal continuous positive airway pressure for obstructive sleep apnoea: a randomised parallel trial. *Lancet* 2002;**359**(9302):204–10.

20. Bazzano LA, Khan Z, Reynolds K, He J. Effect of nocturnal nasal continuous positive airway pressure on blood pressure in obstructive sleep apnea. *Hypertension* 2007;**50**(2):417–23. Epub 2007 Jun 4.

21. Alajmi M, Mulgrew AT, Fox J, Davidson W, Schulzer M, Mak E, Ryan CF, Fleetham J, Choi P, Ayas NT. Impact of continuous positive airway pressure therapy on blood pressure in patients with obstructive sleep apnea hypopnea: a meta-analysis of randomized controlled trials. *Lung* 2007;**185**(2):67–72.

22. Mo L, He QY. [Effect of long-term continuous positive airway pressure ventilation on blood pressure in patients with obstructive sleep apnea hypopnea syndrome: a meta-analysis of clinical trials]. *Zhonghua Yi Xue Za Zhi May 8* 2007;**87**(17):1177–80. Chinese.

23. Haentjens P, Van Meerhaeghe A, Moscariello A, De Weerdt S, Poppe K, Dupont A, Velkeniers B. The impact of continuous positive airway pressure on blood pressure in patients with obstructive sleep apnea syndrome: evidence from a meta-analysis of placebo-controlled randomized trials. *Arch Intern Med* 2007;**167**(8):757–64.

24. Bady E, Achkar A, Pascal S, Orvoen-Frija E, Laaban JP. Pulmonary arterial hypertension in patients with sleep apnoea syndrome. *Thorax* 2000;**55**(11):934–9.

25. Miller MA, Cappuccio FP. Inflammation, sleep, obesity and cardiovascular disease. *Curr Vasc Pharmacol* 2007; **5**(2):93–102.

26. Drager LF, Bortolotto LA, Figueiredo AC, Krieger EM, Lorenzi GF. Effects of continuous positive airway pressure on early signs of atherosclerosis in obstructive sleep apnea. *Am J Respir Crit Care Med* 2007;**176**: 706–12.

27. Arias MA, García-Río F, Alonso-Fernández A, Hernanz A, Hidalgo R, Martínez-Mateo V, Bartolomé S, Rodríguez-Padial L. CPAP decreases plasma levels of soluble tumour necrosis factor-α receptor 1 in obstructive sleep apnoea. *Eur Respir J* 2008;**32**:1009–15.

28. Carneiro G, Togeiro SM, Ribeiro-Filho FF, Truksinas E, Ribeiro AB, Zanella MT, Tufik S. Continuous positive airway pressure therapy improves hypoadiponectinemia in severe obese men with obstructive sleep apnea without changes in insulin resistance. *Metab Syndr Relat Disord* 2009;**7**(6):537–42.

29. West SD, Nicoll DJ, Wallace TM, Matthews DR, Stradling JR. Effect of CPAP on insulin resistance and HbA1c in men with obstructive sleep apnoea and type-2 diabetes. *Thorax* 2007;**62**:969–74.

30. Kohler M, Ayers L, Pepperell JC, Packwood KL, Ferry B, Crosthwaite N, Craig S, Siccoli MM, Davies RJ, Stradling JR. Effects of continuous positive airway pressure on systemic inflammation in patients with

moderate to severe obstructive sleep apnoea: a randomised controlled trial. *Thorax* 2009;**64**:67–73.

31. Partinen M, Kaprio J, Koskenvuo M, Putkonen P, Langinvainio H. Genetic and environmental determination of human sleep. *Sleep* 1983;**6**(3):179–85.

32. Miller MA. Chapter 12 Genetics & Sleep. In: Cappuccio FP, Miller MA, Lockley SW, editors. *Sleep, health and society: from aetiology to public health*. Oxford University Press; 2010. September 23.

33. Leloup JC, Goldbeter A. Modeling the mammalian circadian clock: sensitivity analysis and multiplicity of oscillatory mechanisms. *J Theor Biol* 2004;**230**(4):541–62.

34. Okamura H, Doi M, Yamaguchi Y, Fustin JM. Hypertension Due to Loss of Clock: Novel Insight From the Molecular Analysis of Cry1/Cry2-Deleted Mice. *Curr Hypertens Rep* 2011;**13**(2):103–8. Review.

35. Hardeland R, Cardinali DP, Srinivasan V, Spence DW, Brown GM, Pandi-Perumal SR. Melatonin-A pleiotropic, orchestrating regulator molecule. *Prog Neurobiol* 2011;**93**(2):350–84.

36. Fonken LK, Workman JL, Walton JC, Weil ZM, Morris JS, Haim A, Nelson RJ. Light at night increases body mass by shifting the time of food intake. *Proc Natl Acad Sci USA.* 2010;**107**(43):18664–9. Epub 2010 Oct 11.

37. Sánchez-Barceló EJ, Mediavilla MD, Tan DX, Reiter RJ. Clinical uses of melatonin: evaluation of human trials. *Curr Med Chem* 2010;**17**(19):2070–95.

38. Spiegel K, Tasali E, Leproult R, Van Cauter CE. Effects of poor and short sleep on glucose metabolism and obesity risk. *Nat Rev Endocrinol* 2009;**5**(5):253–61.

39. Cappuccio FP, D'Elia L, Strazzullo P, Miller MA. Quantity and quality of sleep and incidence of type-2 diabetes: a systematic review and meta-analysis. *Diabetes Care* 2010;**33**(2):414–20.

40. Downs SH, Black N. The feasibility of creating a checklist for the assessment of the methodological quality both of randomised and non-randomised studies of health care interventions. *J Epidemiol Community Health* 1998;**52**(6):377–84.

41. Knutson KL, Van Cauter CE, Rathouz PJ, Yan LL, Hulley SB, Liu K, Lauderdale DS. Association between sleep and blood pressure in midlife: the CARDIA sleep study. *Archives of Internal Medicine* 2009;**169**(11): 1055–61.

42. Spiegel K, Knutson K, Leproult R, Tasali E, Van Cauter E. Sleep loss: a novel risk factor for insulin resistance and Type-2 diabetes. *J Appl Physiol* 2005; **99**(5):2008–19.

43. Punjabi NM, Beamer BA. Chapter Sleep Apnea and Metabolic Dysfunction. Principles and Practice of Sleep Medicine. In: Kryger, Roth, Dement, editors. 4th ed. Elevier; 2005.

44. Schwartz MW, Porte Jr D. Diabetes, obesity, and the brain. *Science* 2005;**307**:375–9.

45. Spiegel K, Leproult R, L'hermite-Baleriaux M, Copinschi G, Penev P, Van Cauter E. Leptin levels are dependent on sleep duration: Relationships with sympathovagal balance, carbohydrate regulation, cortisol, and thyrotropin. *Journal of Clinical Endocrinology and Metabolism* 2004;**89**:5762–71.

46. Spiegel K, Tasali E, Penev P, Van Cauter E. Sleep curtailment in healthy young men is associated with decreased leptin levels, elevated ghrelin levels and increased hunger and appetite. *Annals of Internal Medicine* 2004;**141**:846–50.

47. Thomas M, Sing H, Belenky G, Holcomb H, Mayberg H, Dannals R, Wagner H, Thorne D, Popp K, Rowland L, Welsh A, Balwinski S, Redmond D. Neural basis of alertness and cognitive performance impairments during sleepiness. I. Effects of 24 h of sleep deprivation on waking human regional brain activity. *J Sleep Res* 2000;**9**:335–52.

48. Spiegel K, Leproult R, Colecchia EF, L'hermite-Baleriaux M, Nie Z, Copinschi G, Van Cauter E. Adaptation of the 24-h growth hormone profile to a state of sleep debt. *American Journal of Physiology - Regulatory Integrative & Comparative Physiology* 2000;**279**:R874–83.

49. Spiegel K, Leproult R, Van Cauter E. Impact of sleep debt on metabolic and endocrine function. *Lancet* 1999;**354**:1435–9.

50. Van Cauter E, Polonsky KS, Scheen AJ. Roles of circadian rhythmicity and sleep in human glucose regulation. *Endocrine Reviews* 1997;**18**:716–38.

51. Resnick HE, Redline S, Shahar E, Gilpin A, Newman A, Walter R, Ewy GA, Howard BV, Punjabi NM. Sleep Heart Health Study. Diabetes and sleep disturbances: findings from the Sleep Heart Health Study. *Diabetes Care* 2003;**26**(3):702–9.

52. An Bixler EO, Chrousos GP. Sleep apnea is a manifestation of the metabolic syndrome. *Sleep Med Rev* 2005;**9**(3):211–24. Review.

53. Al-Delaimy WK, Manson JE, Willett WC, Stampfer MJ, Hu FB. Snoring as a risk factor for type II diabetes mellitus: a prospective study. *Am J Epidemiol* 2002;**155**(5):387–93.

54. Grunstein RR, Stenlöf K, Hedner J, Sjöström L. Impact of obstructive sleep apnea and sleepiness on metabolic and cardiovascular risk factors in the Swedish Obese Subjects (SOS) Study. *Int J Obes Relat Metab Disord* 1995;**19**(6):410–8.

55. Brooks B, Cistulli PA, Borkman M, Ross G, McGhee S, Grunstein RR, Sullivan CE, Yue DK. Obstructive sleep apnea in obese noninsulin-dependent diabetic patients: effect of continuous positive airway pressure

treatment on insulin responsiveness. *J Clin Endocrinol Metab* 1994;**79**(6):1681—5.

56. Harsch IA, Schahin SP, Radespiel-Tröger M, Weintz O, Jahreiss H, Fuchs FS, Wiest GH, Hahn EG, Lohmann T, Konturek PC, Ficker JH. Continuous positive airway pressure treatment rapidly improves insulin sensitivity in patients with obstructive sleep apnea syndrome. *Am J Respir Crit Care Med* 2004;**169**(2):156—62.

57. Pien GW, Schwab RJ. Sleep disorders during pregnancy. *Sleep Nov 1* 2004;**27**(7):1405—17.

58. Izci-Balserak B, Pien GW. Sleep-disordered breathing and pregnancy: potential mechanisms and evidence for maternal and fetal morbidity. *Curr Opin Pulm Med* 2010;**16**(6):574—82.

59. Goldstein LB, Bushnell CD, Adams RJ, Appel LJ, Braun LT, Chaturvedi S, Creager MA, Culebras A, Eckel RH, Hart RG, Hinchey JA, Howard VJ, Jauch EC, Levine SR, Meschia JF, Moore WS, Nixon JV, Pearson TA on behalf of the American Heart Association Stroke Council; Council on Cardiovascular Nursing; Council on Epidemiology and Prevention; Council for High Blood Pressure Research, Council on Peripheral Vascular Disease, and Interdisciplinary Council on Quality of Care and Outcomes Research. Guidelines for the Primary Prevention of Stroke: A Guideline for Healthcare Professionals From the American Heart Association/American Stroke Association. *Stroke* 2011;**42**(2):517—84. Epub 2010 Dec 2.

22

Roles of Pancreatic Cell Functions, Liver, Skeletal Muscle, and Adipose Tissues in Diabetes and Metabolic Syndrome

Beverly S. Mühlhäusler

FOODplus Research Centre, School of Agriculture, Food and Wine,
The University of Adelaide, Australia

INTRODUCTION

Metabolic syndrome is a constellation of physiological and biochemical abnormalities characterized by insulin resistance or high fasting glucose, central obesity, abnormal cholesterol and triglyceride levels, and hypertension.[1] Individuals with the metabolic syndrome are at increased risk of developing a range of chronic health conditions, in particular type 2 diabetes and cardiovascular disease, and the metabolic syndrome therefore represents a serious health problem. In human populations, the majority of cases are seen in overweight and obese individuals, and the global obesity epidemic has seen a substantial rise in the incidence of metabolic syndrome and type 2 diabetes, particularly in the US and

Nutritional and Therapeutic Interventions for Diabetes and Metabolic Syndrome
DOI: 10.1016/B978-0-12-385083-6.00022-X

other Western countries over the past two decades.[2,3]

Two of the central features of the metabolic disease are insulin resistance and an excessive accumulation of body fat in the abdominal region,[4–6] and the latter is thought to play a central role in the etiology of metabolic dysfunction. This is thought to be the result of the increased release of non-esterified free fatty acids (NEFA) from abdominal adipose cells into the circulation which are then deposited in other peripheral insulin-sensitive tissues, including the liver and skeletal muscle, resulting in impaired insulin action and, ultimately, overt insulin resistance.[7] These fatty acids can also be deposited in the pancreatic β-cell, which impairs β-cell function and reduces the capacity of the pancreas for insulin production.[8]

The purpose of this chapter is to discuss the separate and combined roles of the pancreas, liver, skeletal muscle, and adipose tissue in the pathophysiology of the metabolic syndrome and type 2 diabetes, with a focus on how interactions between these key metabolic tissues result in the characteristic features of metabolic disease, i.e. elevated fasting glucose and NEFA concentrations, peripheral insulin resistance and, in the latter stages of the disease, impaired pancreatic function.

ADIPOSE TISSUE

Type 2 diabetes and its precursor insulin resistance are tightly linked to adipocyte hypertrophy in the abdominal (visceral) adipose tissue in both animals and humans.[9,10] Interestingly, the same is not true of excessive fat storage in peripheral (subcutaneous) fat depots, and in fact individuals who store more fat in these compartments are relatively protected from the metabolic aspects of obesity.[10] This has led to the hypothesis that inadequate deposition of fatty acids in the subcutaneous depots

in the presence of a continuing ability to grow visceral (abdominal) adipocytes is a key factor underlying the development of insulin resistance and type 2 diabetes.[8] In this model, lipid "spills over" to the liver, skeletal muscle, and pancreatic β-cell, resulting in impaired insulin sensitivity and a reduced capacity for insulin production, respectively.[8] It is for this reason that some obese individuals, but in whom adipose tissue is distributed proportionally in visceral and subcutaneous compartments, can be more insulin sensitive (i.e. more metabolically healthy) than individuals who have a much lower body mass index (BMI), but who preferentially accumulate fat in the visceral compartment. Waist circumference is used as a clinical measure of visceral obesity in humans, and has been shown to be a reliable predictor of insulin resistance in several large population-based studies.[11]

WHY IS VISCERAL FAT MORE METABOLICALLY DANGEROUS?

The association between visceral adipose tissue and metabolic risk has been attributed to the increased sensitivity to the lipolytic actions of catecholamines and a decreased sensitivity to the anti-lipolytic effects of insulin in visceral compared to subcutaneous adipocytes.[12] These features result in higher rates of triglyceride turnover and lipid breakdown (lipolysis) in visceral adipose depots, and an increased release of NEFA into the circulation, and these NEFA play a central role in the subsequent development of insulin resistance and type 2 diabetes.

The distinct properties of visceral and subcutaneous adipocytes have been related to differences in gene expression profiles which exist in these two adipocyte populations. Visceral adipocytes have a higher density of β-adrenergic receptors, which explains their increased responsiveness to catecholamine-induced lipolysis.[13] Visceral adipocytes also express more steroid hormone receptors on the cell surface, and are thus more sensitive to the effects of stress hormones, in particular cortisol, compared to subcutaneous adipocytes.[14] Steroid hormones act to promote adipose tissue deposition, and medical conditions in which cortisol concentrations are persistently elevated, including Cushing's syndrome and hyper-secreting adrenal tumors, produce a characteristic increase in central fat deposition.[15] The increased sensitivity to steroids in visceral compared to subcutaneous adipose tissue also explains why exposure to chronic physical or psychological stress can also lead to increased accumulation of abdominal body fat.[15]

The differences between visceral and subcutaneous adipocytes also extend to the relative amounts of the various secreted factors (adipocytokines) which are released from adipocytes into the circulation. Compared with subcutaneous adipocytes, visceral adipocytes produce less leptin, a hormone which plays a central role in regulating energy balance and resisting increases in body fat mass, and adiponectin, which has insulin-sensitizing actions on liver and muscle.[16,17] Visceral adipocytes also release higher amounts of proinflammatory cytokines, including macrophage inflammatory protein-1β (MIP-1β) and interleukins-6 and -7 (IL-6, IL-7), compared with subcutaneous fat.[18] The expression levels of a number of factors implicated in the etiology of cardiovascular disease (CVD), including angiotensinogen, acylation stimulating protein and plasminogen activator inhibitor-1 (PAI-1), are also significantly higher in visceral compared to subcutaneous fat in humans, providing a possible explanation for the relationship between visceral adiposity and increased risk of CVD in humans.[19] Thus, an increased accumulation of visceral fat is associated with reduced circulating concentrations of leptin and adiponectin and increased concentrations of proinflammatory cytokines, which contribute to the dysregulation of energy balance, reduced insulin sensitivity, and

TABLE 22.1 Summary of Differences Between Visceral and Subcutaneous Adipose Tissue

Properties of visceral compared to subcutaneous adipocytes
↑↑ Lipolytic activity
↑ Lipogenic activity
↑↑↑ Sensitivity to steroids
↑↑↑ Sensitivity to catecholamine-induced lipolysis
↑↑ NEFA release into circulation
↑ Proximity to liver
↑ Secretion of proinflammatory cytokines (MIP-1P, IL-6, IL-7)
↓ Secretion of leptin and adiponectin

increased cardiovascular risk. A summary of the key differences between subcutaneous and visceral adipose tissue is shown in Table 22.1.

The anatomical location of the visceral fat depot also contributes to its more pronounced negative metabolic impacts. The visceral fat depots are located in the abdominal compartment and drain directly into the portal vein. Thus, the NEFA released from visceral fat rapidly reach the liver, where they are deposited in hepatic cells and have negative effects on hepatic function.[20] The impact of increased NEFA concentrations on hepatic function will be explored in the next section.

LIVER

The liver is the only tissue in the body that is able to synthesize glucose *de novo* under normal physiological conditions (a process known as gluconeogenesis), and dysregulation of hepatic gluconeogenesis plays an important role in the pathogenesis of insulin resistance and type 2 diabetes.[12] Under normal circumstances, hepatic gluconeogenesis is activated in response to decreases in plasma glucose concentrations in order to return glucose concentrations to normal levels and thus maintain glucose homeostasis.[21] This process is stimulated by glucagon, and inhibited by insulin. However, when the liver becomes insulin resistant, insulin is no longer able to effectively switch off hepatic glucose production, and glucose continues to be released from the liver into the circulation despite the fact that plasma concentrations are normal or above normal.[12] Thus, hepatic insulin resistance contributes to the fasting hyperglycemia which is a characteristic feature of metabolic syndrome and type 2 diabetes.[20]

The development of hepatic insulin resistance has been linked to the increased release of NEFA into the portal circulation, which are taken up by the liver and result in an increase in hepatic lipogenesis and the accumulation of triglycerides in hepatic cells.[22] Over time, excess deposition of lipids in hepatic cells can give rise to a condition known as non-alcoholic fatty liver disease (NAFLD), which refers to hepatic steatosis and consequent decline in hepatic function as a result of increased triglyceride deposition. In recent years, there has been an increasing appreciation of the significance of NAFLD, and it is estimated that this condition affects up to 75% of patients with obesity and type 2 diabetes.[23]

While it is accepted that hepatic fat accumulation is linked to insulin resistance, the exact mechanism is unclear. It has been shown, however, that the excess deposition of fat in the liver, and consequent hepatic insulin resistance, occurs relatively early in the development of metabolic syndrome and type 2 diabetes. Feeding rats a high fat diet for only 3 days is associated with a ~3-fold increase in liver triglyceride and total fatty acyl-CoA content without any significant increase in skeletal muscle fat content, suggesting that the liver is the first port of call for excess dietary fatty acids.[24] The suppression of hepatic glucose production by insulin was diminished in the fat-fed rats, consistent with the development of hepatic insulin resistance.[24]

The ability of fatty acids to impair hepatic insulin responsiveness is largely due to effects on the insulin signalling pathway downstream of the insulin receptor. Under normal circumstances, insulin binding to the receptor activates the receptor-associated insulin receptor substrates (IRS-1 and IRS-2), which then phosphorylates and activates phosphatidylinositol 3 kinase (PI3K).[25] PI3K phosphorylates and activates the serine/threonine protein kinase B (PKB or Akt), which then coordinately activates and inhibits a number of downstream transcription factors, including tuberous sclerosis complex (TSC1 and 2), forkhead Box 01 transcription factor (FOXO1) and glycogen synthase kinase (GSK3) molecules, which results in enhanced protein synthesis, reduced hepatic glucose production and increased hepatic glycogen production, respectively. The accumulation of triglycerides in the liver is associated with impaired insulin-stimulated IRS-1 and IRS-2 tyrosine phosphorylation, and consequently a reduced efficiency of hepatic insulin signalling.[25,26] Ultimately, hepatic fat accumulation decreases insulin activation of glycogen synthase and increases hepatic gluconeogenesis, thus leading to excessive hepatic glucose production and contributing to peripheral hyperglycemia (Figure 22.1).

SKELETAL MUSCLE

Since the skeletal muscle represents the major site of postprandial glucose disposal,[27] it is not surprising that changes in insulin sensitivity within muscle cells has a significant impact on whole-body glucose—insulin metabolism. Randle and colleagues proposed a mechanism more than 40 years ago by which fatty acids could impair insulin-stimulated glucose oxidation in muscle. According to this theory, the oxidation of these fatty acids led to a downregulation of glycolysis in muscle cells, promoted glycogen synthesis, and inhibited the further uptake of glucose into the muscle cell. Thus, in their model, the availability of lipids as a source of fuel generated metabolic signals that impaired the use of glucose through inhibition of the key glycolytic enzymes.[28] More recent

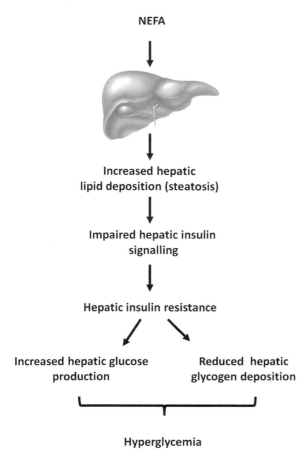

NEFA

Increased hepatic
lipid deposition (steatosis)

Impaired hepatic insulin
signalling

Hepatic insulin resistance

Increased hepatic glucose
production

Reduced hepatic
glycogen deposition

Hyperglycemia

FIGURE 22.1 A summary of the role of the liver in insulin resistance. NEFA released from visceral adipose tissue are deposited in the liver resulting in an increased hepatic lipid content (steatosis). This impairs hepatic insulin signalling, and reduces the capacity of insulin to inhibit hepatic glucose production. As a result, glucose production by the liver increases and more glucose is released into the circulation, contributing to the peripheral hyperglycemia.

transporters are sequestered into vesicles within the cell, and must translocate to the surface of the cell, and insert into cell membrane in order to enable glucose to enter the cell. In healthy individuals, circulating insulin binds to its receptor on the surface of muscle cells, thereby activating the receptor tyrosine kinase activity, with subsequent phosphorylation and activation of IRS1 and PI3K.[27,30] This enzyme, through signalling intermediates, activates Akt2, which phosphorylates and inactivates AS160, a protein that prevents translocation of GLUT4 to the cell membrane. Thus, insulin promotes the docking and fusion of GLUT4-containing vesicles to the plasma membrane.[27] In insulin-resistant and diabetic individuals, however, the tyrosine phosphorylation of IRS1 and associated activation of PI3K are impaired, and the ability of insulin to promote glucose uptake into cells is reduced.[30] As in the liver, this impairment to insulin signalling is the result of excess lipid accumulation in muscle cells. This has been demonstrated in experiments in which human subjects are given lipid infusions. These individuals have a much reduced IRS1-associated PI3K activity in the muscles, indicating that the lipid-induced reduction in insulin-stimulated glucose transport was attributable to a defect in insulin signalling.[31]

Thus, increased deposition of NEFA from visceral adipose tissue in muscle cells impairs the capacity for insulin to promote substrate uptake in the skeletal muscle, the major site of glucose disposal in the body further adds further to the hyperglycemia in insulin resistant and type 2 diabetic subjects (Figure 22.2).

PANCREAS

The pancreatic β-cell plays a fundamental role in the regulation of glucose homeostasis, and is responsible for the synthesis and secretion of insulin in response to increases in plasma

studies, however, have suggested that it is not so much the inhibition of glycolysis, but rather the inhibition of insulin signalling within the muscle cell which results in the reduced glucose uptake.[29]

Insulin-mediated glucose uptake in skeletal muscle cells occurs through the insulin-dependent glucose transporter, GLUT4. In the absence of the insulin stimulus, the GLUT4

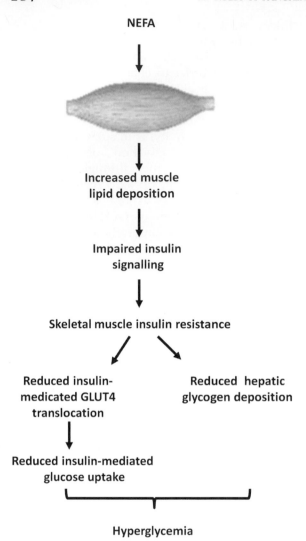

NEFA

↓

Increased muscle
lipid deposition

↓

Impaired insulin
signalling

↓

Skeletal muscle insulin resistance

Reduced insulin-
medicated GLUT4
translocation

Reduced hepatic
glycogen deposition

↓

Reduced insulin-mediated
glucose uptake

Hyperglycemia

FIGURE 22.2 **A summary of the role of the muscle in insulin resistance.** NEFA released from visceral adipose tissue are deposited in the muscle cells and the resulting increase in lipid content in the muscle leads to impaired insulin signalling. The capacity for insulin to promote glucose uptake into muscle is thereby reduced, and contributes to an increase in circulating glucose concentrations.

glucose concentrations. This has been clearly demonstrated in experimental studies in which streptozotocin, a compound which selectively destroys pancreatic β-cells, has been administered to experimental animals. Streptozotocin administration results in an almost complete absence of circulating insulin and a phenotype reflective of type 1 diabetes, i.e. basal and insulin-stimulated hyperglycemia, and is widely used as an animal model of type 1 diabetes.[32]

Whilst type 1 diabetes results from a failure of pancreatic insulin secretion, the initial stages of insulin resistance and type 2 diabetes are characterized by an increased insulin release in an attempt to overcome the lower insulin sensitivity in peripheral tissues.[12] Thus, insulin resistance and type 2 diabetes are typically characterized by both hyperglycemia and hyperinsulinemia[1] (Figure 22.3A). However, over time, this constant drive to increase insulin production leads to pancreatic exhaustion, in which the β-cells lose their capacity to produce insulin.[33] As a result, type 2 diabetes can ultimately progress to a situation in which an individual becomes dependent on exogenous insulin (Figure 22.3B). In addition, NEFA in the circulation which "spill over" from adipose tissues can be deposited directly in the pancreas, and this results in a loss of β-cell function and a consequent decrease in insulin secretory capacity, thereby exacerbating the hyperglycemia and worsening the phenotype.

SUMMARY

Defects in the structure and function of the insulin-producing and insulin-responsive tissues in the body, the pancreas, liver, skeletal muscle and adipose tissue, play a central role in the pathogenesis of metabolic syndrome and type 2 diabetes. In humans, the vast majority of cases of metabolic syndrome, insulin resistance, and type 2 diabetes occur in conjunction with an increased accumulation of body fat, and this has led to the coining of the term, "diabesity" to describe the co-existence of obesity and diabetes in the same individual. An excessive

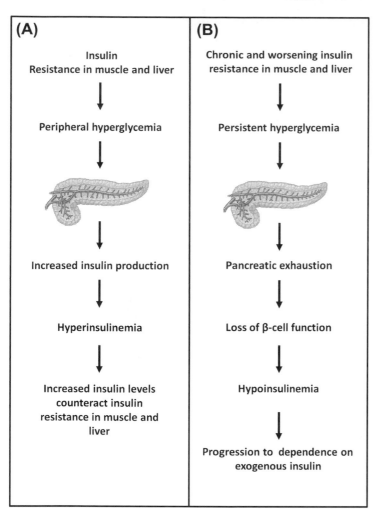

(A)

Insulin
Resistance in muscle and liver

↓

Peripheral hyperglycemia

↓

↓

Increased insulin production

↓

Hyperinsulinemia

↓

Increased insulin levels
counteract insulin
resistance in muscle and
liver

(B)

Chronic and worsening insulin
resistance in muscle and liver

↓

Persistent hyperglycemia

↓

↓

Pancreatic exhaustion

↓

Loss of β-cell function

↓

Hypoinsulinemia

↓

Progression to dependence on
exogenous insulin

FIGURE 22.3 **A summary of the role of the pancreas in insulin resistance:** (A) in the initial stages insulin resistance in the muscle and liver results in peripheral hyperglycemia which stimulates the pancreatic β-cells to increase insulin production, resulting in peripheral hyperinsulinemia in an attempt to counteract the reduction in peripheral insulin sensitivity; (B) if this situation persists, the constant drive to the pancreatic β-cell due as a result of chronic elevations in plasma glucose leads to pancreatic exhaustion, loss of β -cell function and a reduced insulin secretory capacity.

accumulation of adipose tissue in visceral fat depots is regarded as the most important risk factor for the development of insulin resistance in peripheral tissues, and reductions in visceral fat mass have proved effective in reversing insulin resistance and type 2 diabetes in both animals and humans.

This chapter has presented a summary of our current understanding of the mechanisms which link excessive visceral fat accumulation with insulin resistance in liver and muscle, and defects in insulin secretion in pancreatic β-cells.

The study of the molecular mechanisms which underlie these physiological effects remains an active research area, and there is no doubt that these studies have the potential to provide novel targets for intervention to prevent or reverse insulin resistance. There is also considerable interest in examining the possible role of specific dietary factors and environmental toxins in the pathogenesis of insulin resistance in humans, and the potential for such factors to influence metabolic pathways may open up new opportunities for intervention.

KEY CONCEPTS (Figure 22.4)

- In the majority of cases, the development of metabolic syndrome and type 2 diabetes is preceded by an increased accumulation of fat around the abdomen (central obesity).

- Visceral adipose cells are more metabolically active than subcutaneous adipose cells and release more NEFA into the circulation.
- Visceral obesity is associated with an increase in circulating NEFA concentrations.

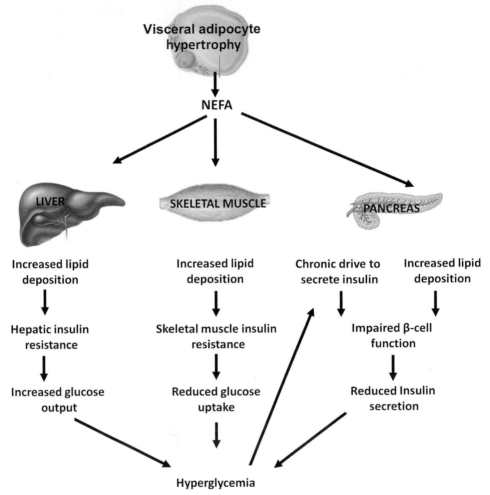

FIGURE 22.4 **Summary of the interactions between visceral adipose tissue, liver, skeletal muscle, and pancreas.** The visceral adipocyte releases NEFA, which are deposited in the liver and skeletal muscle, resulting in the development of insulin resistance in these tissues. This leads to an increase in hepatic glucose secretion and reduced glucose uptake by skeletal muscle, resulting in peripheral hyperglycemia. The elevated glucose levels stimulate the pancreatic β-cells to increase their synthesis and secretion of insulin, leading to peripheral hyperinsulinemia. Over time, this can lead to pancreatic exhaustion and reduce insulin secretary capacity. In addition, NEFA can be deposited directly in the pancreas, resulting in further impairment of β-cell function and insulin secretion.

- These NEFA are deposited in liver and muscle, and result in the development of insulin resistance in these tissues.
- This results in a reduced uptake of circulating glucose into skeletal muscle, and an increase in hepatic glucose output which together result in hyperglycemia.
- This hyperglycemia drives the pancreatic β-cells to increase insulin secretion in order to overcome the peripheral insulin resistance. This ultimately leads to pancreatic exhaustion, in which the pancreas is unable to produce sufficient insulin, and a patient can become dependent on insulin injections.
- NEFA can also be deposited in the pancreatic β-cells and impair β-cell function, which can accelerate the loss of pancreatic function.

Acknowledgments

B. Muhlhausler is supported by a Career Development Award from the National Health and Medical Research Council of Australia (NHMRC). The author wishes to thank John Carragher for editorial assistance.

References

1. Eckel RH, Grundy SM, Zimmet PZ. *The metabolic syndrome* 2005;**365**:1415—28.
2. Ford ES, Giles WH, Dietz WH. *Prevalence of the metabolic syndrome among us adults* 2002;**287**:356—9.
3. Cameron AJ, Shaw JE, Zimmet PZ. The metabolic syndrome: Prevalence in worldwide populations. *Endocrinol Metab Clin North Am* 2004;**33**:351—75.
4. Goralski KB, Sinal CJ. Type 2 diabetes and cardiovascular disease: Getting to the fat of the matter. *Can J Physiol Pharmacol* 2007;**85**:113—32.
5. Smith SR, Lovejoy JC, Greenway F, Ryan D, deJonge L, de la Bretonne J, Volafova J, Bray GA. Contributions of total body fat, abdominal subcutaneous adipose tissue compartments, and visceral adipose tissue to the metabolic complications of obesity. *Metabolism* 2001;**50**:425—35.
6. Ravussin E, Smith SR. Increased fat uptake, impaired fat oxidation, and failure of fat cell proliferation result in ectopic fat storage, insulin resistance, and type 2 diabetes. *Ann N Y Acad Sci* 2002;**967**:363—78.
7. Zimmet P, KBoyko EJ, Collier GR, de Courten M. Etiology of the metabolic syndrome: Potential role of insulin resistance, leptin resistance, and other players. *Ann N Y Acad Sci* 1999;**892**:25—44.
8. Danforth E. Failure of adipocyte differentiation causes type II diabetes mellitus? *Nat Genet* 2000;**26**:13—13.
9. Tarui S, Tokunaga K, Fujioka S, Matsuzawa Y. Visceral fat obesity: Anthropological and pathophysiological aspects. *Int J Obes* 1991;**15**:1—8.
10. Weyer C, Foley JE, Bogardus C, Tataranni PA, Pratley RE. Enlarged subcutaneous abdominal adipocyte size, but not obesity, predicts type II diabetes independent of insulin resistance. *Diabetologia* 2000;**43**:1498—506.
11. Wahrenberg H, Hertel K, Leijonhufvud B-M, Persson L-G r, Toft E, Arner P. *Use of waist circumference to predict insulin resistance: Retrospective study* 2005;**330**:1363—4.
12. Bergman RN, Kim SP, Hsu IR, Catalano KJ, Chiu JD, Kabir M, Richey JM, Ader M. Abdominal obesity: Role in the pathophysiology of metabolic disease and cardiovascular risk. *Am J Med* 2007;**120**:S3—8. discussion S29—32.
13. Alvarez GE, Beske SD, Ballard TP, Davy KP. Sympathetic neural activation in visceral obesity. *Circulation* 2002;**106**:2533—6.
14. Bjorntorp P. Adipose tissue distribution and function. *Int J Obes* 1991;**15**:67—81.
15. Bujalska IJ, Kumar S, Stewart PM. Does central obesity reflect Cushing's disease of the omentum. *Lancet* 1997;**349**:1210—3.
16. Lihn AS, Bruun JM, He G, Pedersen SB, Jensen PF, Richelsen B. Lower expression of adiponectin MRNA in visceral adipose tissue in lean and obese subjects. *Mol Cell Endocrinol* 2004;**219**:9—15.
17. Yamauchi T, Kamon J, Waki H, Terauchi Y, Kubota N, Hara K, Mori Y, Ide T, Murakami K, Tsuboyama-Kasaoka N, Ezaki O, Akanuma Y, Gavrilova O, Vinson C, Reitman ML, Kagechika H, Shudo K, Yoda M, Nakano Y, Tobe K, Nagai R, Kimura S, Tomita M, Froguel P, Kadowaki T. *The fat-derived hormone adiponectin reverses insulin resistance associated with both lipoatrophy and obesity* 2001;**7**:941—6.
18. Lafontan M, Girard J. Impact of visceral adipose tissue on liver metabolism. Part I: Heterogeneity of adipose tissue and functional properties of visceral adipose tissue. *Diabetes Metab* 2008;**34**:317—27.
19. Dusserre E, Moulin P, Vidal H. Differences in MRNA expression of the proteins secreted by the adipocytes in human subcutaneous and visceral adipose tissues. *Biochimica et Biophysica Acta* 2000;**1500**:88—96.
20. Björntorp P. Visceral obesity: A civilization syndrome. *Obes Res* 1993;**1**:206—22.

21. Postic C, Dentin R, Girard J. Role of the liver in the control of carbohydrate and lipid homeostasis. *Diabetes Metab Res Rev* 2004;**30**:398–408.

22. Hellerstein MK. *De novo* lipogenesis in humans: Metabolic and regulatory aspects. *Eur J Clin Nutr* 1999;**53**:S53–65.

23. McCullough AJ. Pathophysiology of nonalcoholic steatohepatitis. *J Clin Gastroenterol* 2006;**40**:S17–29.

24. Samuel VT, Liu Z-X, Qu X, Elder BD, Bilz S, Befroy D, Romanelli AJ, Shulman GI. Mechanism of hepatic insulin resistance in non-alcoholic fatty liver disease. *J Biol Chem* 2004;**279**:32345–53.

25. Samuel VT, Petersen KF, Shulman GI. Lipid-induced insulin resistance: Unravelling the mechanism. *Lancet* 2010;**375**:2267–77.

26. Kabir M, Catalano KJ, Ananthnarayan S, Kim SP, Van Citters GW, Dea MK, Bergman RN. Molecular evidence supporting the portal theory: A causative link between visceral adiposity and hepatic insulin resistance. *Am J Physiol Endocrinol Metab* 2005;**288**:E454–61.

27. Zierler K. Whole body glucose metabolism. *Am J Physiol* 1999;**276**:E409–26.

28. Randle PJ, Priestman DA, Mistry S, Halsall A. Mechanisms modifying glucose oxidation in diabetes mellitus. *Diabetologia* 1994;**37**:S155–61.

29. Kim JY, Nolte LA, Hansen PA, Han DH, Ferguson K, Thompson PA, Holloszy JO. High-fat diet-induced muscle insulin resistance: Relationship to visceral fat mass. *Am J Physiol Regul Integr Comp Physiol* 2000;**279**:R2057–65.

30. Zierath JR, Houseknecht KL, Kahn BB. Glucose transporters and diabetes. *Sem Cell Dev Biol* 1996;**7**:295–307.

31. Dresner A, Laurent D, Marcucci M, Griffin ME, Dufour S, Cline GW, Slezak LA, Andersen DK, Hundal RS, Rothman DL, Petersen KF, Shulman GI. Effects of free fatty acids on glucose transport and IRS-1–associated phosphatidylinositol 3-kinase activity. *J Clin Invest* 1999;**103**:253–9.

32. Wilson GL, Leiter EH. Streptozotocin interactions with pancreatic beta cells and the induction of insulin-dependent diabetes. *Curr Top Microbiol Immunol* 1990;**156**:27–54.

33. Chang-Chen K, Mullur R, Bernal-Mizrachi E. Beta-cell failure as a complication of diabetes. *Rev Endocrine Metabol Disord* 2008;**9**:329–43.

23

Liver Disease: A Neglected Complication of Diabetes Mellitus

Marco Arrese, Juan Pablo Arab, Juan Pablo Arancibia, Roberto Candia, Arnoldo Riquelme, Francisco Barrera

Department of Gastroenterology, School of Medicine, Pontificia Universidad Católica de Chile, Santiago, Chile

INTRODUCTION

Concomitant occurrence of Type 2 diabetes mellitus (T2DM) and chronic liver disease is frequently found in clinical practice.[1,2] Although it is known that cirrhosis can contribute by several mechanisms to the development of T2DM, in recent years it has become evident that diabetes may directly determine the development of advanced liver disease via fatty liver and steatohepatitis and that cirrhosis may be considered a late complication of diabetes.[1,3]

Recent data demonstrate that patients with T2DM are indeed at a significantly higher risk of developing advanced chronic liver disease and its complications than the general population.[4] However, current guidelines for the management of T2DM do not mention the potential risk of chronic liver disease in diabetic patients.[5] This is important since progression to cirrhosis may be potentially halted by pharmacological interventions and, if already present, screening of associated complications such as portal hypertension or hepatocellular carcinoma

Nutritional and Therapeutic Interventions for Diabetes and Metabolic Syndrome
DOI: 10.1016/B978-0-12-385083-6.00023-1

is indicated.[6,7] Thus, liver disease in patients with diabetes may be a potentially overlooked or neglected disease complication.[8] This chapter is devoted to reviewing clinical aspects of non-alcoholic fatty liver disease (NAFLD), the most frequent cause of liver disease in diabetics and a likely cause of advanced liver disease development in this patient population.

NON-ALCOHOLIC FATTY LIVER DISEASE: CURRENT CONCEPTS AND NATURAL HISTORY

NAFLD is defined as an abnormal accumulation of lipids on hepatocytes, conventionally stipulated as more than 5% of fat-laden hepatocytes at light-microscopic examination of liver biopsy, associated with similar histological features to those found in alcoholic liver disease but occurring in subjects with minimal or no alcohol consumption (less than 70 g/week of alcohol for women and less than 140 g/week for men).[9,10] NAFLD is a condition closely associated to overweight and obesity and to insulin resistance and should be differentiated from steatosis, with or without hepatitis, resulting from secondary causes like use of drugs (corticosteroids, amiodarone, tamoxifen, etc.), nutritional alterations (rapid weight loss, parenteral nutrition, bariatric surgery, etc.), metabolic or genetic diseases (lipodystrophy, dysbetalipoproteinemia, acute fatty liver of pregnancy, etc.), and other diseases (inflammatory bowel disease, human inmunodeficiency virus, small bowel diverticulosis with bacterial overgrowth), because these conditions have clearly different pathogenesis and outcomes.[10]

From an epidemiological standpoint, NAFLD is a disease of growing importance and represents a major health burden since it is associated to chronic liver disease development and an increased liver-related mortality.[11, 12] Moreover, NAFLD may have implications far beyond the liver as it is now considered as an independent risk factor for cardiovascular disease.[13] The epidemic of obesity is closely linked to NAFLD and, therefore, NAFLD prevalence has increased recently in parallel with global trends in obesity, T2DM, and metabolic syndrome. Current estimates indicate prevalence figures of 30% of the Western general population[11,14] and 12−24% in Asia.[15]

Conceptually, the term NAFLD is an "umbrella" definition as it refers to a spectrum of histological liver lesions ranging from bland fat accumulation in hepatocytes without concomitant inflammation or fibrosis (simple hepatic steatosis) to hepatic steatosis with a necroinflammatory component [termed non-alcoholic steatohepatitis (NASH)] that may be associated with various degrees of fibrosis.[9,16,17] This is relevant as histological features at the time of presentation relate to prognosis.[11] Thus, while patients with simple steatosis on presentation generally have a benign prognosis, a significant proportion of patients with NASH may develop progressive fibrosis leading to cirrhosis and its complications with an impact on long-term survival.[18] Figures derived from several studies suggest that while the risk of serious liver disease in subjects with simple steatosis is less than 4% over one to two decades,[19] 5−8% of patients with NASH will develop liver cirrhosis in a period of 5 years with an overall progression to liver cirrhosis in up to 20% of patients.[20,21] In addition, while cirrhosis itself is associated with an increased risk of hepatocellular carcinoma, several lines of evidence suggest that the risk could be increased in patients with NASH-associated cirrhosis.[22,23] The complications of NASH, involving cirrhosis and HCC, are expected to increase with the growing epidemic of diabetes and obesity.[22,24]

It has been estimated that between 10 and 30% of subjects with NAFLD have histological features of NASH.[10] Major risk factors associated with NASH include obesity, glucose intolerance or diabetes, hypertriglyceridemia, older age, and T2DM.[10] In particular, diabetic patients are at higher risk of developing hepatic steatosis and NASH compared with non-diabetic individuals.[8,25] This indeed may be related to the recently recognized substantial risk of developing advanced liver disease among T2DM patients.[3,4] The following paragraphs examine current data about NAFLD and diabetes.

Diabetes as a Risk Factor of Non-Alcoholic Steatohepatitis and Chronic Liver Disease

A number of studies indicate that NAFLD is highly prevalent among T2DM patients.[26] The prevalence of NAFLD in T2DM ranges between 40% and 80% depending of the diagnostic tool used. A recent large-scale ultrasound study performed in Scotland reported a prevalence of 42.9% of NAFLD in 939 patients including the full clinical spectrum of T2DM.[27] The use of gold-standard techniques such as magnetic resonance spectroscopy increases the threshold of detection of ectopic fat in the liver, and studies using this technique report NAFLD prevalence of 76% in T2DM patients.[28–30] In addition to being extremely frequent in T2DM patients, NAFLD seems to be more aggressive in this subset of subjects as the prevalence of NASH, the progressive form of the disease, is significantly higher than that seen in non-T2DM patients. In one study, NASH was found in 12.2% of those with T2DM compared to 4.7% among non-diabetics.[31] In other recently published cohort, of 328 adult patients in whom NAFLD was assessed by abdominal ultrasound and a liver biopsy when NAFLD was found, NASH was significantly more frequent in diabetic patients (22.2% vs 10.9% in non-T2DM patients).[32] It is also known that obesity compounds the effects of T2DM, with NAFLD being almost universally present in the obese diabetic and NASH occurring in up to 50% of these patients.[26,31] Thus, these data suggest

that T2DM patients are at risk of developing chronic liver disease. The recent study by Porepa et al.[4] supports this concept. These authors explored the administrative health databases for the province of Ontario (Canada) and assessed outcomes in 438,069 adults with diabetes mellitus. They matched patients to a group of 2,059,708 individuals without known diabetes mellitus. In a median time-frame of 6.4 years of follow-up. The study looked for the occurrence of "serious liver disease", a composite outcome defined as diagnosis of cirrhosis, liver failure, and complications of cirrhosis or being a receptor of a liver graft as a major end point. Results showed that diabetics had a significantly greater risk of liver disease with an unadjusted hazard ratio (HR) of 1.92 (95% CI 1.83–2.01) than controls. The authors performed adjustments for other demographic variables that can influence the risk of liver disease (that is, age, sex, urban vs rural residence, and income level). After those corrections, the association remained significant (HR 1.77, 95% CI 1.68–1.86). No details are provided regarding ethnicity or the proportion of subjects having type 1 diabetes or T2DM, which limits further analysis. Although causality can not be demonstrated in this association study, the currently available basic and clinical data on NAFLD and its risk of progression to advanced fibrosis or cirrhosis suggest a link between NAFLD and the risk of serious liver disease in patients with diabetes mellitus.[3]

Clinical Implications

There are several clinical and practical implications of the above-mentioned concepts and data. First, there is a need for increasing awareness about NAFLD and its implications among health providers involved in diabetes. The concept of NAFLD being a significant risk factor for progressive liver disease and liver-related death in subjects with T2DM is well accepted in the hepatology community but somewhat underestimated among diabetologists. This needs to be corrected in order to proceed with appropriate diagnostic and treatment approaches. Second, diagnosis either of NASH (the progressive form of NAFLD) or the presence of early, previously unrecognized, cirrhosis in a given T2DM patient (which implies the risk of developing cirrhotic complications or hepatocellular carcinoma) represent major clinical challenges. Early diagnosis of NASH is of mainstay importance, not only to reinforce on pharmacologic therapy (diet and exercise) which is the cornerstone in NAFLD therapy[33,34] but to eventually start pharmacological interventions that had demonstrated impact on reducing liver inflammation and fibrosis.[34] Moreover, patients with T2DM with unrecognized liver cirrhosis carry the risk of developing esophageal varices and hepatocellular carcinoma (HCC) and are candidates for endoscopic and imaging surveillance. This would allow beginning primary prevention of variceal bleeding with beta blockers[7] and hepatocellular carcinoma early diagnosis and therapy.[35]

From a diagnostic standpoint, it is important to underline that relying on normal levels of serum aminotransferases to exclude liver disease in patients with T2DM may not be an adequate strategy, as severe fibrosis can be present in this setting.[36] For example, a recent Italian study demonstrated liver fibrosis in 59% of patients who underwent liver biopsy for NAFLD with normal liver enzymes with insulin resistance/glucose intolerance or diabetes being the most important factors associated with severe liver fibrosis (OR = 1.97). Indeed, histological assessment of liver tissue obtained by a liver biopsy is considered the gold standard for the definitive diagnosis of NASH, advanced fibrosis or cirrhosis, if the condition is not evident by other diagnostic methods. However, the invasive nature of liver biopsy limits its use. Thus, the pros and cons of liver biopsy should

be adequately weighed in the individual patient. The use of noninvasive tools to assess liver disease in subjects with NAFLD is gaining relevancy as evidence accumulates.[37] The development of plasma biomarkers (e.g., cytokeratine-18 fragments, IGF-1, IL-6, hyaluronic acid)[38] and improving imaging modalities for evaluating liver fibrosis (e.g., transient elastography, magnetic resonance elastography)[39,40] are promising tools for detecting NAFLD disease patients at risk for development of liver cirrhosis. While available, certain clinical or laboratory clues may be advised to improve detection of NASH patients with significant fibrosis or cirrhosis. Obese patients and/or patients older than 45 years are at increased risk of fibrosis. In this subgroup, particular attention should be given to initial signs of cirrhosis on physical examination (telangiectasias, liver palm, indurated or nodular liver edge, left lobe prominence), laboratory data (low platelet count, elevated GGT, elevated AST/ALT ratio, elevated ferritin, low albumin) and ultrasound evaluation (irregular liver border, caudate lobe prominence, splenomegaly). Subjects presenting with one or more of the features mentioned above should receive further liver evaluation with CT/MRI, transient elastography and/or liver biopsy to diagnose liver fibrosis or cirrhosis. With this information patients should be stratified according to their NAFLD liver status and appropriate intervention should be implemented.

Treatment of NAFLD is an evolving issue that will not be discussed here in detail. The reader is referred to recent review articles for state of the art analysis of current evidence.[41–43] Essentially, multifaceted lifestyle interventions including a balanced diet, exercise, and behavioral counseling are the mainstay of treatment. Pharmacological agents are not highly effective and most of the available evidence comes from uncontrolled, nonrandomized studies with short duration of the intervention and inconsistent outcome measures. Moreover, most of studies exclude patients with diabetes, making it difficult to reach firm conclusions and make recommendations. Among the best-quality trials, the PIVENS study[34,44] explored the effects of high-dose vitamin E (800 IU q.d.) and pioglitazone on patients with NASH and showed that vitamin E significantly reduces steatosis and liver inflammation in these patients.[34] Pioglitazone was also effective although it did not reach significance in the pre-defined outcome. However, pioglitazone had demonstrated positive effects on liver inflammation in other trials,[45–47] but with the important drawback of its association with weight gain. Other pharmacologic interventions (metformin, ursodeoxycholic acid, angiotensin antagonist, statins, fibrates)[8] have not been consistent in improving liver inflammation or fibrosis, although ongoing studies on metformin may bring important results for NASH therapy.[48] Moreover, bariatric surgery has a growing evidence suggesting important results in diminishing liver inflammation in obese patients; this intervention could significantly benefit the subgroup of obese patients who have diabetes and low-grade fibrosis NASH.[49,50] It is important to consider that bariatric surgery has not been demonstrated to reverse liver fibrosis; on the contrary, some studies have shown increments of liver fibrosis at the early weight-losing phase. For this reason it is not currently recommended for patients with high-grade fibrosis or cirrhosis.[38,51]

INTRODUCING LIVER CHECK-UP IN DIABETES

As mentioned above, in spite of compelling data on the risk of liver disease in diabetics, current guidelines on diabetes management do not include liver disease diagnosis and therapy. We suggest that active surveillance for liver disease on routine evaluation of diabetic patients should be incorporated in the same way as the screening of microvascular complications and cardiovascular disease. The diabetes liver check-up must not rely simply on liver enzymes, as they are insufficient for detecting the presence of severe liver fibrosis.[36] Clinical and laboratory factors should be considered and imaging studies used to non-invasively estimate the presence of significant fibrosis or cirrhosis. Liver biopsy should be decided on an individual basis and as part of a team evaluation performed by diabetologists and hepatologists. Figure 23.1 shows a suggested approach to this issue.

CONCLUSIONS AND FUTURE PROSPECTS

1. NAFLD is not always a benign liver disease and can be associated with important liver complications.
2. The association of NAFLD and diabetes is an extremely common and ominous combination.
3. Current diabetes care centers should include liver check-up for staging and providing appropriate therapy for NAFLD, NASH, and cirrhotic patients.
4. The diabetes liver check-up must not simply rely on liver enzymes which are frequently normal in diabetic patients with advanced liver fibrosis.
5. A high level of awareness of NAFLD among healthcare providers of diabetic patients could improve the detection of patients at risk of developing liver fibrosis/cirrhosis and prevent their complications.
6. New diagnosis and staging strategies for NAFLD in diabetic patients should be developed in order to implement cost-effective strategies to adequately manage liver disease in this subset of patients.

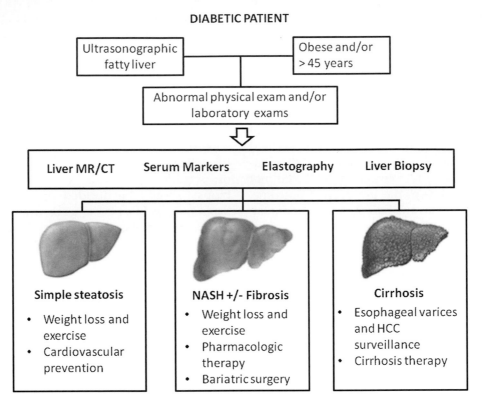

FIGURE 23.1 Suggested diagnostic approach to a T2DM patient with NAFLD. *(See the color plate section at the back of the book.)*

Acknowledgments

This work was partially supported by a grant from the Chilean National Fund for Research in Science and Technology (FONDECYT 1110455 and ACT79 to MA).

References

1. Moscatiello S, Manini R, Marchesini G. Diabetes and liver disease: an ominous association. *Nutr Metab Cardiovasc Dis* 2007;**17**:63−70.
2. Garcia-Compean D, Jaquez-Quintana JO, Gonzalez-Gonzalez JA, Maldonado-Garza H. Liver cirrhosis and diabetes: risk factors, pathophysiology, clinical implications and management. *World J Gastroenterol* 2009;**15**:280−8.
3. Arrese M. Nonalcoholic fatty liver disease: liver disease: an overlooked complication of diabetes mellitus. *Nat Rev Endocrinol* 2010;**6**:660−1.
4. Porepa L, Ray JG, Sanchez-Romeu P, Booth GL. Newly diagnosed diabetes mellitus as a risk factor for serious liver disease. *CMAJ* 2010;**182**:E526−31.
5. Rodbard HW, Blonde L, Braithwaite SS, Brett EM, Cobin RH, Handelsman Y, Hellman R, Jellinger PS, Jovanovic LG, Levy P, Mechanick JI, Zangeneh F. American Association of Clinical Endocrinologists medical guidelines for clinical practice for the management of diabetes mellitus. *Endocr Pract* 2007;**13**(Suppl. 1):1−68.
6. Bolondi L. Screening for hepatocellular carcinoma in cirrhosis. *J Hepatol* 2003;**39**:1076−84.
7. de Franchis R. Revising consensus in portal hypertension: report of the Baveno V consensus workshop on methodology of diagnosis and therapy in portal hypertension. *J Hepatol* 2010;**53**:762−8.
8. Cusi K. Nonalcoholic fatty liver disease in type 2 diabetes mellitus. *Curr Opin Endocrinol Diabetes Obes* 2009;**16**:141−9.

9. Krawczyk M, Bonfrate L, Portincasa P. Nonalcoholic fatty liver disease. *Best Pract Res Clin Gastroenterol* 2010;**24**:695–708.

10. Angulo P. Nonalcoholic fatty liver disease. *N Engl J Med* 2002;**346**:1221–31.

11. Bellentani S, Marino M. Epidemiology and natural history of non-alcoholic fatty liver disease (NAFLD). *Ann Hepatol* 2009;**8**(Suppl. 1):S4–8.

12. Argo CK, Caldwell SH. Epidemiology and natural history of non-alcoholic steatohepatitis. *Clin Liver Dis.* 2009;**13**:511–31.

13. Targher G, Day CP, Bonora E. Risk of cardiovascular disease in patients with nonalcoholic fatty liver disease. *N Engl J Med* 2010;**363**:1341–50.

14. Lazo M, Clark JM. The epidemiology of nonalcoholic fatty liver disease: a global perspective. *Semin Liver Dis* 2008;**28**:339–50.

15. Chitturi S, Farrell GC, Hashimoto E, Saibara T, Lau GK, Sollano JD. Non-alcoholic fatty liver disease in the Asia-Pacific region: definitions and overview of proposed guidelines. *J Gastroenterol Hepatol* 2007; **22**:778–87.

16. Brunt EM. Pathology of nonalcoholic fatty liver disease. *Nat Rev Gastroenterol Hepatol* 2010;**7**:195–203.

17. Brunt EM, Tiniakos DG. Histopathology of nonalcoholic fatty liver disease. *World J Gastroenterol* 2010; **16**:5286–96.

18. Ong JP, Younossi ZM. Epidemiology and natural history of NAFLD and NASH. *Clin Liver Dis* 2007;**11**:1–16. vii.

19. Dam-Larsen S, Franzmann M, Andersen IB, Christoffersen P, Jensen LB, Sorensen TI, Becker U, Bendtsen F. Long term prognosis of fatty liver: risk of chronic liver disease and death. *Gut* 2004;**53**:750–5.

20. Cortez-Pinto H, Baptista A, Camilo ME, De Moura MC. Nonalcoholic steatohepatitis—a long-term follow-up study: comparison with alcoholic hepatitis in ambulatory and hospitalized patients. *Dig Dis Sci* 2003;**48**:1909–13.

21. Matteoni CA, Younossi ZM, Gramlich T, Boparai N, Liu YC, McCullough AJ. Nonalcoholic fatty liver disease: a spectrum of clinical and pathological severity. *Gastroenterology* 1999;**116**:1413–9.

22. Ascha MS, Hanouneh IA, Lopez R, Tamimi TA, Feldstein AF, Zein NN. The incidence and risk factors of hepatocellular carcinoma in patients with nonalcoholic steatohepatitis. *Hepatology* 2010;**51**:1972–8.

23. Siegel AB, Zhu AX. Metabolic syndrome and hepatocellular carcinoma: two growing epidemics with a potential link. *Cancer* 2009;**115**:5651–61.

24. Starley BQ, Calcagno CJ, Harrison SA. Nonalcoholic fatty liver disease and hepatocellular carcinoma: a weighty connection. *Hepatology* 2010;**51**:1820–32.

25. Younossi ZM, Gramlich T, Matteoni CA, Boparai N, McCullough AJ. Nonalcoholic fatty liver disease in patients with type 2 diabetes. *Clin Gastroenterol Hepatol* 2004;**2**:262–5.

26. Adams LA. Nonalcoholic fatty liver disease and diabetes mellitus. *Endocr Res* 2007;**32**:59–69.

27. Williamson RM, Price JF, Glancy S, Perry E, Nee LD, Hayes PC, Frier BM, Van Look LA, Johnston GI, Reynolds RM, Strachan MW. Prevalence of and risk factors for hepatic steatosis and nonalcoholic fatty liver disease in people with type 2 diabetes: the Edinburgh Type 2 Diabetes Study. *Diabetes Care* 2011;**34**:1139–44.

28. Adams LA, Lindor KD. Nonalcoholic fatty liver disease. *Ann Epidemiol* 2007;**17**:863–9.

29. Chen J, Mathew M, Finch J, Cusi K. The prevalence of NAFLD in T2DM is highest among Hispanics and is closely related to hepatic and adipose tissue insulin resistance [abstract]. *Diabetes* 2009;**58**.

30. Cusi K. The role of adipose tissue and lipotoxicity in the pathogenesis of type 2 diabetes. *Curr Diab Rep* 2010;**10**:306–15.

31. Wanless IR, Lentz JS. Fatty liver hepatitis (steatohepatitis) and obesity: an autopsy study with analysis of risk factors. *Hepatology* 1990;**12**:1106–10.

32. Williams CD, Stengel J, Asike MI, Torres DM, Shaw J, Contreras M, Landt CL, Harrison SA. Prevalence of nonalcoholic fatty liver disease and nonalcoholic steatohepatitis among a largely middle-aged population utilizing ultrasound and liver biopsy: a prospective study. *Gastroenterology* 2011;**140**:124–31.

33. St George A, Bauman A, Johnston A, Farrell G, Chey T, George J. Independent effects of physical activity in patients with nonalcoholic fatty liver disease. *Hepatology* 2009;**50**:68–76.

34. Sanyal AJ, Chalasani N, Kowdley KV, McCullough A, Diehl AM, Bass NM, Neuschwander-Tetri BA, Lavine JE, Tonascia J, Unalp A, Van Natta M, Clark J, Brunt EM, Kleiner DE, Hoofnagle JH, Robuck PR. Pioglitazone, vitamin E, or placebo for nonalcoholic steatohepatitis. *N Engl J Med* 2010;**362**:1675–85.

35. Bruix J, Sherman M. Management of hepatocellular carcinoma: an update. *Hepatology* 2011;**53**:1020–2.

36. Fracanzani AL, Valenti L, Bugianesi E, Andreoletti M, Colli A, Vanni E, Bertelli C, Fatta E, Bignamini D, Marchesini G, Fargion S. Risk of severe liver disease in nonalcoholic fatty liver disease with normal aminotransferase levels: a role for insulin resistance and diabetes. *Hepatology* 2008;**48**:792–8.

37. Martinez SM, Crespo G, Navasa M, Forns X. Noninvasive assessment of liver fibrosis. *Hepatology* 2011;**53**:325–35.

38. Hashimoto E, Farrell GC. Will non-invasive markers replace liver biopsy for diagnosing and staging fibrosis in non-alcoholic steatohepatitis? *J Gastroenterol Hepatol* 2009;**24**:501−3.
39. Talwalkar JA, Yin M, Fidler JL, Sanderson SO, Kamath PS, Ehman RL. Magnetic resonance imaging of hepatic fibrosis: emerging clinical applications. *Hepatology* 2008;**47**:332−42.
40. Castera L. Non-invasive diagnosis of steatosis and fibrosis. *Diabetes Metab* 2008;**34**:674−9.
41. Dowman JK, Armstrong MJ, Tomlinson JW, Newsome PN. Current therapeutic strategies in non-alcoholic fatty liver disease. *Diabetes Obes Metab*; 2011.
42. Satapathy SK, Sanyal AJ. Novel treatment modalities for nonalcoholic steatohepatitis. *Trends Endocrinol Metab.* 2010;**21**:668−75.
43. Rafiq N, Younossi ZM. Nonalcoholic fatty liver disease: a practical approach to evaluation and management. *Clin Liver Dis* 2009;**13**:249−66.
44. Chalasani NP, Sanyal AJ, Kowdley KV, Robuck PR, Hoofnagle J, Kleiner DE, Unalp A, Tonascia J. Pioglitazone versus vitamin E versus placebo for the treatment of non-diabetic patients with non-alcoholic steatohepatitis: PIVENS trial design. *Contemp Clin Trials* 2009;**30**:88−96.
45. Belfort R, Harrison SA, Brown K, Darland C, Finch J, Hardies J, Balas B, Gastaldelli A, Tio F, Pulcini J, Berria R, Ma JZ, Dwivedi S, Havranek R, Fincke C, DeFronzo R, Bannayan GA, Schenker S, Cusi K. A placebo-controlled trial of pioglitazone in subjects with nonalcoholic steatohepatitis. *N Engl J Med* 2006;**355**:2297−307.
46. Serfaty L. Pioglitazone: the beginning of a new era for NASH? *J Hepatol* 2007;**47**:160−2.
47. Lang L. Pioglitazone trial for NASH: results show promise. *Gastroenterology* 2007;**132**:836−8.
48. Lavine JE, Schwimmer JB, Molleston JP, Scheimann AO, Murray KF, Abrams SH, Rosenthal P, Sanyal AJ, Robuck PR, Brunt EM, Unalp A, Tonascia J. Treatment of nonalcoholic fatty liver disease in children: TONIC trial design. *Contemp Clin Trials* 2010;**31**:62−70.
49. Mummadi RR, Kasturi KS, Chennareddygari S, Sood GK. Effect of bariatric surgery on nonalcoholic fatty liver disease: systematic review and meta-analysis. *Clin Gastroenterol Hepatol* 2008;**6**:1396−402.
50. Weiner RA. Surgical treatment of non-alcoholic steatohepatitis and non-alcoholic fatty liver disease. *Dig Dis* 2010;**28**:274−9.
51. Chavez-Tapia NC, Tellez-Avila FI, Barrientos-Gutierrez T, Mendez-Sanchez N, Lizardi-Cervera J, Uribe M. Bariatric surgery for non-alcoholic steatohepatitis in obese patients. *Cochrane Database Syst Rev* 2010. CD007340.

PREVENTION AND TREATMENT 1: DIET, EXERCISE, SUPPLEMENTS AND ALTERNATIVE MEDICINES

Antioxidants, Healthy Diet, and Diabetes: Oxidative Stress and Nutrition in Diabetes

Dario Pitocco, Francesca Martini, Francesco Zaccardi, Giovanni Ghirlanda

Diabetes Care Unit, Catholic University School of Medicine, Rome, Italy

Nutritional and Therapeutic Interventions for Diabetes and Metabolic Syndrome
DOI: 10.1016/B978-0-12-385083-6.00024-3

299

INTRODUCTION

Diabetes mellitus is characterized by an increased macrovascular morbidity and mortality, as well as by typical microangiopathic complications (retinopathy, nephropathy, and neuropathy). Oxidative stress is considered the main cause of these complications. Indeed, oxidative stress causes a complex dysregulation of cell metabolism and cell–cell homeostasis that has been implicated in both the pathogenesis of insulin resistance and β-cell dysfunction—the two most relevant mechanisms in the pathophysiology of type 2 diabetes, as well as in the pathogenesis of diabetic complications. Such considerations raise the concept that an antioxidant therapy may be of benefit in these patients. To test this hypothesis, several studies have been done, with conflicting results. In this chapter, we will focus on the effects of an "antioxidant therapy" and a "healthy" diet in diabetic subjects.

WHAT IS OXIDATIVE STRESS? ROS AND RNS

Biological systems living in aerobic conditions are exposed to oxidants. Generally, such oxidants are divided in reactive oxygen and nitrogen species (ROS and RNS, respectively); ROS is a collective term that describes the chemical species that are formed upon incomplete reduction of oxygen and includes the superoxide anion (O^{2-}), hydrogen peroxide (H_2O_2) and the hydroxyl radical (HO•), whereas RNS refers to all oxidation states and reactive adducts of nitric oxide synthase (NOS) products, ranging from nitric oxide (NO) to nitroxyl (NO^-), S-nitrosothiols (RSNOs) and peroxynitrite ($OONO^-$), the product of the reaction between NO and O^{2-}.[1] As ROS and RNS have critical biological functions essential for normal physiology overproduction or deficiency results in impaired homeostasis and associated pathology which is why oxidants are balanced by reductants (antioxidants). Production of ROS and RNS occur in response to a variety of stimuli including nutrients, such as glucose.[2,3] NADPH oxidase,[4] NOS,[5] and mitochondrial electron transfer[6] are the most relevant sources of RS (ROS and RNS), that can react with multiple cellular components (proteins, lipids, nucleic acids), generating reversible or irreversible oxidative modifications. Reactive species (RS) involvement in normal physiological processes involves carefully regulated production in a tight spatial-temporal manner, leading to reversible oxidative modifications. Pathophysiological processes mediated by RS are more likely to involve irreversible modifications of cellular components, as proteins, lipids, or DNA.

Oxidative Stress and Diabetes

Pathogenesis of Diabetes

Oxidative stress has a pivotal role in the pathogenesis of insulin resistance and β-cell dysfunction (Figure 24.1). These are the two most relevant mechanisms in the pathophysiology of type 2 diabetes. A large number of studies have evidenced the pivotal role of oxidative stress in insulin resistance states such as metabolic syndrome, obesity, and type 2 diabetes.[7–9] Decreased antioxidant capacity, increased production of ROS with oxidation products of lipids, DNA, and proteins have been reported in plasma, urine, and various tissues, suggesting systemic and organ-specific oxidative stress. Recent evidence for systemic oxidative stress includes the detection of increased circulating and urinary levels of the lipid peroxidation product F2-isoprostane (8-epi-prostaglandin F2α) in both type 1 and type 2 diabetic patients.[10,11] With regard to the relationship between oxidative stress and β-cell dysfunction, both glucotoxicity and lipotoxicity (that are diabetes-related phenomena that generate oxidative stress) are implicated in the pathogenesis of β-cell dysfunction.[12] Hyperglycemia and hyperlipidemia follow the primary pathogenesis of diabetes and exert

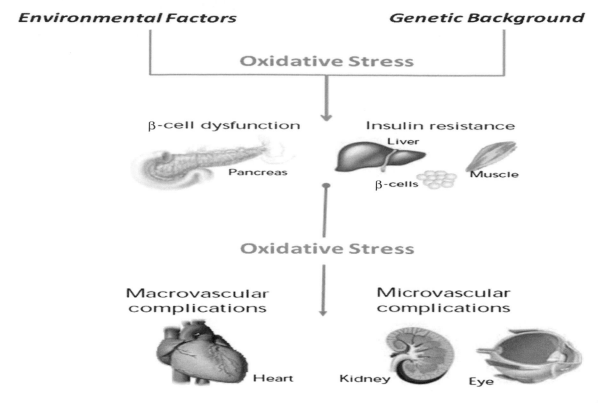

FIGURE 24.1 **Oxidative stress and diabetes.** *(See the color plate section at the back of the book.)*

additional toxic effects on β-cells. Indeed, evidence from *in vitro* and *in vivo* studies indicates that glucose and lipids are harmful to β-cells. Interestingly, some studies reported that lipotoxicity only occurs in the presence of concomitant elevated glucose levels.[13,14] Consequently, hyperglycemia might be a prerequisite for the negative effects of lipotoxicity.

Pathogenesis of Diabetic Complications

Cardiovascular risk factors promote the production of ROS. Imbalance between endogenous oxidants and antioxidants results in oxidative stress, a condition that contributes to impaired NO bioavailability and vascular dysfunction. *In vivo* studies revealed that oxidative stress due to hyperglycemia occurs before late complications become clinically evident.[15] This finding suggests that oxidative stress plays a crucial role in the pathogenesis of late diabetic complications. It has also been documented that endothelial cells in diabetic subjects fail to produce sufficient amount of NO and fail to relax in response to endothelium-dependent vasorelaxants (e.g., acetylcholine, bradykinin, shear stress, etc.).[16] Further clinical data have demonstrated that rapid glycemic swings are associated with an exacerbated degree of oxidant production in human diabetes,[17] and are deleterious to the endothelial function of type 2 diabetic patients.[18] Overall, these data outline the importance of steady glucose control and the potential involvement of oxidative and nitrosative stress in the pathogenesis of complications due to poorly controlled diabetes (Figure 24.1).

GENERAL ASPECTS OF ANTIOXIDANT THERAPY

There are two main approaches to modulate oxidative stress: preventing ROS/RNS or enhancing antioxidant defense. At the cellular level, it is possible to inhibit several sources of oxidative stress [i.e., mitochondrial uncoupling proteins 1 (UCP1), NADPH oxidases, iNOS] or enhance antioxidant defense (lipoic acid, vitamin C and E, GSH, increasing intracellular catalase or SOD activity). Different antioxidants, including vitamins C and E, lipoic acid, and flavanoids, have been shown to attenuate different markers of systemic oxidative stress in a variety of experimental animal models for obesity and diabetes, improving insulin and glucose levels, as well as reducing micro- and macrovascular dysfunction. Human intervention trials are limited to increase antioxidant defense by antioxidant supplementation. Enhanced insulin sensitivity has been demonstrated with lipoic acid,[19] vitamin E,[20] and vitamin C[21] in small-sized, short-term trials; however, these results have not been confirmed in other studies. Late diabetes complications known to associate with metabolic control also do not seem to be positively affected by antioxidant therapy. Consequently, despite some supporting evidence for the ability to improve insulin action with antioxidants, current clinical guidelines do not recommend antioxidant supplementation for the general population of persons with impaired insulin action, like type 2 diabetes.

ANTIOXIDANT MOLECULES AND DIABETES

Vitamin C (Ascorbic Acid)

Vitamin C (ascorbic acid) is a water-soluble vitamin that humans must obtain from the diet. It is a chain-breaking antioxidant that scavenges ROS directly, preventing the reactions that lead to protein glycation. Some prospective studies demonstrate the association between insufficient intake of dietary vitamin C diet and elevated cardiovascular risk, but do not support the hypothesis that its supplementation may reduce cardiovascular events in diabetic or other high-risk individuals.[22] It is possible that genetic differences may influence the effect of vitamin C supplementation on cardiovascular disease. The results of one randomized controlled trial using antioxidant therapy (1,000 mg/day of vitamin C + 800 IU/day of vitamin E), reanalyzed based on haptoglobin genotype showed a higher coronary atherosclerosis in diabetic postmenopausal women with two haptoglobin 1 gene copies but worsening of coronary atherosclerosis in those with two haptoglobin 2 gene copies. The significance of these findings is not clear, but they suggest that there may be a subpopulation of people with diabetes who will benefit from antioxidant therapy.[23]

Biotin

Biotin is a water-soluble that is generally classified as a B-complex vitamin; it is required by all organisms but can be synthesized only by bacteria, yeasts, molds, algae, and some plant species.[24] It is well known that overt biotin deficiency impairs glucose utilization in rats.[25] A human study investigation into blood biotin and glucose levels revealed that biotin was significantly lower in patients with type 2 diabetes than in healthy controls, and there was an inverse correlation between fasting blood glucose and biotin levels.[26] However, studies of the effect of supplemental biotin on blood glucose levels in humans are extremely limited, but they highlight the need for further research.

Niacin

Niacin is a water-soluble vitamin, which is also known as nicotinic acid or vitamin B3.

Nicotinamide is its derivative that is necessary to form nicotinamide adenine dinucleotide (NAD) and nicotinamide adenine dinucleotide phosphate (NADP) coenzymes. Some *in vitro* and animal-based evidences suggest that high nicotinamide levels protect pancreatic β-cells from various damages (such as toxic, inflammatory blood cells or ROS).[27] So, studies using pharmacologic doses of nicotinamide (up to 3 g/day) in nearly onset type 1 diabetes patients found improved β-cell function after 1 year of treatment without any clinical evidence of improved glycemic control.[28] Several studies for the prevention of type 1 diabetes in relatives and ICA-positive relatives of patients with type 1 diabetes yielded conflicting results. Unlike nicotinamide, nicotinic acid has not been found effective in the prevention of type 1 diabetes.[29]

Vitamin D

Vitamin D is a fat-soluble vitamin that is essential for maintaining normal calcium metabolism. Vitamin D3 (cholecalciferol) can be synthesized by humans in the skin upon exposure to ultraviolet-B (UVB) radiation from sunlight, or it can be obtained from the diet. The biologically active form of vitamin D, 1,25-dihydroxyvitamin D, has been found to modulate T-cell responses.[30] Some epidemiological studies have found that the prevalence of autoimmune diseases (and in particular of type 1 diabetes) increases as latitude increases, suggesting that lower exposure to UVB radiation and the resulting decreased endogenous vitamin D synthesis may play a role in the pathology of these diseases.[31] The results of several prospective cohort studies also suggest that adequate vitamin D intake could possibly decrease the risk of autoimmune diseases.[32] Vitamin D may play an immuno-modulatory/anti-inflammatory role reducing β-cells' autoimmune reaction in type 1 diabetes and may decrease insulin resistance in type 2

diabetes-mediated intra/extracellular β-cells' calcium balance. Additional vitamin D intake in childhood may reduce the risk of development of type 1 diabetes, while calcitriol supplementation in nearly onset type 1 diabetes is able to reduce temporally the required daily insulin dose. Vitamin D treatment reduces the risk of development of type 2 diabetes and may improve insulin secretion, glucose tolerance, and metabolic control.[33]

Vitamin E

The term vitamin E describes a family of eight antioxidants: four tocopherols (alpha-, beta-, gamma-, and delta-) and four tocotrienols (alpha-, beta-, gamma-, and delta-). Alpha-tocopherol is the only actively maintained form in the human body and may be found in the largest quantities in blood and tissues. It is a component of the total peroxyl radical antioxidant system that directly reacts with ROS, protecting from lipid peroxidation. Alpha-tocopherol supplementation of individuals with diabetes mellitus has been proposed because of diabetes increased oxidative stress and higher cardiovascular complications risk (heart attack and stroke). Studies of the effect of alpha-tocopherol supplementation on blood glucose control have been contradictory: some studies have shown that vitamin E supplementation improves insulin action and glucose disposal in type 2 diabetic and non-diabetic individuals, while other studies have reported minimal to no improvements in glucose metabolism.[34,35] Increased oxidative stress has also been documented in type 1 diabetes. One study reported that supplementing type 1 diabetic patients with 100 IU/day of synthetic alpha-tocopherol (equivalent to 45 mg RRR-alpha-tocopherol) for 1 month significantly improved both glycosylated hemoglobin and triglyceride levels, but noted non-significant improvements in blood glucose levels. Although there is reason to suspect that alpha-tocopherol supplementation may be beneficial in treatment for type 1 or type 2 diabetes, evidence from well-controlled clinical trials is lacking.[36]

Chromium

The biologically active form of chromium participates in glucose metabolism by enhancing insulin effects. In some controlled studies on impaired glucose tolerance, chromium supplementation (dose of about 200 mcg/day) was found to improve some measure of glucose utilization or to have beneficial effects on blood lipid profiles.[37] Individuals with type 2 diabetes have been found to have higher rates of urinary chromium loss than healthy individuals, especially those with long-lasting duration of disease.[38] Prior to 1997, well-designed studies of chromium supplementation in type 2 diabetes patients showed no improvement in blood glucose control, though they provided some evidence of reduced insulin levels and improved blood lipid profiles.[39] In 1997, a placebo-controlled trial indicated that chromium supplementation might be beneficial in the treatment of type 2 diabetes: participants took either a placebo or chromium picolinate at doses of 200 mcg/day and 1,000 mcg/day. At the end of 4 months, blood glucose levels were 15–19% lower in those who took 1,000 mcg/day compared with placebo and 200 mcg/day groups. Insulin and glycosylated hemoglobin levels were lower in those who took either 200 mcg/day or 1,000 mcg/day of chromium picolinate.[40] A recent review reported that 13 of 15 clinical studies found chromium picolinate improved at least one measure of glycemic control in diabetic patients. However, large-scale randomized controlled trials of chromium supplementation for type 2 diabetes are needed to determine chromium effectiveness in the treatment of type 2 diabetes.[41] The American Diabetes Asssociation (ADA) considers these studies inconclusive for

defining the possible utilization of chromium in diabetes therapy. A few studies have examined the effects of chromium supplementation on gestational diabetes: an observational study in pregnant women did not find serum chromium levels to be associated with measures of glucose tolerance or insulin resistance in late pregnancy, although serum chromium levels may not reflect tissue chromium levels. Women with gestational diabetes whose diets were supplemented with 4 mcg of chromium per kilogram of body weight daily as chromium picolinate for 8 weeks had decreased fasting blood glucose and insulin levels compared with those who took a placebo.[42]

Magnesium

Magnesium depletion is commonly associated with both type 1 and type 2 diabetes mellitus. Between 25% and 38% of diabetics have been found to have decreased serum levels of magnesium (hypomagnesemia). One cause of magnesium depletion may be increased urinary loss related to increased urinary excretion of glucose in poorly controlled diabetes.[43] One study reported that dietary magnesium supplements (400 mg/day) improved glucose tolerance in elderly individuals.[44] More recently, a randomized, double-blind, placebo-controlled study in 63 individuals with type 2 diabetes and hypomagnesemia found that those taking an oral magnesium chloride solution (2.5 g/day) for 16 weeks had improved measures of insulin sensitivity and glycemic control compared to those taking placebo.[45] Yet, a recent meta-analysis concluded that oral supplemental magnesium may lower fasting plasma glucose levels in diabetic individuals.[46] Due to conflicting reports, it is presently unclear whether magnesium supplementation has any therapeutic benefit in type 2 diabetic patients. However, correcting existing magnesium deficiencies may improve glucose metabolism and insulin sensitivity in diabetic individuals. Large-scale, well-controlled studies are needed to determine whether supplemental magnesium is useful in diabetes.[47]

Manganese

Low blood or tissue manganese levels may be associated with several chronic diseases. Manganese deficiency appears to be implicated in glucose intolerance in some animal species, but results about diabetic humans have generated mixed results. Although manganese appears to play a role in glucose metabolism, there is little evidence that manganese supplementation improves glucose tolerance in diabetic or non-diabetic individuals.[48]

Zinc

Moderate zinc deficiency may be relatively common in individuals with diabetes mellitus because of its increased urinary loss. In type 2 diabetics, supplementation with 30 mg/day of zinc for 6 months reduced plasma thiobarbituric acid reactive substances (TBARS), a non-specific measure of oxidative stress, without significantly affecting blood glucose control. Presently, the influence of zinc on glucose metabolism requires further study before high-dose zinc supplementation can be advocated for diabetics.[49]

Coenzyme Q10

Plasma levels of reduced coenzyme Q10 (CoQ10H2) have been found to be lower in diabetic patients than healthy controls when normalized to plasma cholesterol levels. However, supplementation of coenzyme Q10 neither improved glycemic control nor decreased insulin requirements in type 1 diabetics compared to placebo[50] and, similarly, did not improve glycemic control or serum lipid profiles in type 2 diabetics.[51] So, the authors of both studies concluded that coenzyme Q10 supplements could be used safely in diabetic patients as an adjunct therapy for cardiovascular diseases. There are some evidences that long-term coenzyme Q10 supplementation may improve insulin secretion and prevent progressive hearing loss in mitochondrial diabetes.[52]

Essential Fatty Acids

Hypertriglyceridemia is a common lipid abnormality in individuals with type 2 DM, and a number of randomized controlled trials have found that fish oil supplementation significantly lowers serum triglyceride levels in diabetic individuals.[53] A meta-analysis that combined the results of 18 randomized controlled trials in individuals with type 2 DM found that fish oil supplementation decreased serum triglycerides by 31 mg/dl compared to placebo, but had no effect on serum cholesterol, fasting glucose, or hemoglobin A1c concentrations; however, fish oil supplementation has been associated with a slight increase in LDL cholesterol levels. Moreover, there is little evidence that daily eicosapentaenoic acid and docosahexaenoic acid (EPA + DHA) intakes of less than 3 g/day adversely affect long-term glycemic control in diabetics.[54] The American Diabetes Association recommends that diabetic individuals increase omega-3 fatty acid consumption by consuming two to three 3-oz servings of fish weekly.[55]

Alpha Lipoic Acid

There is limited evidence that high doses of alpha lipoic acid (LA) can improve glucose utilization in individuals with type 2 DM. A small clinical trial in 13 patients with type 2 DM found that a single intravenous infusion of 1000 mg of racemic LA improved insulin-stimulated glucose disposal (insulin sensitivity) by 50% compared to a placebo infusion.[56] A placebo-controlled study of 72 patients with type 2 DM found that oral administration of racemic LA at doses of 600 mg/day, 1200 mg/day, or 1,800 mg/day improved insulin sensitivity by 25% after 4 weeks of treatment.[57] There were no significant differences among the three doses of LA, suggesting that 600 mg/day may be the maximum effective dose. Data from animal studies suggest that the R-isomer of LA may be more effective in improving insulin sensitivity than the S-isomer, but this possibility has not been tested in any published human trials.[58,59] The effect of LA supplementation on long-term blood glucose (glycemic) control has not been well-studied. Intravenous and oral LA are approved for the treatment of diabetic neuropathy. A meta-analysis that combined the results of four randomized controlled trials, including 1,258 diabetic patients, found that treatment with 600 mg/day of intravenous racemic LA for 3 weeks significantly reduced the symptoms of diabetic neuropathy to a clinically meaningful degree.[60] The efficacy of oral LA in the treatment of diabetic neuropathy is less clear. A large clinical trial randomly assigned more than 500 patients with type 2 DM and symptomatic peripheral neuropathy to one of the following treatments: (1) 600 mg/day of intravenous racemic LA for 3 weeks followed by 1,800 mg/day of oral racemic LA for 6 months; (2) 600 mg/day of intravenous racemic LA for 3 weeks followed by oral placebo for 6 months; or (3) intravenous placebo for 3 weeks followed by oral placebo for 6 months.[61] Although symptom scores did not differ significantly from baseline in any of the groups, assessments of sensory and motor deficits by physicians improved significantly after 3 weeks of intravenous LA therapy. Motor and sensory deficits were also somewhat improved at the end of 6 months of oral LA therapy, but the trend did not reach statistical significance. Another neuropathic complication of diabetes is cardiovascular autonomic neuropathy, which occurs in as many as 25% of diabetic patients. In a randomized controlled trial of 72 patients with type 2 DM and reduced heart rate variability, oral supplementation with 800 mg/day of racemic LA for 4 months resulted in significant improvement in two out of four measures of heart rate variability compared to placebo.[62] Overall, the available research suggests that treatment with 600 mg/day of intravenous LA for 3 weeks significantly reduces the symptoms of diabetic peripheral neuropathy, but the benefit of long-term oral LA supplementation is less clear: there are some evidences to suggest that oral LA may be beneficial in the treatment of diabetic peripheral neuropathy (600–1,800 mg/day) and cardiovascular autonomic neuropathy (800 mg/day). Both *in vivo* and *in vitro* studies have demonstrated the efficacy of alpha lipoic acid in the prevention of retina ischemia-reperfusion injuries, one of the most frequent causes of visual loss in diabetes.[63]

HEALTHY DIET

Type 2 diabetes is a complex metabolic disease in which lifestyle factors act on a gene-involved predisposition. However, there are conditions characterized by a dysregulation of glucose homeostasis that precede the onset of diabetes mellitus: these conditions include the impaired fasting glucose (IFG) and impaired glucose tolerance (IGT), in which the progression to diabetes is favored by obesity, reduced physical activity, and sedentary lifestyle. Overweight has been identified as the single most predictive factor for the development of type 2 diabetes while insulin resistance has been identified as a causative factor for type 2 diabetes. Several epidemiological and intervention studies have demonstrated the efficacy of the Mediterranean diet in the prevention and treatment of type 2 diabetes mellitus, also proving its effectiveness in the prevention of vascular complications (myocardial infarction), despite its carbohydrate content. One possible explanation is based on the consideration that these carbohydrates derive from low glycemic index/glycemic load ratio foods (whole and unrefined grains, rich in fiber).

Traditional Mediterranean diet is based on:

- High intake of vegetables (< 250 g/die);
- Legumes/fruit/nuts;
- Cereals (in particular whole grain, rich in fiber);
- Animal sources of proteins (primary fish, while red meat, poultry and eggs are consumed in moderate amounts);
- Olive oil as main fat source (containing vitamin E and monounsaturated fatty acid);
- Low to moderate milk and dairy products consumption;
- Low alcohol consumption (almost exclusively red wine during meals).[64]

In most clinical studies the adherence to the Mediterranean diet is assessed by a score, as suggested by Trichopoulou *et al.*, that evaluates protective (such as monounsaturated fatty acid, whole grain, vegetables, fish) *vs* non-protective (such as meat and dairy products) food intake.[65]

Regarding diabetes prevention, adherence to a Mediterranean diet has been shown both in cross-sectional and in prospective studies to lower the incidence of diabetes, also in patients with a recent myocardial infarction.[66,67] Regarding glycemic control and insulin sensitivity (assessed by HOMA index) in type 2 diabetes mellitus patients, a cross-sectional analysis showed an inverse association between adherence to Mediterranean diet and post-prandial glucose levels, as well as mean HbA1c concentration and a direct correlation with insulin sensitivity.[68] In particular, Esposito *et al.* demonstrate in nearly diagnosed type 2 diabetes patients a decreased fasting glucose and HbA1c levels effect, as well as lower HOMA index in Mediterranean diet compared with low-fat diet group.[69] Regarding the effects of the Mediterranean diet on cardiovascular risk in type 2 diabetes patients, several trials demonstrate an improvement of traditional cardiovascular risk factors (such as systolic blood pressure, HDL- and LDL-cholesterol) in patients receiving Mediterranean-type compared with a control diet.[70] In a short-term intervention trial the Mediterranean diet has been shown to reduce after 3 months, several causes of inflammation, such as monocytes adhesion molecules expression in patients with type 2 diabetes and at least three cardiovascular risk factors.[71] However, there are no prospective and controlled trials that have specifically investigated the role of the Mediterranean diet in the prevention of cardiovascular events and mortality in diabetes. A trial that includes a significant portion of diabetic patients demonstrates a benefit of Mediterranean diet in post-myocardial infarction reducing cardiovascular events.[72]

Nutritional therapy is proving able to compensate for about a third of diabetics; it poses several objectives, including:

1. Maintain normal blood glucose levels or close to normal lipid and blood pressure profile that ensures a low risk of cardiovascular disease.
2. Prevention and possible treatment of diabetes complications.
3. Improve healthy status through the modification of lifestyle and quality of food ingested.
4. Achieving the objectives above according with the personal choices, food preferences and usual lifestyle.

In specific conditions nutritional therapy may be permitted:

- To ensure optimal levels of nutrients for growth for young subjects with type 1 diabetes;
- To stimulate change in lifestyle to ensure an acceptable level of physical activity in young people with type 2 diabetes.
- For pregnant or breastfeeding women providing the right amount of nutrients for proper development of the pregnancy or breastfeeding;
- For subjects receiving insulin or oral insulin secretagogues to make sure they are well educated in hypoglycemia prevention;

- For individuals at risk of developing diabetes to encourage an increase in physical activity and a change in dietary habits aimed at a moderate weight loss or maintenance.[73,74]

Carbohydrates

Carbohydrate should be around 50–55% of the total energy requirement per day. Studies in healthy subjects and those at risk of developing diabetes have shown the importance of regularly consuming carbohydrates, in particular those derived from grain and cereals, fruit, vegetables, and low-fat milk: these recommendations are also valid for patients with type 1 diabetes and type 2 diabetes. Carbohydrates induce a response in terms of insulin production which may vary depending on the amount, the type (glucose, fructose, sucrose, lactose) and food preparation/processing of carbohydrate ingested. As is well known, carbohydrates evoke different responses depending on their chemical composition; the total amount of carbohydrates consumed is more important than source or type. Sucrose, although not prohibited, should be replaced by other carbohydrate sources. The use of fructose as a sweetener is not recommended. The use of fiber-rich foods should be encouraged in people with diabetes as well as in the general population. At least seven large prospective studies have found that higher whole-grain intakes are associated with significant reductions in the risk of developing type 2 diabetes mellitus. In the studies conducted in the US, those who consumed an average of about three daily servings of whole-grain foods had a risk of type 2 DM that was 21–30% lower than those who rarely or never consumed them.[73,75,76]

Legumes

Legumes are excellent sources of protein, low-glycemic index carbohydrates, essential micronutrients, and fiber. Low-glycemic load diets have been associated with reduced risk of developing type 2 diabetes in several large prospective studies.[77] Numerous clinical trials have shown that the consumption of low-glycemic index foods delays the return of hunger, decreases subsequent food intake, and increases the sensation of fullness compared to high-glycemic index foods.[78] Thus, diets rich in legumes may decrease the risk of type 2 diabetes by improving blood glucose control, decreasing insulin secretion, and delaying the return of hunger after a meal.

Proteins

The daily protein needs of healthy people are between 15 and 20% of the total energy, with variations according to age or some specific physiological states such as pregnancy. In diabetes patients there is no evidence to suggest changing (increase or decrease) the amount of protein consumption. A moderate decrease in protein intake was effective in combating diabetic nephropathy and should therefore be planned in diabetic patients with this complication.[73]

Fat

A major target in the diet of diabetics is reducing saturated fat and cholesterol intake. Diets low in saturated fat and high in carbohydrates cause a general improvement in lipid profile, while diets high in monounsaturated fat have proved to be effective in lowering LDL cholesterol levels. Although data are still scarce, diets rich in polyunsaturated fats appear to be very effective in lowering LDL cholesterol levels but do not show significant effects on blood glucose levels. In people with diabetes, saturated fat should provide no more than 10% of the total energy, 7% if LDL cholesterol is greater than 100 mg/dl. The cholesterol introduced with the diet should not exceed 300 mg per day, 200 if the level of LDL cholesterol is greater than 100 mg/dl. Polyunsaturated fatty acids should provide approximately 10% of daily energy.[73]

Alcohol

A recent meta-analysis of 15 prospective cohort studies concluded that moderate alcohol consumption reduces risk of type 2 diabetes by about 30%, but heavy alcohol consumption does not offer protection against the disease. With the exception of pregnant diabetic women and diabetic subjects in which there is simultaneously the presence of a disease or condition incompatible with alcohol, moderate amounts of alcohol (wine) may be consumed. In subjects who consume alcohol, sugar content should be taken into consideration in calculating the total carbohydrate ingested during the day.[79]

Fruits and Vegetables

Dietary patterns characterized by high intakes of fruits and vegetables are consistently associated with significant reductions in cardiovascular disease risk and type 2 diabetes mellitus.[80] Some studies suggest that higher intakes of fruits and vegetables are associated with improved blood glucose control and lower risk of developing type 2 diabetes.[81] Possible compounds in fruits and vegetables that may enhance glucose control include fiber and magnesium. Daily consumption of 2 cups (4 servings) of fruit and 2½ cups (5 servings) of vegetables are recommended for people who consume 2,000 kcal/day, while 1.5 cups of fruit (3 servings) and 2 cups (4 servings) of vegetables are recommended for people who consume 1,600 kcal/day. In both cases, consumption of a variety of different fruits and vegetables is recommended, including dark green, red, orange, yellow, blue, and purple fruits and vegetables, as well as legumes (peas and beans), onions, and garlic.[73]

Coffee

Studies demonstrate an inverse correlation between coffee consumption and both insulin sensitivity and diabetes risk. Evidences suggest that caffeine induces acute increases in β-cell insulin secretion with acute reduction of insulin sensitivity; this short-term effect may reflect acute decreased glucose storage due to epinephrine action. Studies using decaffeinated coffee led to similar results, suggesting the possible involvement of other substances contained in coffee such as chlorogenic acid and lignans.[82]

References

1. D'Autreaux B, Toledano MB. ROS as signalling molecules: mechanisms that generate specificity in ROS homeostasis. *Nat Rev Mol Cell Biol* 2007 Oct;**8**(10):813–24. Review.
2. Kanda M, Ihara Y, Murata H, Urata Y, Kono T, Yodoi J, Seto S, Yano K, Kondo T. Glutaredoxin modulates platelet-derived growth factor-dependent cell signaling by regulating the redox status of low molecular weight protein-tyrosine phosphatase. *J Biol Chem* 2006;**281**:28518–28.
3. Sundaresan M, Yu ZX, Ferrans VJ, Irani K, Finkel T. Requirement for generation of H2O2 for platelet-derived growth factor signal transduction. *Science* 1995;**270**:296–9.
4. Bedrad K, Krause KH. The NOX family of ROS-generating NADPH oxidases: physiology and pathophysiology. *Physiol Rev* 2007;**87**:245–313.
5. Pacher P, Beckman JS, Liaudet L. Nitric oxide and peroxynitrite in health and disease. *Physiol Rev* 2007;**87**:315–424.
6. Zhang DX, Gutterman DD. Mitochondrial reactive oxygen species-mediated signaling in endothelial cells. *Am J Physiol Heart Circ Physiol* 2007;**292**:H2023–31.
7. Atabek ME, Vatansev H, Erkul I. Oxidative stress in childhood obesity. *J Pediatr Endocrinol Metab* 2004;**17**:1063–8. 50-52.
8. Baynes JW. Role of oxidative stress in development of complications in diabetes. *Diabetes* 1991;**40**:405–12.
9. Block G, Dietrich M, Norkus EP, Morrow JD, Hudes M, Caan B, Packer L. Factors associated with oxidative stress in human populations. *Am J Epidemiol* 2002;**156**:274–85.
10. Davi G, Chiarelli F, Santilli F, Pomilio M, Vigneri S, Falco A, Basili S, Ciabattoni G, Patrono C. Enhanced lipid peroxidation and platelet activation in the

early phase of type 1 diabetes mellitus: role of inter-
leukin-6 and disease duration. *Circulation* 2003;
107:3199—203.

11. Davi G, Ciabattoni G, Consoli A, Mezzetti A, Falco A,
Santarone S, Pennese E, Vitacolonna E, Bucciarelli T,
Costantini F, Capani F, Patrono C. In vivo formation of
8-isoprostaglandin F2alpha and platelet activation in
diabetes mellitus: effects of improved metabolic
control and vitamin E supplementation. *Circulation*
1999;**99**:224—9.

12. Poitout V, Robertson RP. Glucolipotoxicity: fuel excess
and beta-cell dysfunction. *Endocr Rev* 2008;**29**(3):
351—66.

13. El-Assaad W, Buteau J, Peyot ML, Nolan C, Roduit R,
Hardy S, Joly E, Dbaibo G, Rosenberg L, Prentki M.
Saturated fatty acids synergize with elevated glucose
to cause pancreatic beta-cell death. *Endocrinology*
2003;**144**:4154—63.

14. Harmon JS, Gleason CE, Tanaka Y, Poitout V,
Robertson RP. Antecedent hyperglycemia, not hyperlipidemia, is associated with increased islet triacylglycerol content and decreased insulin gene
mRNA level in Zucker diabetic fatty rats. *Diabetes*
2001;**50**:2481—6.

15. Pitocco D, Zaccardi F, Di Stasio E, Romitelli F,
Martini F, Scaglione GL, Speranza D, Santini S,
Zuppi C, Ghirlanda G. Role of asymmetric-dimethyl-
larginine (ADMA) and nitrite/nitrate (NOx) in the
pathogenesis of oxidative stress in female subjects with
uncomplicated type 1 diabetes mellitus. *Diabetes Res
Clin Pract* 2009;**86**(3):173—6.

16. Avogaro A, Fadini GP, Gallo A, Pagnin E, de
Kreutzenberg S. Endothelial dysfunction in type 2
diabetes mellitus. *Nutr Metab Cardiovasc Dis*
2006;**16**(Suppl. 1):S39—45.

17. Monnier L, Mas E, Ginet C, Michel F, Villon L,
Cristol JP, Colette C. Activation of oxidative stress by
acute glucose fluctuations compared with sustained
chronic hyperglycemia in patients with type 2 diabetes. *JAMA* 2006;**295**(14):1681—7.

18. Ceriello A, Esposito K, Piconi L, Ihnat MA, Thorpe JE,
Testa R, Boemi M, Giugliano D. Oscillating glucose is
more deleterious to endothelial function and oxidative
stress than mean glucose in normal and type 2 diabetic
patients. *Diabetes* 2008;**57**(5):1349—54.

19. Evans JL, Goldfine ID. Alpha-Lipoic acid: a multifunctional antioxidant that improves insulin sensitivity
in patients with type 2 diabetes. *Diabetes Technol Ther*
2000;**2**:401—13.

20. Paolisso G, Di Maro G, Galzerano D, Cacciapuoti F,
Varricchio G, Varricchio M, D'Onofrio F. Pharmacological doses of vitamin E and insulin action in elderly
subjects. *Am J Clin Nutr* 1994;**59**:1291—6.

21. Hirashima O, Kawano H, Motoyama T, Hirai N,
Ohgushi M, Kugiyama K, Ogawa H, Yasue H.
Improvement of endothelial function and insulin
sensitivity with vitamin C in patients with coronary
spastic angina: possible role of reactive oxygen species.
J Am Coll Cardiol 2000;**35**:1860—6.

22. MRC/BHF Heart Protection Study of antioxidant
vitamin supplementation in 20,536 high-risk individuals: a randomized placebo-controlled trial. *Lancet*
2002;**360**(9326):23—33.

23. Levy AP, Friedenberg P, Lotan R, Ouyang P,
Tripputi M, Higginson L, Cobb FR, Tardif JC, Bittner V,
Howard BV. The effect of vitamin therapy on the
progression of coronary artery atherosclerosis varies
by haptoglobin type in postmenopausal women. *Diabetes Care* 2004;**27**(4):925—30.

24. Fernandez-Mejia C. Pharmacological effects of biotin.
J Nutr Biochem 2005;**1**:424—7.

25. Yoshikawa H, Tajiri Y, Sako Y, Hashimoto T,
Umeda F, Nawata H. Effects of biotin on glucotoxicity or lipotoxicity in rat pancreatic islets. *Metabolism*
2002 Feb;**51**(2):163—8.

26. Singer GM, Geohas J. The effect of chromium picolinate
and biotin supplementation on glycemic control in
poorly controlled patients with type 2 diabetes mellitus:
a placebo-controlled, double-blinded, randomized trial.
Diabetes Technol Ther 2006 Dec;**8**(6):636—43.

27. Al-Mohaissen MA, Pun SC, Frohlich JJ. Niacin: from
mechanisms of action to therapeutic uses. *Mini Rev
Med Chem* 2010 Mar;**10**(3):204—17. Review.

28. Lampeter EF, Klinghammer A, Scherbaum WA,
Heinze E, Haastert B, Giani G, Kolb H. The Deutsche
Nicotinamide Intervention Study: an attempt to
prevent type 1 diabetes. DENIS Group. *Diabetes*
1998;**47**(6):980—4.

29. Greenbaum CJ, Kahn SE, Palmer JP. Nicotinamide's
effects on glucose metabolism in subjects at risk for
IDDM. *Diabetes* 1996 Nov;**45**(11):1631—4.

30. Maruotti N, Cantatore FP. Vitamin D and the immune
system. *J Rheumatol* 2010 Mar;**37**(3):491—5. Epub 2010
Jan 15. Review.

31. Grant WB. Hypothesis—ultraviolet-B irradiance and
vitamin D reduce the risk of viral infections and thus
their sequelae, including autoimmune diseases and
some cancers. *Photochem Photobiol.* 2008 Mar-
Apr;**84**(2):356—65. Epub 2008 Jan 7. Review.

32. Pelajo CF, Lopez-Benitez JM, Miller LC. Vitamin D and
autoimmune rheumatologic disorders. *Autoimmun Rev.*
2010 May;**9**(7):507—10. Epub 2010 Feb 8. Review.

33. Danescu LG, Levy S, Levy J. Vitamin D and diabetes
mellitus. *Endocrine* 2009;**35**:11—7.

34. Paolisso G, D'Amore A, Giugliano D, Ceriello A,
Varricchio M, D'Onofrio F. Pharmacologic doses of

vitamin E improve insulin action in healthy subjects and non-insulin-dependent diabetic patients. *Am J Clin Nutr* 1993;**57**(5):650—6.

35. Paolisso G, D'Amore A, Galzerano D, Balbi V, Giugliano D, Varricchio M, D'Onofrio F. Daily vitamin E supplements improve metabolic control but not insulin secretion in elderly type II diabetic patients. *Diabetes Care* 1993;**16**(11):1433—7.

36. Jain SK, McVie R, Jaramillo JJ, Palmer M, Smith T. Effect of modest vitamin E supplementation on blood glycosylated hemoglobin and triglyceride levels and red cell indices in type I diabetic patients. *J Am Coll Nutr* 1996;**15**(5):458—61.

37. Mertz W. Chromium in human nutrition: a review. *J Nutr* 1993;**123**(4):626—33.

38. Morris BW, MacNeil S, Hardisty CA, Heller S, Burgin C, Gray TA. Chromium homeostasis in patients with type II (NIDDM) diabetes. *J Trace Elem Med Biol* 1999;**13**(1—2):57—61.

39. Hellerstein MK. Is chromium supplementation effective in managing type II diabetes? *Nutr Rev* 1998; **56**(10):302—6.

40. Anderson RA, Cheng N, Bryden NA, Polansky MM, Chi J, Feng J. Elevated intakes of supplemental chromium improve glucose and insulin variables in individuals with type 2 diabetes. *Diabetes* 1997;**46**(11): 1786—91.

41. Broadhurst CL, Domenico P. Clinical studies on chromium picolinate supplementation in diabetes mellitus—a review. *Diabetes Technol Ther* 2006;**8**(6): 677—87.

42. Gunton JE, Hams G, Hitchman R, McElduff A. Serum chromium does not predict glucose tolerance in late pregnancy. *Am J Clin Nutr* 2001;**73**(1):99—104.

43. Tosiello L. Hypomagnesemia and diabetes mellitus. A review of clinical implications. *Arch Intern Med* 1996;**156**(11):1143—8.

44. Paolisso G, Sgambato S, Gambardella A, Pizza G, Tesauro P, Varricchio M, D'Onofrio F. Daily magnesium supplements improve glucose handling in elderly subjects. *Am J Clin Nutr* 1992;**55**(6):1161—7.

45. Rodriguez-Moran M, Guerrero-Romero F. Oral magnesium supplementation improves insulin sensitivity and metabolic control in type 2 diabetic subjects: a randomized double-blind controlled trial. *Diabetes Care* 2003;**26**(4):1147—52.

46. Yokota K, Kato M, Lister F, Ii H, Hayakawa T, Kikuta T, Kageyama S, Tajima N. Clinical efficacy of magnesium supplementation in patients with type 2 diabetes. *J Am Coll Nutr* 2004;**23**(5):506S—9S.

47. Song Y, He K, Levitan EB, Manson JE, Liu S. Effects of oral magnesium supplementation on glycemic control in Type 2 diabetes: a meta-analysis of randomized double-blind controlled trials. *Diabet Med* 2006;**23**(10):1050—6.

48. Kazi TG, Afridi HI, Kazi N, Jamali MK, Arain MB, Jalbani N, Kandhro GA. Copper, chromium, manganese, iron, nickel, and zinc levels in biological samples of diabetes mellitus patients. *Biol Trace Elem Res* 2008;**122**(1):1—18.

49. Anderson RA, Roussel AM, Zouari N, Mahjoub S, Matheau JM, Kerkeni A. Potential antioxidant effects of zinc and chromium supplementation in people with type 2 diabetes mellitus. *J Am Coll Nutr* 2001;**20**(3): 212—8.

50. Henriksen JE, Andersen CB, Hother-Nielsen O, Vaag A, Mortensen SA, Beck-Nielsen H. Impact of ubiquinone (coenzyme Q10) treatment on glycaemic control, insulin requirement and well-being in patients with Type 1 diabetes mellitus. *Diabet Med* 1999;**16**(4): 312—8.

51. Eriksson JG, Forsen TJ, Mortensen SA, Rohde M. The effect of coenzyme Q10 administration on metabolic control in patients with type 2 diabetes mellitus. *Biofactors* 1999;**9**(2—4):315—8.

52. Suzuki S, Hinokio Y, Ohtomo M, Hirai M, Hirai A, Chiba M, Kasuga S, Satoh Y, Akai H, Toyota T. The effects of coenzyme Q10 treatment on maternally inherited diabetes mellitus and deafness, and mitochondrial DNA 3243 (A to G) mutation. *Diabetologia* 1998;**41**(5):584—8.

53. Montori VM, Farmer A, Wollan PC, Dinneen SF. Fish oil supplementation in type 2 diabetes: a quantitative systematic review. *Diabetes Care* 2000; **23**(9):1407—15.

54. Hartweg J, Farmer AJ, Perera R, Holman RR, Neil HA. Meta-analysis of the effects of n-3 polyunsaturated fatty acids on lipoproteins and other emerging lipid cardiovascular risk markers in patients with type 2 diabetes. *Diabetologia* 2007;**50**(8):1593—602.

55. Franz MJ, Bantle JP, Beebe CA, Brunzell JD, Chiasson JL, Garg A, Holzmeister LA, Hoogwerf B, Mayer-Davis E, Mooradian AD, Purnell JQ, Wheeler M. American Diabetes Association. Evidence-based nutrition principles and recommendations for the treatment and prevention of diabetes and related complications. *Diabetes Care* 2003;**26**(Suppl. 1): S51—61.

56. Jacob S, Henriksen EJ, Schiemann AL, Simon I, Clancy DE, Tritschler HJ, Jung WI, Augustin HJ, Dietze GJ. Enhancement of glucose disposal in patients with type 2 diabetes by alpha-lipoic acid. *Arzneimittelforschung* 1995;**45**(8):872—4.

57. Jacob S, Rett K, Henriksen EJ, Haring HU. Thioctic acid—effects on insulin sensitivity and glucose-metabolism. *Biofactors* 1999;**10**(2—3):169—74.

58. Estrada DE, Ewart HS, Tsakiridis T, Volchuk A, Ramlal T, Tritschler H, Klip A. Stimulation of glucose uptake by the natural coenzyme alpha-lipoic acid/thioctic acid: participation of elements of the insulin signaling pathway. *Diabetes* 1996;**45**(12):1798–804.

59. Streeper RS, Henriksen EJ, Jacob S, Hokama JY, Fogt DL, Tritschler HJ. Differential effects of lipoic acid stereoisomers on glucose metabolism in insulin-resistant skeletal muscle. *Am J Physiol* 1997;**273**(1 Pt 1): E185–91.

60. Ziegler D, Nowak H, Kempler P, Vargha P, Low PA. Treatment of symptomatic diabetic polyneuropathy with the antioxidant alpha-lipoic acid: a meta-analysis. *Diabet Med* 2004;**21**(2):114–21.

61. Ziegler D, Hanefeld M, Ruhnau KJ, Hasche H, Lobisch M, Schütte K, Kerum G, Malessa R. Treatment of symptomatic diabetic polyneuropathy with the antioxidant alpha-lipoic acid: a 7-month multicenter randomized controlled trial (ALADIN III Study). ALADIN III Study Group. Alpha-Lipoic Acid in Diabetic Neuropathy. *Diabetes Care* 1999; **22**(8):1296–301.

62. Ziegler D, Schatz H, Conrad F, Gries FA, Ulrich H, Reichel G. Effects of treatment with the antioxidant alpha-lipoic acid on cardiac autonomic neuropathy in NIDDM patients. A 4-month randomized controlled multicenter trial (DEKAN Study). Deutsche Kardiale Autonome Neuropathie. *Diabetes Care* 1997;**20**(3):369–73.

63. Johnsen-Soriano S, Garcia-Pous M, Arnal E, Sancho-Tello M, Garcia-Delpech S, Miranda M, Bosch-Morell F, Diaz-Llopis M, Navea A, Romero FJ. Early lipoic acid intake protects retina of diabetic mice. *Free Radic Res* 2008 Jul;**42**(7):613–7.

64. Biesalski HK. Diabetes preventive components in the Mediterranean diet. *Eur J Nutr* 2004 Mar;**43**(Suppl. 1): I/26–30. Review.

65. Trichopoulou A, Costacou T, Bamia C, Trichopoulos D. Adherence to a Mediterranean diet and survival in a Greek population. *N Engl J Med* 2003 Jun 26;**348**(26):2599–608.

66. Martínez-González MA, de la Fuente-Arrillaga C, Nunez-Cordoba JM, Basterra-Gortari FJ, Beunza JJ, Vazquez Z, Benito S, Tortosa A, Bes-Rastrollo M. Adherence to Mediterranean diet and risk of developing diabetes: prospective cohort study. *BMJ* 2008 Jun 14;**336**(7657):1348–51. Epub 2008 May 29.

67. Mozaffarian D, Marfisi R, Levantesi G, Silletta MG, Tavazzi L, Tognoni G, Valagussa F, Marchioli R. Incidence of new-onset diabetes and impaired fasting glucose in patients with recent myocardial infarction and the effect of clinical and lifestyle risk factors. *Lancet* 2007 Aug 25;**370**(9588):667–75.

68. Esposito K, Maiorino MI, Di Palo C, Giugliano D. Campanian Postprandial Hyperglycemia Study Group. Adherence to a Mediterranean diet and glycaemic control in Type 2 diabetes mellitus. *Diabet Med* 2009 Sep;**26**(9):900–7.

69. Esposito K, Maiorino MI, Ciotola M, Di Palo C, Scognamiglio P, Gicchino M, Petrizzo M, Saccomanno F, Beneduce F, Ceriello A, Giugliano D. Effects of a Mediterranean-style diet on the need for antihyperglycemic drug therapy in patients with newly diagnosed type 2 diabetes: a randomized trial. *Ann Intern Med* 2009 Sep 1;**151**(5):306–14. Erratum in: *Ann Intern Med* 2009 Oct 20;151(8):591.

70. Elhayany A, Lustman A, Abel R, Attal-Singer J, Vinker S. A low carbohydrate Mediterranean diet improves cardiovascular risk factors and diabetes control among overweight patients with type 2 diabetes mellitus: a 1-year prospective randomized intervention study. *Diabetes Obes Metab* 2010 Mar;**12**(3):204–9.

71. Llorente-Cortés V, Estruch R, Mena MP, Ros E, González MA, Fitó M, Lamuela-Raventós RM, Badimon L. Effect of Mediterranean diet on the expression of pro-atherogenic genes in a population at high cardiovascular risk. *Atherosclerosis* 2010 Feb;**208**(2):442–50. Epub 2009 Aug 8.

72. Panagiotakos DB, Dimakopoulou K, Katsouyanni K, Bellander T, Grau M, Koenig W, Lanki T, Pistelli R, Schneider A, Peters A. AIRGENE Study Group. Mediterranean diet and inflammatory response in myocardial infarction survivors. *Int J Epidemiol* 2009 Jun;**38**(3):856–66. Epub 2009 Feb 24.

73. ADA. Nutrition principles and recommendations in diabetes. *Diabetes Care* January 2004;**27**(S36). doi:10.2337/diacare.27.2007.S36.

74. Franz MJ, Powers MA, Leontos C, Holzmeister LA, Kulkarni K, Monk A, Wedel N, Gradwell E. The evidence for medical nutrition therapy for type 1 and type 2 diabetes in adults. *J Am Diet Assoc* 2010 Dec;**110**(12):1852–89. Review.

75. de Munter JS, Hu FB, Spiegelman D, Franz M, van Dam RM. Whole grain, bran, and germ intake and risk of type 2 diabetes: a prospective cohort study and systematic review. *PLoS Med* 2007; **4**(8):e261.

76. Pegklidou K, Nicolaou I, Demopoulos VJ. Nutritional overview on the management of type 2 diabetes and the prevention of its complications. *Curr Diabetes Rev* 2010 Nov;**6**(6):400–9. Review.

77. Krishnan S, Rosenberg L, Singer M, Hu FB, Djoussé L, Cupples LA, Palmer JR. Glycemic index, glycemic load, and cereal fiber intake and risk of type 2

diabetes in US black women. *Arch Intern Med* 2007;**167**(21):2304—9.

78. Ludwig DS. Dietary glycemic index and the regulation of body weight. *Lipids* 2003;**38**(2):117—21.

79. Koppes LL, Dekker JM, Hendriks HF, Bouter LM, Heine RJ. Moderate alcohol consumption lowers the risk of type 2 diabetes: a meta-analysis of prospective observational studies. *Diabetes Care* 2005;**28**(3):719—25.

80. Winer N, Sowers JR. Epidemiology of diabetes. *J Clin Pharmacol* 2004;**44**(4):397—405.

81. Hamer M, Chida Y. Intake of fruit, vegetables, and anti-oxidants and risk of type 2 diabetes: systematic review and meta-analysis. *J Hypertens* 2007;**25**(12):2361—9.

82. van Dam RM, Hu FB. Coffee consumption and risk of type 2 diabetes: a systematic review. *JAMA* 2005;**294**(1): 97—104.

Molecular Mechanisms of Diabetes Prevention by Structurally Diverse Antioxidants

Lucyna A. Wozniak*, Katarzyna Cypryk†, Marzena Wojcik*

*Department of Structural Biology, Faculty of Biomedical Sciences and Postgraduate Education, Medical University of Lodz, Lodz, Poland †Diabetology and Metabolic Diseases Department, Medical University of Lodz, Poland

INTRODUCTION

Reactive oxygen species (ROS) are highly reactive molecules possessing one or more unpaired electrons, which are generated in living systems in the presence of molecular oxygen (dioxygen, O_2) as an electron acceptor by, among others, four endogenous sources: mitochondria,

Nutritional and Therapeutic Interventions for Diabetes and Metabolic Syndrome
DOI: 10.1016/B978-0-12-385083-6.00025-5

phagocytic cells (neutrophils, eosinophils, macrophages), peroxisomes, and cytochrome P450 enzymes. ROS include either oxygen radicals like superoxide ($^{\bullet}O_2^-$), hydroxyl ($HO^{\bullet}$), hydroperoxyl ($HROO^{\bullet -}$), peroxyl ($ROO^{\bullet}$), or non-radical species such as hydrogen peroxide (H_2O_2) or singlet oxygen ($^1O_2$). Besides ROS in aerobic organisms, there are reactive nitrogen species (RNS) including free radicals, such as nitric oxide ($^{\bullet}NO$) and nitrogen dioxide ($^{\bullet}NO_2^-$), as well as non-radicals like peroxynitrite ($ONOO^-$), nitrous oxide (HNO_2) and alkyl peroxynitrates (RONOO).

Under physiological conditions, ROS/RNS may play a dual function in humans. Their beneficial effects occur at low-to-moderate concentrations and include participation in both defense against infectious agents and cell signal transduction cascades, leading to activation of several transcription factors responsible for the expression regulation of genes relevant for cell growth and differentiation. In contrast,

when there is simultaneous ROS/RNS overproduction and impaired antioxidant defense mechanisms, including superoxide dismutase (SOD), catalase (CAT), glutathione peroxidase (GPx), or glutathione reductase (GSR) activity, a state of oxidative/nitrosative stress exists. This imbalance between ROS/RNS formation and their elimination triggers various physiological and pathological responses in cells either resulting in damage of cellular biomolecules such as DNA, proteins, and lipids or alteration of specific signaling pathways [e.g., mitogen-activated protein kinases (MAPKs), the phosphoinositide 3-kinase (PI3K)/protein kinase B (Akt) pathway, protein kinase C (PKC)], and transcription factors [(e.g., nuclear factor κB (NF-κB), activator protein 1 (AP-1), nuclear factor erythroid 2-related factor 2 (Nrf2), FOXO proteins, hypoxia-inducible factors (HIF)], leading to changes in gene expression, and ultimately, to the development of numerous chronic diseases (Figure 25.1).[1,2] Among them,

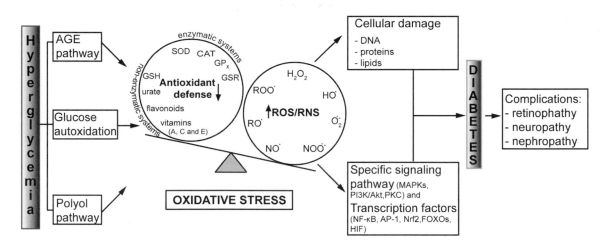

FIGURE 25.1 **Hyperglycemia-induced oxidative stress in diabetes and its complications.** Chronic hyperglycemia induces oxidative stress, i.e. an imbalance between excess formation and/or impaired removal of ROS/RNS by the antioxidant defense system, through various mechanisms, involving glycation-formation of AGE products, glucose autoxidation, or activation of polyol pathway. Hyperglycemia-induced oxidative stress exerts a range of pathophysiological responses in cells either as a result of cellular damage of DNA, proteins and lipids or by altering specific signaling pathways and/or activity several transcription factors, leading to diabetes and its complications (i.e. neuropathy, nephropathy, and retinopathy).

diabetes mellitus (DM) is one of the most abundant worldwide metabolic diseases, resulting in both morbidity and mortality that affected approximately 171 million people in 2000 and is expected to double by 2030.[3] At present, a large body of experimental evidence supports the idea that the increased oxidative stress resulting from hyperglycemia is one of the major mechanisms contributing to the development and progression of DM with and without diabetes-associated complications like neuropathy, nephropathy, and retinopathy.[4]

The mechanisms of hyperglycemia-induced ROS production in diabetes are partly known, including: (i) glucose autoxidation resulting in generation of $HO^{\bullet}$ radicals; (ii) enhanced glucose metabolism through the polyol pathway (also known as the sorbitol-aldose reductase pathway) accompanied by an increase in $O_2^{\bullet-}$ level; and (iii) increased formation of advanced glycation end products (AGEs) as a consequence of a non-enzymatic glucose reaction with proteins (Figure 25.1). In light of the knowledge that hyperglycemia-induced oxidative stress may result in the pathogenesis of diabetes and its complications, it has been presumed that an antioxidant strategy might be an effective approach in reducing oxidative stress in diabetes. To this end, the potential therapeutic value of several antioxidants has been demonstrated in many systems. These studies suggest that some antioxidants, particularly α-lipoic acid (LA) and polyphenolic green tea catechins (GTCs), have the potential to become promising new therapeutic agents for diabetes treatment, although further studies of the molecular mechanisms of their action are required.

This chapter is divided into sections, each discussing a specific aspect of the signal transduction pathways of response to oxidative stress in diabetes, and postulates the molecular mechanisms by which natural antioxidants like LA and GTCs, especially epigallocatechin gallate (EGCG), may act as antidiabetic agents.

ROS-MEDIATED MECHANISMS OF T2DM

Unlike type 1, type 2 diabetes mellitus (T2DM) is characterized by insulin resistance in peripheral tissues (i.e. the liver, skeletal muscle, and adipose tissue) and either accelerated apoptosis or dysfunction of the pancreatic β-cells. Although the pathogenesis of T2DM is not completely understood, the role of increased ROS production in the progression of insulin resistance as well as pancreatic β-cell dysfunction has been implicated.[5] For example, studies by Tirosh et al.[6] on the cellular mechanisms by which oxidative stress disrupts insulin action in 3T3-L1 adipocytes, disclosed that excess ROS impaired the compartment-specific activation of phosphatidylinositol 3-kinase (PI3K), insulin receptor substrate-1 (IRS-1) redistribution, and protein kinase B (PKB) activation induced by insulin, leading to impaired insulin-stimulated glucose transporter 4 (GLUT4) translocation and glucose transport. Additionally, in diabetic patients, treatment with the antioxidant LA improved insulin resistance, implying that ROS are involved in vivo in the progression of insulin resistance.[7] This section includes a brief summary of recently published and interesting findings with respect to some of the underlying mechanisms by which oxidative stress under diabetic conditions triggers pathological responses in the pancreatic β-cells and muscle cells.

ROS and the Progression of β-Cell Dysfunction

Several lines of evidence have implicated oxidative stress contribution in the progression of β-cell dysfunction in T2DM. It is well established that elevated glucose concentration may generate excessive levels of ROS resulting in adverse structural and functional changes, i.e. glucose toxicity, in the pancreatic β-cells. For example, chronic exposure of the β-cell line

HIT-T15 to high glucose concentrations diminished insulin gene expression, insulin content, and glucose-induced insulin secretion. Moreover, these parameters were linked to decreased post-transcriptional levels of pancreas duodenum homeobox-1 (PDX1) and MafA, respectively, being two critical insulin promoter transcription factors.[8,9]

In Zucker diabetic fatty (ZDF) rats, a relationship was observed between increased hyperglycemia and defects in PDX1 and MafA binding to DNA, as well as decreased insulin mRNA levels, insulin content, and glucose-induced insulin secretion.[9] In order to confirm whether these effects occur as a result of increased ROS production, ZDF rats were treated with two antioxidants: N-acetylcysteine (NAC) and aminoguanine (AG). It was found that both NAC and AG prevented an increase in formation of the oxidative stress markers in blood and ameliorated development of hyperglycemia, glucose intolerance, and defective insulin secretion as well as decrements in β-cell insulin content, insulin gene expression, and PDX1 binding to the insulin gene promoter.[8] Thus, these results clearly indicate that chronic oxidative stress is the major mechanism for glucose toxicity in the pancreatic β-cells. In a diabetic state, the islets are at a high risk of oxidative damage by ROS since β-cells, which express the glucose transporter 2 (GLUT2) responsible for glucose uptake, are defenseless to ROS due to low levels and activities of antioxidant enzymes like CAT and GPx.[10]

Interestingly, with regard to the beneficial effects evoked by antioxidants in the protection of β-cells against glucose toxicity, Shao et al.[11] found that candesartan, an angiotensin II type 1 receptor blocker (ARB), improved glucose tolerance with an increased serum insulin level in db/db mice, and these changes were accompanied by an increase in β-cell mass and a decrease in both expression of NAD(P)H oxidase and ROS markers in β-cells. Thus, candesartan intervention might reduce ROS levels and eventually protect β-cells against their progressive damage, confirming the hypothesis that ROS are involved in β-cell glucose toxicity found in diabetes.

Apart from elevated glucose level, increased levels of free fatty acids (FFAs) in blood (i.e. lipotoxicity) may also induce ROS formation leading to a reduction of insulin secretion and β-cell dysfunction, implicating lipotoxicity in T2DM.[12] However, it has been suggested that while lipotoxicity requires concomitant hyperglycemia to damage the islet's function, glucose toxicity can exert harmful effects on the islet in the absence of elevated circulating triglycerides.[9] The c-Jun N-terminal kinase (JNK) pathway and the p38 MAPK pathway, the major MAPK pathways activated by oxidative stress, have been shown to involve β-cell dysfunction. The mechanism by which both hyperglycemia- and/or hyperlipidemia-mediated ROS can affect β-cell dysfunction has been reported to occur through activation of the JNK pathway, leading to stimulation of PDX1 translocation from the nucleus to the cytoplasm. This nucleocytoplasmic PDX1 translocation causes a reduction of the PDX1 activity and subsequently, suppression of insulin gene transcription, resulting in reduction of biosynthesis and secretion of insulin (Figure 25.2).[13,14] However, the precise mechanism by which the JNK pathway induces nuclear export of PDX1 is still unknown. Newer insights into the molecular mechanisms of the JNK-induced deterioration of β-cell function was provided by Kawamori et al.,[15] whose studies revealed that the forkhead transcription factor Foxo1 (previously known as FKHR), playing a key role in apoptosis, cellular proliferation, differentiation and glucose metabolism through regulating the transcription of various target genes, appears to be a mediator between the JNK pathway and PDX-1 in pancreatic β-cells. The authors reported that Foxo1 may be involved in the oxidative stress-induced, JNK pathway-mediated nucleocytoplasmic

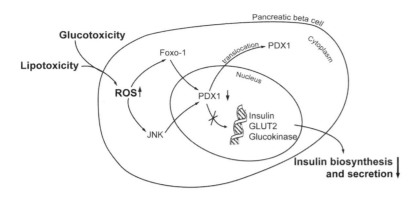

FIGURE 25.2 **Progression of pancreatic β-cell dysfunction in type 2 diabetes induced by ROS.** ROS induced by hyperglycemia (glucotoxicity) or hyperlipidemia (lipotoxicity) under diabetic conditions, cause activation of the JNK and Foxo 1 pathways in pancreatic β-cells. ROS and the activated JNK pathway stimulate the Foxo 1 induced nucleocytoplasmic translocation of PDX1, which leads to the reduction of PDX1 activity resulting in suppression of insulin biosynthesis and secretion.

translocation of PDX1 and, moreover, this transcription factor can directly affect the nuclear expression of PDX1 by altering the intracellular localization of PDX1.[15] However, the precise mechanism of the Foxo1-induced PDX1 translocation under oxidative stress conditions remains to be clarified. Thus, the molecular mechanism for β-cell dysfunction in diabetic state might be explained, at least partially, through the oxidative stress-induced nuclear translocation of Foxo1 through activation of the JNK pathway, leading to the nucleocytoplasmic translocation of PDX1.

It should be noted, with respect to the JNK pathway in pancreatic β-cells, that there are yet many unanswered questions concerning identification of the β-cell-specific roles of JNK, and the molecular mechanisms of JNK function in β-cells that contribute to the etiology of T2DM. Nevertheless, it can be concluded that a successful suppression of the JNK pathway could improve insulin resistance and glucose intolerance. Since both the JNK and IkappaB kinase β (IKK) pathways are activated by several factors including ROS, endoplasmic reticulum (ER) stress, FFAs, and inflammatory cytokines like TNF-α, they are implicated in the development of insulin resistance found in T2DM. Therefore, it is likely that activation of stress signaling *via* the JNK and IKK pathways is involved in the development of insulin resistance and that

such pathways could be therapeutic targets for diabetes.[16,17]

ROS and Muscle Cells

ROS are produced by several different pathways under diabetic conditions and involved in the deterioration of function of various cells. Hyperglycemia induces ROS through activation of the glycation reaction and electron transport chain in mitochondria. In addition, AGEs, insulin, and angiotensin II induce ROS through activation of NADPH oxidase. Their elevated concentrations lead to development of atherosclerosis. It has been shown that the membrane-bound NADPH oxidase is one of the major sources of ROS in muscles and that NADPH oxidase-derived ROS play a critical role in the development of atherosclerosis. Indeed, it has been reported that ROS production in atherosclerotic human coronary arteries is associated with NADPH oxidase subunit p22 phox.[18] NADPH oxidase is activated by various factors such as AGEs, insulin, and angiotensin II. Moreover, it was shown that high glucose levels stimulate ROS production through the activation of NADPH oxidase and that they are associated with significant increases in p22 phox level in rat and human diabetic arteries.[19] Therefore, it is possible that such increased expression of p22 phox contributes to the development of atherosclerosis.

ROS cause the increased expression of various adhesion molecules such as intercellular adhesion molecule 1 (ICAM-1) and vascular cell adhesion molecule 1 (VCAM-1), which leads to inflammatory cell recruitment. The molecules decrease nitric oxide levels, which leads to endothelial cell dysfunction. ROS modulate expression of various growth factors and several growth related protooncogenes such as c-Myc, c-Fos and c-Jun.[20] High concentration of ROS causes the increased expression of growth factors and activates various stress signaling such as JNK and Pim-1, which leads to proliferation of smooth muscle cells.[21]

MOLECULAR MECHANISMS AND THERAPEUTIC POTENTIAL OF CHOSEN ANTIOXIDANTS

Given that the oxidative stress mediated through hyperglycemia-induced production of ROS/RNS contributes to development and progression of DM and its complications, the numerous efforts of many researchers have been focused on searching for naturally occurring antioxidants, including LA and polyphenolic green tea catechins, that might effectively protect humans against oxidative stress and reduce its role in the pathogenesis of this disease. Even though these antioxidants represent natural compounds, they are considered as potential pharmacological agents and, therefore, certain criteria must be met for them to be effective in experimental cell-based systems and the clinical setting, i.e. ROS scavenging, metal chelation, bioavailability, low toxicity, and interaction with other antioxidants. The present section describes the antioxidant properties of structurally varied compounds like LA and polyphenolic green tea catechins and their antidiabetic mechanisms proposed based on studies in tissue cultures, animal models, and human epidemiological trials.

α-Lipoic Acid (LA)

α-Lipoic acid [known as (R)-5-(1,2-dithiolan-3-yl)pentanoic or thioctic acid], along with its reduced form, dihydrolipoic acid (DHLA), are the eight-carbon dithiol compounds exhibiting an amphiphilic character. Their structural hallmark is the presence of one asymmetric carbon, thereby they exist in the R- and S-enantiomeric forms (the R-LA and the S-LA). Of these two isomers, only the R-LA is synthesized in mitochondria of plants and animals from octanoic acid and cysteine as a sulfur source.[22] Endogenously, the R-LA plays an essential role in energy metabolism as a cofactor covalently bound to mitochondrial α-ketoacid dehydrogenases involved in oxidative metabolism.[23] As opposed to the endogenous R-LA form, there are exogenous LA sources like leafy green vegetables and meats, where R-LA is covalently bound to the ε-amino moiety of lysine residues in proteins (the complex called lipollysine), and a nutritional supplement containing R-LA or, most commercially available, a racemic mixture of R-LA and S-LA (the R,S-LA).

The potencies of the R-LA and S-LA isomers appear to be different. For example, Breithaupt-Grögler et al.[24] found that the oral administration of LA (at single doses of 50–600 mg) in healthy volunteers resulted in about 40–50% higher maximum plasma concentrations (C_{max}) of R-LA than the S-LA. In addition, the R-LA sodium salt displays significantly higher C_{max} and area under the curve (AUC) values than an equivalent dose of the pure R,S-LA or R-LA.[25] The pharmacokinetics of orally administrated LA, especially as supplement, are well characterized. Generally, most studies using animal models show that: (i) LA is rapidly transported into the bloodstream from the gastrointestinal system, and subsequently it is equally rapidly cleared, reflecting both uptake into tissue (e.g., liver, brain, heart, and skeletal muscle) as well as glomerular filtration and renal excretion;[26] (ii) various carrier proteins are probably involved in LA uptake into cells, e.g., the monocarboxylate and the Na^+-dependent multivitamin transporters responsible for intestinal and gastrointestinal uptake of LA, respectively;[27,28] (iii) in cells, LA is extensively catabolized into 12 major metabolites including β-oxidation as the major metabolic outcome *in vivo*, accompanied by oxidation of the dithiolane ring;[29] and (iv) food intake declines the bioavailability of LA, apparently by competition with other dietary components,[30] and therefore it is recommended to be taken 1 h before a meal.

With respect to the antioxidant properties of LA, there exist numerous studies *in vitro* demonstrating the distinct advantage of this compound as a potential therapeutic agent over other antioxidants (Figure 25.3). The most important advantage, besides amphiphilic properties, is the low standard reduction potential ($E_0 = -32$ V) of the DHLA/LA redox couple, enabling DHLA to scavenge ROS/RNS as well as reduce the oxidized form of other antioxidants (e.g., glutathione, vitamins C and E), and

chelation of transition metals.[31] Interestingly, some studies provide compelling evidence that LA, despite the oxidized state of its sulfhydryl groups, appears to be an ROS/RNS quencher, as is DHLA; both LA and DHLA are capable of scavenging hydrogen peroxide, hydroxyl radicals, nitric oxide radicals, peroxynitrite, and hypochlorous acid; moreover LA, unlike DHLA, is able to quench a singlet oxygen. Since LA is a powerful antioxidant, many studies, including tissue culture, animal models, and human epidemiological trials, have been performed to evaluate its therapeutic potential in diabetes prevention and treatment. There are several general issues with regard to beneficial effects of LA in diabetes and their complications described below.

LA and Oxidative Stress

At early stages of LA research, an inverse correlation between LA and oxidative stress in diabetes was proposed. Indeed, a reduction of oxidative stress in diabetic patients, even with

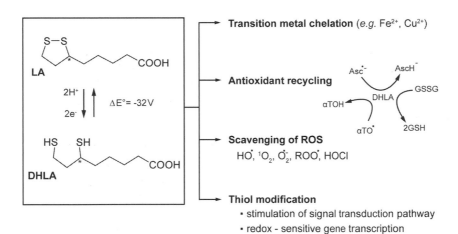

FIGURE 25.3 The proposed biological roles of LA and its reduced form, DHLA. Both LA and DHLA (which have one chiral center denoted by an asterisk) can act on cell functions through direct scavenging of ROS, chelation of transition metals (e.g., Fe^{2+}, Cu^{2+}), and activation of certain signaling pathways and redox-sensitive genes. In addition, DHLA as a strong reductant can convert ascorbyl ($Asc^{\bullet-}$) and α-tocopheroxyl ($\alpha TO^{\bullet-}$) radicals into ascorbate monoanion ($AscH^-$) and α-tocopherol (αTOH), respectively, as well as the oxidized disulfide form of glutathione (GSSG) into the reduced thiol (GSH).

poor glycemic control and albuminuria was observed after LA treatment (600 mg/day for >3 months).[32] Additionally, the antioxidant properties of LA in the diet seem to prevent an increase in the oxidative stress through a decrease in the superoxide anion (O_2^-) production in aortic vessels as well as through the preservation of GPx activity in the plasma of chronically glucose-fed rats; this compound would appear to be capable of exerting the antihypertensive and hypoglycemic effects, thus attenuating the elevation of blood pressure and the development of insulin resistance.[33]

LA and Glucose Uptake

LA treatment of ZDF rats and streptozotocin (STZ)-induced diabetic rats markedly enhanced insulin-stimulated glucose uptake into the muscles, as well as reduced plasma glucose levels.[34,35] The studies concentrated on mechanisms by which LA stimulates glucose uptake revealed the engagement of LA in the insulin signaling pathway. It has been shown that this compound increased tyrosine phosphorylation of IRS-1 and activated both PI3K and the serine/threonine kinase Akt1, resulting in GLUT1 and GLUT4 translocation to the plasma membrane in L6 muscle cells and 3T3-L1 adipocytes.[36,37] However, the GLUT4 translocation is not sufficient itself to cause a maximum stimulation of glucose uptake. To achieve effective glucose transport, LA has to stimulate the intrinsic activity of GLUT4 *via* a p38 MAPK-dependent pathway in addition to GLUT4 translocation.[38] Taken together, stimulation of glucose uptake by LA comprises two mechanisms: the IRS-1/PI3K/Akt-dependent translocation of GLUT4 to the plasma membrane and p38 MAPK-dependent stimulation of their intrinsic activity. Recently, computer modeling studies by Diesel *et al.*[39] identified a binding site for LA at the tyrosine kinase domain of IR, confirming, along with the above-described results, that LA is insulin mimetic.

Besides the direct function of LA on IR, this compound was also shown to oxidize critical cysteine thiol groups in tyrosine phosphatase B1 (PTPB1) resulting in suppression of its catalytic activity and, in consequence, inhibition of the IR dephosphorylation and elevated glucose uptake into cells.[40] Moreover, it has been revealed that LA-treated ZDF rats exhibit improved insulin action on skeletal muscle glucose transport activity related to significantly enhanced IRS-1 protein expression and insulin-mediated phosphotyrosine IRS-1 associated with the p85 subunit of PI3K.[41] Moreover, substantial evidence exists supporting the beneficial metabolic effects of LA on glucose uptake in muscle through the stimulation of peripheral AMP-activated protein kinase (AMPK), the protein playing a critical role in the stimulation of glucose transport in response to hypoxia and inhibition of oxidative phosphorylation.[28] In this regard, two LA-stimulated AMPK-dependent cellular mechanisms are considered. The first assumes that LA induces the phosphorylation of IRS-1 Ser789 and stimulation of the IRS-1/PI3K signaling through AMPK, whereas the second includes activation of GLUT4 translocation by inhibition of the Akt substrate of 160 kDa (AS160) independently of the IRS-1/PI3K/Akt signaling cascade.[28] Finally, it is well established that LA positively affects signal transduction cascades related to glucose transport into cells, thereby improving glucose disposal, as observed in patients with T2DM.[7,34]

LA and Diabetic Polyneuropathies

There is a growing body of clinical evidence that LA is an effective agent for treatment of diabetic neuropathy (DN), i.e. pathophysiological nerve dysfunction, caused by changes in endoneuronal blood flow and distal nerve conduction, associated with both T1DM and T2DM. There are several randomized, double-blind, placebo-controlled studies, including the so-called ALA-DIN (Alpha Lipoic Acid in Diabetic Neuropathy: ALADIN, ALADIN II, ALADIN III) trials and the

OPRIL (Oral Pilot) study, that have revealed the positive effects of LA in symptomatic DN. For example, in the short-term ALADIN study, where LA (up to 1,200 mg/day) was administered intravenously (i.v.) to patients with T2DM exhibiting peripheral neuropathies, a significant improvement of clinical symptoms of neuropathy (pain, numbness, and paresthesias) at the higher doses (600 and 1,200 mg/day) was found.[42] Analogously, a significant improvement in peripheral nerve conduction was observed in the long-term ALADIN II trial, where patients with T1DM and T2DM were treated with either 600 or 1,200 g/day i.v. once daily for five consecutive days and subsequently the same doses of LA were administered orally for 2 years. The ALADIN III study, a combination of short- and long-term LA supplementation where T2DM patients treated with 600 or 1,200 mg LA/day for 3 weeks, followed by 1,800 mg/day LA for 6 months, demonstrated a trend towards improved neurological pain.[42] These findings indicate that intravenous LA is more efficacious compared to the oral LA, although there are trials (e.g., the OPRIL study) confirming health benefits after LA administered orally. It should be noted that LA appears to be both an attractive and relevant compound since it is already approved as treatment in pharmacotherapy for DN in Germany.

Polyphenols

Polyphenols are a broad and heterogeneous group of compounds, divided into 10 different classes based on their chemical structure, which are present in plant-based foods and beverages like tea, coffee, wine, fruits, and vegetables. An important class of phenolic compounds are the flavonoids, which are composed of flavonols, flavones, flavanols, flavanones, anthocyanidins, and isoflavones. Polyphenols are known for their antioxidant properties, which have been evaluated in a number of ROS-associated diseases, such as diabetes, cancer, cardiovascular, and neurodegenerative diseases.[2] Regarding diabetes, a variety of polyphenolic extracts of plants, including berries (strawberries, raspberries, blueberries, and blackcurrants), vegetables (pumpkin, beans, maize, and eggplant), and beverages rich in polyphenols, such as green and black tea, and red wine have been demonstrated to affect carbohydrate homeostasis through several different pathways like inhibition of carbohydrate digestion and glucose absorption in the intestine, stimulation of insulin secretion from the pancreatic β-cells, modulation of glucose release from liver, activation of insulin receptors and glucose uptake in the insulin-sensitive tissues, or modulation of hepatic glucose output.[43] Of polyphenols, green tea catechins and resveratrol (described in Chapter 5, section 33) have received special attention as agents in protection against diabetes. This section is limited to recent studies of effects of green tea polyphenols (GTPs), particularly catechins, on oxidative stress, and carbohydrate and lipid metabolism based on various *in vitro* and *in vivo* studies.

Green Tea Catechins

Catechins are the predominant form of flavanols, which along with flavonols, are the most abundant polyphenols in green tea. There are four catechins identified in green tea leaves: epigallocatechin gallate (EGCG), epigallocatechin (EGC), epicatechin gallate (ECG), and epicatechin (EC) (Figure 25.4). The major polyphenolic constituent of green tea, EGCG, is considered to be a powerful antioxidant and the most pharmacologically active of the catechins with multiple beneficial health effects, including its role in preventing cancer, cardiovascular disease, and the risk of developing diabetes. It should be noted that EGCG is unique among GTCs, whose structure consists of three aromatic rings with different numbers of hydroxyl groups, because its structure contains the largest number of

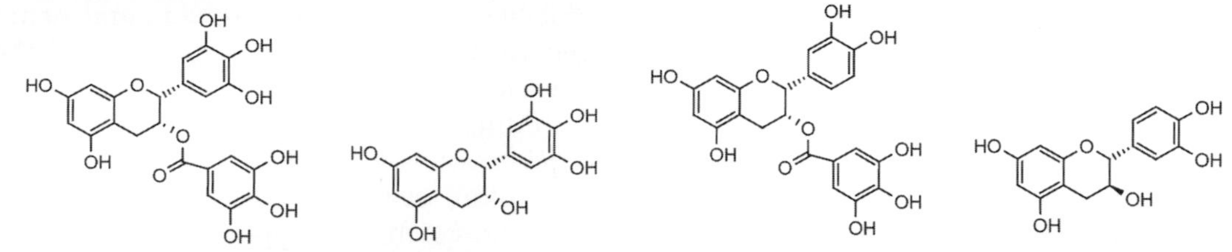

FIGURE 25.4   The chemical structures catechins present in green tea.

hydroxyl moieties, which may participate in hydrogen bonding, and both gallyl and galloyl groups, which confer conformational flexibility. Thus, the structural aspect of EGCG might be taken into account in the case when EGCG interacts with some biomolecules (e.g., enzymes) engaged in carbohydrate and lipid metabolism, independent of antioxidant activity.

Concerning the evaluation of bioavailability, safety, and tolerability of EGCG *in vivo*, a controlled clinical investigation assessing the plasma kinetic behavior of single oral doses (in range of 50–1,600 mg) of EGCG under fasting conditions in 60 healthy male volunteers revealed that the plasma pharmacokinetics of EGCG in humans are dose-dependent, with the C_{max} and the AUC values increasing, and moreover, that single oral doses of EGCG up to 1,600 mg are safe and well tolerated.[44]

Effect on Oxidative Stress

There is conclusive evidence from *in vivo* studies about antioxidant properties of GTCs. For example, Hininger-Favier *et al.*[45] reported that green tea extract (GTEs) intake decreases such oxidative stress parameters as plasma lipid peroxidation, sulfhydryl (SH) group oxidation, and DNA oxidative damage in the animal model of insulin resistance (Wistar rats on a high-fructose diet). In addition to antioxidant effects, GTE consumption is linked to a reduction in glycemia, insulinemia, and

triglyceridemia, thereby protecting against insulin resistance. The earlier studies revealed that GTE intake causes a significant decrease in lipid peroxidation products, in particular malondialdehyde (MDA)—a marker of oxidative stress—as well as an increase in GPx and GSR activity[46] and, moreover, it enhances CAT expression in the aorta.[47] Thus, these findings imply that catechins may act either directly as antioxidants on a reduction of oxidative stress markers, or indirectly, increasing activity or expression of the enzymes involved in cellular protection against ROS.

Effect on Carbohydrate Metabolism

Since GTCs have exhibited antioxidant properties, they have attracted much attention as dietary supplements which might improve glucose tolerance and a decrease of oxidative status.[45] The antidiabetic effect of EGCG in H4IIE rat hepatoma cells has been reported by Waltner-Law *et al.*,[48] who observed a significant decrease of hepatic glucose production at high levels (25–50 μM) of EGCG. Interestingly, they showed that EGCG mimics insulin, thereby enhancing tyrosine phosphorylation of IR and IRS-1, and inhibiting the expression of gluconeogenic genes like phosphoenolpyruvate carboxykinase (PEPCK) and G6Pase in a PI3K-dependent manner. However, the authors suggest that EGCG, unlike insulin, may regulate the expression of these genes by modifying the redox state of hepatic cells, since pretreatment of SOD and N-acetylcysteine for 30 min completely reverses the antigluconeogenic effect of EGCG, but not insulin, in H4IIE cells. These studies have also revealed that EGCG enhances the activities of PI3K, MAPK, and p70[s6k].[48] Recently, Collins et al.[49] confirmed that EGCG indeed suppresses hepatic gluconeogenesis, but not at the 10 μM or higher concentrations that are cytotoxic to liver cells, rather at the relatively low concentrations (≤ 1 μM) reachable by ingestion of green tea or pure EGCG. Nevertheless, EGCG at low concentrations does not activate Akt and IRS-1, which are required for insulin inhibition of hepatic gluconeogenesis, but instead activates AMPK mediated by Ca^{2+}/calmodulin-dependent protein kinase (CaMKK) and ROS. However, it is still unclear how EGCG exactly activates CaMKK through production of ROS. Regardless of the mechanism by which EGCG exerts beneficial effects on liver cells, it should be borne in mind that higher intake of this catechin may exert acute cytotoxicity in these cells.

A deeper insight into the EGCG-mediated repression of gluconeogenic genes such as PEPCK reveals that this catechin is capable of inducing Foxo1 phosphorylation through a similar, but not identical, mechanism to insulin, which inhibits the function of Foxo1 through Akt/PKB-mediated phosphorylation and nuclear exclusion, and thereby suppresses hepatic gluconeogenesis.[50]

Considerable experimental evidence also exists highlighting the antidiabetic properties of green tea, GTEs, and EGCG in human and animal-based studies. For example, GTE administration by alloxan (which destroys pancreatic β-cells) to diabetic rats led to reduced serum glucose levels,[51] implying that catechins participate in glucose metabolism. Tsuneki et al.[52] provided evidence that green tea promotes glucose metabolism in healthy humans, and generates an antihyperglycemic effect in diabetic mice, which may result from the promotion of insulin action in peripheral tissues,

such as skeletal muscles and adipocytes. In this context, Wu et al.[53] demonstrated that green tea supplementation for 12 weeks ameliorates insulin resistance and increases GLUT4 content in Sprague–Dawley rats fed a fructose-rich diet (i.e. the fructose-fed rat model resembling the human T2DM). Further identification of potential targets regulated by green teas within the GLUT family, and insulin transduction pathway in rats fed a fructose-rich diet, revealed that GTE significantly increased the mRNA levels of GLUT4 in the muscle and glycogen synthase kinase 3β (Gsk3b) in the liver; it was also found to increase the levels of Irs2, PI3K and catalytic β (Pik3cb) but lowered Src homology 2 domain-containing transforming protein 1(Shc1) mRNA levels in the liver and enhanced Irs1, Shc1, and son of sevenless 1 (Sos1) mRNA levels in the muscle.[54] These results indicate that supplementation with green tea or its extract may regulate gene expression in the glucose uptake and the insulin signal transduction pathways; thereby it might affect glucose disposal, insulin resistance, diabetes and obesity.

Besides the antihyperglycemic effect, GTCs modulate insulin secretion and insulin sensitivity action. In the in vitro study, EGCG was shown to have insulin-stimulating properties in rat epididymal adipocytes.[55] In addition, an enhancement of insulin binding to adipocytes and, subsequently, an increase in insulin-stimulated adipocyte glucose uptake, as well as a decrease in fasting plasma levels of glucose, insulin, triglyceride (TG), and FFA were observed in Sprague–Dawley rats fed GTE and polyphenols for 12 weeks, suggesting that green tea supplementation results in higher insulin sensitivity.[56] However, elsewhere, green tea was found to significantly reduce glucose uptake, decrease translocation of GLUT4 in the adipose tissue of male Wistar rats, as well as stimulate glucose uptake with GLUT4 translocation in skeletal muscle.[57] The discrepancy in adipose tissue behavior is somewhat surprising, but it may result from various experimental conditions. The molecular mechanisms of green tea and/or EGCG as modulators of insulin sensitivity in adipocytes and muscle cells have not yet been established, although a recent study by Li et al.[58] revealed that EGCG specifically and allosterically inhibits glutamate dehydrogenase (GDH) with a nanomolar ED_{50} value. This enzyme plays a major role in the regulation of insulin secretion, leading to suppression of insulin secretion by rat pancreatic β-cells. Interestingly, EGCG acts in an allosteric manner independent of its antioxidant activity.

Although studies in experimental models demonstrate that green tea rich in EGCG beneficially affects glucose homeostasis, clinical evidence of its application is not comprehensive. In general, most human intervention studies reveal an improvement of glucose levels in response to GTCs, although there are reports of a lack of association between blood glucose in T2DM patients and green tea supplementation.[59] These contrary conclusions may well result from both different doses of green tea (or EGCG) being consumed and different end points being assessed in the studied populations.

Effect on Lipid Metabolism

It is now well accepted that obesity, i.e. an increased number of fat cells and lipid accumulation due to mitogenesis and differentiation, is a risk factor for development of T2DM. There is growing evidence from in vivo animal studies that green tea catechins, in particular EGCG, can be used to treat metabolic dyslipidemia by modulating different pathways resulting in reduction of food uptake and lipid absorption. Moreover, GTCs decrease blood TG, FFA, and total cholesterol levels, and stimulate energy expenditure, fat oxidation, high-density lipoprotein levels, and fecal lipid excretion. Interestingly, a recent report on the antiobesity and antidiabetic effects of GTCs in the fructose fed hypertriglyceridemic, insulin-resistant hamsters disclosed that the tea extract supplementation

of these animals led to a reduction of body, liver, and adipose tissue weight. In addition, a significant increase in expression of hepatic peroxisome proliferator-activated receptors (PPAR)-α and -γ, which are ligand-dependent transcription factors participating in lipid (uptake and oxidation of fatty acid, lipolysis) and glucose (glucose production and disposal) metabolism, was observed. It is likely that tea catechins acting as agonists of these ligand-dependent transcription factors ameliorate the fructose-induced hypertriglyceridemia and the insulin-resistant state.[60]

These antiobesity effects of green tea catechins in vivo can be explained, at least partially, by the following in vitro data: (i) green tea reduced body fat accretion and increased energy expenditure in obese rats through the β-adrenoreceptor activation of thermogenesis in brown adipose tissue (BAT) (the effect on fat oxidation); (ii) GTE rich in EGCG suppressed the enzymes involved in lipid digestion, such as gastric and pancreatic lipases (i.e. the effect on lipolytic enzyme); (iii) GTCs inhibited the activity and/or expression of lipogenic enzymes, such as acetyl-CoA carboxylase (ACC: the rate-limiting enzyme in fatty acid synthesis that catalyzes a conversion of acetyl-CoA to malonyl-CoA), fatty acid synthase (FAS: the enzyme catalyzing the conversion of malonyl-CoA to fatty acyl-CoA), malic enzyme (ME: the enzyme that, along with G6PDH, generates NADPH for fatty acid biogenesis), glucose-6-phosphate dehydrogenase (G6PDH), glycerol-3-phosphate dehydrogenase (G3PDH: participates in triglyceride biosynthesis), and stearoyl-CoA desaturase-1 (SCD1: the rate-limiting enzyme in the synthesis of monounsaturated fatty acids) (e.g., the effect on lipogenic enzyme); (iv) EGCG inhibited lipid peroxidation enzymes such as lipoxygenase, suppressed radical reaction of apolipoprotein B-100, and ameliorated LDL receptor expression in HepG2 (i.e. the effect on lipoproteins); (v) EGCG inhibited, in a dose- and time-dependent manner, the mitogenic effect of insulin on preadipocytes (i.e. the antimitogenic effect).[61] Recently, the study by Ku et al.[62] provided an in-depth analysis of the role of EGCG on the insulin regulation of preadipocyte mitogenesis. As reported, EGCG inhibited insulin action in a dose- and time-dependent manner through its suppressive effects on insulin-stimulated phosphorylation of the insulin receptor-β, IRS-1, IRS-2, and MAPK pathway proteins, RAF-1, MEK-1/2, and ERK-1/2. Furthermore, EGCG inhibited the association of IR with the IRS-1 and IRS-2 proteins, but not with the IRS-4 protein. Taken together, these results suggest that EGCG selectively affects particular types of IRS and MAPK family members.

Despite numerous epidemiological observations and clinical trials of the antiobesity and hypolipidemic effects of GTCs, their results are ambiguous. These discrepancies between clinical studies may result from the different protocols employed, the purity of GTEs, the period of administration, the physiological condition of the subjects and the caffeine content in tea.[59,61] Moreover, recent data suggest that low EGCG (300 mg) as well as 200 mg caffeine increases postprandial fat oxidation in obese men, while a high dose of EGCG (600 mg) does not trigger this effect. Additionally, no synergic action of low EGCG and 200 mg caffeine in vivo was observed.[63]

Effect on Nephropathy

The activity of GTCs has received a lot of attention in regard to nephropathy, a serious complication that frequently accompanies diabetes due to microvascular dysfunction or impairment. There are reports that GTCs improve the kidney function of STZ-induced diabetic rats resulting from their antithrombogenic action, which in turn controls the arachidonic acid cascade system.[64] Additionally, the antioxidative function of GTCs on reduction of the blood nitrogen level, as well as a decrease of the MDA level and an increase of the CAT activity in renal tissue were observed, suggesting their beneficial role in reduction of oxidative stress in the kidney.[65]

CONCLUSIONS

In recent years, numerous studies have confirmed that oxidative stress, mediated mainly by hyperglycemia-induced generation of free radicals, contributes to development and progression of diabetes and its complications. Therefore, a decrease in oxidative stress with the use of wide-spectrum antioxidants has become an alternative approach in the prevention and treatment of diabetes and its complications. To date, many beneficial effects of both LA and GTEs, particularly EGCG, on glucose and lipid homeostasis in tissue cultures and animal models have been reported. It should be highlighted that these antioxidants not only change the redox state but also trigger signaling cascades that result in a redox-independent regulation of transcriptional activity. Therefore, further studies on the identification of both redox-dependent and independent specific new targets will lead to additional progress in understanding how the above-mentioned antioxidants may prevent diabetes. The clinical trials conducted to date, except LA studies in diabetic neuropathy, have provided mixed results without a definitive conclusion. However, the positive trends and antidiabetic and antiobesity effects of these antioxidants have been observed. Further well-controlled long-term human studies should provide additional data for the potential therapeutic roles for LA and EGCG on diabetes and its complications.

References

1. Valko M, Leibfritz D, Moncol J, Cronin MT, Mazur M, Telser J. Free radicals and antioxidants in normal physiological functions and human disease. *Int J Biochem Cell Biol* 2007;**39**:44—84.

2. Wojcik M, Burzynska-Pedziwiatr I, Wozniak LA. A review of natural and synthetic antioxidants important for health and longevity. *Curr Med Chem* 2010;**17**:3262−88.

3. Wild S, Roglic G, Green A, Sicree R, King H. Global prevalence of diabetes. *Diabetes Care* 2004;**27**:1047−53.

4. Pan HZ, Zhang H, Chang D, Li H, Sui H. The change of oxidative stress products in diabetes mellitus and diabetic retinopathy. *Br J Ophthalmol* 2008;**92**:548−51.

5. Evans JL, Goldfine ID, Maddux BA, Grodsky GM. Oxidative stress and stress-activated signaling pathways: a unifying hypothesis of type 2 diabetes. *Endocrine Reviews* 2002;**23**:599−622.

6. Tirosh A, Potashnik R, Bashan N, Rudich A. Oxidative stress disrupts insulin-induced cellular redistribution of insulin receptor substrate-1 and phosphatidylinositol 3-kinase in 3T3-L1 adipocytes: a putative cellular mechanism for impaired protein kinase B activation and GLUT4 translocation. *J Biol Chem* 1999;**274**:10595−602.

7. Konrad T, Vicini P, Kusterer K, Höflich A, Assadkhani A, Böhles HJ, Sewell A, Tritschler HJ, Cobelli C, Usadel KH. α-Lipoic acid treatment decreases serum lactate and pyruvate concentrations and improves glucose effectiveness in lean and obese patients with type 2 diabetes. *Diabetes Care* 1999;**22**:280−7.

8. Robertson RP, Harmon JS. Diabetes, glucose toxicity, and oxidative stress: A case of double jeopardy for the pancreatic islet beta cell. *Free Radic Biol Med* 2006;**41**:177−84.

9. Robertson RP. Oxidative stress and impaired insulin secretion in type 2 diabetes. *Curr Opin Pharmacol* 2006;**6**:615−9.

10. Tanaka Y, Tran POT, Harmon J, Robertson RP. A role of glutathione peroxidase in protecting pancreatic β cells against oxidative stress in a model of glucose toxicity. *Proc Natl Acad Sci U S A* 2002;**99**:12363−8.

11. Shao J, Iwashita N, Ikeda F, Ogihara T, Uchida T, Shimizu T, Uchino H, Hirose T, Kawamori R, Watada H. Beneficial effects of candesartan, an angiotensin II type 1 receptor blocker, on β-cell function and morphology in db/db mice. *Biochem Biophys Res Commun* 2006;**344**:1224−33.

12. Oprescu AI, Bikopoulos G, Naassan A, Allister EM, Tang C, Park E, Uchino H, Lewis GF, Fantus IG, Rozakis-Adcock M, Wheeler MB, Giacca A. Free fatty acid-induced reduction in glucose-stimulated insulin secretion: evidence for a role of oxidative stress *in vitro* and *in vivo*. *Diabetes* 2007;**56**:2927−37.

13. Kaneto H, Katakami N, Matsuhisa M, Matsuoka TA. Role of reactive oxygen species in the progression of type 2 diabetes and atherosclerosis. *Mediators Inflamm* 2010. doi:10.1155/2010/453892.

14. Kaneto H, Xu G, Fujii N, Kim S, Bonner-Weir S, Weir GC. Involvement of c-Jun N-terminal kinase in oxidative stress-mediated suppression of insulin gene expression. *J Biol Chem* 2002;**277**:30010−8.

15. Kawamori D, Kaneto H, Nakatani Y, Matsuoka TA, Matsuhisa M, Hori M, Yamasaki Y. The forkhead transcription factor Foxo1 bridges the JNK pathway and the transcription factor PDX-1 through its intracellular translocation. *J Biol Chem* 2006;**281**:1091−8.

16. Cai D, Yuan M, Frantz DF, Melendez PA, Hansen L, Lee J, Shoelson SE. Local and systemic insulin resistance resulting from hepatic activation of IKK-β and NF-κB. *Nat Med* 2005;**11**:183−90.

17. Arkan MC, Hevener AL, Greten FR, Maeda S, Li ZW, Long JM, Wynshaw-Boris A, Poli G, Olefsky J, Karin M. IKK-β links inflammation to obesity-induced insulin resistance. *Nat Med* 2005;**11**:191−8.

18. Azumi H, Inoue N, Ohashi Y, Terashima M, Mori T, Fujita H, Awano K, Kobayashi K, Maeda K, Hata K, Shinke T, Kobayashi S, Hirata K, Kawashima S, Itabe H, Hayashi Y, Imajoh-Ohmi S, Itoh H, Yokoyama M. Superoxide generation in directional coronary atherectomy specimens of patients with angina pectoris: important role of NAD(P)H oxidase. *Arterioscler Thromb Vasc Biol* 2002;**22**:1838−44.

19. Inoguchi T, Li P, Umeda F, Yu HY, Kakimoto M, Imamura M, Aoki T, Etoh T, Hashimoto T, Naruse M, Sano H, Utsumi H, Nawata HT. High glucose level and free fatty acid stimulate reactive oxygen species production through protein kinase C-dependent activation of NAD(P)H oxidase in cultured vascular cells. *Diabetes* 2000;**49**:1939−45.

20. Madamanchi NR, Vendrov A, Runge. MS. Oxidative stress and vascular disease. *Arterioscler Thromb Vasc Biol* 2005;**25**:29−38.

21. Guzik TJ, Mussa S, Gastaldi D, Sadowski J, Ratnatunga C, Pillai R, Channon KM. Mechanisms of increased vascular superoxide production in human diabetes mellitus: role of NAD(P)H oxidase and endothelial nitric oxide synthase. *Circulation* 2002;**105**:1656−62.

22. Morikawa T, Yasuno R, Wada H. Do mammalian cells synthesize lipoic acid? Identification of a mouse cDNA encoding a lipoic acid synthase located in mitochondria. *FEBS Lett* 2001;**498**:16−21.

23. Reed L. Multienzyme complexes. *Acc Chem Res* 1974;**7**:40−6.

24. Breithaupt-Grögler K, Niebch G, Schneider E, Erb K, Hermann R, Blume HH, Schug BS, Belz GG. Dose-proportionality of oral thioctic acid−coincidence of assessments *via* pooled plasma and individual data. *Eur J Pharm Sci* 1999;**8**:57−65.

25. Carlson DA, Smith AR, Fischer SJ, Young KL, Packer L. The plasma pharmacokinetics of R-(+)-lipoic acid administered as sodium R-(+)-lipoate to healthy human subjects. *Altern Med Rev* 2007;**12**:343−51.

26. Harrison EH, McCormick DB. The metabolism of dl-(1,6-14C)lipoic acid in the rat. *Arch Biochem Biophys* 1974;**160**:514−22.

27. Takaishi N, Yoshida K, Satsu H, Shimizu M. Trans-epithelial transport of alpha-lipoic acid across human intestinal Caco-2 cell monolayers. *J Agric Food Chem* 2007;**55**:5253−9.

28. Shay KP, Moreau RF, Smith EJ, Smith AR, Hagen TM. Alpha-lipoic acid as a dietary supplement: molecular mechanisms and therapeutic potential. *Biochim Biophys Acta* 2009;**1790**:1149−60.

29. Schupke H, Hempel R, Peter G, Hermann R, Wessel K, Engel J, Kronbach T. New metabolic pathways of α-lipoic acid. *Drug Metab Dispos* 2001;**29**:855−62.

30. Gleiter CH, Schug BS, Hermann R, Elze M, Blume HH, Gundert-Remy U. Influence of food intake on the bioavailability of thioctic acid enantiomers. *Eur J Clin Pharmacol* 1996;**50**:513−4.

31. Bast A, Haenen GR. Lipoic acid: a multifunctional antioxidant. *Biofactors* 2003;**17**:207−13.

32. Borcea V, Nourooz-Zadeh J, Wolff SP, Klevesath M, Hofmann M, Urich H, Wahl P, Ziegler R, Tritschler H, Halliwell B, Nawroth PP. α-Lipoic acid decreases oxidative stress even in diabetic patients with poor glycemic control and albuminuria. *Free Radic Biol Med* 1999;**26**:1495−500.

33. EI Midaoui A, de Champlain J. Prevention of hypertension, insulin resistance, and oxidative stress by α-lipoic acid. *Hypertension* 2002;**39**:303−7.

34. Jacob S, Henriksen EJ, Tritschler HJ, Augustin HJ, Dietze GJ. Improvement of insulin-stimulated glucose-disposal in type 2 diabetes after repeated parenteral administration of thioctic acid. *Exp Clin Endocrinol Diabetes* 1996;**104**:284−8.

35. Khamaisi M, Potashnik R, Tirosh A, Demshchak E, Rudich A, Tritschler H, Wessel K, Bashan N. Lipoic acid reduces glycemia and increases muscle GLUT4 content in streptozotocin-diabetic rats. *Metabolism* 1997;**46**:763−8.

36. Yaworsky K, Somwar R, Ramlal T, Tritschler HJ, Klip A. Engagement of the insulin-sensitive pathway in the stimulation of glucose transport by alpha-lipoic acid in 3T3-L1 adipocytes. *Diabetologia* 2000;**43**:294−303.

37. Estrada DE, Ewart HS, Tsakiridis T, Volchuk A, Ramlal T, Tritschler H, Klip A. Stimulation of glucose uptake by the natural coenzyme alpha-lipoic acid/thioctic acid: participation of elements of the insulin signaling pathway. *Diabetes* 1996;**45**:1798−804.

38. Konrad D, Somwar R, Sweeney G, Yaworsky K, Hayashi M, Ramlal T, Klip A. The antihyperglycemic drug alpha-lipoic acid stimulates glucose uptake *via* both GLUT4 translocation and GLUT4 activation: potential role of p38 mitogen-activated protein kinase in GLUT4 activation. *Diabetes* 2001;**50**:1464−71.

39. Diesel B, Kulhanek-Heinze S, Höltje M, Brandt B, Höltje HD, Vollmar AM, Kiemer AK. Alpha-lipoic acid as a directly binding activator of the insulin receptor: protection from hepatocyte apoptosis. *Biochemistry* 2007;**46**:2146−55.

40. Cho KJ, Moini H, Shon HK, Chung AS, Packer L. Alpha-lipoic acid decreases thiol reactivity of the insulin receptor and protein tyrosine phosphatase 1B in 3T3-L1 adipocytes. *Biochem Pharmacol* 2003;**66**:849−58.

41. Saengsirisuwan V, Perez FR, Sloniger JA, Maier T, Henriksen EJ. Interactions of exercise training and alpha-lipoic acid on insulin signaling in skeletal muscle of obese Zucker rats. *Am J Physiol Endocrinol Metab* 2004;**287**:E529−36.

42. Singh U, Jialal I. Alpha-lipoic acid supplementation and diabetes. *Nutr Rev* 2008;**66**:646−57.

43. Hanhineva K, Törrönen R, Bondia-Pons I, Pekkinen J, Kolehmainen M, Mykkänen H, Poutanen K. Impact of dietary polyphenols on carbohydrate metabolism. *Int J Mol Sci* 2010;**11**:1365−402.

44. Lambert JD, Lee MJ, Lu H, Meng X, Hong JJJ, Seril DN, Sturgill MG, Yang CS. Epigallocatechin-3-gallate is absorbed but extensively glucuronidated following oral administration to mice. *J Nutr* 2003;**133**:4172−7.

45. Hininger-Favier I, Benaraba R, Coves S, Anderson RA, Roussel AM. Green tea extract decreases oxidative stress and improves insulin sensitivity in an animal model of insulin resistance, the fructose-fed rat. *J Am Coll Nutr* 2009;**28**:355−61.

46. Skrzydlewska E, Ostrowska J, Farbiszewski R, Michalak K. Protective effect of green tea against lipid peroxidation in the rat liver, blood serum and the brain. *Phytomedicine* 2002;**9**:232−8.

47. Negishi H, Xu JW, Ikeda K, Njelekela M, Nara Y, Yamori Y. Black and green tea polyphenols attenuate blood pressure increases in stroke-prone spontaneously hypertensive rats. *J Nutr* 2004;**134**:38−42.

48. Waltner-Law ME, Wang XL, Law BK, Hall RK, Nawano M, Granner DK. Epigallocatechin gallate, a constituent of green tea, represses hepatic glucose production. *J Biol Chem* 2002;**277**:34933−40.

49. Collins QF, Liu HY, Pi J, Liu Z, Quon MJ, Cao W. Epigallocatechin-3-gallate (EGCG), a green tea polyphenol, suppresses hepatic gluconeogenesis through 5'-AMP-activated protein kinase. *J Biol Chem* 2007;**282**:30143−9.

50. Anton S, Melville L, Rena G. Epigallocatechin gallate (EGCG) mimics insulin action on the transcription factor FOXO1a and elicits cellular responses in the presence and absence of insulin. *Cell Signal* 2007;**19**:378—83.

51. Sabu MC, Smitha K, Kuttan R. Anti-diabetic activity of green tea polyphenols and their role in reducing oxidative stress in experimental diabetes. *J Ethnopharmacol* 2002;**83**:109—16.

52. Tsuneki H, Ishizuka M, Terasawa M, Wu JB, Sasaoka T, Kimura I. Effect of green tea on blood glucose levels and serum proteomic patterns in diabetic mice and on glucose metabolism in healthy humans. *BMC Pharmacol* 2004;**4**:18.

53. Wu LY, Juan CC, Hwang LS, Hsu YP, Ho PH, Ho LT. Green tea supplementation ameliorates insulin resistance and increases glucose transporter IV content in a fructose-fed rat model. *Eur J Nutr* 2004;**43**:116—24.

54. Cao H, Hininger-Favier I, Kelly MA, Benaraba R, Dawson HD, Coves S, Roussel AM, Anderson RA. Green tea polyphenol extract regulates the expression of genes involved in glucose uptake and insulin signaling in rats fed a high fructose diet. *J Agric Food Chem* 2007;**55**:6372—8.

55. Anderson RA, Polansky MM. Tea enhances insulin activity. *J Agric Food Chem* 2002;**50**:7182—6.

56. Wu LY, Juan CC, Ho LT, Hsu YP, Hwang LS. Effect of green tea supplementation on insulin sensitivity in Sprague-Dawley rats. *J Agric Food Chem* 2004;**52**:643—8.

57. Ashida H, Furuyashiki T, Nagayasu H, Bessho H, Sakakibara H, Hashimoto T, Kanazawa K. Anti-obesity actions of green tea: possible involvements in modulation of the glucose uptake system and suppression of the adipogenesis-related transcription factors. *Biofactors* 2004;**22**:135—40.

58. Li RW, Douglas TD, Maiyoh GK, Adeli K, Theriault AG. Green tea leaf extract improves lipid and glucose homeostasis in a fructose-fed insulin-resistant hamster model. *J Ethnopharmacol* 2006;**104**:24—31.

59. Thielecke F, Boschmann M. The potential role of green tea catechins in the prevention of the metabolic syndrome—A review. *Phytochemistry* 2009;**70**:11—24.

60. Li RW, Douglas TD, Maiyoh GK, Adeli K, Theriault AG. Green tea leaf extract improves lipid and glucose homeostasis in a fructose-fed insulin-resistant hamster model. *J Ethnopharmacol* 2006;**104**:24—31.

61. Kao YH, Chang HH, Lee MJ, Chen CL. Tea, obesity, and diabetes. *Mol Nutr Food Res* 2006;**50**:188—210.

62. Ku HC, Chang HH, Liu HC, Hsiao CH, Lee MJ, Hu YJ, Hung PF, Liu CW, Kao YH. Green tea (-)-epigallocatechin gallate inhibits insulin stimulation of 3T3-L1 preadipocyte mitogenesis *via* the 67-kDa laminin receptor pathway. *Am J Physiol Cell Physiol* 2009;**297**:C121—32.

63. Thielecke F, Rahn G, Bohnke J, Adams F, Birkenfeld AL, Jordan J, Boschmann M. Epigallocatechin-3-gallate and postprandial fat oxidation in overweight/obese male volunteers: a pilot study. *Eur J Clin Nutr* 2010;**64**:704—13.

64. Rhee SJ, Choi JH, Park MR. Green tea catechin improves microsomal phospholipase A2 activity and the arachidonic acid cascade system in the kidney of diabetic rats. *Asia Pac J Clin Nutr* 2002;**11**:226—31.

65. Yokozawa T, Nakagawa T, Lee KI, Cho EJ, Terasawa K, Takeuchi S. Effects of green tea tannin on cisplatin-induced nephropathy in LLC-PK1 cells and rats. *J Pharm Pharmacol* 1999;**51**:1325—31.

CHAPTER

26

Cardioprotective Roles of Selenium in Diabetes

Belma Turan*, Guy Vassort[†]

Department of Biophysics, Faculty of Medicine, Ankara University, Ankara, Turkey [†]Laboratoire de Physiopathologie Cardiovasculaire, INSERM U-1046, CHU Arnaud de Villeneuve, Montpellier, France

INTRODUCTION: SELENIUM AND SELENOPROTEINS

Selenium, chemically discovered in 1817, was long considered a dangerous poison. Selenium toxicity in livestock that consumed selenium-accumulator plants such as Astralagus or Xylorrhiza, can be traced back to Marco Polo and was first described in animals in the 1930s.[1] It took almost one-and-a-half centuries until it became recognized that selenium plays a role in biology beyond threatening life, as indicated above. Selenium compounds exert their biological effects either directly or by being incorporated

Nutritional and Therapeutic Interventions for Diabetes and Metabolic Syndrome
DOI: 10.1016/B978-0-12-385083-6.00026-7

into enzymes and other bio-active proteins. The main two inorganic dietary forms of selenium are primarily sodium selenite (Na_2SeO_3) and sodium selenate (Na_2SeO_4). In the organic forms selenomethionine and selenocysteine, a selenium atom is present in the position occupied by a sulfur atom in the amino acids methionine and cysteine. *In vitro*, selenite, selenium dioxide, and diselenides react with thiols, such as glutathione, producing superoxide and other reactive oxygen species. Methylation of selenium by both plants and animals serves to detoxify selenium by generating methylselenides. The catalytic prooxidant attribute of some selenium compounds appears to account for their toxicity when such activity exceeds plant and animal methylation reactions and antioxidant defenses. This prooxidant activity may also account for cellular apoptosis and is used for pharmaceutical application of selenium compounds as antibacterial, antiviral, antifungal, and anticancer agents. The health benefits of selenium in the mammalian body are summarized in Figure 26.1. In the body, selenium is incorporated into proteins to make important antioxidant enzymes called selenoproteins. The antioxidant properties of selenoproteins help prevent cellular damage from free radicals scavenging them and reducing them to water and other harmless molecules.

The first selenium deficiency syndrome in humans, indeed a childhood cardiomyopathy known as Keshan disease, was reported back in 1937 by an anonymous group of Chinese scientists.[2] Patients with Keshan disease showed low activity of glutathione peroxidase-1 (GSH-Px-1), which suggested that dysfunctional GSH-Px-1 may play a role in the pathogenesis of Keshan disease[3] besides the early recognized selenium-deficient activation of Coxsackie B virus triggering the onset of this disease.[2] Chronic selenium deficiency may also occur in individuals with malabsorption and long-term selenium-deficient parenteral nutrition. Moreover hypozincemia and hyposelenemia are commonly observed in elderly[4] and in CHF patients.[5-8] Plasma selenium concentration decreased with higher BMI which is one of the stronger diabetes risk factors,[9] in agreement with a recent study showing that patients with diabetes demonstrate significantly lower levels of selenoalbumine.[10] The potential relevance of selenium deficiency to human health was supported only by epidemiological studies for a long time, which suggested a protective role

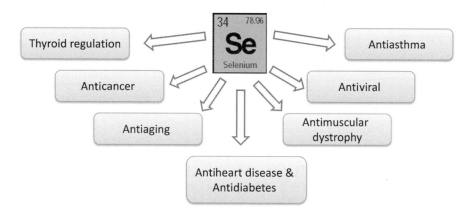

FIGURE 26.1 **Some examples of the health benefits of selenium in mammalian body.** Selenium basically detoxifies cancer-causing agents, stabilizes DNA and preserves DNA integrity, reduces cellular as well as motochondrial oxidative stress, and has antioxidant effects as selenoenzymes which have vital roles in the body. (*See the color plate section at the back of the book*).

of selenium against cancer and cardiovascular diseases.[11] The recommended dietary allowance for selenium is 55 µg/d for healthy adults in the US, although to allow full expression of seleno-proteins, an intake of 75 µg selenium/d as sele-nomethionine is suggested as an optimal value.[12] Selenium supplementation results in a significant increase in plasma selenium and glutathione peroxidase (GSH-Px) activity, and decrease lipid peroxidation (LPO).[13–15] Some reports have suggested that selenium may be beneficial in treating diabetes.[16,17] Other studies indicate that selenium supplementation has no overall benefit in prevention of cardiovascular diseases,[18] or even that high serum selenium levels are positively associated with the preva-lence of diabetes.[19]

Besides GSH-Px, some other selenoproteins have been identified in the heart tissues, such as selenoprotein W and selenoprotein K, SelW and SelK, respectively,[20] besides selenoprotein P that incorporated about 60% of selenium present in plasma. Overexpression of SelK decreases the reactive oxygen species (ROS) level in cultured cardiomyocytes and protects cells from oxidative stress-induced toxicity.[21]

SELENIUM EFFECTS ON THE CONTROL OF CARDIAC ACTIVITY

Control of Cardiac Activity by Selenium

Selenium provides a classic example of dichotomy of effects and has generated concerns at both ends of its supply spectrum. Selenium, originally recognized as a toxic element, was initially shown in 1957, along with vitamin E, to be essential for prevention in liver necrosis.[22] In heart, either low- or high-selenium diet induced dysfunction.[23] Selenium compounds are known to play an antioxidant role. However, selenium may have opposite effects.[24] Thus, although selenium at low essen-tial levels (nM) is required for the synthesis of

redox active selenoenzymes such as GSH-Px and Trx-R, in higher toxic levels (> 5–10 mM) selenite can react with essential thiol groups on enzymes to form RS—Se—SR adducts with resultant inhibition of enzyme activity. Also toxic effects could be directly or indirectly related to increased endogenous release of hydrogen peroxide,[25] or to a reduced binding of nuclear factor kappa B (NF-κB) to nuclear responsive element.[26]

In selenium-deficient rats, the contractile force of electrically stimulated left atria and Langendorff-perfused hearts were not altered.[27] Also, in rats fed with selenium and vitamin E-deficient diet that halved the plasma and tissue selenium and vitamin E contents, the contractile force of papillary muscles was not modified.[23] Moreover, the papillary muscle preparations demonstrated marked diminished β-adrenergic responses with no change in EC_{50}, implying a reduced number of β-adrenergic receptors or/and an impaired signal transduction.[23,28] A later study showed that selenium-deficient mice, either at basal or after isoprenaline stimula-tion, have both a reduction in atria frequency and cAMP content but a higher iNOS activity that suggests a negative cross-talk between inducible nitric oxide synthase (iNOS) and adenylyl cyclase in these mice.[29]

As a selenium-dependent enzyme, GSH-Px-1 has an important protective role by partici-pating in the detoxification of H_2O_2 and a wide range of organic peroxides with reduced glutathione.[30] Protective effects of the seleno-enzyme GSH-Px were early suggested by the observation that Langendorff-perfused sele-nium-deficient hearts demonstrate much higher H_2O_2 sensitivity of diastolic dysfunction and relaxation rate than controls.[27] GSH-Px-1$^{-/-}$ mice are highly sensitive to the oxidant para-quat and developed myocarditis on infection with the benign strain of coxsackievirus B3.[31,32] In contrast, GSH-Px-1 transgenesis confers protection against ischemia/reperfusion damage, left-ventricular remodeling, and heart failure after myocardial infarction in mice.[32,33] GSH-Px-1 transgenic mice also showed increased resistance to doxorubicin-induced acute cardiac dysfunction.[34] Thus a reduced selenium tissue level or a lowered GSH-Px activity increases tissue sensitivity to oxidative stress.

Sodium selenite supplementation for 4 weeks to control rats increased blood glucose and lowered plasma insulin.[35] GSH-Px but not SOD activity was increased, leading to a significant increase (70%) in GSSG level associated with a limited decrease in GSH. This treatment also caused a slight prolongation in action potential with no significant effect on spontaneous contraction parameters or in intracellular Ca^{2+} transients. I_{CaL} or I_{to} kinetic, but not density, showed marked alterations resulting in, respectively, a $\approx$ 50% increase or decrease in total charges carried by Ca^{2+} or K^+ currents of the selenium-supplemented rat cardiomyocytes.[35]

Acute Effects of Selenium Exposure *In Vitro*

The classical idea that selenium is toxic to the heart at levels higher than available in a balanced diet is not always supported by experimental work. In the dog isolated ventricular segment perfused with blood, the acute administration of sodium selenite caused a positive inotropic effect.[36] Indeed, rather than correcting selenium deficiency, a positive influence of sodium selenite is observed on hearts that have been acutely stressed by oxygen lack, ouabain, or 2,4-dinitrophenol. In a later study on rat papillary muscles, it was shown that selenite applied in the millimolar range had biphasic contractile effects.[37] The initial transient increase in force, attributable to Ca^{2+}-sensitization of the myofilaments, is later on counterbalanced by a reduction of the Ca^{2+} current and Ca^{2+} transient associated with an increased diastolic Ca^{2+} level. These effects occurred mainly through oxidative alteration

of protein thiols since the disulfide-reducing agent DTT restored control observations. These cardiomyocytes acutely exposed to selenite demonstrate significant decreases in both reduced glutathione and protein thiols levels.[37] The increase in resting tension and decrease in contractile force induced by selenite were protected by adding ATP to the bathing solution.[38] Furthermore, millimolar selenite, by reducing the Na^+ current, shortens the action potential recorded on rat isolated papillary muscles, without affecting resting membrane potential.[39]

Selenite addition to the perfusion medium was found to exert significant protective effects on H_2O_2-induced alterations in both LVDP (17-fold decrease) and LVEDP (18-fold increase) of isolated hearts perfused either with xanthine plus xanthine oxidase, an oxyradical-generating system or H_2O_2, a potent oxidant. In addition, sodium selenite prevented the large changes occurring in $+dP/dt$ and $-dP/dt$.[40]

EFFECTS OF SELENIUM SUPPLEMENTATION IN DIABETIC HEARTS

Cardiovascular Alterations in Diabetes: A Summary

Cardiovascular complications, the leading cause for the mortality of diabetic individuals, result from multiple parameters including glucotoxicity, lipotoxicity, fibrosis, and mitochondrial uncoupling. Diabetic cardiomyopathy was originally described as a specific diabetes-form of myocardial dysfunction often starting as diastolic dysfunction.[41] In diabetic subjects, oxidative stress arises from an imbalance between the production of ROS and reactive nitrogen species (RNS) and the capability of the system to readily detoxify reactive intermediates. With ROS production becoming excessive, oxidative and nitrosative stress will develop and cause functional alterations of biological tissues.[42,43] With respect to healthy subjects, patients with diabetes demonstrate significant lower plasma levels of GSH-Px and selenoalbumin that are negatively correlated to fasting plasma glucose.[10] A number of ways have been suggested in which the damaging effect of hyperglycemia can be mediated or enhanced by ROS. Basically, alterations in the redox status appear to be a common link in diabetic cardiomyopathy. Several antioxidant strategies have been developed and reviewed recently.[44,45]

General Effects of Selenium Supplementation

Experimental studies showed that in streptozotocin-induced diabetic rats, daily sodium selenate treatment reduced or normalized high blood glucose level and restored left ventricular pressure parameters without any positive effect on low insulin level.[16] Selenite treatment of diabetic rats significantly restored the altered activities of glutathione-S-transferase (GS-T), glucose-6-phosphate dehydrogenase (G-6-PD), 6-phosphogluconate dehydrogenase (6-PGA), superoxide dismutase (SOD), glutathione reductase (GR), and GSH-Px, which are involved in the glutathione metabolism. Selenium treatment also slightly but significantly decreased the high blood glucose level and reduced the high levels of LPO and NOPs.[46,47] Selenite treatment could prevent the loss of myofibrils and Z-lines, the reduction of cardiomyocyte diameter and the alterations of the *discus intercalaris* seen in heart tissue of diabetic rats, as well as it could reverse the increased platelet aggregation and thromboxane B2 level to the control levels.[48,49] More recent studies demonstrate that sodium selenate administration for 4 weeks also reduced the oxidized protein sulfhydryl and nitrite concentrations via reducing MMP-2 activation and therefore reducing the degradation of two of its target proteins, troponin I and α-actinin.[50]

Ion Homeostasis under Selenium Supplementation

Sodium selenite treatment reversed the prolongation in both action potential duration and twitch duration of the diabetic rats by restoring both fast transient, I_{to} and sustained, I_{ss} K^+ currents[51] while treatment of cardiomyocytes from diabetic rats with GSH, like insulin application, have been shown to upregulate I_{to} density.[52]

Plasma deficiency of Zn^{2+}, a complex antioxidant and a potent inducer of metallothionein (MT), is a risk factor for the development of diabetes with Zn^{2+} supplementation having beneficial effects and preventing the development of cardiomyopathy in STZ-induced diabetic mice.[53] Sodium selenite treatment (4 weeks) of the diabetic rats caused a significant normalization of cationic homeostasis. Thus selenite treatment restored basal $[Zn^{2+}]_i$ and $[Ca^{2+}]_i$ values and normalized Ca^{2+} transients of cardiomyocytes isolated from diabetic rats.[46] A schematic summary related with preventive effects of selenium treatment on diabetes-induced cardiac dysfunction is given in Figure 26.2. Selenite treatment, besides preventing the diabetic-induced increase in $[Zn^{2+}]_i$ also restores the decreased metallothionein, MT content.[46] MT is a potent antioxidant protein and binds seven Zn^{2+} with sulfur ligands. Redox reagents are asymmetrically involved in both directions of Zn^{2+} transfer from MT to thionein.[54] Reduced glutathione mediates Zn^{2+} transfer from enzymes to thionein, whereas glutathione disulfide oxidizes MT with enhanced release and transfer of Zn^{2+} to apoenzymes. This pathway seems true for our model study due to increased GSSG and MT and decreased GSH. Restoring controlled MT content is of importance in connection with the protective function to cells by reducing damage from ROS and inhibiting ROS production.[46,55]

Previous studies showed that inhibition of aldose reductase normalized Na^+ and Ca^{2+}

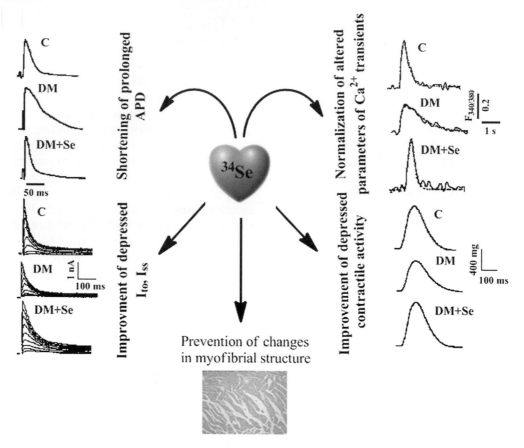

FIGURE 26.2 Beneficial effects of selenium treatment on function and structure of heart in diabetic rat. Either sodium selenite or sodium selenate treatment of diabetic rats for 4 weeks had beneficial effects on both mechanical and electrical activities of heart preparations. Diabetes induced a marked depression in both left ventricular developed pressure and electrically stimulated isometric contraction, and significant prolongation in intracellular action potential duration (APD) in isolated papillary muscle strips. Reduced amplitudes of transient (I_{to}) and steady state (I_{ss}) outward K^+ currents, alterations in the parameters of $[Ca^{2+}]_i$ transients obtained with electrical-field stimulation and increase in the basal $[Ca^{2+}]_i$ level in isolated cardiomyocytes from diabetic rat heart were recorded at the cellular level. All these alterations, in most part due to increased ROS, were prevented by a 4-week selenium treatment.

levels in ischemic-reperfused hearts by normalizing Na^+/K^+-ATPase activity.[56] The authors postulated that during ischemic-reperfusion, polyol pathway activity increases NADH/NAD$^-$ ratio, leading to the activation of protein kinase C, PKC and inhibition of Na^+/K^+-ATPase activity. Since NADH/NAD$^-$ ratio is also increased in high glucose-treated hearts because of polyol pathway activity, activation of PKC and reduction of Na^+/K^+-ATPase activity might also be a potential contributory factor for the abnormal Ca^{2+} signalling in the acute hyperglycemic hearts. Presently no data are available in cardiac tissues; however, it was reported that selenium supplementation resulted in a complete normalization of the Na^+/K^+ pump activity in diabetic aorta homogenates.[57]

Could Selenium Supplementation Restore NF-κB Activity in Diabetes?

The nuclear factor NF-κB is a transcription factor that regulates a number of cellular genes, such as those encoding iNOS. Reactive oxygen species enhance the signal transduction pathways for NF-κB activation in the cytoplasm and translocation into the nucleus.[58] In contrast, the DNA binding activity of oxidized NF-κB is significantly diminished, and that activity is restored by reducing enzymes, such as thioredoxin or redox factor 1 and by antioxidants.[59] In the diabetic heart, enhanced NF-κB activity can be anticipated that results from increased oxidative stress but also from degradation of lipids or proteins by free radical attack. Through its role in LPO, selenium supplementation could be efficient to reduce NF-κB activity in the diabetic heart as it was shown to reduce the 80% increased in NF-κB activity in peripheral blood mononuclear cells of diabetic patients.[14] Also, NF-κB blockade mitigates oxidative stress and improves mitochondrial structural integrity directly, through downregulation of increased oxygen-free radicals, thereby increasing ATP synthesis and thus restoring cardiac function in type 2 diabetes.[60] Similar restoring effects of selenium were reported in ischemic/reperfusion-mediated cardiac dysfunction on the elevated ratios of NF-κB in particulate and cytosolic fractions and of phosphorylated NF-κB and total NF-κB in hearts.[40]

CONCLUDING REMARKS

Diabetes mellitus is a disorder resulting in impaired control of blood glucose levels by either impaired insulin release (Type 1) or impaired insulin function or insulin resistance (Type 2). Selenium has been reported to exert insulin-like cellular functions both *in vivo* and *in vitro*. Addition of selenium as sodium selenate to isolated primary rat adipocytes stimulated glucose transport.[61] In STZ-induced diabetic rats, sodium selenate was shown to improve glucose homeostasis.[16,62,63] In these rats, selenium partly reversed abnormal expression of liver glycolytic (i.e. glucokinase and pyruvate kinase) and gluconeogenic (phosphoenolpyruvate carboxykinase) enzymes[62]; and glucose-6-phosphate dehydrogenase and fatty acid synthase.[64] However, insulin release in response to a glucose challenge is markedly reduced in control selenate-treated rats but not diabetic selenium-treated rats,[16] despite selenium potentially promoting an overall improvement in islet function.[65] Selenium stimulates glucose transport and antilipolysis by stimulating the tyrosine kinases involved in the distal signalling of the insulin signalling cascade but independent of insulin receptor activation.[66] Thus selenium exerts both insulin-like and non-insulin-like actions in cells.

The results of selenium supplementation are likely dependent on the dose and form of selenium used given the variations in the reported observations. Selenium was equally well retained by infants from both selenite and selenate despite apparent selenium absorption and urinary excretion being higher for selenite.[67] Selenomethionine was more effective in raising blood selenium concentrations than selenate, but both selenomethionine and selenate were equally effective in raising GSH-Px activities in whole blood, erythrocytes and plasma, indicating a similar bioavailability for the two forms, consistent with the incorporation of selenium from selenomethionine into a general tissue protein pool while selenate is directly available for GSH-Px synthesis.[68] However, in another more recent study, the beneficial effects on GSH-Px activity appeared more prominent when selenium was supplemented as selenomethionine.[69] Also, it should be noted that selenomethionine did not have a significant effect on phosphorylation of NF-κB p65 on chondrocytes while high doses of selenite have been shown to inhibit NF-κB activity in macrophages.[70,71]

To conclude, despite the fact that the importance of selenium for heart physiology has been known since the Roman era (following Pliny the elder, who said that those patients with spasticity and heart palpitations should eat from the "hyena heart", an organ rich in protein, vitamin B12 and selenium),[72] its dietary supplementation has been popularized for its beneficial effects in general health only recently.[73] Much work is still needed to understand its multiple effects and the numerous pathways that are implicated. The effects of selenium are dependent upon its concentration and chemical form of supplementation, but also they are markedly dependent on the status of the tissues, particularly its redox status. Also it should be considered that part of the selenium-dependent beneficial effects could result from its chelating properties of the deleterious heavy metals. No doubt selenium will be the subject of several studies to better delineate its cardioprotective effects in the coming years.

References

1. Spallholz JE. On the nature of selenium toxicity and carcinostatic activity. *Free Radic Biol Med* 1994;**17**:45–64.
2. Li GS, Wang F, Kang D, Li C. Keshan disease: an endemic cardiomyopathy in China. *Hum Pathol* 1985;**16**:602–9.
3. Lei C, Niu X, Wei J, Zhu J, Zhu Y. Interaction of glutathione peroxidase-1 and selenium in endemic dilated cardiomyopathy. *Clin Chim Acta* 2009;**399**:102–8.
4. Savarino L, Granchi D, Ciapetti G, Cenni E, Ravaglia G, Forti P, Maioli F, Mattioli R. Serum concentrations of zinc and selenium in elderly people: results in healthy nonagenarians/centenarians. *Exp Gerontol* 2001;**36**:327–39.
5. Arroyo M, Laguardia SP, Bhattacharya SK, Nelson MD, Johnson PL, Carbone LD, Newman KP, Weber KT. Micronutrients in African-Americans with decompensated and compensated heart failure. *Transl Res* 2006;**148**:301–8.
6. Beaglehole R, Jackson R, Watkinson J, Scragg R, Yee RL. Decreased blood selenium and risk of myocardial infarction. *Int J Epidemiol* 1990;**19**:918–22.
7. de Lorgeril M, Salen P. Selenium and antioxidant defenses as major mediators in the development of chronic heart failure. *Heart Fail Rev* 2006;**11**:13–7.
8. Suadicani P, Hein HO, Gyntelberg F. Serum selenium concentration and risk of ischaemic heart disease in a prospective cohort study of 3000 males. *Atherosclerosis* 1992;**96**:33–42.
9. Laclaustra M, Navas-Acien A, Stranges S, Ordovas JM, Guallar E. Serum selenium concentrations and diabetes in U.S. adults: National Health and Nutrition Examination Survey (NHANES) 2003-2004. *Environ Health Perspect* 2009;**117**:1409–13.
10. Roman M, Lapolla A, Jitaru P, Sechi A, Cosma C, Cozzi G, Cescon P, Barbante C. Plasma selenoproteins concentrations in type 2 diabetes mellitus—a pilot study. *Transl Res* 2010;**156**:242–50.
11. Neve J. Selenium as a risk factor for cardiovascular diseases. *J Cardiovasc Risk* 1996;**3**:42–7.
12. Xia Y, Hill KE, Li P, Xu J, Zhou D, Motley AK, Wang L, Byrne DW, Burk RF. Optimization of selenoprotein P and other plasma selenium biomarkers for the assessment of the selenium nutritional requirement: a placebo-controlled, double-blind study of selenomethionine supplementation in selenium-deficient Chinese subjects. *Am J Clin Nutr* **92**, 525–31.
13. Brown BG, Zhao XQ, Chait A, Fisher LD, Cheung MC, Morse JS, Dowdy AA, Marino EK, Bolson EL, Alaupovic P, Frohlich J, Albers JJ. Simvastatin and niacin, antioxidant vitamins, or the combination for the prevention of coronary disease. *N Engl J Med* 2001;**345**:1583–92.
14. Faure P, Ramon O, Favier A, Halimi S. Selenium supplementation decreases nuclear factor-kappa B activity in peripheral blood mononuclear cells from type 2 diabetic patients. *Eur J Clin Invest* 2004;**34**:475–81.
15. Xia Y, Hill KE, Byrne DW, Xu J, Burk RF. Effectiveness of selenium supplements in a low-selenium area of China. *Am J Clin Nutr* 2005;**81**:829–34.
16. Battell ML, Delgatty HL, McNeill JH. Sodium selenate corrects glucose tolerance and heart function in STZ diabetic rats. *Mol Cell Biochem* 1998;**179**:27–34.
17. Faure P. Protective effects of antioxidant micronutrients (vitamin E, zinc and selenium) in type 2 diabetes mellitus. *Clin Chem Lab Med* 2003;**41**:995–8.
18. Stranges S, Marshall JR, Trevisan M, Natarajan R, Donahue RP, Combs GF, Farinaro E, Clark LC, Reid ME. Effects of selenium supplementation on cardiovascular disease incidence and mortality: secondary analyses in a randomized clinical trial. *Am J Epidemiol* 2006;**163**:694–9.
19. Bleys J, Navas-Acien A, Guallar E. Serum selenium and diabetes in U.S. adults. *Diabetes Care* 2007;**30**:829–34.
20. Yeh JY, Beilstein MA, Andrews JS, Whanger PD. Tissue distribution and influence of selenium status on levels of selenoprotein. W. *FASEB J* 1995;**9**:392–6.

21. Lu C, Qiu F, Zhou H, Peng Y, Hao W, Xu J, Yuan J, Wang S, Qiang B, Xu C, Peng X. Identification and characterization of selenoprotein K: an antioxidant in cardiomyocytes. *FEBS Lett* 2006;**580**:5189−97.

22. Papp LV, Lu J, Holmgren A, Khanna KK. From selenium to selenoproteins: synthesis, identity, and their role in human health. *Antioxid Redox Signal* 2007;**9**:775−806.

23. Turan B, Hotomaroglu O, Kilic M, Demirel-Yilmaz E. Cardiac dysfunction induced by low and high diet antioxidant levels comparing selenium and vitamin E in rats. *Regul Toxicol Pharmacol* 1999;**29**:142−50.

24. Oldfield JE. The two faces of selenium. *J Nutr* 1987;**117**:2002−8.

25. Simmons TW, Jamall IS, Lockshin RA. The effect of selenium deficiency on peroxidative injury in the house fly, Musca domestica. A role for glutathione peroxidase. *FEBS Lett* 1987;**218**:251−4.

26. Kim IY, Stadtman TC. Inhibition of NF-kappaB DNA binding and nitric oxide induction in human T cells and lung adenocarcinoma cells by selenite treatment. *Proc Natl Acad Sci U S A* 1997;**94**:12904−7.

27. Konz KH, Haap M, Hill KE, Burk RF, Walsh RA. Diastolic dysfunction of perfused rat hearts induced by hydrogen peroxide. Protective effect of selenium. *J Mol Cell Cardiol* 1989;**21**:789−95.

28. Sayar K, Ugur M, Gurdal H, Onaran O, Hotomaroglu O, Turan B. Dietary selenium and vitamin E intakes alter beta-adrenergic response of L-type Ca-current and beta-adrenoceptor-adenylate cyclase coupling in rat heart. *J Nutr* 2000;**130**:733−40.

29. Gomez RM, Pacienza N, Schattner M, Habarta A, Levander OA, Sterin-Borda L. Decreased beta-adrenoceptor chronotropic response in selenium-deficient mice: negative crosstalk between iNOS activity and cAMP accumulation. *Biol Trace Elem Res* 2007;**117**:127−38.

30. Yang MS, Chan HW, Yu LC. Glutathione peroxidase and glutathione reductase activities are partially responsible for determining the susceptibility of cells to oxidative stress. *Toxicology* 2006;**226**:126−30.

31. Beck MA, Esworthy RS, Ho YS, Chu FF. Glutathione peroxidase protects mice from viral-induced myocarditis. *FASEB J* 1998;**12**:1143−9.

32. de Haan JB, Bladier C, Griffiths P, Kelner M, O'Shea RD, Cheung NS, Bronson RT, Silvestro MJ, Wild S, Zheng SS, Beart PM, Hertzog PJ, Kola I. Mice with a homozygous null mutation for the most abundant glutathione peroxidase, Gpx1, show increased susceptibility to the oxidative stress-inducing agents paraquat and hydrogen peroxide. *J Biol Chem* 1998;**273**:22528−36.

33. Shiomi T, Tsutsui H, Matsusaka H, Murakami K, Hayashidani S, Ikeuchi M, Wen J, Kubota T, Utsumi H, Takeshita A. Overexpression of glutathione peroxidase prevents left ventricular remodeling and failure after myocardial infarction in mice. *Circulation* 2004;**109**:544−9.

34. Xiong Y, Liu X, Lee CP, Chua BH, Ho YS. Attenuation of doxorubicin-induced contractile and mitochondrial dysfunction in mouse heart by cellular glutathione peroxidase. *Free Radic Biol Med* 2006;**41**:46−55.

35. Ayaz M, Ozdemir S, Yaras N, Vassort G, Turan B. Selenium-induced alterations in ionic currents of rat cardiomyocytes. *Biochem Biophys Res Commun* 2005;**327**:163−73.

36. Aviado DM, Drimal J, Watanabe T, Lish PM. Cardiac effects of sodium selenite. *Cardiology* 1975;**60**:113−20.

37. Turan B, Desilets M, Acan LN, Hotomaroglu O, Vannier C, Vassort G. Oxidative effects of selenite on rat ventricular contractility and Ca movements. *Cardiovasc Res* 1996;**32**:351−61.

38. Ugur M, Turan B. Adenosine triphosphate alters the selenite-induced contracture and negative inotropic effect on cardiac muscle contractions. *Biol Trace Elem Res* 2001;**79**:235−45.

39. Ugur M, Ayaz M, Ozdemir S, Turan B. Toxic concentrations of selenite shortens repolarization phase of action potential in rat papillary muscle. *Biol Trace Elem Res* 2002;**89**:227−38.

40. Turan B, Saini HK, Zhang M, Prajapati D, Elimban V, Dhalla NS. Selenium improves cardiac function by attenuating the activation of NF-kappaB due to ischemia-reperfusion injury. *Antioxid Redox Signal* 2005;**7**:1388−97.

41. Solang L, Malmberg K, Ryden L. Diabetes mellitus and congestive heart failure. Further knowledge needed. *Eur Heart J* 1999;**20**:789−95.

42. Ceriello A. New insights on oxidative stress and diabetic complications may lead to a "causal" antioxidant therapy. *Diabetes Care* 2003;**26**:1589−96.

43. Pacher P, Obrosova IG, Mabley JG, Szabo C. Role of nitrosative stress and peroxynitrite in the pathogenesis of diabetic complications. Emerging new therapeutical strategies. *Curr Med Chem* 2005;**12**:267−75.

44. Turan, B. Role of antioxidants in redox regulation of diabetic cardiovascular complications. *Curr Pharm Biotechnol* 2010;**11**:819−36.

45. Vassort, G. and Turan, B. Protective role of antioxidants in diabetes-induced cardiac dysfunction. *Cardiovasc Toxicol* 2010;**10**:73−86.

46. Ayaz M, Turan B. Selenium prevents diabetes-induced alterations in [Zn^{2+}]i and metallothionein level of rat heart via restoration of cell redox cycle. *Am J Physiol Heart Circ Physiol* 2006;**290**:H1071−80.

47. Ulusu NN, Turan B. Beneficial effects of selenium on some enzymes of diabetic rat heart. *Biol Trace Elem Res* 2005;**103**:207−16.

48. Ayaz M, Can B, Ozdemir S, Turan B. Protective effect of selenium treatment on diabetes-induced myocardial structural alterations. *Biol Trace Elem Res* 2002;**89**:215−26.

49. Ersoz G, Yakaryilmaz A, Turan B. Effect of sodium selenite treatment on platelet aggregation of streptozotocin-induced diabetic rats. *Thromb Res* 2003;**111**:363−7.

50. Aydemir-Koksoy A, Bilginoglu A, Sariahmetoglu M, Schulz R, Turan B. Antioxidant treatment protects diabetic rats from cardiac dysfunction by preserving contractile protein targets of oxidative stress. *J Nutr Biochem* 2010;**21**:827−33.

51. Ayaz M, Ozdemir S, Ugur M, Vassort G, Turan B. Effects of selenium on altered mechanical and electrical cardiac activities of diabetic rat. *Arch Biochem Biophys* 2004;**426**:83−90.

52. Xu Z, Patel KP, Lou MF, Rozanski GJ. Up-regulation of K(+) channels in diabetic rat ventricular myocytes by insulin and glutathione. *Cardiovasc Res* 2002;**53**:80−8.

53. Wang J, Song Y, Elsherif L, Song Z, Zhou G, Prabhu SD, Saari JT, Cai L. Cardiac metallothionein induction plays the major role in the prevention of diabetic cardiomyopathy by zinc supplementation. *Circulation* 2006;**113**:544−54.

54. Haase H, Maret W. A differential assay for the reduced and oxidized states of metallothionein and thionein. *Anal Biochem* 2004;**333**:19−26.

55. Cai L, Wang J, Li Y, Sun X, Wang L, Zhou Z, Kang YJ. Inhibition of superoxide generation and associated nitrosative damage is involved in metallothionein prevention of diabetic cardiomyopathy. *Diabetes* 2005;**54**:1829−37.

56. Ramasamy R, Liu H, Oates PJ, Schaefer S. Attenuation of ischemia induced increases in sodium and calcium by the aldose reductase inhibitor zopolrestat. *Cardiovasc Res* 1999;**42**:130−9.

57. Aydemir-Koksoy A, Turan B. Selenium inhibits proliferation signaling and restores sodium/potassium pump function of diabetic rat aorta. *Biol Trace Elem Res* 2008;**126**:237−45.

58. Schreck R, Albermann K, Baeuerle PA. Nuclear factor kappa B: an oxidative stress-responsive transcription factor of eukaryotic cells (a review). *Free Radic Res Commun* 1992;**17**:221−37.

59. Li N, Karin M. Is NF-kappaB the sensor of oxidative stress? *FASEB J* 1999;**13**:1137−43.

60. Mariappan N, Elks CM, Sriramula S, Guggilam A, Liu Z, Borkhsenious O, Francis J. NF-kappaB-induced oxidative stress contributes to mitochondrial and cardiac dysfunction in type II diabetes. *Cardiovasc Res* 2010;**85**:473−83.

61. Ezaki O. The insulin-like effects of selenate in rat adipocytes. *J Biol Chem* 1990;**265**:1124−8.

62. Becker DJ, Reul B, Ozcelikay AT, Buchet JP, Henquin JC, Brichard SM. Oral selenate improves glucose homeostasis and partly reverses abnormal expression of liver glycolytic and gluconeogenic enzymes in diabetic rats. *Diabetologia* 1996;**39**:3−11.

63. McNeill JH, Delgatty HL, Battell ML. Insulinlike effects of sodium selenate in streptozocin-induced diabetic rats. *Diabetes* 1991;**40**:1675−8.

64. Berg EA, Wu JY, Campbell L, Kagey M, Stapleton SR. Insulin-like effects of vanadate and selenate on the expression of glucose-6-phosphate dehydrogenase and fatty acid synthase in diabetic rats. *Biochimie* 1995;**77**:919−24.

65. Li S, Li X, Li YL, Shao CH, Bidasee KR, Rozanski GJ. Insulin regulation of glutathione and contractile phenotype in diabetic rat ventricular myocytes. *Am J Physiol Heart Circ Physiol* 2007;**292**:H1619−29.

66. Heart E, Sung CK. Insulin-like and non-insulin-like selenium actions in 3T3-L1 adipocytes. *J Cell Biochem* 2003;**88**:719−31.

67. Van Dael P, Davidsson L, Ziegler EE, Fay LB, Barclay D. Comparison of selenite and selenate apparent absorption and retention in infants using stable isotope methodology. *Pediatr Res* 2002; **51**:71−5.

68. Thomson CD, Robinson MF, Butler JA, Whanger PD. Long-term supplementation with selenate and selenomethionine: selenium and glutathione peroxidase (EC 1.11.1.9) in blood components of New Zealand women. *Br J Nutr* 1993;**69**:577−88.

69. Erbayraktar Z, Yilmaz O, Artmann AT, Cehreli R, Coker C. Effects of selenium supplementation on antioxidant defense and glucose homeostasis in experimental diabetes mellitus. *Biol Trace Elem Res* 2007;**118**:217−26.

70. Cheng AW, Stabler TV, Bolognesi M, Kraus VB. Selenomethionine inhibits IL-1beta inducible nitric oxide synthase (iNOS) and cyclooxygenase 2 (COX2) expression in primary human chondrocytes. *Osteoarthritis Cartilage*

71. Shin KM, Shen L, Park SJ, Jeong JH, Lee KT. Bis-(3-hydroxyphenyl) diselenide inhibits LPS-stimulated iNOS and COX-2 expression in RAW 264.7 macrophage cells through the NF-kappaB inactivation. *J Pharm Pharmacol* 2009;**61**:479−86.

72. van Tellingen C. Quibus cor palpitet: hyena cor. *Int J Cardiol* 2007;**122**:164−7.

73. Rayman MP. The importance of selenium to human health. *Lancet* 2000;**356**:233−41.

27

Exercise and Physical Activity in the Prevention of Diabetes and Metabolic Syndrome

Cheri L. Gostic, Dawn Blatt

Division of Rehabilitation Sciences, School of Health Technology and Management
Stony Brook University, NY, USA

DIABETES

The prevalence of diabetes in the US has risen by epidemic proportions over recent decades due to type 2 diabetes' underlying association with escalating rates of obesity in this country. In 2010, the CDC estimated that 8.3% of the US population had diabetes, affecting 25.8 million people at a total cost in 2007 of $174 billion.[1] The CDC released a startling report in 2010

Nutritional and Therapeutic Interventions for Diabetes and Metabolic Syndrome
DOI: 10.1016/B978-0-12-385083-6.00027-9

that indicated that the prevalence of type 2 diabetes could double or triple over the next 40 years if current trends continue, with 33% of the population to be diagnosed with diabetes by 2050.[2] This prediction highlights the need for effective population-based interventions to prevent this impending national health crisis.

PREDIABETES

Type 2 diabetes is usually preceded by a period of years in which a person has elevated blood glucose levels but does not meet diagnostic criteria for diabetes. This state referred to as "prediabetes". Individuals with prediabetes can exhibit impaired glucose tolerance (IGT) or impaired fasting glucose (IFG), or both. NHANES data from 2005 to 2008 indicate that 35% of adults 20 years or older and, remarkably, 50% of adults ages 65 or older in the US had pre-diabetes.[1] Without intervention, approximately one-third of individuals with either IGT or IFG and two-thirds of individuals with both will develop diabetes within 6 years.[3] The goal of identifying and treating prediabetes is clearly to prevent the development of type 2 diabetes and its associated complications.

INSULIN RESISTANCE

Insulin resistance, a reduction in the ability of the body to clear a glucose load from the bloodstream in response to circulating insulin, is characteristic of prediabetes and type 2 diabetes. When people are insulin resistant, their muscle, fat, and liver cells do not respond adequately to normal levels of insulin in the blood. As a result, their bodies require higher levels of insulin to adequately transport glucose into cells for energy production. Normally, 75% of ingested glucose is utilized by skeletal muscle for energy,[4] but in persons with insulin resistance, glucose disposal into skeletal muscle is reduced

by as much as 50%.[5] Physical activity is important in regulating plasma glucose levels, decreasing excess fat deposition, and reducing the risk of insulin resistance. Insulin resistance is often precipitated by lifestyle factors such as excess food intake and physical inactivity,[6,7] and significantly increases the risk of developing type 2 diabetes and cardiovascular disease. Obesity often predisposes individuals to type 2 diabetes through the deposition of excess triglycerides and fat into specific regions of the body including visceral adipose tissue, the liver, and skeletal muscle. This accumulation of adipose tissue is associated with an increased production of free fatty acids and adipokines (molecules and hormones released by adipocytes) that interfere with insulin receptor signaling in muscle, adipose tissue, and the liver, and leads to decreased glucose transport in genetically predisposed individuals. Adipokines are also associated with a proinflammatory effect and endothelial dysfunction that increases the risk for metabolic dysfunction and cardiovascular disease.[8,9]

EVIDENCE ON THE ROLE OF LIFESTYLE INTERVENTIONS IN THE PREVENTION OF TYPE 2 DIABETES

Because excess adiposity drives the underlying pathology of type 2 diabetes, it seems intuitive that an intervention that combines caloric restriction with an increase in exercise or physical activity is the most effective approach to prevent progression to diabetes in high-risk individuals. In fact, the principal modifiable risk factors associated with type 2 diabetes, which accounts for 90–95% of all diagnosed cases of diabetes in adults, are obesity and sedentary lifestyle.[10] Studies consistently indicate that an increased body mass index (BMI) is one of the strongest risk factors for the development of diabetes and, additionally, an increased waist-to-hip ratio significantly increases a person's risk.[11] A review of 10 prospective cohort studies indicates that people with an active lifestyle have about a 30% lower risk of diabetes than individuals who are sedentary.[12] The research clearly supports the benefit of weight loss and physical activity in the prevention of type 2 diabetes.[4]

There is an extensive body of evidence that supports the value of lifestyle interventions such as a healthy diet and physical activity in delaying or preventing the onset of diabetes in high-risk groups of individuals. The results of the Finnish Diabetes Prevention Study (DPS) provided the first such evidence from a properly randomized controlled trial. The study randomly assigned 522 middle-aged overweight subjects with IGT to an intensive lifestyle intervention group or a control group. The control group received general dietary and exercise advice at baseline only. During the first year, those in the intervention group received individualized counseling aimed at reducing weight, total intake of fat, and intake of saturated fat, and at increasing intake of fiber and physical activity. After a mean duration of follow-up of 3.2 years, the overall incidence of diabetes was reduced by 58% in the intervention group, and almost 100% in those patients meeting all the goals of the intervention.[13] Weight loss was significantly associated with the achievement of each of the other four lifestyle goals and, accordingly, success score was strongly and inversely correlated with weight reduction.[14] After an additional 3 years of follow-up without further lifestyle counseling, the intervention group demonstrated a 36% reduction in the relative risk of diabetes. This demonstrated that the lifestyle changes that had been achieved by participants in the intervention group yielded long-term benefits after the discontinuation of the intervention.[15] *Post hoc* analyses of the role of leisure-time physical activity (LTPA) in preventing type 2 diabetes in the participants of the DPS revealed that individuals who increased moderate to vigorous LTPA, or strenuous, structured LTPA were 63–65% less likely to develop diabetes. Low-intensity LTPA and walking was also found to confer benefits, consistent with the finding that the change in total physical activity was the most important factor in reducing the incidence of type 2 diabetes among participants. Both endurance LTPA and resistance training practiced at a moderate or higher intensity appeared to protect against progression from IGT to diabetes.[16]

In the US Diabetes Prevention Program (DPP), 3,234 overweight or obese subjects with IFG and IGT were randomized to standard lifestyle recommendations plus metformin (an insulin-sensitizing drug), standard lifestyle recommendations plus placebo, or to intensive lifestyle modification involving dietary and exercise counseling. The standard lifestyle group received written material and an annual individual counseling session emphasizing the benefits of a healthy lifestyle. Those in the intensive lifestyle intervention group set goals to lose at least 7% of initial body weight via a low-fat diet and to participate in moderate intensity physical activity for at least 150 min/week. After a mean follow-up period of 2.8 years, intensive lifestyle modification had reduced the incidence of type 2 diabetes by 58% relative to the standard lifestyle modification plus placebo group. Those receiving standard lifestyle modification with metformin saw a reduction in the incidence of diabetes of 31%.[17] Weight loss was the dominant predictor of reduced diabetes incidence in the DPP, as every kilogram of weight lost was associated with a 16% reduction in diabetes risk, adjusted for changes in diet and physical activity. Increased physical activity and a decrease in percentage of calories ingested from fat were predictive of weight loss, and increased physical activity was found to be important to sustain weight loss. Achievement of the physical activity goal of 150 min/week, though, was substantially and independently related to the development of diabetes among the 495 participants in the intensive lifestyle modification group who did not meet the weight loss goal at year 1, and resulted in a 46% reduction in the incidence of diabetes.[18] When weight loss proves difficult, research demonstrates that exercise alone can reduce diabetes risk by increasing insulin-mediated glucose disposal to muscle.[19] In the 10-year follow-up to the DPP, the advantage of lifestyle intervention remained, with the intensive lifestyle group exhibiting the lowest cumulative incidence of diabetes.[20]

Similar benefits of lifestyle interventions were found in studies conducted in other countries. A Japanese trial included 458 men with IGT randomized to receive either intensive lifestyle intervention or standard intervention. The goals of intensive intervention included body weight reduction, consumption of large amounts of vegetables with a 10% reduction of other foods, reduction of fat and alcohol intake and physical activity of greater than 30–40 min/day. The cumulative 4-year incidence of type 2 diabetes in the intensive lifestyle intervention group was 67% lower than in the standard intervention group.[21] In the Indian Diabetes Prevention Program (IDPP), 531 individuals with IGT were randomized into four groups: control, lifestyle modification, metformin, and lifestyle modification with metformin. After a median 30-month follow-up, relative risk reduction was 28.5% with lifestyle modification, 26.4% with metformin, and 28.2% with lifestyle modification plus metformin, compared to the control group. Although lifestyle modification or metformin reduced the incidence of diabetes, no added benefit was observed from the combination of a lifestyle and pharmacological approach.

A prospective European population-based cohort study involving 24,155 participants aged 40–79 quantified the association between the achievement of the five lifestyle goals previously established by the DPS and the incidence of diabetes during a 4.6-year follow-up. The incidence of type 2 diabetes was inversely related to the number of goals achieved. None of the participants who *met* all five goals developed diabetes, whereas the risk of diabetes was highest in participants who did not meet any of the goals. Only 20% of the participants met three or more diabetes prevention behavior goals, 10% achieved no goals, and only 1% achieved all five goals. The diabetes prevention goals which appeared to confer the most protection against the development of type 2 diabetes were a BMI $< 25 \text{ kg/m}^2$ and, secondly, at least 4 h/week of physical activity, a goal achieved by 76% of the participants. These findings confirm that healthy lifestyle modifications in the general population may significantly reduce future incidence of type 2 diabetes.[22]

A review of 20 longitudinal cohort studies by Gill and Cooper and a systematic review of 10 prospective cohort studies by Jeon *et al.* also support the protective effect of regular physical activity in substantially reducing the risk of type 2 diabetes. Regular physical activity of moderate or vigorous intensity was found to confer a 20–30% risk reduction after adjustments for confounding factors such as age, health status (including family history), BMI and the presence of other diabetes risk factors.[23] After adjustment for BMI, the reduction in diabetes risk remained substantial (17%) for both moderately intense activity and walking, confirming the benefits of physical activity even in the absence of weight loss.[12] It is evident from the extensive literature available that long-term effects of lifestyle interventions are beneficial and that associated long-term costs of prevention are relatively very low.[24]

THE EFFECT OF EXERCISE ON INSULIN RESISTANCE

Exercise and physical activity have been shown to clearly improve insulin sensitivity and influence the pathophysiological conditions underlying the development of type 2 diabetes. Research demonstrates that adults with insulin resistance and type 2 diabetes possess a lower percentage of type I fibers, an increased proportion of type IIb fibers and a diminished capillary density, suggesting a decreased capacity to metabolize glucose and lipids using oxidative pathways.[4] Aerobic exercise increases the lipid oxidative capacity of muscle cells, decreases the amount of lipid products stored in skeletal muscle, increases glucose uptake by muscle during physical activity and promotes the storage of glucose in muscle after exercise.[25] Glucose uptake into skeletal muscle has been shown to increase up to 20-fold[26] during lower extremity exercise and is facilitated by an increase in blood flow to exercising muscles. Studies demonstrate a significant increase in glucose utilization and translocation of GLUT4 (the insulin-regulated glucose transporter protein 4) to the skeletal muscle cell membrane in both healthy individuals as well as in individuals with type 2 diabetes with exercise.[27,28] Studies reveal that an improvement in insulin sensitivity is observed for several hours up to a few days after a single session of exercise in both healthy individuals as well as those with type 2 diabetes and obesity.[29,30] Conversely, several days without physical activity significantly decreases insulin sensitivity.[31]

Houmard et al. examined the impact of exercise volume and intensity of training on insulin action among sedentary, overweight or obese men and women. After 6 months of training, the low-volume/moderate-intensity group and high-volume/high-intensity group improved insulin sensitivity by about 85% compared with the control group. This was twice the improvement demonstrated by the low-volume/high-intensity group, suggesting that cumulative exercise time, independent of exercise intensity, is an important factor in improving insulin sensitivity in high-risk individuals. Total exercise duration should thus be considered when designing training programs with the intent of enhancing insulin action.[32] Greater benefits are likely to be achieved if more than the minimum recommended amount of activity is accumulated, but most importantly, physical activity must become an integral part of an individual's lifestyle to preserve its benefits. For individuals who have lost a significant amount of weight, studies generally support the need for 60–90 min of moderate-intensity physical activity/day to prevent weight regain.[33–35] Individuals should establish realistic goals that allow adequate time to steadily progress to this recommended level of daily physical activity.

Protective mechanisms conferred by exercise and physical activity in preventing the onset of type 2 diabetes include both acute and chronic adaptations. Acute responses involve an increase in glucose uptake, transport, and/or disposal that occur during and appear to last for 12–48 h post physical activity, depending on overall energy expenditure.[36] Chronic adaptations include improved endothelial function and capillarization,[37] increased mitochondrial biogenesis and fiber ratios,[38] improved muscular respiratory capacity and fatty acid oxidation,[39] and the increased synthesis of GLUT4 and enzymes that control the uptake and metabolism of glucose in skeletal muscle.[40]

THE ROLE OF AEROBIC AND RESISTIVE EXERCISE IN PREVENTING DIABETES

Exercise and physical activity play a crucial role in preventing or delaying the development of type 2 diabetes in those at risk, by improving insulin sensitivity and, indirectly, by producing beneficial changes in body mass and body composition.[41,42] Both aerobic and resistive exercise have therapeutic value in preventing type 2 diabetes, largely independent of weight loss, and are both valuable components of an exercise program. Aerobic activity decreases adiposity, particularly in the visceral region, even in the absence of weight loss, and has greater effects on cardiorespiratory fitness.[43] Resistive training increases muscle mass, elevates the resting metabolic rate, increases GLUT4 protein content, and improves glucose metabolism through increased glycogen synthase activity within the trained muscle. In addition to improving muscle quality and insulin sensitivity, strength training was shown to reduce free fatty acids and C-reactive protein, while increasing serum adiponectin (an adipokine associated with a reduced risk of type 2 diabetes), all findings associated with improved metabolic control.[44]

METABOLIC SYNDROME

Metabolic syndrome is a cluster of metabolically related abnormalities and cardiovascular risks, defined differently by various health organizations by criteria that generally include obesity, hypertriglyceridemia, high density lipidemia, hypertension, and elevated fasting glucose levels. Table 27.1 outlines the diagnostic criteria endorsed by the World Health Organization (WHO), as well as the American Heart Association (AHA) and National Heart, Lung, and Bone Institute (NHLBI). In the early stages of metabolic syndrome, there may be mild and varying degrees of abnormal insulin, glucose, and lipid metabolism, hypertension and overweight, which commonly progress to diabetes and atherosclerosis. With the growing epidemic of overweight and obesity, metabolic syndrome represents an extremely important health issue requiring immediate attention.

Depending on the criteria used, between one in three or one in five adults in the US can be labeled as having metabolic syndrome.[45] This

TABLE 27.1 Two Common Definitions for Metabolic Syndrome

The World Health Organization Criteria[a]	American Heart Association and National Heart, Lung and Bone Institute Criteria[b]
Insulin resistance (defined by either type 2 diabetes, IFG or IFT)	Positive diagnosis if ≥ 3 of the following:
AND two of the following:	Poor glucose regulation (fasting glucose ≥ 100 mg/dl or treatment for the condition)
Central obesity (waist:hip ratio > 0.9 in men, > 0.85 in women) and/or BMI > 30 kg/m^2	Overweight or obesity/Abdominal obesity (waist circumference in inches > 40 in men and > 35 in women)
Plasma triglycerides > 150 mg/dl and/or HDL cholesterol < 35 mg/dl in men or < 39 mg/dl in women	Hypertriglyceridemia (≥ 150 mg/dl or treatment for the condition)
Hypertension (≥ 140 mmHg systolic or ≥ 90 mmHg diastolic), or on antihypertensive medication	Low HDL cholesterol (< 40 mg/dl for men or < 50 mg/dl for women or treatment for the condition)
Urinary albumin excretion rate ≥ 20 µg/min or albumin:creatinine ratio ≥ 30 mg/g	Hypertension (blood pressure ≥ 130 mmHg systolic, ≥ 85 mmHg diastolic or treatment for the condition)

[a]Alberti K. G. and Zimmet P. Z. (1998) Definition, diagnosis and classification of diabetes mellitus and its complications. Part 1. Diagnosis and classification of diabetes mellitus: provisional report of a WHO consultation. Diabet. Med. **15**, 539–553.
[b]Grundy S. M., Cleeman J. I., Daniels S., Donato K. A., Eckel R. H., Franklin B. A., Gordon D. J., Krauss R. M., Savage P. J., Smith S. C., Spertus J. A. and Costa F. (2005) Diagnosis and management of the metabolic syndrome. Circulation **112**, 2735–2752.

diagnosis increases the risk of coronary heart disease two-fold, and all-cause mortality by 40%.[46] Lifestyle habits of smoking, alcohol, family history of cardiac disease, diabetes, and premature cardiovascular disease are all associated with metabolic syndrome.[47] Those diagnosed have been found to be susceptible to polycystic ovary disease, cholesterol gallstones, fatty liver, asthma, sleep disturbances, and certain forms of cancer.[48] There is speculation on the possible pathogenesis for this syndrome, with three etiological categories: obesity and disorders of adipose tissue, insulin resistance, or a constellation of independent factors (hepatic, vascular, and immunologic origin). Other contributing factors such as aging, hormonal changes, and a proinflammatory state have been proposed.[49] Adults who have no leisure time physical activity (LTPA) were found to be 45% more likely to be diagnosed when compared with active counterparts.[50]

EVIDENCE ON THE ROLE OF EXERCISE AND PHYSICAL ACTIVITY IN THE PREVENTION OF METABOLIC SYNDROME

There is an inverse relationship between increasing LTPA and the diagnosis of metabolic syndrome. Churilla and Fitzhugh utilized a measurement of MET (metabolic equivalent)* min/wk to quantify LTPA.[50] Defining activity requirements in this manner provides greater flexibility in an individual's exercise regimen. They found that individuals who achieved between 393 and 736 MET*min/wk of LTPA were 30% less likely to meet WHO criteria for metabolic syndrome and those achieving between 736 and 1,360 MET*min/wk were 35% less likely to meet AHA/NHLBI criteria when compared with inactive adults. It was also confirmed that higher doses of exercise led to an increased level of protection from metabolic syndrome.[50]

A prospective study by Laaksonen *et al.* that followed middle-aged men and their lifestyle physical activity, found that men who met the American College of Sports Medicine (ACSM) recommendations were half as likely to be diagnosed with metabolic syndrome compared with those who participated in less than 60 min of moderate intensity exercise/week.[51] Ekelund *et al.* found that middle-aged men who engaged in brisk walking for 1 h/day significantly decreased their risk of metabolic syndrome.[52]

Exercise can have a significant impact on the criteria of metabolic syndrome, even eliminating the diagnosis. Katzmarzyk *et al.* trained a group of individuals with sedentary lifestyles, increasing the supervised sessions to 45 min/day, 3 days/week for a 20-week training period. Of those subjects originally diagnosed with metabolic syndrome, 30.5% reversed the diagnosis by the end of the training period, demonstrating the positive impact of aerobic training for this condition.[53]

Dumortier *et al.* found that even low-intensity exercise in sedentary individuals over a 2-month time-frame led to an increased ability to oxidize lipids, decrease body weight and fat, and decrease insulin resistance. They trained a group of overweight and obese sedentary individuals over 8 weeks, 40 min/session, three times per week using an ergometer. This low-intensity exercise program was intended as a first-phase program, but itself had a positive effect on participants in the exercise group.[54] Johnson *et al.* randomly assigned sedentary adults who were overweight to moderately obese to three exercise groups (low amount/moderate intensity, low amount/vigorous intensity and high amount/vigorous intensity) and a control group for a 6-month training period. The low amount/moderate intensity group walked approximately 10—11 miles/week over an average of 170 min/wk, with a significant improvement noted in metabolic criteria relative to the control group. This finding demonstrated that a modest amount (low amount/moderate intensity) of exercise can produce significant health benefits and is in line with the ACSM recommendation of 30 min of moderate-intensity activity on most, preferably all, days of the week.[55,56] The group with the higher amount of vigorous exercise (jogging approximately 17 miles/wk) had greater, more widespread health benefits (greater improvement in more metabolic syndrome criteria), than all other groups, suggesting an exercise-dose effect.[55]

Low levels of physical activity have been associated with the development of metabolic syndrome. A study in Korea examined the LTPA of 11,925 participants in a cross-sectional study, and found that the prevalence of metabolic syndrome in the middle- and top-thirds of the group with higher LTPA was significantly lower compared to the those with no physical activity. Cho et al. found a linear relationship between duration and intensity of LTPA and decreased risk of diagnosis. Participating in any amount of LTPA led to a reduction in odds of diagnosis of metabolic syndrome, a decrease of 34% in women and 15% in men. This study quantified LTPA as a total MET score, intensity (METs)* duration of activity (min)* frequency (days/wk), and found a significant decrease in men's diagnosis with moderate and vigorous activity total MET scores $\geq$ 1,515 MET*min/wk compared to the group with no physical activity.[57] The current ACSM physical activity recommendation translates to a score of 735 MET-min/week, or 3.5 METs*30 min *7 days/week, and provides another method to educate the public on ways to meet their weekly physical activity requirement.

Levels of LTPA can impact metabolic syndrome criteria independent of body weight and weight loss. The SMART Study examined LTPA over the course of a year, classifying subjects into three categories: 0 METs (no physical activity), 1–14.9 MET/h/week (moderate physical activity), and > 15 MET/h/week (vigorous physical activity). There was 36% less prevalence of metabolic syndrome among those

in the >15 MET group compared to the 0 MET group. As LTPA increased, there was also a decrease in fasting glucose levels, hypertriglyceridemia, and abdominal obesity. The only criterion not impacted by increasing levels of LTPA was hypertension.[58]

Studies indicate that participating in a regular exercise program has a positive impact on blood pressure, decreasing one of the common criteria for metabolic syndrome. Welton et al. reviewed 54 randomized, controlled studies on aerobic exercise and its effect on blood pressure and found that physical inactivity led to a 30–50% increased risk for hypertension. Physical activity was found to decrease blood pressure in hypertensive and normotensive persons. Aerobic exercise led to a decrease in blood pressure for those with normal BMI scores as well. In addition, all forms of exercise appeared to have a positive impact on blood pressure measurements. Blood pressure was noted to decrease in trials independent of change in body weight.[59]

A review of randomized, controlled trials by Leon and Sanchez examined the effect of 12 weeks or more of exercise on hyperlipidemia. They found that programs consisting of moderate to vigorous intensity levels, three to five days/week, for at least 30 min/session resulted in an increase in HDL-C levels in half of the studies. Low pretraining HDL-C levels were a moderately strong predictor for a positive training response. They also noted a dose–response relationship in the observational studies. Overall, there were inconsistencies in blood lipid changes with endurance exercise training in the studies with the exception of HDL-C.[60]

EXERCISE PRESCRIPTION

Prior to the initiation of an exercise program, risk factors, medical history, and medications should be assessed and, when indicated, medical clearance obtained from a physician. The

Physical Activity Readiness Questionnaire (PAR-Q) has been recommended by the ACSM as a minimal standard for participation in a moderate-intensity exercise program.[61] ACSM has developed risk stratification guidelines based on age, health status, coronary artery disease risk factors, and symptoms that can be utilized to determine the need for a medical exam and exercise testing prior to the initiation of an exercise program.[62] Heart rate parameters derived from an exercise stress test should be incorporated into the exercise prescription. It is recommended that healthcare professionals follow these individuals' progress on a regular basis to improve compliance.

Information regarding an individual's previous level of activity, exercise preferences, physical impairments and time constraints should be ascertained. Exercise should be pain-free, convenient, and enjoyable to the participant to facilitate long-term compliance.

An exercise prescription should incorporate a warm-up, training, and cool-down program and include guidelines for progression of intensity, duration, and frequency of exercise. The warm-up and cool-down portion should be designed to address impairments in body function and structures that may contribute to activity limitations, while also serving to prevent injuries and sudden changes in heart rate and blood pressure. Warm-up and cool-down exercises can include flexibility, resistive, or balance exercises tailored to address any impairments an individual may have.

Based on the literature, the American Heart Association, the American College of Sports Medicine and the American Diabetes Association recommend that individuals engage in moderate-intensity aerobic exercise or physical activity for at least 150 min/week, or vigorous-intensity aerobic exercise for at least 90 min/week. Parameters that can be utilized to define moderate- and vigorous-intensity exercise levels are listed in Table 27.2. In addition, individuals should exercise at least 3 days/wk with no more than 2 consecutive days without physical activity.[56,63] Exercise does not need to be accomplished in one continuous session each day, but can be accrued in short bouts of 10 min or longer throughout the course of the day, and can include a variety of physical activities beyond structured exercise. A comparison of the effects of performing multiple 10-min bouts of exercise throughout the day with a single, longer bout in overweight subjects revealed greater adherence by those exercising in short bouts, with no negative impact on long-term weight loss or fitness.[64] Cumulative exercise time is important, independent of exercise intensity, for improving insulin sensitivity.

TABLE 27.2 Indicators of Moderate and Vigorous Intensity Exercise

Moderate intensity	Vigorous intensity
Borg Rating of Perceived Exertion Scale 12—14 ("somewhat hard")[a]	Borg Rating of Perceived Exertion Scale 14—16 ("hard")[a]
55—69% Maximum Heart Rate[b]	70—89% Maximum Heart Rate[b]
3.0 to 6.0 METs[c]	> 6.0 METs[c]

[a]Borg G. A. (1982) Psychophysical bases of perceived exertion. Med. Sci. Sports Exerc. **14**, 377—381.
[b]Pollock M. L., Gaesser G. A., Butcher J. D., Despres J. P., Dishman R. K., Franklin B. A. and Garber C. E. (1998) The recommended quantity and quality of exercise for developing and maintaining cardiorespiratory and muscular fitness, and flexibility in healthy adults. Med. Sci. Sports Exerc. **30**, 975—991.
[c]Pate R. R., Pratt M., Blair S. N., Haskell W. L., Macera C. A., Bouchard C., Buchner D., Ettinger W., Heath G. W., King A. C., Kriska A., Leon A. S., Marcus B. H., Morris J., Paffenbarger R. S., Patrick K., Pollack M. L., Rippe J. M., Sallis J. and Wilmore J. H. (1995) Physical activity and public health: a recommendation from the CDC and the ACSM. JAMA **273**, 402—407.

Individuals should be encouraged to gradually increase the intensity of their exercise from low to moderate and, if desired, to vigorous over time. Both moderate and vigorous intensity physical activity have been shown to be effective in reducing the risk of type 2 diabetes and metabolic syndrome. A gradual increase in duration and frequency of exercise should be implemented as well, based upon the individual's tolerance and prior activity level.

In accordance with the literature, individuals with metabolic syndrome or at risk of developing type 2 diabetes should include resistive exercises in their exercise regimen three times per week, targeting all major muscle groups and progressing to three sets of eight to 10 repetitions. The AHA recommendations for resistance training for persons without cardiovascular disease are as follows:[65]

- training a minimum of 2 days/week, progressing to 3 days/week;
- training of eight to 10 major muscle groups, including back, abdomen, thighs, lower legs, chest, shoulders, and arms;
- train with weights of moderate intensity, defined as 30–40% of one repetition maximum for upper extremities, 50–60% for lower extremities;
- when 12–15 repetitions can be accomplished with little difficulty, increase the weight gradually.

SUMMARY

The literature strongly supports the benefits of exercise and physical activity in the prevention of metabolic syndrome and type 2 diabetes. Exercise and physical activity enhance insulin sensitivity and glycemic control, reduce blood pressure, improve dyslipidemia and are crucial components of weight reduction.

The challenge in combating diabetes and metabolic syndrome appears to lie in developing effective public health approaches that support individuals in their attempt to incorporate the necessary lifestyle changes into their daily routine and maintain these changes for life. Recent data from the Medical Expenditure Panel survey indicate that less than 50% of individuals with three or more risk factors for diabetes received advice from a healthcare professional to exercise.[66] The WHO Global Strategy on Diet, Physical Activity and Health suggests that patients' and families' routine contact with healthcare providers should include practical advice on the benefits of healthy diets and increased levels of physical activity as well as support to assist the patient to initiate and maintain healthy behaviors. Governments should consider incentives to encourage such preventive services and identify opportunities for prevention within existing clinical services, including an improved financial structure to encourage and enable health professionals to dedicate more time to prevention.[67]

References

1. 2005–2008 National Health and Nutrition Examination Survey (NHANES). Hyattsville, (MD). US Department of Health and Human Services, Centers for Disease Control and Prevention. *National Center for Health Statistics*. Available at, http://www.cdc.gov/diabetes/pubs/pdf/ndfs_2011.pdf; 2010. accessed on May 8, 2011.
2. Boyle JP, Thompson TJ, Gregg EW, Barker LE, Williamson DF. Projection of the year 2050 burden of diabetes in the US adult population: dynamic modeling of incidence, mortality, and prediabetes prevalence. *Popul Health Metr* 2010;**8**:29.
3. de Vegt F, Dekker JM, Jager A, Hienkens E, Kostense PJ, Stehouwer CD, Nijpels G, Bouter LM, Heine RJ. Relation of impaired fasting and postload glucose with incident type 2 diabetes in a Dutch population: the Hoorn Study. *JAMA* 2001;**285**:2109–13.
4. Stump CS, Henriksen EJ, Yongzhong W, Sowers JR. The metabolic syndrome: role of skeletal muscle metabolism. *Ann Med* 2006;**38**:389–402.
5. Defronzo RA, Gunnarsson R, Bjorkman O, Olsson M, Wahren J. Effects of insulin on peripheral and splanchnic glucose metabolism in noninsulin-dependent (type II) diabetes mellitus. *J Clin Invest* 1985;**76**:149–55.

6. Albright A, Franz M, Hornsby G, Kriska A, Marrero D, Ullrich I, Verity LS. American College of Sports Medicine position stand. Exercise and type 2 diabetes. *Med Sci Sports Exerc* 2000;**32**:1345−60.

7. Sigal RJ, Kenny GP, Wasserman DH, Castaneda-Sceppa C, White RD. Physical activity/exercise and type 2 diabetes: a consensus statement from the American Diabetes Association. *Diabetes Care* 2006;**29**:1433−8.

8. Bluher M. Adipose tissue dysfunction in obesity. *Exp Clin Endocrinol Diabetes* 2009;**117**:241−50.

9. McCall A, Raj R. Exercise for prevention of obesity and diabetes in children and adolescents. *Clin Sports Med* 2009;**28**:393−421.

10. Hu G, Lakka TA, Kilpelainen TO, Tuomilehto J. Epidemiological studies of exercise in diabetes prevention. *Appl Physiol Nutr Metab* 2007;**32**:583−95.

11. Kaye SA, Folsom AR, Sprafka JM, Prineas RJ, Wallace RB. Increased indicence of diabetes mellitus in relation to abdominal adiposity in older women. *J Clin Epidemiol* 1991;**44**:329−34.

12. Jeon CY, Lokken RP, Hu FB, van Dam RM. Physical activity of moderate intensity and risk of type 2 diabetes: a systematic review. *Diabetes Care* 2007;**30**:744−52.

13. Tuomilehto J, Lindstrom MS, Eriksson JG, Valle TT, Hamalainen H, Ilanne-Parikka P, Keinanen-Klukaanniemi S, Laakso M, Louheranta A, Rastas M, Salminen V, Aunola S, Cepaitis Z, Moltchanov V, Hakumaki M, Mannelin M, Martikkala V, Uusitupa M, for the Finnish Diabetes Prevention Study Group. Prevention of type 2 diabetes mellitus by changes in lifestyle among subjects with impaired glucose tolerance. *N Engl J Med* 2001;**344**:1343−50.

14. Lindstrom J, Peltonen M, Eriksson J, Aunola S, Hamalainen H, Ilanne-Parikka P, Keinanen-Kiukaanniemi S, Uusitupa M, Tuomilehto J, for the Finnish Diabetes Prevention Study Group. Determinants for the effectiveness of lifestyle intervention in the Finnish Diabetes Prevention Study. *Diabetes Care* 2008;**31**:857−62.

15. Lindstrom J, Ilanne-Parikka P, Peltonen M, Aunola S, Eriksson JG, Hemio K, Hamalainen H, Harkonen P, Keinanen-Klukaanniemi S, Laakso M, Louheranta A, Mannelin M, Paturi M, Sundvall J, Valle TT, Uusitupa M, Tuomilehto J, for the Finnish Diabetes Prevention Study Group. Sustained reduction in the incidence of type 2 diabetes by lifestyle intervention: follow-up of the Finnish Diabetes Prevention Study. *Lancet* 2006;**368**:1673−9.

16. Laaksonen DE, Lindström J, Lakka TA, Eriksson JG, Niskanen L, Wikström K, Aunola S, Keinänen-Kiukaanniemi S, Laakso M, Valle TT, Ilanne-Parikka P, Louheranta A, Hämäläinen H, Rastas M, Salminen V, Cepaitis Z, Hakumäki M, Kaikkonen H, Härkönen P, Sundvall J, Tuomilehto J, Uusitupa M, for the Finnish Diabetes Prevention Study Group. Physical activity in the prevention of type 2 diabetes, The Finnish Diabetes Prevention Study. *Diabetes* 2005;**54**:158−65.

17. Knowler WC, Barrett-Connor E, Fowler SE, Hamman RF, Lachin JM, Walker EA, Nathan DM, Diabetes Prevention Program Research Group. Reduction in the incidence of type 2 diabetes with lifestyle intervention or metformin. *N Engl J Med* 2002;**346**:393−403.

18. Hamman R, Wing R, Edelstein S, Lachin J, Bray G, Delahanty L, Hoskin M, Kriska A, Mayer-Davis E, Pi-Sunyer X, Regensteiner J, Venditti B, Wylie-Rosett J. Effect of weight loss with lifestyle intervention on risk of diabetes. *Diabetes Care* 2006;**29**:2102−7.

19. Horowitz JF. Exercise-induced alterations in muscle lipid metabolism improve insulin sensitivity. *Exerc Sport Sci Rev* 2007;**35**:192−6.

20. Knowler WC, Fowle r SE, Hamman RF, Christophi CA, Hoffman HJ, Brenneman AT, Brown-Friday JO, Goldberg R, Venditti E, Nathan DM, for the Diabetes Prevention Program Research Group. 10-year follow-up of diabetes incidence and weight loss in the Diabetes Prevention Program Outcomes Study. *Lancet* 2009;**374**:1677−86.

21. Kosaka K, Noda M, Kuzuya T. Prevention of type 2 diabetes by lifestyle intervention: a Japanese trial in IGT males. *Diabetes Res Clin Pract* 2005;**67**:152−62.

22. Simmons RK, Harding AH, Jakes RW, Welch A, Wareham NJ, Griffin SJ. How much might achievement of diabetes prevention behaviour goals reduce the incidence of diabetes if implemented at the population level? *Diabetologia* 2006;**49**:905−11.

23. Gill JM, Cooper AR. Physical activity and prevention of type 2 diabetes mellitus. *Sports Med* 2008;**38**: 807−24.

24. Herman WH, Hoerger TJ, Brandle M, Hicks K, Sorensen S, Zhang P, Hamman R, Ackermann RT, Engelgau MM, Ratner RE. The cost-effectiveness of lifestyle modification or metformin in preventing type 2 diabetes in adults with impaired glucose tolerance. *Ann Intern Med* 2005;**42**:323−32.

25. Turcotte LP, Fisher JS. Skeletal muscle insulin resistance: role of fatty acid metabolism and exercise. *Phys Ther* 2008;**88**:1279−96.

26. Wahren J, Felig P, Ahlborg G, Jorfeldt L. Glucose metabolism during leg exercise in man. *J Clin Invest* 1971;**50**:2715−25.

27. Martin KK, Katz A, Wahren J. Splanchnic and muscle metabolism during exercise in NIDDM patients. *Am J Physiol* 1995;**269**:E583−90.

28. Kennedy JW, Hirshman MF, Gervino EV, Ocel JV, Forse RA, Hoenig SJ, Aronson D, Goodyear LJ, Horton ES. Acute exercise induces GLUT4 translocation in skeletal muscle of normal human subjects and subjects with type 2 diabetes. *Diabetes* 1999;**48**:1192–7.

29. Cartee GD, Young DA, Sleeper MD, Zierath J, Wallberg-Henriksson H, Holloszy JO. Prolonged increase in insulin-stimulated glucose transport in muscle after exercise. *Am J Physiol* 1989;**256**:E494–9.

30. Devlin JT, Hirschman M, Horton ED, Horton ES. Enhanced peripheral and splanchnic insulin sensitivity in NIDDM men after single bout of exercise. *Diabetes* 1987;**36**:434–9.

31. Dela F, Mikines KJ, von Linstow M, Secher NH, Galbo H. Effect of training on insulin-mediated glucose uptake in human muscle. *Am J Physiol* 1992;**263**:E1134–43.

32. Houmard J, Tanner C, Slentz C, Duscha BD, McCartney JS, Kraus WE. Effect of the volume and intensity of exercise training on insulin sensitivity. *J Appl Physiol* 2004;**96**:101–6.

33. American College of Sports Medicine. *ACSM's Guidelines for Exercise Testing and Prescription*. 7th ed. Philadelphia: Lippincott Williams & Wilkins; 2006 [chapter 1].

34. Schoeller DA, Shay K, Kushner RF. How much physical activity is needed to minimize weight gain in previously obese women? *Am J Clin Nutr* 1997;**66**:551–6.

35. Weinsier RL, Hunter GR, Desmond RA, Byrne MN, Zuckerman PA, Darnell BE. Free-living activity energy expenditure in women successful and unsuccessful at maintaining a normal body weight. *Am J Clin Nutr* 2002;**75**:499–504.

36. Magkos F, Tsekouras Y, Kavouras SA, Mittendorfer B, Sidossis LS. Improved insulin sensitivity after a single bout of exercise is curvilinearly related to exercise energy expenditure. *Clin Sci* 2008;**114**:59–64.

37. De Filippis E, Cusi K, Ocampo G, Berria R, Buck S, Consoli A, Mandarino LJ. Exercise-induced improvement in vasodilatory function accompanies increased insulin sensitivity in obesity and type 2 diabetes mellitus. *J Clin Endocrinol Metab* 2006;**91**:4903–10.

38. Kelley DE, He J, Menshikova EV, Ritov VB. Dysfunction of mitochondria in human skeletal muscle in type 2 diabetes. *Diabetes* 2002;**51**:2944–50.

39. Schrauwen P, van Aggel-Leijssen DP, Hul G, Wagenmakers AJ, Vidal H, Saris WH, van Baak MA. The effect of a 3-month low-intensity endurance training program on fat oxidation and acetyl-CoA carboxylase-2 expression. *Diabetes* 2002;**51**:2220–6.

40. Gulve EA. Exercise and glycemic control in diabetes: benefits, challenges, and adjustments to pharmacotherapy. *Phys Ther* 2008;**88**:1297–321.

41. Boule N, Haddad E, Kenny G, Wells G, Sigal R. The effects of exercise on glycemic control and body mass in type 2 diabetes. *JAMA* 2001;**285**:1218–27.

42. Hawley JA. Exercise as a therapeutic intervention for the prevention and treatment of insulin resistance. *Diabetes Metab Res Rev* 2004;**20**:383–93.

43. Ross R, Bradshaw AJ. The future of obesity reduction: beyond weight loss. *Nat Rev Endocrinol* 2009;**5**:319–25.

44. Brooks N, Layne JE, Gordon PL, Roubenoff R, Nelson ME, Castaneda-Sceppa C. Strength training improves muscle quality and insulin sensitivity in Hispanic older adults with type 2 diabetes. *Int J Med Sci* 2007;**4**:19–27.

45. Clurilla JR, Fitz EC, Thompson DF. The metabolic syndrome: how definition impacts the prevalence and risk in US adults: 1999–2004 NHANES. *Metab Syndr Rel Disord* 2007;**5**:331–41.

46. Malik S, Wong ND, Franklin SS, Kamath TV, L'Italien GJ, Pio JR, Williams GR. Impact of the metabolic syndrome on mortality from coronary heart disease, cardiovascular disease, and all causes in United States adults. *Circulation* 2004;**110**:1245–50.

47. Haskell WL, Lee IM, Pate RR, Powell KE, Blair SN, Franklin BA, Macera CA, Heath GW, Thompson PD, Bauman A. Physical activity and public health: updated recommendations for adults from ACSM and the AHA. *Circulation* 2007;**116**:1081–93.

48. Grundy SM, Brewer B, Cleeman JI, Smith SC, Lenfant C. Definition of metabolic syndrome: report of NHLBI/AHA conference on scientific issues related to definition. *Circ* 2004;**109**:433–8.

49. Grundy SM, Hansen B, Smith SC, Cleeman JI, Kahn RA. Clinical management of metabolic syndrome: report of the AHA/NHLBI/ADA conference on scientific issues related to management. *Circ* 2004;**109**:551–6.

50. Churilla JR, Fitzhugh EC. Relationship between leisure-time physical activity and metabolic syndrome using varying definitions: 1999–2004 NHANES. *Diab and Vasc Dis* 2009;**6**:100–9.

51. Laaksonen DE, Lakka HM, Salonen JT, Niskanen LK, Rauramaa R, Laaka TA. Low levels of leisure-time physical activity and cardiorespiratory fitness predict development of the metabolic syndrome. *Diabetes Care* 2002;**25**:1612–8.

52. Ekelund U, Brage S, Franks PW, Hennings S, Emms S. Physical activity energy expenditure predicts progression toward the metabolic syndrome independently of aerobic fitness in middle-aged healthy caucasions: the medical research council ely study. *Diabetes Care* 2005;**25**:1195–200.

53. Katzmarzyk PT, Leon A, Wilmore JH, Skinner JS, Rao DC, Tankinen T, Bouchard C. Targeting the

metabolic syndrome with exercise: evidence from the HERITAGE family study. *Med Sci Sports Exerc* 2003;**35**:1703–9.

54. Dumortier M, Brandou F, Perez-Martin A, Fedou C, Mercier J, Brun JF. Low intensity endurance exercise targeted for lipid oxidation improves body composition and insulin sensitivity in patients with the metabolic syndrome. *Diab Metab* 2003;**29**:509–18.

55. Johnson JL, Slentz CA, Houmard JA, Samsa GP, Duscha BD, Aiken LB, McCartney JS, Tanner CJ, Kraus WE. Exercise training amount and intensity effects on metabolic syndrome (from studies of a targeted risk reduction intervention through defined exercise). *Am J Cardiol* 2007;**100**:1759–66.

56. Haskell WL, Lee IM, Pate RP, Powell KE, Blair SN, Franklin BA, Macera CA, Heath GW, Thompson PD, Bauman A. Physical activity and public health: updated recommendation for adults from the American College of Sports Medicine and the American Heart Association. *Med Sci Sports Exerc* 2007;**39**:1423–34.

57. Cho ER, Shin A, Jeongseon K, Jee SH, Sung J. Leisure-time physical activity is associated with a reduced risk for metabolic syndrome. *Annal Epidemiol* 2009;**19**:784–92.

58. Brouwer BG, Visseren FL, van der Graaf Y. The effect of leisure-time physical activity on the presence of metabolic syndrome in patients with manifest arterial disease. The SMART study. *Amer Heart J* 2007;**154**:1146–52.

59. Whelton SP, Chin A, Xin X, He J. Effect of aerobic exercise on blood pressure: a meta analysis of randomized, controlled trials. *Annals Int Med* 2002;**136**:493–503.

60. Gaesser GA, Sanchez OA. Response of blood lipids to exercise training alone or combined with dietary intervention. *Med Sci Sports Exerci* 2001;**33**:S502–15.

61. Canadian Society for Exercise Physiology. PAR-Q and you, Revised 2002, www.csep.ca/cmfiles/publications/parq/par-q.pdf. Accessed April 22, 2011.

62. Guthrie J. Cardiorespiratory and health-related physical fitness assessments. In: Ehrman JK, et al., editors. *ACSM's Resource Manual for Guidelines for Exercise Testing and Prescription*. 6th ed. Philadelphia: Lippincott Williams & Wilkins; 2010 (chapter 1. 19).

63. American Diabetes Association. Standards of medical care in diabetes-2007. *Diabetes Care* 2007;**30**(Suppl. 1):S4–41.

64. Jakicic JM, Wing RR, Butler BA, Robertson RJ. Prescribing exercise in multiple short bouts versus one continuous bout: effects on adherence, cardiorespiratory fitness, and weight loss in overweight women. *Int J Obes Relat Metab Disord* 1995;**19**:893–901.

65. Braith RW, Stewart KJ. Resistance exercise training: Its role in the prevention of cardiovascular disease. *Circulation.* 2006;**113**:2642–50.

66. Morrato EH, Hill JO, Wyatt HR, Ghushchyan MA, Sullivan PW. Are health care professionals advising patients with diabetes or at risk for developing diabetes to exercise more? *Diabetes Care* 2006;**29**:543–8.

67. World Health Organization. Global strategy on diet, physical activity and health. Available at, http://www.who.int/dietphysicalactivity/en/. Accessed April 8, 2011.

28

An Overview on Nutraceuticals and Herbal Supplements for Diabetes and Metabolic Syndrome

Wadie I. Najm

University of California, Irvine School of Medicine, Family Medicine & Geriatrics, Orange, CA, USA

INTRODUCTION

Information about the use of nutraceuticals and herbals supplements in the management of diabetes (DM) and metabolic syndrome (MetS) is sparse. Data from the 2002 National Health Interview Survey revealed that the use of any Complementary and Alternative Medicine (CAM) modality did not differ significantly by diabetic status (47.6 *vs* 47.9%, p = 0.81). Individuals with diabetes were more likely to use prayer (OR 1.19, 95% CI 1.05, 1.36), and less

Nutritional and Therapeutic Interventions for Diabetes and Metabolic Syndrome
DOI: 10.1016/B978-0-12-385083-6.00028-0

likely to use herbs (OR 0.86, 95% CI 0.75, 0.99), or vitamins (OR 0.82, 95% CI 0.72, 0.93) compared to people without diabetes after controlling for relevant covariate.[1,2] Age, duration of diabetes, degree of complications and self-monitoring of blood glucose were among the characteristics which influence CAM use.[3] Variations of CAM use were also observed across groups in the correlation with race/ethnicity and socioeconomic status. A survey of patients diagnosed with diabetes in Taiwan reported that Chinese herbals and nutritional supplements were the most commonly used modalities before and after diagnosis (8 *vs* 27.9% and 8.6 *vs* 41.1%; p < 0.001, respectively).[4] Among Mexican patients with diabetes who use CAM therapies, 94.2% used herbal remedies, while the remaining 5.8% used other treatments.[5] Similar findings were also reported by other surveys across the world with differences in the herbs and supplements used based on the cultural and regional variation.

An overview of nutraceuticals and herbal supplements commonly used in the management of diabetes is given in Table 28.1.

BITTER MELON (MOMORDICA CHARANTIA)

Bitter melon is a long, slender vine, with long-stalked leaves and very bitter fruit, grown in tropical and subtropical areas of Asia, South America, Africa, and the Caribbean. The fruit has been used as a food and medicine. Parts of the fruit have been used as an antibacterial agent, hypoglycemic agent, and to treat high lipid levels.

Animal studies report that the active ingredient charantin (steroidal saponins) can decrease gluconeogenesis, increase glucose metabolism and tolerance, increase the number of β-cells, leading to a reduction in blood glucose level and increased concentration of plasma insulin.[6,7] Proposed mechanisms of action include activation of the AMP-activated

protein kinase system,[5] expression of the peroxisome proliferator-activated receptors α and gamma (PPARα and PPARgamma) which may mitigate insulin resistance[8] and a protein extract that exerted both insulin secretagogue and insulin-mimetic activities.[9]

A 2010 Cochrane review[10] of clinical evidence found three randomized clinical trials (RCTs) of up to 3 months' duration and investigating 350 participants that met their inclusion criteria. Two RCTs compared the effect of preparations from different parts of the *Momordica charantia* plants and placebo on the glycemic control in type 2 diabetes (T2DM). There was no statistically significant difference compared to placebo. In contrast, the effects of the preparation from the leaves of the plant and glibenclamide were comparable in the third study. Several small controlled trials and case series with small numbers of subjects (eight to 100) reported statistical improvement in blood glucose levels.[11] The largest trial was a 2-day study of 100 subjects with T2DM given bitter melon extract 1 h before an oral glucose tolerance test (OGTT); the patients' mean fasting glucose level and 2-h blood glucose level were significantly different from those of the previous day (p < 0.001).[6]

Bitter melon is offered in different forms. For the encapsulated extract, the suggested dose is 100−200 mg three times daily. For the liquid form, the dosage is 50−100 ml/day and for the dry powder, 3−15 g daily has been given.

Bitter melon is generally safe. Side effects include abdominal discomfort, pain, and diarrhea. Caution should be used to avoid potential interaction with hypoglycemic drugs. Two case reports of hypoglycemic coma in children have been described.[12]

CINNAMON (CINNAMOMUM CASSIA)

Cinnamon trees are grown in tropical areas. Sticks of bark from the tree are used as a spice

TABLE 28.1 Overview of Nutraceuticals and Herbal Supplements Commonly Used in the Management of Diabetes

Herbal supplement	Proposed action	Potential interactions and contraindications	Side effects	Level of evidence
Bitter melon (*Momordica charantia*)	• ↓ Gluconeogenesis, • ↑ Glucose metabolism and tolerance, • ↑ Number of β-cells	• Hypoglycemic agents • Pregnancy	• Abdominal discomfort • Diarrhea	B1
Cinnamon (*Cinnamomum Cassia*)	• ↑ Insulin sensitivity • ↓ Absorption of glucose	• Hepatotoxicity • Hypoglycemic agents • Hepatotoxic medications	• None reported	B1
Fenugreek (*Trigonella foenum-graecum*)	• ↓ Glucose absorption • ↑ Insulin secretion • ↑ Peripheral glucose utilization	• Hypoglycemic agents • Pregnancy • Anticoagulant drugs • MAO inhibitors	• Diarrhea • Flatulence	B1
Ginseng (*Panax ginseng*)	• Unknown • Antioxidant • ↓ Inflammation • ↓ Body weight	• Hypoglycemic agents • Corticosteroids • Oral contraceptives • Anticoagulant drugs • Digoxin • MAOI and tricyclic antidepressants • Diuretics	• Hypertension • Epistaxis • Headache • Nervousness • Vomiting	B2
Gymnema (*Gymnema sylvestre*)	• ↑ Glucose uptake • ↑ Insulin secretion • ↑ Beta cells	Hypoglycemic agents	Toxic hepatitis (1 case)	B1
Nopal	• ↓ Glucose absorption • ↓ Insulin level	Hypoglycemic agents	• Abdominal bloating • Diarrhea • Nausea	B1

Level of evidence: Efficacy: A = Excellent; B = Equivocal; C = Poor; // Safety: 1 = Safe; 2 = Equivocal; 3 = Unsafe.
↑ = *Increase*; ↓ = *Decrease*.

and in several cultures as traditional treatment of different health problems such as digestive concerns, menstrual problems, and common colds.

Animal studies suggest that cinnamon extract may exert a blood glucose-suppressing effect by improving insulin sensitivity or slowing absorption of carbohydrates in the small intestine. Cinnamon extract significantly increased insulin sensitivity, reduced serum and hepatic lipids, and improved hyperglycemia and hyperlipidemia possibly by regulating the PPAR-mediated glucose and lipid metabolism.[13,14]

In animals fed a high fat/high fructose diet (an animal model of metabolic syndrome) to induce insulin resistance, treatment with polyphenols from cinnamon altered body composition, improved insulin sensitivity, prevented a reduction in pancreatic mass, and decreased mesenteric white fat accumulation.[15]

Clinical trials suggest that cinnamon has a possible modest effect in lowering blood sugar. However, the studies were limited by small sample size, and short duration of follow-up. In a small RCT 60 subjects with diabetes and hyperlipidemia were divided into six groups, groups 1—3 were given 1, 3, or 6 g of cinnamon while the other groups received placebo. All three doses of cinnamon reduced the mean fasting glucose (18—29%), triglycerides (23—30%), low-density lipoprotein (LDL; 7—27%), and total cholesterol (12—26%) after 40 days of treatment, while no changes were noted in the placebo groups.[16] Another double-blind placebo-controlled trial randomized 79 subjects with T2DM to 1 g three times per day of cinnamon (aqueous cinnamon extract TC112) or placebo. After 4 months, a significant difference in the blood sugar was noted in both groups when pre- and post-intervention measurements were compared. The mean percentage difference in blood sugar was 10.3% in the cinnamon group and 3.37% in the placebo group (p = 0.046). However, no statistical differences between groups were noted for hemoglobin A1c, and lipid profile.[17]

Cinnamon is generally well tolerated and is believed to be safe. Large doses (7 g/day) may cause hepatotoxicity due to the coumarin content. Caution should be used in subjects with liver disease, those on hypoglycemic agents (additive effect) and/or hepatotoxic medications.

FENUGREEK (*TRIGONELLA FOENUM-GRAECUM*)

Fenugreek is an annual herb native to western Asia and southeastern Europe but cultivated worldwide. Traditionally it is used as a food flavor and in traditional medicine (Ayurvedic and Oriental) to treat indigestion, to induce labor, as a lactation stimulant, as a general tonic, and for high blood sugar.

Fenugreek has several constituents such as fiber, iron, phenolic acid, saponins, and alkaloids. Several laboratory and animal studies indicate that the amino acid 4-hydroxyisoleucine in fenugreek can raise the rate of insulin release,[18–20] improve insulin resistance by increasing peripheral glucose utilization, and decrease glucose utilization.[20,21] A water-soluble extract (GII) was reported to decrease the lipid content of liver and stimulate the enzymes of glycolysis (except glucokinase) and inhibit enzymes of gluconeogenesis in the liver resulting in a reduction of fasting blood glucose (FBG), and significantly attenuating the area under the curve (AUC) following a glucose tolerance test (GTT) in sub-diabetic and moderately diabetic rabbits.[22] The soluble dietary fiber fraction of fenugreek seeds was also found to exert antidiabetic effects through inhibition of carbohydrate digestion and absorption and enhancement of peripheral insulin action.[18]

A few small trials evaluated the clinical effects in subjects with type 1 DM (T1DM) or T2DM. One study explored the effects of 100 g defatted fenugreek seed powder given twice daily to 10 subjects with T1DM over 10 days.[23] In this study, the fasting blood glucose, serum total cholesterol, LDL, and very low density lipoprotein (VLDL) were reduced and GTT was improved. Other trials used fenugreek alone or in combination with other nutraceuticals for management of subjects with T2DM. A randomized clinical trial of 25 subjects newly diagnosed with T2DM were given 1 g/day hydroalcoholic extract of fenugreek seeds *vs* usual care and followed over 2 months.[24] After 2 months there was no statistical difference between groups for fasting blood glucose and blood glucose levels following 2-h post-glucose challenge. But a significant decrease in percent β-cell secretion, AUC of blood glucose, triglycerides, and an increase in percent insulin sensitivity was seen in the fenugreek-treated group. A review of several small studies shows similar mild to moderate beneficial effect.[25]

Different studies reviewed used different doses and preparations of fenugreek. Fenugreek is most commonly used as 25–100 g of seed powder or capsules given as 1–6 g daily.

Although fenugreek is thought to be safe, caution should be exercised in subjects with allergy to fenugreek, pregnant women (oxytocic effect), and subjects using hypoglycemic and/or antithrombotic medications (enhances activity). High doses may cause diarrhea and flatulence.

GYMNEMA (GYMNEMA SYLVESTRE)

Gymnema is a woody climbing plant found in central and southern India, tropical Africa, and Australia. It has been used traditionally in Ayurvedic medicine for the treatment of "honey urine". Extracts from the leaves contain alkaloids, phenols, tannins, flavonoids, and saponin.

The hypoglycemic effect of gymnema has been recognized in early animal experiments and re-confirmed over the last decades. Ethanol and water extracts (high in saponin) reduced blood glucose levels in normal and glucose-infused rats.[26] Earlier studies reported that the hypoglycemic activity was due to an increase in insulin levels secondary to regeneration of endocrine pancreas[27–29] and enhanced secretion.[29]

A systematic review of RCTs identified only two efficacy studies, both of poor methodological quality.[30] Significant reductions in blood glucose and hemoglobin A1c were noted in 22 subjects with T2DM who were given a combination of 400 mg of gymnema extract and standard treatment daily for over 18 months.[31] Similar results were also seen in 27 patients with T1DM given 400 mg of gymnema extract, who exhibited reduced A1c and increased C-peptide levels.[32]

A small clinical study (11 subjects diagnosed with T2DM) using an aqueous alcohol extract of gymnema leaves (Om Santi Adivasi) 500 mg twice daily given over 60 days reported a statistically significant reduction of fasting blood glucose, postprandial blood glucose, and an associated increase in circulating levels of insulin and C-peptide.[29]

Overall, clinical evidence is suggestive of a beneficial effect but remains insufficient due to the poor quality of studies.

The dose commonly reported is an ethanol extract from gymnema labeled GS4 given as 200–400 mg twice daily.

Gymnema extract appears to be safe. Caution should be used when taken along with antidiabetic medications (additive effect). Caution should be used in pregnant and breastfeeding women since the effects have not been evaluated. A recent case reported toxic hepatitis, in a 60-year-old woman with T2DM, secondary to Gymnema sylvestre taken over 10 days, as a tea, three times daily.[33] The exact mechanism of the injury is unknown, although the authors indicate that diabetes and non-alcoholic fatty liver disease could be predisposing factors.

PRICKLY PEAR CACTUS (NOPAL SPECIES) (OPUNTIA STREPTACANTHA AND FULGINOSA)

Nopal is a large cactus prickly pear native to arid areas of South and North America. It is traditionally used among Mexicans as a food and medicinally as an anti-inflammatory, laxative, for alcohol hangover, to manage abdominal pain, and for high blood sugar.

The exact mechanism of the blood-sugar-lowering property of Nopal is unknown although it has a high soluble fiber and pectin content which may affect glucose uptake. Prior studies, however, dispute the role of fiber in reducing blood glucose in animal studies but do not offer an alternative mechanism.[34] Use of *Opuntia* extract (1 mg/kg body weight) in combination with insulin for 7 weeks followed by *Opuntia* extract alone was capable of rapidly returning blood glucose to the levels of the non-diabetic rats. A recent animal study explored the effect of a liquid extract and a filtered extract of *Opuntia streptacantha* in streptozoto-cin (STZ)-diabetic rats.[35] The extracts failed to produce a hypoglycemic effect. However when given prior to an OGTT it produced an antihyperglycemic effect suggesting possible mechanism through blocking the hepatic glucose output.

Several small ($N = 7–32$) published clinical trials (all conducted by the same research group) using different forms and doses of *Opuntia* species confirm mild to moderate bene-ficial effect in subjects with T2DM.[36–39]

The most common form of Nopal used in the studies was the broiled stem of *Opuntia streptacantha* given as a 100–500 g daily dose.

Nopal should be avoided in pregnant and nursing women and in people with kidney disease. Side effects may include abdominal bloating, diarrhea, and nausea. It should be used with caution in subjects on antidiabetic medications (one case report).[40]

OTHER NUTRACEUTICALS USED FOR THE MANAGEMENT OF DIABETES AND METABOLIC SYNDROME

Chromium

A detailed review of chromium can be found in another chapter. Chromium is an essential trace element commonly used in products mar-keted for diabetes and weight loss. Chromium deficiency can be associated with symptoms similar to those of diabetes.[41] Chromium defi-ciency impairs the body's ability to use glucose. A meta-analysis of 20 studies ($N = 618$) assessing the effect of chromium on glucose, insulin, or glycosylated hemoglobin (HbA1c) showed no effect of chromium on glucose or insulin concentrations in non-diabetic subjects.[42] The data for subjects with diabetes are inconclusive.

A meta-analysis (10 trials) exploring the effect of chromium picolinate on reducing body weight suggested a relatively small effect of chromium picolinate compared with placebo for reducing body weight.[43] The clinical relevance of the effect is debatable.

Panax Ginseng (Korean or Asian Ginseng)

Panax ginseng is traditionally used as tonic. It has many active chemicals of which ginseno-sides, a group of steroidal saponins, is consid-ered the active component. Interest in its effect on blood sugar and body weight has led to a few animal and clinical studies. Obese diabetic mice receiving daily intraperitoneal injections of Panax ginseng's berry extract (150 mg/kg) over 12 days showed improved glucose tolerance associated with a reduction in serum insulin.[44] The extract-treated mice lost a significant amount of weight (p < 0.01) and had signifi-cantly reduced plasma cholesterol (p < 0.01).

Few small studies explored the clinical role of Panax ginseng in the management of T2DM. A double-blind placebo-controlled trial (DBPCT) of 36 subjects with T2DM treated for 8 weeks with 100–200 mg *vs* placebo reported that ginseng reduced fasting blood glucose, hemoglobin A1c, and body weight.[45] In another RDBPCT (cross-over design) 19 subjects with T2DM received Korean ginseng 2 g/meal (6 g/day) in combination with their usual antidiabetic agents over 12 weeks.[46] No change in HbA1c was noted, although a decrease in FBG, OGTT, and plasma insulin was noted. Despite encouraging results, addi-tional studies regarding doses, effectiveness, and safety remain to be conducted.

Panax Quinquefolius (American Ginseng)

American ginseng has also been evaluated for its hypoglycemic potential. Laboratory studies using water extract of ginseng root given as intraperitoneal injection (300 mg/kg) to obese diabetic mice over 12 days found a statistically significant effect on fasting blood glucose, glucose tolerance test, and body weight.[47] This effect was attributed to the antioxidant actions of American ginseng. Other studies propose a protective effect of β-cells from apoptosis by decreasing the level of uncoupling protein-2 and increasing ATP in the mitochondria.[48,49]

A clinical study evaluating the effect of dosing and timing of American ginseng on postprandial glycemia (25 g oral glucose challenge) in 12 healthy subjects reported that all three doses (1, 2, and 3 g of ginseng) decreased glycemia, and no differences were seen between doses.[50] Time of administration (40 min prior to glucose challenge) was the only significant factor that affected postpraudial glycemia.

Based on the above reviews it seems that ginsing (Panax and American) could be beneficial for the management of diabetes. However, additional work is needed to identify the appropriate dose, active component(s), time of administration, and mechanism of action.

Alpha Lipoic Acid (Thioctic Acid)

Alpha lipoic acid (ALA) is found in foods such as red meat, organ meats, spinach, broccoli, and yeast. It is both fat- and water-soluble. The proposed mechanisms of action of ALA are as an antioxidant, scavenging of free radicals, and metal ion chelation. ALA is approved in Germany for the management of diabetes-associated polyneuropathies. In experimental animal models of diabetes, ALA treatment improves neural blood flow, endoneural glucose uptake and metabolism and nerve conduction.[51] ALA administered intravenously, 600 mg daily for 3 weeks, improved symptoms of diabetic neuropathy pain.[52] Similar findings were also reported with oral doses of ALA.[53] One hundred and eighty-one subjects were randomized to receive once-daily oral doses of 600 mg, 1200 mg, and 1800 mg of ALA, or placebo over 5 weeks. Significant improvements favoring all three ALA groups were reported for stabbing and burning pain, and the patients' global assessment of efficacy.

Common oral doses of 600–1800 mg/day were often used in clinical trials, while 600 mg/day intravenously was used for peripheral neuropathy.

Few side effects have been reported following use of ALA, consisting mainly of skin rash and mild gastrointestinal upset. Caution should also be used for pregnant or breastfeeding women, people taking thyroid medications (dosing adjustment), and people with thiamine deficiency (alcohol use) due to increased risk of toxicity.

Vitamin D

Recently there has been a mounting interest in the effect of vitamin D on diabetes. Several studies suggested that vitamin D may have an effect on: (i) pancreatic β-cell function mediated through the direct effect of 1-25 OH-D on β-cell vitamin D receptor,[54] β-cell function could also be mediated by vitamin D through the flux of intra- and extra-cellular calcium;[55] (ii) insulin resistance by stimulating the expression of insulin receptor and enhancing responsiveness,[56] via regulation of intra-/extra-cellular calcium influx and its impact on insulin resistance in peripheral tissue;[57–59] and (iii) modulating the effect of cytokines leading to decreased inflammation and subsequently decreased insulin resistance.[60,61]

A review of seven RCTs testing the effects of a variety of formulations of vitamin D on subjects with T2DM reported no effect on glycemic measures (FBG, HbA1c) in five studies.[62] Another study using a combination of 700 IU vitamin D3 and calcium 500 mg/day reported attenuation in FBG in subjects with impaired glucose but not in those with normal blood sugars. The Women Health Initiative trial found no effect when 400 IU of vitamin D3 was combined with 1,000 mg calcium per day.

Data from the Nurses' Health Study found that higher levels of plasma 25-OHD were associated with a lower risk for T2DM.[63] The odds ratio for incident of type diabetes in the top (median 25-OHD, 33.4 ng/ml) *vs* the bottom (median 25-OHD, 14.4 ng/ml) quartile was 0.52 (95% CI 0.33–0.83). The associations were consistent across subgroups of baseline BMI, age, and calcium intake.

A review of available observational studies and clinical trials to examine the association between vitamin D status, including the effect of vitamin D supplementation, and cardiometabolic outcomes in generally healthy adults reported uncertain association. Trials showed no clinically significant effect of vitamin D supplementation at the dosages given.

Beta-Glucan

Beta-glucan is a soluble fiber used classically to boost the immune system and to treat high lipids.

Beta-glucan can modulate the autoimmune mechanisms directed to pancreatic islets and inhibit the development of diabetes in BB rats.[64] Intravenous administration of beta-glucan 1 mg/kg for 1 week decreased the cumulative incidence of diabetes from 43.3% to 6.7% (p < 0.005) and the incidence of insulitis from 82.4 to 26.3% at the age of 20 weeks (p < 0.002). Eight of nine rats were free from diabetes for 5 weeks after stopping beta-1,6;1,3 D-glucan at the age of 20 weeks.

The high viscosity of beta-glucan may also contribute to delayed gastrointestinal absorption causing a decrease in blood glucose.[65] A 50% reduction in glycemic peak can be achieved with a concentration of 10% beta-glucan included in breakfast cereal. A significant lowering of plasma LDL cholesterol concentrations can also be anticipated with the daily consumption of ≥ 3 g of beta-glucan.

Several small RCTs with methodological limitations support the use of beta-glucan for glycemic control, however larger well-designed studies are needed to confirm these findings.[66] Several controlled trials examining the effect of beta-glucan on cholesterol reported a small reduction in LDL-cholesterol but not for triglycerides.

CONCLUSION

Several nutraceuticals and dietary supplements reviewed show great promise and potential, either alone or in combination with diet or mainstream medications, for treatment of T2DM and metabolic syndrome. A general limitation is the methodological weakness of clinical trials that restricts the ability to translate results into clinical application.

References

1. Bell RA, Suerken CK, Grzywacz JG, Lang W, Quandt SA, Arcury TA. Complementary and alternative medicine use among adults with diabetes in the United States. *Altern Ther Health Med* 2006; **12**:16–22.
2. Garrow D, Egede LE. National patterns and correlates of complementary and alternative medicine use in adults with diabetes. *J Altern Complement Med* 2006;**12**:895–902.
3. Chang HY, Wallis M, Tiralongo E. Use of complementary and alternative medicine among people living with diabetes: literature review. *J Adv Nurs* 2007;**58**:307–19.
4. Chang HY, Wallis M, Tiralongo E. Use of Complementary and Alternative Medicine among People

with Type 2 Diabetes in Taiwan: A Cross-Sectional Survey. *Evid Based Complement Alternat Med*; 2011. pii: 983792.

5. Cheng HL, Huang HK, Chang CI, Tsai CP, Chou CH. A cell-based screening identifies compounds from the stem of Momordica charantia that overcome insulin resistance and activate AMP-activated protein kinase. *J Agric Food Chem* 2008;**56**:6835−43.

6. Ahmed I, Chandranath I, Sharma AK, Adeghate E, Pallot DJ, Singh J. Mechanism of hypoglycemic action of Momordica charantia fruit juice in normal and diabetic rats. *J Physiol* 1999;**520**:25.

7. Han C, Hui Q, Wang Y. Hypoglycaemic activity of saponin fraction extracted from Momordica charantia in PEG/salt aqueous two-phase systems. *Nat Prod Res* 2008;**22**:1112−9.

8. Shih CC, Lin CH, Lin WL. Effects of Momordica charantia on insulin resistance and visceral obesity in mice on high-fat diet. *Diabetes Res Clin Pract* 2008;**81**:134−43.

9. Yibchok-anun S, Adisakwattana S, Yao CY, Sangvanich P, Roengsumran S, Hsu WH. Slow acting protein extract from fruit pulp of Momordica charantia with insulin secretagogue and insulinomimetic activities. *Biol Pharm Bull* 2006;**29**:1126−31.

10. Ooi CP, Yassin Z, Hamid TA. Momordica charantia for type 2 diabetes mellitus. *Cochrane Database Syst Rev*; 2010:CD007845.

11. Leung L, Birtwhistle R, Kotecha J, Hannah S, Cuthbertson S. Anti-diabetic and hypoglycaemic effects of Momordica charantia (bitter melon): a mini review. *Br J Nutr* 2009;**102**:1703−8.

12. Raman A, Lau C. Anti-diabetic properties and phyto-chemistry of Momordica charantia L. (Cucurbitaceae). *Phytomedicine* 1996;**2**:349−62.

13. Kim SH, Choung SY. Antihyperglycemic and anti-hyperlipidemic action of Cinnamomi Cassiae (Cinnamon bark) extract in C57BL/Ks db/db mice. *Arch Pharm Res* 2010;**33**:325−33.

14. Kim SH, Choung SY. Antihyperglycemic and anti-hyperlipidemic action of Cinnamomi Cassiae (Cinnamon bark) extract in C57BL/Ks db/db mice. *Arch Pharm Res* 2010;**33**:325−33.

15. Couturier K, Batandier C, Awada M, Hininger-Favier I, Canini F, Anderson RA, Leverve X, Roussel AM. Cinnamon improves insulin sensitivity and alters the body composition in an animal model of the metabolic syndrome. *Arch Biochem Biophys* 2010;**501**:158−61.

16. Khan A, Safdar M, Ali Khan MM, Khattak KN, Anderson RA. Cinnamon improves glucose and lipids of people with type 2 diabetes. *Diabetes Care* 2003;**26**:3215−8.

17. Mang B, Wolters M, Schmitt B, Kelb K, Lichtinghagen R, Stichtenoth DO, Hahn A. Effects of a cinnamon extract on plasma glucose, HbA, and serum lipids in diabetes mellitus type 2. *Eur J Clin Invest* 2006;**36**:340−4.

18. Hannan JM, Ali L, Rokeya B, Khaleque J, Akhter M, Flatt PR, Abdel-Wahab YH. Soluble dietary fibre fraction of Trigonella foenum-graecum (fenugreek) seed improves glucose homeostasis in animal models of type 1 and type 2 diabetes by delaying carbohydrate digestion and absorption, and enhancing insulin action. *Br J Nutr* 2007;**97**:514−21.

19. Xue WL, Li XS, Zhang J, Liu YH, Wang ZL, Zhang RJ. Effect of Trigonella foenum-graecum (fenugreek) extract on blood glucose, blood lipid and hemorheo-logical properties in streptozotocin-induced diabetic rats. *Asia Pac J Clin Nutr* 2007;**16**:422−6.

20. Haeri MR, Izaddoost M, Ardekani MR, Nobar MR, White KN. The effect of fenugreek 4-hydroxy-isoleucine on liver function biomarkers and glucose in diabetic and fructose-fed rats. *Phytother Res* 2009;**23**:61−4.

21. Broca C, Breil V, Cruciani-Guglielmacci C, Manteghetti M, Rouault C, Derouet M, Rizkalla S, Pau B, Petit P, Ribes G, Ktorza A, Gross R, Reach G, Taouis M. Insulinotropic agent ID-1101 (4-hydroxy-isoleucine) activates insulin signaling in rat. *Am J Physiol Endocrinol Metab* 2004;**287**:E463−71.

22. Moorthy R, Prabhu KM, Murthy PS. Mechanism of anti-diabetic action, efficacy and safety profile of GII purified from fenugreek (Trigonella foenum-graceum Linn.) seeds in diabetic animals. *Indian J Exp Biol* 2010;**48**:1119−22.

23. Sharma RD, Raghuram TC, Rao NS. Effect of fenu-greek seeds on blood glucose and serum lipids in type I diabetes. *Eur J Clin Nutr* 1990;**44**:301−6.

24. Gupta A, Gupta R, Lal B. Effect of Trigonella foenum-graecum (fenugreek) seeds on glycaemic control and insulin resistance in type 2 diabetes mellitus: a double blind placebo controlled study. *J Assoc Physicians India* 2001;**49**:1057−61.

25. Srinivasan K. Plant foods in the management of dia-betes mellitus: spices as beneficial antidiabetic food adjuncts. *Int J Food Sci Nutr* 2005;**56**:399−414.

26. Yadav M, Lavania A, Tomar R, Prasad GB, Jain S, Yadav H. Complementary and comparative study on hypoglycemic and antihyperglycemic activity of various extracts of Eugenia jambolana seed, Momordica charantia fruits, Gymnema sylvestre, and Trigonella foenum graecum seeds in rats. *Appl Biochem Biotechnol* 2010;**160**:2388−400.

27. Shanmugasundaram K, Panneerselvam C, Samudam P, Shanmugasundaram E. E. Enzyme changes and glucose

utilisation in diabetic rabbits: The effect of Gymnema sylvestre. *R Br J Ethnopharmacol* 1983;**7**:205–34.

28. Shanmugasundaram ER, Gopinath KL, Shanmugasundaram KR, et al. Possible regeneration of the islets of Langerhams in streptozocin-diabetic rats given Gymnema sylvestre leaf extracts. *J Ethnopharmacol* 1990;**30**:265–79.

29. Al-Romaiyan A, Liu B, Asare-Anane H, Maity CR, Chatterjee SK, Koley N, Biswas T, Chatterji AK, Huang GC, Amiel SA, Persaud SJ, Jones PM. A novel Gymnema sylvestre extract stimulates insulin secretion from human islets in vivo and in vitro. *Phytother Res* 2010;**24**:1370–6.

30. Leach MJ. Gymnema sylvestre for diabetes mellitus: A systematic review. *The Journal of Alternative and Complementary Medicine* 2007;**13**:977–83.

31. Baskaran K, Kizar Ahamath B, Radha Shanmugasundaram K, Shanmugasundaram E. Antidiabetic effect of a leaf extract from Gymnema sylvestre in non-insulin-dependent diabetes mellitus patients. *J Ethnopharmacol* 1990;**30**:295–305.

32. Shanmugasundaram ER, Rajeswari G, Baskaran K, Rajesh Kumar BR, Radha Shanmugasundaram K, Kizar Ahmath B. Use of Gymnema sylvestre leaf extract in the control of blood glucose in insulin-dependent diabetes mellitus. *J Ethnopharmacol* 1990;**30**:281–94.

33. Shiyovich A, Sztarkier I, Nesher L. Toxic hepatitis induced by Gymnema sylvestre, a natural remedy for type 2 diabetes mellitus. *Am J Med Sci* 2010;**340**:514–7.

34. Trejo-González A, Gabriel-Ortiz G, Puebla-Pérez AM, Huízar-Contreras MD, Munguía-Mazariegos MR, Mejía-Arreguín S, Calva E. A purified extract from prickly pear cactus (Opuntia fuliginosa) controls experimentally induced diabetes in rats. *J Ethnopharmacol* 1996;**55**:27–33.

35. Andrade-Cetto A, Wiedenfeld H. Anti-hyperglycemic effect of Opuntia streptacantha Lem. *J Ethnopharmacol* 2011;**133**:940–3.

36. Frati-Munari AC, Fernandez-Harp JA, Banales-Ham M, Ariza-Andraca CR. Decreased blood glucose and insulin by nopal (Opuntia sp.). *Arch Invest Med (Mex)* 1983;**14**:269–74.

37. Frati AC, Xilotl Díaz N, Altamirano P, Ariza R, López-Ledesma R. The effect of two sequential doses of Opuntia streptacantha upon glycemi. *Arch Invest Med (Mex)* 1991;**22**:333–6.

38. Frati-Munari AC, Gordillo BE, Altamirano P, Ariza CR. Hypoglycemic effect of Opuntia streptacantha Lemaire in NIDDM. *Diabetes Care* 1988;**11**:63–6.

39. Frati AC, Gordillo BE, Altamirano P, Ariza CR, Cortés-Franco R, Chávez-Negrete A, Islas-Andrade S. Influence of nopal intake upon fasting glycemia in type II

diabetics and healthy subjects. *Arch Invest Med (Mex)* 1991;**22**:51–6.

40. Sobieraj DM, Freyer CW. Probable hypoglycemic adverse drug reaction associated with prickly pear cactus, glipizide, and metformin in a patient with type 2 diabetes mellitus. *Ann Pharmacother* 2010;**44**:1334–7.

41. Liu VJ, Abernathy RP. Chromium and insulin in young subjects with normal glucose tolerance. *Am J Clin Nutr* 1982;**35**:661–7.

42. Althuis MD, Jordan NE, Ludington EA, Wittes JT. Glucose and insulin responses to dietary chromium supplements: a meta-analysis. *Am J Clin Nutr* 2002;**76**:148–55.

43. Pittler MH, Stevinson C, Ernst E. Chromium picolinate for reducing body weight: meta-analysis of randomized trials. *Int J Obes Relat Metab Disord* 2003;**27**:522–9.

44. Attele AS, Zhou YP, Xie JT, Wu JA, Zhang L, Dey L, Pugh W, Rue PA, Polonsky KS, Yuan CS. Antidiabetic effects of Panax ginseng berry extract and the identification of an effective component. *Diabetes Care* 2002;**51**:1851–8.

45. Sotaniemi EA, Haapakoski E, Rautio A. Ginseng therapy in non-insulin-dependent diabetic patients. *Diabetes Care* 1995;**18**:1373–5.

46. Vuksan V, Sung MK, Sievenpiper JL, Stavro PM, Jenkins AL, Di Buono M, Lee KS, Leiter LA, Nam KY, Arnason JT, Choi M, Naeem A. Korean red ginseng (Panax ginseng) improves glucose and insulin regulation in well-controlled, type 2 diabetes: results of a randomized, double-blind, placebo-controlled study of efficacy and safety. *Nutr Metab Cardiovasc Dis* 2008;**18**:46–56.

47. Xie JT, Wang CZ, Li XL, Ni M, Fishbein A, Yuan CS. Anti-diabetic effect of American ginseng may not be linked to antioxidant activity: comparison between American ginseng and Scutellaria baicalensis using an ob/ob mice model. *Fitoterapia* 2009;**80**:306–11.

48. Wu Z, Luo JZ, Luo L. American ginseng modulates pancreatic beta cell activities. *Chin Med* 2007;**2**:11.

49. Luo JZ, Luo L. American ginseng stimulates insulin production and prevents apoptosis through regulation of uncoupling protein-2 in cultured beta cells. *Evid Based Complement Alternat Med* 2006;**3**:365–72.

50. Vuksan V, Sievenpiper JL, Wong J, Xu Z, Beljan-Zdravkovic U, Arnason JT, Assinewe V, Stavro MP, Jenkins AL, Leiter LA, Francis T. American ginseng (*Panax quinquefolius L.*) attenuates postprandial glycemia in a time-dependent but not dose-dependent manner in healthy individuals. *Am J Clin Nutr* 2001;**73**:753–8.

51. Smith AR, Shenvi SV, Widlansky M, Suh JH, Hagen TM. Lipoic acid as a potential therapy for chronic diseases associated with oxidative stress. *Curr Med Chem* 2004;**11**:1135–46.

52. Ziegler D, Nowak H, Kempler P, Vargha P, Low PA. Treatment of symptomatic diabetic polyneuropathy with the antioxidant alpha-lipoic acid: a meta-analysis. *Diab Med* 2004;**21**:114–21.

53. Ziegler D, Ametov A, Barinov A, Dyck PJ, Gurieva I, Low PA, Munzel U, Yakhno N, Raz I, Novosadova M, Maus J, Samigullin R. Oral treatment with alpha-lipoic acid improves symptomatic diabetic polyneuropathy: the SYDNEY 2 trial. *Diabetes Care* 2006;**29**:2365–70.

54. Bland R, Markovic D, Hills CE, Hughes SV, Chan SL, Squires PE, Hewison M. Expression of 25-hydroxyvitamin D3-1alpha-hydroxylase in pancreatic islets. *J Steroid Biochem Mol Biol* 2004;**89-90**:121–5.

55. Milner RD, Hales CN. The role of calcium and magnesium in insulin secretion from rabbit pancreas studied in vitro. *Diabetologia* 1967;**3**:47–9.

56. Maestro B, Campión J, Dávila N, Calle C. Stimulation by 1,25-dihydroxyvitamin D3 of insulin receptor expression and insulin responsiveness for glucose transport in U-937 human promonocytic cells. *Endocr J* 2000;**47**:383–91.

57. Draznin B, Sussman KE, Eckel RH, Kao M, Yost T, Sherman NA. Possible role of cytosolic free calcium concentrations in mediating insulin resistance of obesity and hyperinsulinemia. *J Clin Invest* 1988;**82**:1848–52.

58. Draznin B. Intracellular calcium, insulin secretion, and action. *Am J Med Sci* 1988;**85**:44–58.

59. Segal S, Lloyd S, Sherman N, Sussman K, Draznin B. Postprandial changes in cytosolic free calcium and glucose uptake in adipocytes in obesity and non-insulin-dependent diabetes mellitus. *Horm Res* 1990;**34**:39–44.

60. Pittas AG, Harris SS, Stark PC, Dawson-Hughes B. The effects of calcium and vitamin D supplementation on blood glucose and markers of inflammation in nondiabetic adults. *Diabetes Care* 2007;**30**:980–6.

61. Pittas AG, D.-H.B., Li T, Van Dam RM, Willett WC, Manson JE, Hu FB. Vitamin D and calcium intake in relation to type 2 diabetes in women. *Diabetes Care* 2006;**29**:650–6.

62. Pittas AG, Dawson-Hughes B. Vitamin D and diabetes. *J Steroid Biochem Mol Biol* 2010;**121**:425–9.

63. Pittas AG, Sun Q, Manson JE, Dawson-Hughes B, Hu FB. Plasma 25-hydroxyvitamin D concentration and risk of incident type 2 diabetes in women. *Diabetes Care* 2010;**33**:2021–3.

64. Kida K, Inoue T, Kaino Y, Goto Y, Ikeuchi M, Ito T, Matsuda H, Elliott RB. An immunopotentiator of beta-1,6;1,3 D-glucan prevents diabetes and insulitis in BB rats. *Diabetes Res Clin Pract* 1992;**17**:75–9.

65. Würsch P, Pi-Sunyer FX. The role of viscous soluble fiber in the metabolic control of diabetes. A review with special emphasis on cereals rich in beta-glucan. *Diabetes Care* 1997;**20**:1774–80.

66. Natural Standard. Natural Standard Database,

Therapeutic Effect of Fucoxanthin on Metabolic Syndrome and Type 2 Diabetes

Kazuo Miyashita, Show Nishikawa, Masashi Hosokawa

Faculty of Fisheries Sciences, Hokkaido University, Hakodate, Hokkaido, Japan

INTRODUCTION

Diabetes is one of the most common endocrine disorders affecting more than 285 million people globally with 90% of the cases diagnosed as type 2 diabetes.[1] Type 2 diabetes is known to show disease-specific complications such as blindness and renal failure. It is a disease characterized by an inadequate β-cell response to the progressive insulin resistance that typically accompanies advancing age, inactivity, weight gain, and genetic disorders. The prevalence of type 2 diabetes is increasing worldwide, not only in developed countries, but also in developing countries.

Diabetes causes approximately 5% of all deaths globally each year and its incidence is

Nutritional and Therapeutic Interventions for Diabetes and Metabolic Syndrome
DOI: 10.1016/B978-0-12-385083-6.00029-2

predicted to increase by over 50% in the next 10 years.[2] People with diabetes develop cardiovascular diseases (CVD) at an earlier age and are two to four times more likely to suffer strokes than healthy subjects, and approximately 73% of adults with diabetes are considered prehypertensive. Thus, diabetes is one of the leading causes of death worldwide and healthcare expenditures for diabetes are expected to increase year after year. Estimates on the global trend of the diabetes are generally based on diagnosed cases only, and few studies have screened the general population with undiagnosed diabetes, prediabetes. However, it is likely that the proportion of people at the prediabetic phase is much bigger than that at the diagnosed stage. Prediabetes is also a possible risk factor for CVD and other diseases.

The majority of patients with type 2 diabetes are obese[3] and have several modifiable cardiovascular factors, emphasizing the need for lifestyle modification as an essential component of metabolic syndrome care. Several clinical trials have demonstrated the benefits of lifestyle modification in reducing type 2 diabetes morbidity and mortality.[4] Lifestyle interventions, mainly diet and/or physical activity, are effective in delaying or preventing metabolic syndrome, and then type 2 diabetes.

Increased availability of refined foods, which are often cheaper than traditional foods, and limited physical activity, which is typical of modern civilizations, have been recognized as the main causes of the great number of type 2 diabetes.[5] Thus, initial nutritional approach to protection against metabolic syndrome and type 2 diabetes has been focused on reversing its root causes of atherogenetic diet, sedentary lifestyle, and overweight or obesity. Epidemiologic evidence suggests a lower prevalence of the metabolic syndrome associated with dietary patterns rich in fruit, vegetables, whole grains, dairy products, and polyunsaturated fats.[6,7] Several nutraceuticals have also been shown to reduce the risk of diabetes mellitus and metabolic syndrome and their complications, and to favorably modulate a number of biochemical and clinical end points. These compounds include antioxidant vitamins, such as vitamins A, C, and E, carotenoids, flavonoids, vitamin D, conjugated linoleic acid, omega-3 fatty acids, minerals such as chromium and magnesium, α-lipoic acid, phytoestrogens, and dietary fibers.[8]

Most desirable nutraceuticals to fight against metabolic syndrome and type 2 diabetes are those to improve a clustering of metabolic abnormalities that is characterized by abdominal obesity, impaired insulin sensitivity, hypertension, dyslipidemia, hyperglycemia and a systemic proinflammatory state. Interest in functionality of marine nutraceuticals continues to grow year by year, due to the fact that prevention against the lipid metabolism abnormalities through marine dietary means has been better understood and recognized by the public. Marine lipids, especially omega-3 polyunsaturated fatty acids such as eicosapentaenoic acid (EPA) and docosahexaenoic acid (DHA), have drawn increased interest due to several health benefits they afford. Major interest has also been paid to fucoxanthin, a characteristic carotenoid found in brown seaweeds, as fucoxanthin has been reported to show antiobesity effects and improvement of insulin resistance on the basis of certain molecular mechanisms. This chapter focuses on the physiological activity of fucoxanthin.

FUCOXANTHIN AND ITS ABSORPTION MECHANISM

Carotenoids including fucoxanthin have been implicated as important dietary nutrients having antioxidant potential. The antioxidant properties of carotenoids have been suggested as being the main mechanism by which they afford their beneficial health effects. However, it would be difficult to explain all the physiological effects of carotenoids only by their antioxidant activity. Other mechanisms of action that are independent of the antioxidant activity are likely to be of more interest to the scientific community. Although there are several reports published on the antioxidant activity of fucoxanthin,[9,10] the main mechanism for the physiological actions of fucoxanthin is its modulatory effects on specific gene and protein expression in biological systems. The physiological effect of fucoxanthin depends on its characteristic chemical structure including allenic bonds and other polar groups.

Dietary fucoxanthin is hydrolyzed to fucoxanthinol in the gastrointestinal tract by digestive enzymes such as lipase and cholesterol esterase,[11] and then converted to amarouciaxanthin A in the liver[12] (Figure 29.1). Both metabolites have the same structure of one side of the end ring, that contains one allenic bond and two hydroxyl groups. Although fucoxanthinol and amarouciaxanthin A have been detected in plasma and all tissues of mice given fucoxanthin,[11–14] most of the fucoxanthin metabolites preferentially accumulate as amarouciaxanthin A in the visceral white adipose tissue (WAT).[13] Recent study showed that more than 80% of fucoxanthin metabolites accumulated in visceral WAT[15] of obese/diabetes model mice (KK-A^y) (Figure 29.2). A total of three kinds of fucoxanthin metabolites detected in the WAT lipids was calculated to be 11.486 mg/mg protein, while those in all other tissue lipids was 2.127 mg/mg protein. This preferential accumulation of fucoxanthin metabolites in visceral WAT should be strongly related to its characteristic physiological activity such as antiobesity and antidiabetic effect.

ANTIOBESITY EFFECT OF FUCOXANTHIN

Type 2 diabetes and CVD are twin epidemics that are escalating globally. Metabolic syndrome is a cluster of risk factors of both diseases. Thus,

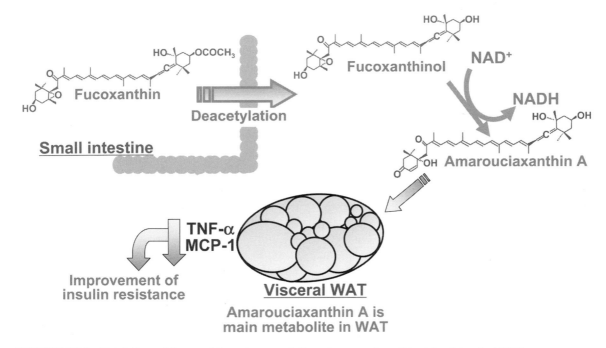

FIGURE 29.1 Metabolism of fucoxanthin and accumulation of amarouciaxanthin A in abdominal WAT.

FIGURE 29.2 Concentration of fucoxanthin metabolites in mice fed fucoxanthin (FX) (0.1%) for 4 weeks. *(Adapted from Reference 15.)*

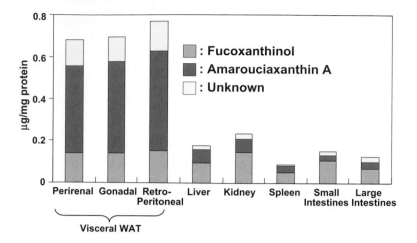

enormous numbers of publications have been devoted to the metabolic syndrome and several prestigious scientific organizations have tried to define the climes of the metabolic syndrome.[16] Although criteria for diagnosing the metabolic syndrome have still not been shared by all, the following should be included: abdominal obesity (as estimated by an increased waist circumference), a high blood triacyglycerol (TG) and a low high-density lipoprotein (HDL) cholesterol concentration, elevated blood pressure, insulin-resistant/glucose intolerance.

Abdominal obesity is the most obvious symptom of the metabolic syndrome. Other medical conditions associated with obesity include type 2 diabetes, several forms of cancer, renal and liver diseases, polycystic ovarian syndrome, sleep apnea, chronic inflammation, and atherosclerosis.[17] Although not all overweight/obese individuals are insulin resistant,[16] the increasing global prevalence of type 2 diabetes is tied to rising rates of obesity.[18] The prevalence of overweight and obesity in the US has increased dramatically over the past two decades to one in three adults. More than 80% of diabetes cases could have been prevented by only avoiding an overweight or obese status.[5]

Recent studies showed the antiobesity effect of fucoxanthin. Nutrigenomic study reveals that fucoxanthin induces uncoupling protein 1 (UCP1) expression in WAT mitochondria leading to oxidation of fatty acids and heat production in WAT (19,20). UCP1, usually expressed only in brown adipose tissue (BAT), is a key molecule for antiobesity. UCP1 expression in BAT is recognized as a significant component of whole body energy expenditure and its dysfunction contributes to the development of obesity. However, adult humans have very little BAT and most fat is stored in WAT. Considered as breakthrough discoveries for an ideal therapy of obesity, induction of UCP1 expression in tissues other than BAT by food constituent would be important. From this viewpoint, the antiobesity effect of the edible seaweed carotenoid, fucoxanthin, is very interesting, as its activity depends on the protein and gene inductions of UCP1 in WAT.[19]

Earlier studies using animal models indicated that more than 100 mg/kg weight fucoxanthin has been insufficient to show antiobesity effects.[15,19–22] However, recent study demonstrated a significant reduction of body fat in obese female volunteers by intake of fucoxanthin at less than 0.024 mg/kg weight.[23] This difference in the effectiveness between rodents and humans may be due to the different absorption rate and/or to different sensitivity to fucoxanthin.

Although chemical synthesis of fucoxanthin is possible, it is very expensive and its yield is very low. Several brown seaweeds contain more than 0.3–1.0% fucoxanthin.[24] This content is exceptionally high as compared with those of carotenoids in other natural products. Abidov et al.[23] reported that at most 2.4 mg fucoxanthin intake per day significantly increased energy expenditure of obese female volunteers (100 kg average weight) and decreased body weight, body fat, plasma TG, and liver lipid contents. Judging from this human trial, the fucoxanthin levels of several brown seaweed lipids will be sufficient for their antiobesity activity, when these materials are applied to general foods.

LOWERING EFFECT OF FUCOXANTHIN ON BLOOD GLUCOSE

When fucoxanthin is given to obese/diabetes model mice (KK-A^y), it markedly attenuates the gain of visceral WAT weight in KK-A^y mice with increasing UCP1 expression compared with the control mice. In addition, fucoxanthin significantly decreased the blood glucose and plasma insulin concentrations as compared with the control KK-A^y mice.[20] Similar results have also been obtained in normal mice (c57Bl/6J mice).[21] In this study, the mice were fed high-fat or normal-fat diets. Body weight and visceral WAT weight of high-fat dietary group were higher than those of the normal-fat dietary group. The fucoxanthin-containing diet significantly suppressed body weight and WAT weight gain induced by the high-fat diet. Dietary administration of high-fat diet resulted in hyperglycemia, hyperinsulinemia, and hyperleptinemia in the mouse model, while these perturbations were completely normalized in the fucoxanthin feeding group.

The antidiabetic effect of fucoxanthin found in obese/diabetes model mice (KK-A^y) and in high-fat-diet mice is mainly due to the regulatory effect of fucoxanthin and its metabolites accumulated in visceral WAT on releasing biologically active mediators termed adipokines. Adipose tissue has been recognized as an active endocrine organ in addition to its role as the main storage depot for triglycerides. An increasing number of obesity-derived secretory factors, adipokines, are described as the central role of adipose tissue in regulating whole body energy homeostasis, not only by partitioning lipids into various depots, but also through adipokine-mediated modulation of a number of signaling cascades in target tissues. It is well-established that individuals that are obese and/or suffer from the metabolic syndrome display a characteristic imbalance of their adipokine profile.[25] This altered adipokine profile leads to profound changes in insulin sensitivity and other biochemical alterations of metabolites, making an individual more prone to metabolic disorders.

With the exception of adiponectin and adipsin (complement factor D), most other adipokines have been implicated in obesity, type 2 diabetes, hypertension, inflammation, and CVD.[25] Fucoxanthin intake has been reported to downregulate the over-expressions of these adipokines. In obese/diabetes model mice (KK-A^y), leptin and tumor necrosis factor-α (TNF-α) mRNA expression in WAT were significantly decreased by fucoxanthin intake.[20] Increased expression of monocyte chemoattractant protein-1 (MCP-1) mRNA expression was observed in high-fat-feeding normal mice, but was normalized by fucoxanthin intake.[21]

Under normal conditions leptin is an important factor in regulating food intake, energy expenditure, and TNF-α secretion from WAT. However, during situations of chronic hyperleptinemia and leptin resistance, this hormone may function pathophysiologically for the development of insulin resistance, hypertension and cardiac and renal diseases. Adipose tissue secretes a number of inflammatory factors such as TNF-α and MCP-1. These adipokines appear to play an essential role not only in inflammatory-metabolic cross talk but in development of insulin resistance. Thus, downregulation of these adipokines found in animals given fucoxanthin will be one of the main mechanisms underlying its suppression effect on blood glucose level of diabetes models.

TNF-α, IL-6, MCP-1, AND PAI-1 AS TARGET ADIPOKINES OF FUCOXANTHIN

Through their autocrine, paracrine, and endocrine functions, adipokines influence a number of organs critical for energy homeostasis. The changes in each individual adipokine are the result of a coordinated change of specific transcriptional programs that affect entire groups of adipocyte gene products as well as post-translational mechanisms that affect the release of specific proteins differentially. Deng and Schherer[25] reviewed adipokines to have four major functions, namely, metabolism,

proinflammatory factors and acute phase reactants, extracellular matrix components, promitogenic and proangiogenic factors. The dysregulation in these adipokines secretions induces several potential pathophysiologic conditions, which contribute to the cardiometabolic consequences of abdominal obesity, inflammatory state, and ectopic excess fat deposition in the visceral WAT.

The overproduction of pro-inflammatory adipokines in obese WAT has an important role in the pathogenesis of insulin resistance and obesity-related type 2 diabetes. It is well known that pro-inflammatory adipokines such as TNF-α and IL-6 are strongly correlated to insulin resistance found in obesity (Figure 29.3). Development of obesity induces macrophage infiltration into the visceral WAT, causing a chronic low-grade inflammation characterized by the upregulation of pro-inflammatory adipokines, such as TNF-α and downregulation of an anti-inflammatory adiponectin. During the obesity development, saturated fatty acid and TNF-α derived from adipocytes and

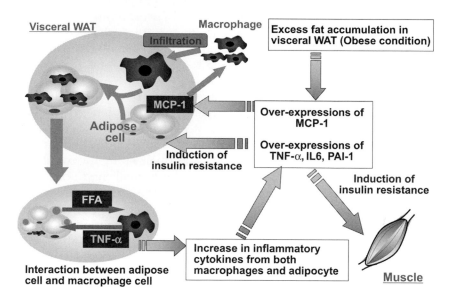

FIGURE 29.3 Involvement of inflammatory cytokines from both macrophages and adipocytes in insulin resistance. (*See the color plate section at the back of the book.*)

macrophages, respectively, organize a paracrine loop that lead to inflammation in the adipose (Figure 29.3).[26]

Among these adipokines, adiponectin has sometimes been regarded as one of the most potent molecules with respect to its insulin-sensitizing activity.[25,27] However, the nature of the key adipokines that are involved in the pathogenesis of type 2 diabetes and metabolic syndrome is as yet unclear. Although numerous adipokines have been reported, with their biological importances,[25,28] four of them have been reported to be regulated by fucoxanthin. They are pro-inflammatory adipokines, TNF-α, interleukin-6 (IL-6), MCP-1, and plasminogen activator inhibitor-1 (PAI-1). Several animal studies have clearly shown that fucoxanthin intake markedly reduces these adipokine mRNA expressions and secretions.[20–22]

TNF-α

TNF-α is a cytokine that links inflammation in adipocytes with obesity-induced insulin resistance. The importance of TNF-α in the development of insulin resistance has been confirmed by the fact that knockout mice for TNF-α or its receptors are protected from insulin resistance and exhibit improved insulin signaling in WAT and skeletal muscle.[29]

IL-6

IL-6 is another important inflammatory factor that is secreted from visceral WAT. Similar to TNF-α, IL-6 levels in plasma are correlated positively with adiposity.[30] Increase in IL-6 levels is found in insulin-resistant states and administration of IL-6 to rodents induces insulin resistance in the liver and skeletal muscle.[31]

MCP-1

MCP-1 is secreted by adipose tissue and recruits these macrophages to adipose tissue in obese mice[32] and humans[33] (Figure 29.3). Consistent with this role of MCP-1, adipose tissue of lean subjects usually consists of approximately 5–10% macrophages, whereas in obese patients, macrophage content in adipose tissue can be as high as 50% of the total number of cells.[34] Targeted ablation of MCP-1 or its receptor reduces adipose tissue macrophage infiltration, and improves insulin sensitivity without inducing weight loss.[35,36] Conversely, insulin resistance and increased macrophages of adipose tissue are observed in models of MCP-1 overexpression.[37]

PAI-1

PAI-1 is a member of the serine protease inhibitor (serpin) superfamily. PAI-1 inhibits fibrinolysis through its inhibition of plasminogen activator.[31] Increased PAI-1 is linked to not only thrombosis and fibrosis, but also to obesity, and insulin resistance.[38] Mice lacking functional PAI-1 are protected from obesity and insulin resistance.[38] Plasma levels of PAI-1 are elevated in human obesity and insulin resistance.[31] Obesity and obesity-related complications, including type 2 diabetes and CVD, may be modulated by PAI-1, making it an attractive therapeutic target.

REGULATORY EFFECT OF FUCOXANTHIN ON PRO-INFLAMMATORY ADIPOKINES

Antidiabetic effect of fucoxanthin is strongly related to the downregulation of pro-inflammatory adipokines secreted from visceral WAT.[22] When 0.2% fucoxanthin was given to two kinds of mice models, diabetic/obese KK-A^y mice and lean C57BL/6J mice, WAT weight gain was reduced by fucoxanthin intake as expected, although it was not affected in lean C57BL/6J mice (Figure 29.4A). Fucoxanthin intake also markedly decreased blood glucose level of

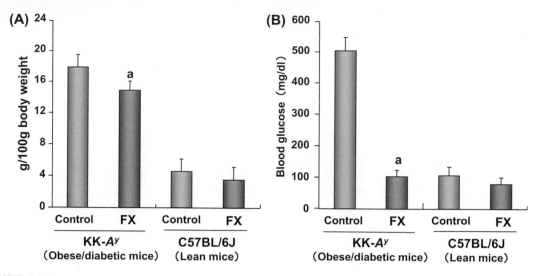

FIGURE 29.4 Effects of fucoxanthin (FX) on abdominal WAT weight (A) and blood glucose levels (B) of KK-A^y and C57BL/6J mice fed control or fucoxanthin diets. Mice were fed either control or fucoxanthin diets for 4 weeks. Values represent the mean $\pm$ SEM of six mice per group. [a]Significantly different from each control ($P < 0.05$). (*Adapted from Reference 22.*)

obese/diabetic mice to the same level as that in control C57BL/6J mice, whereas fucoxanthin did not affect blood glucose levels in C57BL/6J lean mice (Figure 29.4B). Furthermore, mRNA expression levels of TNF-α. MCP-1, MCP-1, and PAI-1, which are considered to induce insulin resistance, were markedly reduced by fucoxanthin intake compared to control mice (Figure 29.5). In contrast to KK-A^y mice, fucoxanthin did not alter MCP-1 and TNF-α mRNA expression levels in the WAT of lean C57BL/6J mice.[22]

It is likely that the antidiabetic effect of fucoxanthin is derived from the downregulation of TNF-α, IL-6, MCP-1, and PAI-1 mRNA in the visceral WAT of obese condition. This effect may be based on the inhibitory effect of fucoxanthin on the infiltration of macrophages into adipose tissue. As shown in Figure 29.6, a decrease in F4/80-positive macrophages was clearly confirmed in perigonadal WAT of KK-A^y mice fed fucoxanthin diet.[22] Obese adipose tissue is characterized by an increased infiltration of macrophages (Figure 29.3).

Suganami *et al.* further demonstrated a paracrine loop involving TNF-α and free fatty acids (FFA) between infiltrated macrophages and adipocytes (Figure 29.3).[26] Adipose cells and macrophages secrete large amounts of TNF-α. TNF-α and other pro-inflammatory adipokines promote lipolysis of triacylglycerols and releasing FFA. These FFA activate macrophages infiltrated into WAT, and then again enhance TNF-α production.[39] Fucoxanthin effectively stops this adverse circulation between adipose cells and macrophages.[22]

3T3-F442A preadipocytes differentiate to adipocytes at a high ratio. *In vitro* study using the preadipocytes showed that fucoxanthinol, one of main fucoxanthin metabolites, reduced TNF-α mRNA expression and protein production in RAW264.7 macrophage-like cells treated with palmitic acid.[22] However, fucoxanthinol also reduced the mRNA and the protein expressions of MCP-1 and IL-6 in differentiating 3T3-F442A cells stimulated with TNF-α, which is an inflammatory cytokine produced by both macrophages and adipocytes (Figure 29.3).

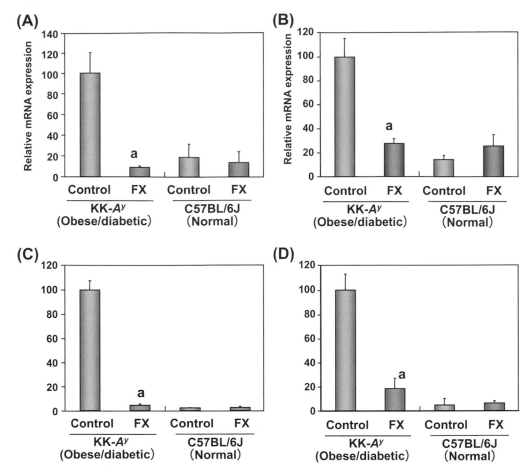

FIGURE 29.5 Effects of fucoxanthin on adipocytokine mRNA expression level in WAT of KK-A^y and C57BL/6J mice. Mice were fed either control or fucoxanthin diets for 4 weeks. TNF-α (A), IL-6 (B), MCP-1 (C), and PAI-1 (D) mRNA expression levels are expressed relative to control KK-A^y mice set as 100. Values represent the mean $\pm$ SEM of six mice per group. [a]Significantly different from each control ($P < 0.05$). *(Adapted from Reference 22.)*

In addition, fucoxanthinol decreases inducible nitric oxide synthase (iNOS) and cyclooxygenase-2 (COX-2) mRNA expression in RAW264.7 cells stimulated by palmitic acid.[22] iNOS is an enzyme that produces NO, which is a free radical molecule related to the pathogenesis of inflammation. Overexpression of iNOS mRNA has been observed in the WAT of obese mice and adipocytes.[40,41] Treatment of diabetic db/db mice with an iNOS inhibitor reversed hyperglycemia and improved insulin sensitivity, therefore the downregulation of iNOS mRNA in macrophages is suggested to be the molecular target for the prevention and improvement of type 2 diabetes.[40] COX-2 is an inducible enzyme that produces prostaglandin E2 (PGE2). Pharmacologic inhibition of COX-2 reduces IL-6 in WAT.[42] The downregulation of COX-2 and iNOS mRNAs found in macrophages with fucoxanthinol may contribute to suppress or ameliorate the increased inflammation in WAT and insulin resistance.

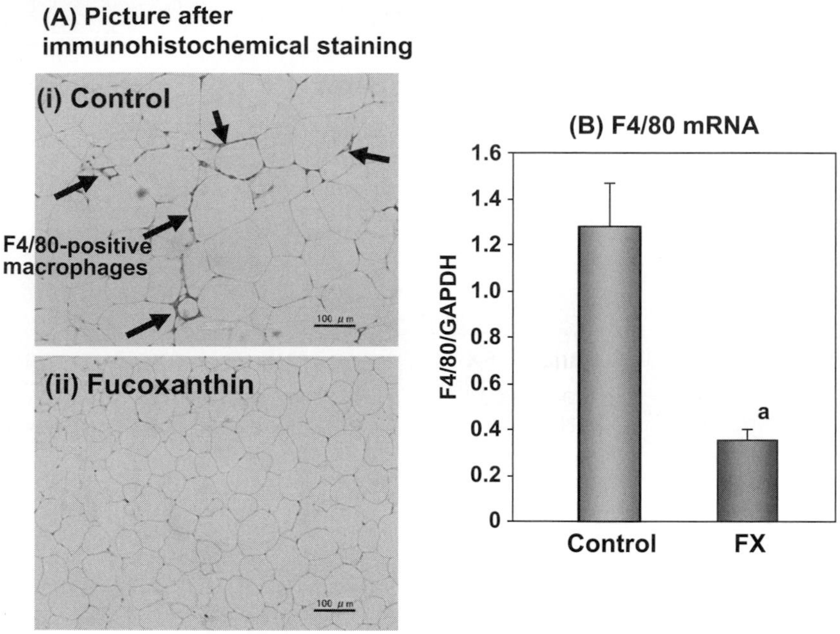

FIGURE 29.6   Macrophage infiltration in perigonadal WAT of KK-A^y mice. The infiltration was analyzed by perigonadal WAT by immunohistochemical staining with the anti-F4/80 antibody (A), and F4/80 mRNA expression (B). Mice were fed either control or fucoxanthin diets for 28 days. [a]Significantly different from each control ($P < 0.05$). (Adapted from Reference 22.)

EFFECT OF FUCOXANTHIN ON GLUT4 EXPRESSION IN MUSCLE

Insulin increases the uptake of glucose into a fat or muscle cells through a function of glucose transport protein to be redistributed at the cell's surface. The protein is the specialized sugar carrier glucose transport 4 (GLUT4), which is greatly enriched in muscle and fat cells. Following the discovery of GLUT4, the mechanisms regulating the expression of the GLUT4 gene have been intensively studied over the past decade. Studies using transgenic mouse models demonstrate that modifying the expression of GLUT4 profoundly affects whole-body insulin action and, consequently, glucose and lipid metabolism.[43,44] Mice with overexpression of the GLUT4 gene in skeletal muscle or adipose tissue showed enhanced insulin responsiveness and peripheral glucose utilization.[45] Thus, the regulation of the GLUT4 gene is of clinical relevance for whole-body glucose homeostasis and insulin sensitivity.

Skeletal muscle accounts for nearly 40% of body mass. A significant reduction in GLUT4 protein and mRNA levels in skeletal muscle is found in high-fat-diet cases.[46,47] Indeed, when mice were fed high-fat (HF) or normal-fat (NF) diets, the HF group resulted in hyperglycemia, hyperinsulinemia, and hyperleptinemia with a significant decrease in GLUT4 mRNA levels in skeletal muscle as compared to the NF group.[21] However, these perturbations were completely normalized by the addition of fucoxanthin to the HF diet and GLUT4 mRNA levels in the HF group fed fucoxanthin were restored to levels observed in the NF group. Thus, regulatory effect of fucoxanthin on GLUT4 expression found in muscle of normal mice fed high-fat diet[21] is related to the antidiabetic activity of fucoxanthin.

Skeletal muscle is an important site of glucose utilization. However, in contrast to the adipose tissue, the levels of muscle GLUT4 protein and mRNA remained almost unchanged.[48] Similarly, increasing adiposity does not seem to activate inflammatory cascades in skeletal muscle. DeFronze[49] reported that GLUT4 levels are lower in fat cells from diabetic people, while the amount of GLUT4 in muscle cells in such people changes little. Cai et al.[50] reported that neither muscle-specific ablation of IKK-β nor muscle-specific inhibition of nuclear factor-κB (NF-κB) improves insulin resistance in obese mice. Therefore, it may be appropriate to think of the skeletal muscle as a target for inflammation-induced insulin resistance rather than as a site of its initiation.

Another important aspect is the translocation level of GLUT4 molecules to cell membranes. Insulin stimulation of glucose uptake into muscle and fat cells requires movement of GLUT4-containing vesicles from intracellular compartments to the membrane. Accordingly, insulin-derived signals must arrive at and be recognized by the appropriate intracellular GLUT4 pools. Fucoxanthin may activate the movement of GLUT4 to the cell surface (unpublished data). More research is needed to make clear the effect of fucoxanthin intake on the glucose metabolism in muscle cells.

CONCLUSIONS

Fucoxanthin, a marine carotenoid found in edible brown seaweeds, is an effective natural compound for the prevention of obesity and its related type 2 diabetes. The antiobesity effect of fucoxanthin is mainly based on the increase in energy expenditure. Fucoxanthin promotes lipid metabolism in adipose tissue through the UCP1 upregulation in the mitochondria leading to oxidation of fatty acids and heat production. However, fucoxanthin downregulates expressions of proinflammatory adipokines involved in insulin resistance. These effects of fucoxanthin are specific in the obese phenotype and are not found in the lean normal model. Fucoxanthin is mainly metabolized to fucoxanthinol and amarouciaxanthin A. The key structure of fucoxanthin metabolites for the expression of antiobesity effect and antidiabetic effect is the end ring of the polyene chromophore containing an allenic bond and two hydroxyl groups.

The ability to store energy as a lipid depot is necessary to maintain immune and other systems for animals to survive at times of low nutrient availability. Energy storage, effective energy utilization, and strong immune response are among the most basic requirements to maintain the animal body. However, a chronic metabolic overload induces overweight or obesity leading to immune imbalance. The immune disorders in turn worsen the metabolic conditions. Thus, the most important therapy for the metabolic and immune disorders is to reduce the excess accumulation of body fat, especially fat in visceral WAT. However, in normal conditions over-fat expenditure or decreased-fat intake should be avoided. Fucoxanthin is effective in subjects with obesity and with metabolic disorders, and is devoid of any activity in lean subjects. In addition, the molecular mechanisms underlying the effects of fucoxanthin have been characterized and its biological effect can be improved by the selective accumulation of fucoxanthin metabolites in the target organ, visceral WAT. Fucoxanthin will be a desirable nutraceutical to alleviate obesity and metabolic disorders.

References

1. Cantrell RA, Alatorre CI, Davis EJ, Zarotsky V, Nestour EL, Carter GC, Goetz I, Paczkowski R, Sierra-Johnson J. A review of treatment response in type 2 diabetes: assessing the role of patient heterogeneity. Diabetes Obes Metab 2010;12:845—57.

2. Saha S, Gerdtham UG, Johansson P. Economic evaluation of lifestyle interventions for preventing diabetes and cardiovascular diseases. *Int J Environ Res Public Health* 2010;7:3150—95.

3. Leibson CL, Williamson DF, Melton LJ, Palumbo PJ, Smith SA, Ransom JE, Schilling PL, Narayan KMV. Temporal trends in BMI among adults with diabetes. *Diabetes Care* 2001;24:1584—9.

4. Bloomgarden ZT. Approaches to treatment of prediabetes and obesity and promising new approaches to type 2 diabetes. *Diabetes Care* 2008;31:1461—6.

5. Bruno G, Landi A. Epidemiology and costs of diabetes. *Transplant Proc* 2011;43:327—9.

6. Abete I, Astrup A, Martinez JA, Thorsdottir I, Zulet MA. Obesity and the metabolic syndrome: role of different dietary macronutrient distribution patterns and specific nutritional components on weight loss and maintenance. *Nutr Rev* 2010;68:214—31.

7. Rudkowska I. Functional foods for health: focus on diabetes. *Maturitas* 2009;62:263—9.

8. Davì G, Santilli F, Patrono C. Nutraceuticals in diabetes and metabolic syndrome. *Cardiovasc Ther* 2010;28:216—26.

9. Hosokawa M, Okada T, Mikami N, Konishi I, Miyashita K. Bio-functions of marine carotenoids. *Food Sci Biotechnol* 2009;18:1—11.

10. Sachindra NM, Sato E, Maeda H, Hosokawa M, Niwano Y, Kohno M, Miyashita K. Radical scavenging and singlet oxygen quenching activity of marine carotenoid fucoxanthin and its metabolites. *J Agric Food Chem* 2007;55:8516—22.

11. Asai A, Sugawara T, Ono H, Nagao A. Biotransformation of fucoxanthinol into amarouciaxanthin A in mice and HepG2 cells: formation and cytotoxicity of fucoxanthin metabolites. *Drug Metab Dispo.s* 2004;32:205—11.

12. Sugawara T, Baskaran V, Tsuzuki W, Nagao A. Brown algae fucoxanthin is hydrolyzed to fucoxanthinol during absorption by Caco-2 human intestinal cells and mice. *J Nutr* 2002;132:946—51.

13. Hashimoto T, Ozaki Y, Taminato M, Das SK, Mizuno M, Yoshimura K, Maoka T, Kanazawa K. The distribution and accumulation of fucoxanthin and its metabolites after oral administration in mice. *Br J Nutr* 2009;102:242—8.

14. Tsukui T, Baba T, Hosokawa M, Sashima T, Miyashita K. Enhancement of hepatic docosahexaenoic acid and arachidonic acid contents in C57BL/6J mice by dietary fucoxanthin. *Fisheries Sci* 2009;75:261—3.

15. Airanthi MKWA, Sasaki N, Iwasaki S, Baba N, Abe M, Hosokawa M, Miyashita K. Effect of brown seaweed lipids on fatty acid composition and lipid hydroperoxide levels of mouse liver. *J Agric Food Chem* 2011;59:4156—63.

16. Reaven GM. The metabolic syndrome: time to get off the merry-go-round? *J Intern Med* 2010;269:127—36.

17. Gade W, Schmit J, Collins M, Gade J. Beyond obesity: the diagnosis and pathophysiology of metabolic syndrome. *Clin Lab Sci* 2010;23:51—61.

18. Teixeira ME, Budd GM. Obesity stigma: A newly recognized barrier to comprehensive and effective type 2 diabetes management. *J Am Acad Nurse Pract* 2010;22:527—33.

19. Maeda H, Hosokawa M, Sashima T, Funayama K, Miyashita K. Fucoxanthin from edible seaweed, Undaria pinnatifida, shows antiobesity effect through UCP1 expression in white adipose tissues. *Biochem Biophys Res Commun* 2005;332:392—7.

20. Maeda H, Hosokawa M, Sashima T, Miyashita K. Dietary combination of fucoxanthin and fish oil attenuates the weight gain of white adipose tissue and decrease blood glucose in obese/diabetic KK- A^y mice. *J Agric Food Chem* 2007;55:7701—6.

21. Maeda H, Hosokawa M, Sashima T, Murakami-Funayama K, Miyashita K. Anti-obesity and anti-diabetic effects of fucoxanthin on diet-induced obesity conditions in a murine model. *Mol Med Rep* 2009;2:897—902.

22. Hosokawa M, Miyashita T, Nishikawa S, Emi S, Tsukui T, Beppu F, Okada T, Miyashita K. Fucoxanthin regulates adipocytokine mRNA expression in white adipose tissue of diabetic/obese KK-Ay mice. *Arch Biochem Biophys* 2010;504:17—25.

23. Abidov M, Ramazanov Z, Seifulla R, Grachev S. The effects of Xanthigen™ in the weight management of obese premenopausal women with non-alcoholic fatty liver disease and normal liver fat. *Diab Obes Met* 2010;12:72—81.

24. Terasaki M, Baba Y, Yasui H, Saga N, Hosokawa M, Miyashita K. Evaluation of recoverable functional lipid components with special reference to fucoxanthin and fucosterol contents of several brown seaweeds of Japan. *J Phycol* 2009;45:974—80.

25. Deng Y, Scherer PE. Adipokines as novel biomarkers and regulators of the metabolic syndrome. *Ann NY Acad Sci* 2010;1212:E1—19.

26. Suganami T, Nishida J, Ogawa Y. A paracrine loop between adipocytes and macrophages aggravates inflammatory changes: role of free fatty acids and tumor necrosis factor a. *Arterioscler Thromb Vasc Biol* 2005;25:2062—8.

27. Kadowaki T, Yamauchi T, Kubota N, Hara K, Ueki K, Tobe K. Adiponectin and adiponectin receptors in insulin resistance, diabetes, and the metabolic syndrome. *J Clin Invest* 2006;116:1784—92.

28. Rosen ED, Spiegelman BM. Adipocytes as regulators of energy balance and glucose homeostasis. *Nature* 2006;444:847—53.

29. Uysal KT, Wiesbrock SM, Marino MW, Hotamisligil GS. Protection from obesity induced insulin resistance in mice lacking TNF-a function. *Nature* 1997;**389**:610—4.

30. Fernandez-Real JM, Vayreda M, Richart C, Gutierrez C, Broch M, Vendrell J, Ricart W. Circulating interleukin 6 levels, blood pressure, and insulin sensitivity in apparently healthy men and women. *J Clin Endocrinol Metab* 2001;**86**:1154—9.

31. Kershaw EE, Flier JS. Adipose tissue as an endocrine organ. *J Clin Endocrinol Metab* 2004;**89**:2548—56.

32. Xu H, Barnes GT, Yang Q, Tan G, Yang D, Chou CJ, C.J., Sole J, Nichols A, Ross JS, Tartaglia LA, Chen H. Chronic inflammation in fat plays a crucial role in the development of obesity-related insulin resistance. *J Clin Invest* 2003;**112**:1821—30.

33. Curat CA, Miranville A, Sengenès C, Diehl M, Tonus C, Busse R, Bouloumié A. From blood monocytes to adipose tissue-resident macrophages: induction of diapedesis by human mature adipocytes. *Diabetes* 2004;**53**:1285—92.

34. Weisberg SP, McCann D, Desai M, Rosenbaum M, Leibel RL, Ferrante Jr AW. Obesity is associated with macrophage accumulation in adipose tissue. *J Clin Invest* 2003;**112**:1796—808.

35. Weisberg SP, Hunter D, Huber R, Lemieux J, Slaymaker S, Vaddi K, Charo I, Leibel RL, Anthony W, Ferrante Jr AW. CCR2 modulates inflammatory and metabolic effects of high-fat feeding. *J Clin Invest* 2006;**116**:115—24.

36. Kanda H, Tateya S, Tamori Y, Kotani K, Hiasa K, Kitazawa R, Kitazawa S, Miyachi H, Maeda S, Egashira K, Kasuga M. MCP-1 contributes to macrophage infiltration into adipose tissue, insulin resistance, and hepatic steatosis in obesity. *J Clin Invest* 2006;**116**:1494—505.

37. Guilherme A, Virbasius JV, Puri V, Czech MP. Adipocyte dysfunctions linking obesity to insulin resistance and type 2 diabetes. *Nat Rev Mol Cell Biol* 2008;**9**:367—77.

38. Ma LJ, Mao SL, Taylor KL, Kanjanabuch T, Guan Y, Zhang Y, Brown NJ, Swift LL, McGuinness OP, Wasserman DH, Vaughan DE, Fogo AB. Prevention of obesity and insulin resistance in mice lacking plasminogen activator inhibitor 1. *Diabetes* 2004;**53**:336—46.

39. Kennedy A, Martinez K, Chuang CC, LaPoint K, McIntosh M. Saturated fatty acid-mediated inflammation and insulin resistance in adipose tissue: mechanisms of action and implications. *J Nutr* 2008;**139**:1—4.

40. Fujimoto M, Shimizu N, Kunii K, Martyn JA, Ueki K, Kaneki M. A role for iNOS in fasting hyperglycemia and impaired insulin signaling in the liver of obese diabetic mice. *Diabetes* 2005;**54**:1340—8.

41. Nozaki M, Fukuhara A, Segawa K, Okuno Y, Abe M, Hosogai N, Matsuda M, Komuro R, Shimomura I. Nitric oxide dysregulates adipocytokine expression in 3T3-L1 adipocytes. *Biochem Biophys Res Commun* 2007;**364**:33—9.

42. Ogston NC, Karastergiou K, Hosseinzadeh-Attar MJ, Bhome R, Madani R, Stables M, Gilroy D, Flachs P, Hensler M, Kopecky J, Mohamed-Ali V. Low-dose acetylsalicylic acid inhibits the secretion of interleukin-6 from white adipose tissue. *Int J Obes* 2008;**32**:1807—15.

43. Charron MJ, Katz EB. Metabolic and therapeutic lessons from genetic manipulation of GLUT4. *Mol Cell Biochem* 1998;**182**:143—52.

44. Minokoshi Y, Kahn CR, Kahn BB. Tissue-specific ablation of the GLUT4 glucose transporter or the insulin receptor challenges assumptions about insulin action and glucose homeostasis. Tissue-specific ablation of the GLUT4 glucose transporter or the insulin receptor challenges assumptions about insulin action and glucose homeostasis. *J Biol Chem* 2003;**278**:33609—12.

45. Charron MJ, Ellen B, Katz EB, Olson AL. GLUT4 gene regulation and manipulation. *J Biol Chem* 1999;**274**:3253—6.

46. Kahn BB, Pedersen O. Suppression of GLUT4 expression in skeletal muscle of rats that are obese from high fat feeding but not from high carbohydrate feeding or genetic obesity. *Endocrinology* 1993;**132**:13—22.

47. Kim Y, Tamura T, Iwashita S, Tokuyama K, Suzuki M. Effect of high-fat diet on gene expression of and insulin receptor in soleus muscle. *Biochem Biophys Res Commun* 1994;**202**:519—26.

48. Armoni M, Harel C, Karnieli E. Transcriptional regulation of the GLUT4 gene: from PPAR-gamma and FOXO1 to FFA and inflammation. *Trends Endocr Metab* 2007;**18**:100—7.

49. Morris J, Birnbaum MJ. Dialogue between muscle and fat. *Nature* 2001;**409**:672—3.

50. Cai D, Frantz JD, Tawa Jr NE, Melendez PA, Oh B-C, Lidov HGW, Hasselgren P-O, Frontera WR, Lee J, Glass DJ, Steven E, Shoelson SE. IKKbeta/NF-kappaB activation causes severe muscle wasting in mice. *Cell* 2004;**119**:285—98.

30

Beneficial Effects of Chromium(III) and Vanadium Supplements in Diabetes

John B. Vincent

Department of Chemistry, The University of Alabama, Tuscaloosa, AL, USA

INTRODUCTION

Chromium and vanadium are neighboring first row transition metals in the periodic table. While having quite distinct chemical properties, both have been proposed for use in treating the symptoms of type 1 and type 2 diabetes. Both elements are ubiquitous in the environment and in foods at very low concentrations. Vanadium compounds are toxic, while chromium(III)

compounds (with a few exceptions) are essentially non-toxic so that estimating safety limits is difficult. While both have been proposed to be essential trace elements in mammals, vanadium has never been formally recognized as essential and probably has no role in normal mammalian biology. In contrast, chromium has been accepted as an essential trace element for three decades; however, this status has received serious challenge such that chromium will

Nutritional and Therapeutic Interventions for Diabetes and Metabolic Syndrome
DOI: 10.1016/B978-0-12-385083-6.00030-9

probably be removed from the list of essential elements for mammals. The proposed mechanisms for the biological activity of the elements are distinct. Vanadium appears to serve as an insulin mimetic, while chromium(III) apparently can amplify insulin sensitivity. This chapter describes the current status of the potential use of chromium and vanadium compounds as pharmacological agents to treat the symptoms of diabetes, most notably type 2 diabetes.

CHROMIUM

Essential Element?

Chromium was proposed to be an essential trace element for mammals just over 50 years ago. Rats fed a diet with Torula yeast as the sole protein source developed an apparent inability to properly dispose of glucose after a glucose challenge.[1] Adding high doses of a variety of chromium(III) complexes (200 μg Cr/kg diet), but not over 50 different elements to the diet restored this ability. Similarly, the addition of Brewer's yeast or porcine kidney powder, both rich in chromium, also apparently reversed the condition. Unfortunately, the study was flawed. For example, the rats were kept in metal cages, and the Cr content of diet was never measured. Additionally, large doses of chromium(III) have subsequently been shown to have pharmacological effects on rodents.[2]

In 1980, the Food and Nutritional Board of the National Academy of Science (USA) determined that chromium was an essential element and set an Estimated Safe and Adequate Daily Dietary Intake (ESSADI) of 50–200 μg.[3] In 2002, this was changed to an Adequate Intake (AI) of 30 μg per day.[4]

Recently, providing rats a diet with as little chromium as reasonably possible has been shown to not have any deleterious effects.[5] Rats were provided the AIN-93 G purified diet with added chromium in the mineral mix (< 20 μg Cr/kg diet) and were kept in cages with no access to metal for 6 months. This Cr content is similar to that of a human consuming 30 μg Cr daily (the AI value). No differences in body mass, insulin sensitivity, or response to a glucose challenge were observed compared to rats on the complete AIN-93 G diet (with 1,000 μg Cr/kg). Adding additional Cr(III) to the diet (200 μg/kg or 1,000 μg/kg), clearly supra-nutritional or pharmacological doses, also had no effects on body mass but resulted in increased insulin sensitivity.[5]

Other data have been proposed to support chromium being an essential trace element in humans and other mammals. Most notable are studies on effects of chromium supplementation of rats on high-sugar[6] or high-fat diets,[7] or humans on total parenteral nutrition (TPN) that developed diabetes-type symptoms.[8] In these cases, the animals had altered carbohydrate and lipid metabolism that was at least partially restored by supplementation with high, supra-nutritional doses of chromium. These actually only provide evidence for a pharmacological role for chromium, not one as an essential trace element.[2]

Additional evidence for a potential role for Cr comes from studies of chromium absorption as a function of chromium intake. Anderson and coworkers have reported that for humans absorption varies inversely with intake; low intakes (~15 μg/day) lead to "high" rates of absorption (~2%) while high intake (~35 μg/day) reduces absorption to ~0.4%.[9] However, the effects were only observed for female subjects; no dependence of absorption as a function of dose was observed for male subjects. The greater number of female subjects resulted in an effect being observed when all subjects were considered. Close scrutiny of this work suggests that propagation of error analysis needs to be carefully performed with these results. Studies of this type are not trivial to perform, and the error associated with the results is probably easily as large as the apparently observed effects. The study also needs to be reproduced. Recently, Kottwitz et al.[10] demonstrated in rats that absorption of chromium from oral $CrCl_3$ was independent of dose over seven different doses in the range of 0.01–20 μg Cr.

Consequently, unless additional evidence should appear, chromium can no longer be considered an essential trace element.[2]

Chromium Conditionally Essential?

Humans and rodents with type 1 or type 2 diabetes excrete larger quantities of chromium in their urine than their healthy counterparts (for example, see Ref.[10]). This has been taken as evidence that diabetic subjects could become chromium deficient, leading to exacerbation of the symptoms of their diabetes, and that chromium should be considered a conditionally essential element. However, the intake of chromium in these subjects had not been adequately addressed.

Dietary chromium is absorbed via passive diffusion with an efficiency of about 1%.[11] Recently, studies have shown that Zucker diabetic fatty rats (a type 2 diabetes model)[12] and rats with streptozotocin-induced diabetes (a type 1 diabetes model)[13] absorb more chromium from the diet. The increased urinary chromium loss is simply a reflection of the increased chromium intake. Thus, increased urinary chromium loss should not lead to chromium deficiency and exacerbation of diabetic symptoms. Thus, chromium can not be considered a conditionally essential element.

"Glucose Tolerance Factor"

In the original studies from the 1950s, the component that was believed to be missing from the Torula yeast diet and was responsible for the inability to properly handle a glucose challenge was named "glucose tolerance factor" or GTF.[1] Based on the original proposal, GTF was equated with Cr^{3+}. However, to have a biological effect, chromium must bind to some biomolecule. As the addition of Brewer's yeast to the Torula yeast diet was reported to lead to restoration of glucose tolerance, attempts were made to identify a bioactive chromium-organic species from Brewer's yeast. The term GTF was used to name the initial product of this search, reported by Mertz and coworkers in 1977.[14] After this paper appeared, the term GTF was generally used for the product of this isolation, not for Cr^{3+}. Unfortunately, this research is rife with problems. For example, the isolation procedure included harsh procedures such as an 18-h reflux in 5 M HCl, which would hydrolyze any proteins, complex carbohydrates, or nucleic acids. Thus, the chances that the form of Cr recovered after the treatment resembles the form in the yeast are remote. Nicotinic acid was apparently sublimed from the material and identified (although no data were presented). Amino acid analyses indicated the presence of glycine, glutamic acid, and cysteine as well as other amino acids, although the relative amounts were not reported. The results were interpreted to indicate that "GTF" was a complex of Cr, nicotinate, glycine, cysteine, and glutamate. Yet, in subsequent paper chromatography experiments, the material on which the studies above were performed produced several Cr-containing bands, only one of which was active in bioassays. (The bioassays measured the ability of a material to activate the metabolism of glucose by adipose tissue from rats on the *Torula* yeast diet in the presence of insulin.) The Cr in the active band represented only 6% of the total Cr. Hence, the characterization of a chromium-containing fraction from yeast was performed on a mixture that contained multiple Cr-containing species and other components; the characterization, thus, can not be assumed to reflect the identity of the active component. Still Cr^{3+} has been demonstrated repeatedly to be separable from agents in yeast responsible for *in vitro* stimulation of glucose metabolism in adipocytes (reviewed in Ref.[15]). Thus, the component of Brewer's yeast that is active in the bioassays apparently *does not contain Cr*. Glucose tolerance factor is an artifact; the use of this term should be abandoned.[15]

Effects of Chromium Supplementation on Rodent Models of Diabetes

In rodent models of diabetes and obesity-related insulin resistance resulting from mutations in the genes encoding for the hormone leptin or its receptor, chromium appears to have beneficial effects on insulin resistance, marginally beneficial effects on blood glucose, and effects on the grossly elevated plasma lipid levels (for a recent review, see Ref.[16]). Unfortunately, only a tiny percentage of human type 2 diabetes cases are the result of mutations in leptin or its receptor.

Effects of Chromium Supplementation on Type 2 Diabetes

Human studies have used considerably lower doses (in terms of µg Cr/kg body mass) than rodent studies and tend to be negative or at best ambiguous. In response to a request from a nutraceutical company, the US Food and Drug Administration (FDA) examined the relationship between chromium and insulin resistance, cardiovascular disease, type 2 diabetes, and other conditions related to high glucose levels.[17] The FDA issued a letter of enforcement discretion allowing only one qualified health claim for the labeling of dietary supplements: "One small study suggests that chromium picolinate may reduce the risk of type 2 diabetes. FDA concludes that the existence of such a relationship between chromium picolinate and either insulin resistance or type 2 diabetes is highly uncertain".[17] The small study was performed by Cefalu and coworkers.[18] This study was a placebo-controlled, double-blind trial examining 1,000 µg/day of Cr as chromium

picolinate in 29 obese subjects with a family history of type 2 diabetes; while no effects of the supplement were found on body mass or body fat composition or distribution, a significant increase in insulin sensitivity was observed after 4 and 8 months of supplementation.

As part of the investigation, the FDA commissioned a meta-analysis of studies on the effects of chromium on glucose and insulin metabolism in healthy subjects, subjects with compromised carbohydrate metabolism, and subjects with type 2 diabetes.[19] The studies were generally found to tend to have small subject pools and not be well designed. No benefit from chromium supplementation was identified for healthy individuals. No effects were noted on glycated hemoglobin, fasting glucose, low-density lipoprotein (LDL) or high-density lipoprotein (HDL) cholesterol, or triglycerides as only one study reported a significant effect on one of these variables. Chromium supplementation was found to statistically improve glycemic control in type 2 diabetics. The effects were quite small but significant overall. When broken down by chromium source, the effects were small but significant for subjects on yeast and [Cr(pic)$_3$] but not CrCl$_3$. Yet, the authors determined the results were not definitive because of the poor quality and heterogeneity of the studies. Overall chromium did not affect lipid levels, while [Cr(pic)$_3$] lowered glycated hemoglobin levels. However, lower glycated hemoglobin levels were only observed in three interventions out of 14, two of which came from a single, large study. Among fasting glucose studies, a trend was observed that industry-sponsored studies were more likely to observe beneficial effects. The authors also expressed concerns that the brewer's yeast results suggested that another component in the yeast may be having an effect because effects were observed at lower doses of chromium. As a bottom line the authors concluded that chromium supplementation "may have a modest effect" on glucose metabolism in type 2 diabetics but that "the large heterogeneity and the overall poor quality limit the strength of our conclusions" and that more randomized trials are required.[19]

The one well-designed study that dominated the statistics examined 185 adult-onset diabetic Chinese patients in which decreases in the concentration of fasting serum glucose, insulin, hemoglobin A_{1C} and total cholesterol and decreased glucose and insulin levels in response to glucose challenges were observed as a result of Cr supplementation in a dose-responsive manner.[20] Unfortunately, attempts to reproduce these results on other populations, including Western populations, have been unsuccessful. No controlled follow-up studies have been performed in China.

Consequently, the American Diabetes Association's position has been consistent for over a decade and is that "Benefit from chromium supplementation in people with diabetes or obesity has not been conclusively demonstrated and, therefore, cannot be recommended".[21] If Cr(III) complexes are found to have beneficial effects on subjects with altered glucose and lipid metabolism, the effects would be small compared to treatment with insulin or current diabetes medications. Cr supplementation would potentially then have a role as an inexpensive treatment to allow the use of lower doses of current medications (which have potentially severe side effects) or to treat subjects at the early stages of type 2 diabetes to potentially delay the continued onset of the disease.

A recent study may have potentially provided a path through the morass of human studies. In a preliminary report, Cefalu and coworkers[22] have suggested that only a subgroup of type 2 diabetic subjects respond positively to Cr supplementation. The trick for future studies is whether subjects of the subgroup can be identified before chromium supplementation and then effects observed in this group compared to appropriate controls from chromium supplementation.

Proposed Mechanism of Action of Chromium

Numerous pathways by which a Cr biomolecule could manifest its effects have been proposed. However, in vivo research results are contradictory such that the state of the field is not immediately clear.[2] Attention has been focused on two sites of action in the insulin signaling cascade as the potential sites of Cr action: insulin receptor and Akt. However, the results from the various research groups using different cell types or Cr compounds are irreconcilable at the current time. For example, one group does not observe any effects from chromium(III) compounds on the insulin signaling system but has proposed an effect on lipid processing.[2] The problem is straight forward—applying solutions of Cr(III) compounds to cultured cells in general does not present Cr(III) to the cells in a comparable fashion to that by which Cr(III) is presented to cells in the body; the difference may be crucial to the results and interpretation of the study.

Toxicity

Toxicity of chromium(III) supplements has been a long-standing concern, particularly for the most popular supplement chromium picolinate. Recent studies have shown that chromium picolinate is a potent genotoxic and possible carcinogen for cultured cells and fruit flies; however, when taken orally by mammals, the supplement is not toxic.[2] In the most notable study sponsored by the National Toxicology Program (NTP) of the National Institutes of Health (NIH) (USA), supplementation with chromium picolinate as to 5% of the diet (by mass) of rats and mice for up to 2 years found no harmful effects on female rats or mice and at most ambiguous data for one type of carcinogenicity in male rats (along with no changes in body mass in either sex of rats or mice).[23] This leads to a No-Observed-Adverse-Effect Level (NOAEL) of 300 mg Cr/kg body mass/day or 5 mg Cr/day for an average 60 kg adult. Fortuitously, the supplement hydrolyzes in the gastrointestinal tract, releasing the chromium before the intact complex can be absorbed to an appreciable level, in contrast to the cell studies where the very stable, neutral complex could be absorbed intact.[2] The World Health Organization and the European Food Safety Authority consider chromium supplementation of 250 µg Cr/day to be without safety concerns, while the Expert Group on Vitamins and Minerals (UK) has indicated that a daily dose of 10 mg Cr/day would be anticipated to be without adverse effects.[24]

Future Research

To resolve issues on whether chromium(III) compounds have potential as pharmaceuticals to treat symptoms of type 2 diabetes and related conditions, much research is still needed. Most notably clearly controlled and well-designed human studies using doses of 7−10 mg Cr per day are required to determine whether increasing the dosage to doses approximately those in rodent model studies can result in reproducible beneficial effects; these studies will require rigorous protocols for monitoring the health of participants. The use of chromium compounds that are well characterized is also important. Although the review of chromium nutritional supplements was beyond the scope of this review, the chromium compounds most popular currently in nutritional supplements are poorly absorbed with ~1−2% efficiency. Well-characterized chromium(III) compounds that are absorbed with 40 times more efficiency are now known; use of these compounds would potentially further increase chances of observing beneficial effects from supplementation of diabetic subjects.

Mechanistic studies need to be done on well-characterized complexes whose stability in growth media, etc. has been elucidated. A comprehensive study of the effects of chromium(III) compounds on cultured cells is required in which the effects of the identity of the Cr(III) compound, media, cell type, exposure time, and chromium concentration, and other related variables are systematically examined. Only in this manner can the currently irreconcilable results potentially be resolved and the mechanism or mechanisms of chromium action at a molecular level be elucidated.

VANADIUM

Nutritional Status and Toxicity

No AI or estimated average requirement (EAR) has been set for vanadium in contrast to chromium, and no biological role for vanadium in mammals has been established.[4] A few isolated reports of vanadium deficiency in rats and goats have been reported (e.g., Refs [25,26]); however, distinguishing between nutritional and pharmacological effects is difficult,[27] as vanadium has a distinct pharmacological effect on glucose metabolism. As with chromium, the literature must be treated with care; for example in Ref.[25] the vanadium content of the basal diet could not be determined because of matrix effects. Human dietary intake is normally in the range of 5−20 µg V/day.[28,29] An upper tolerable level (UL) for vanadium has been established at 1.8 mg/day, about 100 times the average intake.[4] The amount of vanadium used in diabetes studies is far in excess of the UL, which is allowable for clinical studies with careful safety monitoring.[4] Vanadium is less toxic to humans than rodents. While acute vanadium poisoning has not been noted for humans, adverse effects in humans are primarily gastrointestinal effects including cramping, diarrhea, and loose stools.[4]

Absorption and Transport

Absorption of dietary vanadium, similar to chromium, is very small, being about 1%. Under physiological conditions, vanadium converts to the vanadium(IV) species, VO^{2+}, although this species can potentially be in equilibrium with a variety of other vanadium(IV) and vanadium(V) species. In the bloodstream, VO^{2+} binds to the iron transport protein transferrin (see Ref.[30] and references therein). Transferrin contains two metal ion metal sites, and VO^{2+} binds to both with relatively similar affinity. The binding of metal ions to transferrin requires a synergistic anion, usually bicarbonate under physiological conditions, although other anions such as citrate can be used as well. If vanadium concentrations could exceed 10 μM, then the binding of VO^{2+} to serum albumin could potentially be significant.[30] Given the toxicity of vanadium, the biotransformations and biodistribution of vanadium-containing drugs are particularly important. A drug that would not readily hydrolyze in the gastrointestinal tract when given orally and could potentially be directed to specific tissues might be able to overcome certain deleterious side effects. The fate of vanadium drugs in the body is an area of significant current research.[31]

Mode of Action

In terms of pharmacological effects, the primary mode of action of vanadium seems reasonably clear, although definite *in vivo* experiments are still lacking. As vanadate, $VO_4{}^{3-}$, vanadium inhibits the active sites of phosphatases and related enzymes involved in the hydrolysis of phosphate esters. This is not unexpected as vanadate is a structural analog of the product phosphate, $PO_4{}^{3-}$ (although this ion is protonated to varying degrees at physiological pHs). Kinase activation does not appear to be involved with the pharmacological effects of vanadium, at least for autophosphorylation of insulin receptors, other phosphotyrosine phosphatases, or PI-3 kinase.[32–34] Treatment of diabetic rats with vanadium compounds has been shown to inhibit the activity of multiple phosphatases.[35–37] Particular attention has been focused on phosphotyrosine phosphatase (PTP) 1B,[38] which is believed to be responsible for the dephosphorylation of autophosphorylated insulin receptors and is upregulated in type 2 diabetics. Vanadium as vanadate, $VO_4{}^{3-}$, is a competitive inhibitor of PTP-1B binds to its active site; the X-ray structure of the enzyme with the bound inhibitor has been solved to 2.2 angstrom resolution.[38] The vanadium in the active site has a trigonal bipyramidal geometry. The three equatorial sites are filled by oxide oxygens, while one apical site is filled by an oxide oxygen and the other apical site is filled by the hydroxyl oxygen from a serine residue. In rat adipocytes pretreated with vanadate, insulin-stimulated insulin receptor kinase activity is augmented, as is the autophosphorylation of insulin receptor.[39] In high-glucose-treated rat adipocytes (that are insulin resistant), vanadate stimulation of insulin receptor autophosphorylation and insulin receptor kinase activity are enhanced, as is Akt serine phosphorylation.[40] Thus, vanadium appears to serve as an insulin mimetic. While vanadium is able to inhibit PTP-1B, it also basically inhibits all phosphatases, although the K_i values can differ considerably. Given the range of functions regulated by phosphatase enzymes and that vanadate administration could potentially affect them all to some degree, the potential for side effects from vanadium treatments is easily understood. Additionally, the involvement of other phosphatases or related enzymes could be important contributors to the biological activity of vanadium.[41]

Animal Models

Oral administration of inorganic vanadium compounds to rodent models of type 1 (streptozotocin-treated rats) and type 2 diabetes [Zucker fatty (*fa/fa*) rats and *db/db* and *ob/ob* mice] has reproducibly resulted in the improvement of diabetic symptoms, although in some cases side effects were noted. The vanadium was generally provided in the drinking water. Improvements were particularly noted in plasma glucose levels and response to oral glucose challenges (for reviews, see Refs [42,43]).

Vanadium Chelates

To attempt to increase the efficacy of and decrease the adverse side effects from vanadium administration, the use of a number of vanadium complexes has been examined.[44,45] Attention has been focused on the use of chelating ligands which should not as readily be exchanged by water or water-derived ligands (oxo/hydroxo), potentially altering the absorption, transport, and distribution of the vanadium. One compound, bis(maltolato)-oxovanadium(VI) where maltol is 3-hydroxy-4-pyrone, has been by far the most popular choice in these studies. This compound is absorbed with much greater efficiency, 38%, than dietary vanadium.[46] In vitro the compound is a nonselective inhibitor of PTPs including PTP-1B ($K_i = 0.90\ \mu M$), similar to vanadate.[38] The compound can inhibit PTP-1B in HEK293 cells overexpressing PTP-1B; and in rats pretreated with the compound, insulin receptor activation in response to insulin (but not in the absence of exogenous insulin) is increased.[38] Treating crystals of PTP-1B with an aqueous solution of the compound results in vanadate binding in the enzyme active site in an identical fashion to adding a solution of vanadate to the crystals; this result has been interpreted to suggest that uncomplexed vanadium is still the bioactive form of vanadium, despite the use of the chelated vanadium compound.[38] However, studies with the compound are also consistent phosphatases or related enzymes being important contributors to the biological activity of vanadium.[47] Bis(maltolato)oxovanadium(VI) at a comparable dose to inorganic vanadium compounds generates less toxic effects and exhibits greater lowering of blood glucose in rodent models.[42] Recent studies have suggested that at high concentrations in the blood, some of the ligand of the compound and other vanadyl-organic chelate complexes might be retained when the vanadium binds to transferrin, forming ternary species.[48] The formation of these species could potentially alter biodistribution, although these results need to be tested in vivo. A derivative of this compound is the only vanadium-organic ligand complex to be tested in clinical trials (vide infra).

Clinical Trials

Results of human clinical trials with vanadium must be treated with great care, as with trials with chromium. A systemic review reported in 2008 identified studies with vanadium compounds with type 2 diabetic subjects.[49] However, when the very reasonable criteria that the trials were placebo-controlled, were of at least 2 months' duration, and possessed at least 10 subjects per arm were applied, none of the studies met the inclusion criteria! The authors determined that "there is no good evidence that oral vanadium supplementation improves glycemic control in type 2 diabetes".[49] When the criteria were lowered to any clinical trial with oral vanadium supplementation of adults with diabetes, five studies were identified, all using vanadyl sulfate (between 75 and 150 mg daily). None of the studies was double-blind, while four studies measured glycated hemoglobin levels despite treatment being 6 weeks or less. All the studies using 100 mg or greater daily reported statistically significant improvement in fasting blood glucose and glycated hemoglobin, although 75 mg was found in one study not to lead to a significant change in fasting blood glucose. All the studies reported a high incidence of adverse gastrointestinal side effects.[49] Individual variation in response to vanadyl was surprisingly large, although large variations in effects have also been noted in rodent studies.[50]

The first results of a phase I and phase IIa clinical trials using a vanadium chelate complex, bis(ethylmaltolato)oxovanadium(IV), have recently been reported.[31,50] In the phase I trial, 40 adult volunteers participated. In part of the study, four individuals were administered a single oral dose of the compound (10 mg) followed by an escalating dose study using four dose levels: 25, 35, 60, and 90 mg; no adverse effects were observed.[31] The phase IIa trial examined the safety and efficacy of a daily oral dose of the compound (20 mg) for 28 days with type 2 diabetic subjects with a 14-day non-treatment follow-up; seven subjects received the compound, while two subjects received a placebo.[50] The study was single-blinded, with the subjects unaware of whether they were receiving treatment or placebo. Unfortunately, these small numbers of subjects prevent any meaningful statistical analysis. For the treatment group, five of the seven subjects had decreased fasting plasma glucose levels, while the levels increased in both subjects receiving placebo. Area under the curve for an oral glucose challenge increased 5% on average for the placebo subjects but decreased 10% on average for the treatment subjects. The percentage of glycated hemoglobin increased in the placebo group but decreased or was unchanged in five of the seven subjects in the treatment group.[50] The compound was "consistently well tolerated".[50] While perhaps suggestive, clearly larger, better-designed clinical studies are required before any meaningful assessment of effects of administration of chelated vanadium compounds on symptoms of type 2 diabetes can be made.

Future Research

The potential of vanadium compounds to treat type 2 diabetes is still an open question. Ideally to avoid or at least minimize adverse side effects, chelated vanadium compounds need to be developed that can be directed to insulin-sensitive tissues (adipocytes, hepatocytes, and skeletal muscle). Partial or complete hydrolysis of the chelate ligands in these tissues could release the bioactive form locally. While this type of research has started appearing, very detailed studies on the absorption, distribution, and speciation of vanadium from the chelate complexes are desperately needed. Larger, better designed clinical studies are required before any meaningful assessment of effects of administration of chelated vanadium compounds on symptoms of type 2 diabetes can be made, particularly given the apparent diversity of response to vanadyl administration. Whether the tight rope between adverse effects and beneficial effects can be walked is very far from being determined.

References

1. Schwarz K, Mertz W. Chromium(III) and the glucose tolerance factor. *Arch Biochem Biophys* 1959;**85**:292–5.
2. Vincent JB. Chromium: Celebrating 50 years as an essential element? *Dalton Trans* 2010;**39**:3878–3794.
3. National Research Council. *Recommended Dietary Allowances, 9th Ed. Report of the Committee on Dietary Allowances, Division of Biological Sciences, Assembly of Life Science, Food and Nutrition Board, Commission on Life Science, National Research.* Washington, DC: National Academy Press; 1980.
4. National Research Council. *Dietary Reference Intakes for Vitamin A, Arsenic, Boron, Chromium, Copper, Iodine, Iron, Manganese, Molybdenum, Nickel, Silicon, Vanadium, and Zinc. A Report of the Panel on Micronutrients, Subcommittee on Upper Reference Levels of Nutrients and of Interpretations and Uses of Dietary Reference Intakes, and the Standing Committee on the Scientific Evaluation of Dietary Reference Intakes.* Washington, DC: National Academy of Sciences; 2002.
5. Di Bona KR, Love S, Rhodes NR, McAdory D, Sinha SH, Kern N, Kent J, Strickland J, Wilson A, Beaird J, Ramage J, Rasco JF, Vincent JB. Chromium is not an essential trace element for mammals: Effects of a "low-chromium" diet. *J Biol Inorg Chem* 2011;**16**:381–90.
6. Striffler JS, Law JS, Polansky MM, Bhathena SJ, Anderson RA. Chromium improves insulin response to glucose in rats. *Metabolism* 1995;**44**:1314–20.
7. Striffler JS, Polansky MM, Anderson RA. Dietary chromium decreases insulin resistance in rats fed

a high fat mineral imbalanced diet. *Metabolism* 1998;**47**:396−400.

8. Jeejeebhoy KN. Chromium and parenteral nutrition. *J Trace Elem Exp Med* 1999;**12**:85−9.

9. Anderson RA, Kozlovsky AS. Chromium intake, absorption and excretion of subjects consuming self-selected diets. *Am J Clin Nutr* 1985;**41**:1177−83.

10. Morris BW, Kemp GJ, Hardisty CA. Plasma chromium and chromium excretion in diabetes. *Clin Chem* 1985;**31**:334−5.

11. Dowling HJ, Offenbacher EG, Pi-Sunyer FX. Absorption of inorganic, trivalent chromium from the vascularly perfused rat small intestine. *J Nutr* 1989;**119**:1138−45.

12. Rhodes NR, McAdory D, Love S, DiBona KR, Chen Y, Ansorge K, Hira J, Kent J, Lara P, Rasco JF, Vincent JB. Urinary chromium loss associated with diabetes is offset by increases in absorption. *J Inorg Biochem* 2010;**104**:790−7.

13. Feng W, Ding W, Qian Q, Chai Z. Use of the enriched stable isotope Cr-50 as a tracer to study the metabolism of chromium(III) in normal and diabetic rats. *Biol Trace Elem Res* 1998;**63**:129−38.

14. Toepfer EW, Mertz W, Polansky MM, Roginski EE, Wolf WR. Preparation of chromium-containing material of glucose tolerance factor activity from brewer's yeast extracts and by synthesis. *J Agric Food Chem* 1977;**25**:162−162.

15. Vincent JB. The bioinorganic chemistry of chromium. *Polyhedron* 2001;**20**:1−26.

16. Vincent JB, Stearns DM. *The bioinorganic chemistry of chromium: essentiality, therapeutic agent, toxin, carcinogen?* Chichester: Wiley-Blackwell; 2011.

17. Food and Drug Administration. Qualified Health Claims: Letter of Enforcement Discretion—Chromium Picolinate and Insulin Resistance (Docket No. 2004Q-0144), 2005. http://www.fda.gov/Food/LabelingNutrition/Label Claims/QualifiedHealthClaims/ucm073017.htm

18. Cefalu WT, Bell-Farrow AD, Stegner J, Wang ZQ, King T, Morgan T, Terry JG. Effect of chromium picolinate on insulin sensitivity *in vivo*. *J Trace Elem Exp Med* 1999;**12**:71−83.

19. Balk EM, Tatsioni A, Lichenstein AH, Lau J, Pittas AG. Effect of chromium supplementation on glucose metabolism and lipids: a systematic review of randomized controlled trials. *Diabetes Care* 2007;**30**:2154−63.

20. Anderson RA, Cheng NC, Bryden NA, Polansky MM, Cheng N, Chi J, Feng J. Elevated levels of supplemental chromium improve glucose and insulin variables in individuals with type 2 diabetes. *Diabetes* 1997;**46**:1786−91.

21. American Diabetes Association. Standards of medical care in diabetes—2010. *Diabetes Care* 2010;**23** (Suppl. 1):S11−61.

22. Cefalu WT, Rood J, Pinsonat P, Qin J, Sereda O, Levitan L, Abderson RA, Zhang XH, Martin JM, Wang ZQ, Newcomer B. Characterization of the metabolic and physiological response to chromium supplementation in subjects with type 2 diabetes mellitus. *Metabolism* 2010;**59**:755−62.

23. Stout MD, Nyska A, Collins BJ, Witt KL, Kissling GE, Malarkey DE, Hooth MJ. Chronic toxicity and carcinogenicity studies of chromium picolinate monohydrate administered in feed to F344/N rats and B6C3F1 mice for 2 years. *Food Chem Toxicol* 2009;**47**:729−33.

24. European Food Safety Authority. Scientific opinion on the safety of trivalent chromium as a nutrient added for nutritional purposes to foodstuffs for particular nutritional uses and foods intended for the general population (including food supplement) *EFSA J* 2010;**8**:1−46.

25. Schwarz K, Milne DB. Growth effects of vanadium in the rat. *Science* 1971;**4007**:426−8.

26. Uthus EO, Nielsen FH. Effect of vanadium, iodine and their interaction on growth, blood variables, liver trace elements and thyroid status indices in rats. *Magnes Trace Elem* 1990;**9**:219−26.

27. Nielsen FH. Nutritional requirements for boron, silicon, vanadium, nickel, and arsenic: current knowledge and speculation. *FASEB J* 1991;**5**:2661−7.

28. Myron DR, Zimmerman TJ, Shuler TR, Klevay LM, Lee DM, Nielsen FH. Intake of nickel and vanadium by humans. A survey of selected diets. *Am J Clin Nutr* 1978;**31**:527−31.

29. Pennington JA, Jones JW. Molybdenum, nickel, cobalt, vanadium, and strontium in total diets. *J Am Diet Assoc* 1987;**87**:1644−50.

30. Sanna D, Buglyo P, Micera G, Garribba E. A quantitative study of the biotransformation of insulin-enhancing VO^{2+} compounds. *J Biol Inorg Chem* 2010;**15**:825−39.

31. Thompson KH, Orvig C. Vanadium in diabetes: 100 years from Phase 0 to Phase I. *J Inorg Biochem* 2006;**100**:1925−35.

32. Mohammad A, Bhanot S, McNeill JH. *In vivo* effects of vanadium in diabetic rats are independent of changes in PI-3 kinase activity in skeletal muscle. *Mol Cell Biochem* 2001;**223**:103−8.

33. Shisheva A, Shechter Y. Quercetin selectively inhibits insulin receptor function *in vitro* and the bioresponses of insulin and insulinomimetic agents in rat adipocytes. *Biochemistry* 1992;**31**:8059−63.

34. Vankatesan N, Avidan A, Davidson MB. Antidiabetic action of vanadyl in rats independent of *in vivo* insulin-receptor kinase activity. *Diabetes* 1991;**40**:492−8.

35. Meyerovitch J, Baker JM, Kahn CR. Hepatic phospho-tyrosine phosphatase activity and its alterations in diabetic rats. *J Clin Invest* 1989;**84**:976—83.

36. Pugazhenthi S, Tanha F, Dahl B, Khandelwal RL. Decrease in protein tyrosine phosphatase activities in vanadate-treated obese Zucker (fa/fa) rat liver. *Mol Cell Biochem* 1995;**153**:125—9.

37. Mohammad A, Wang J, McNeill JH. Bis(maltolato) oxovanadium(IV) inhibits the activity of PTP1B in Zucker rat skeletal muscle *in vivo*. *Mol Cell Biochem* 2002;**229**:125—8.

38. Peters KG, Davis MG, Howard BW, Pokross M, Rastogi V, Diven C, Greis KD, Eby-Wilkens E, Maier M, Evdokimov Λ, Soper S, Genbauffe F. Mechanism of insulin sensitization by BMOV (bis maltolato oxo vanadium); unliganded vanadium (VO_4) as the active component. *J Inorg Biochem* 2003;**96**:321—30.

39. Fantus IG, Ahmad F, Deragon G. vanadate augments insulin-stimulated insulin receptor kinase activity and prolongs insulin action in rat adipocytes: evidence for transduction of amplitude of signaling into duration of response. *Diabetes* 1994;**43**:375—83.

40. Lu B, Ennis D, Lai R, Bogdanovic E, Nikolov R, Salamon L, Fantus, Le-Tien C, Fantus IG. Enhanced sensitivity of insulin-resistant adipocytes to vanadate is associated with oxidative stress and decreased reduction of vanadate (+5) to vanadyl (+4). *J Biol Chem* 2001;**276**:35589—98.

41. Medhi MZ, Pandey SK, Theberge J-F, Srivastava AK. Insulin signal mimicry as a mechanism for the insulin-like effect of vanadium. *Cell Biochem Biophys* 2006;**44**:73—81.

42. Srivastava AK, Mehdi MZ. Insulin-mimetic and anti-diabetic effects of vanadium compounds. *Diabet Med* 2005;**22**:2—13.

43. Shechter Y, Goldwaser I, Mironchik M, Fridkin M, Gefel D. Historic perspective and recent developments on the insulin-like actions of vanadium; towards developing vanadium-based drugs for diabetes. *Coord Chem Rev* 2003;**237**:3—11.

44. Thompson KH, Orvig C. Vanadium compounds in the treatment of diabetes. *Met Ions Biol Syst* 2004; **41**:221—52.

45. Thompson KH, Orvig C. Coordination chemistry of vanadium in metallopharmaceutical candidate compounds. *Coord Chem Rev* 2001;**219—221**:1033—53.

46. Setyawati IA, Thompson KH, Yiuen VG, Sun Y, Battell M, Lyster DM, Vo C, Ruth J, Zeisler S, McNeill JH, Orvig C. Kinetic analysis and comparison of uptake, distribution, and excretion of [48]V-labeled compounds in the rat. *J Appl Physiol* 1998;**84**:569—75.

47. Vardatsikos G, Medhi MZ, Srivastava AK. Bis(maltolato)-oxovanadium(IV)-induced phosphorylation of PKB, GSK-3 and FOX01 contributes to its glucoregulatory responses (Review). *Int J Mol Med* 2009;**24**:303—9.

48. Sanna D, Micera G, Garribba E. New developments in the comprehension of the biotransformation and transport of insulin-enhancing vanadium compounds in blood serum. *Inorg Chem* 2010; **49**:174—87.

49. Smith DM, Pickering RM, Lewith GT. A systematic review of vanadium oral supplements for glycaemic control in type 2 diabetes mellitus. *Q J Med* 2008;**101**:351—8.

50. Thompson KH, Lichter J, LeBel C, Scaife MC, McNeill JH, Orvig C. Vanadium treatment of type 2 diabetes: A view to the future. *J Inorg Biochem* 2009;**103**:554—8.

31

Role of n-6 and n-3 Polyunsaturated Fatty Acids in Type 2 Diabetes

Jose E. Galgani, Pamela Rojas

Department of Nutrition, Faculty of Medicine, University of Chile, Santiago, Chile

INTRODUCTION

Diet and physical activity patterns have changed drastically in both industrialized and developing countries, with a corresponding rapid increase in obesity-related chronic diseases such as type 2 diabetes.[1] It is well recognized that sustained changes in diet and physical activity, which promote better health, are difficult to achieve without aggressive and targeted interventions. Nutritionists have focused on several dietary characteristics, such as fat quality, that could contribute to the adverse consequences of obesity.

Total fat intake has increased in the last two centuries along with consumption of saturated (SFA) and n-6 polyunsaturated (n-6 PUFA) fat, whereas n-3 polyunsaturated fat (n-3 PUFA)

Nutritional and Therapeutic Interventions for Diabetes and Metabolic Syndrome
DOI: 10.1016/B978-0-12-385083-6.00031-0

intake has been reduced.[2] Based on well-demonstrated effects of specific fatty acids on fuel metabolism-related gene expression[3] as well as the role of altered lipid metabolism on the etiology of type 2 diabetes,[4] dietary fat quality might play a role on the rapid emergence of type 2 diabetes. Therefore, manipulating dietary ingredients or the fatty acid composition of the traditional fats consumed may contribute to treating obesity-related co-morbidities such as type 2 diabetes. Here we discuss the evidence supporting the relationship between fat quality, especially PUFA, and type 2 diabetes.

NUTRITIONAL AND BIOCHEMICAL BASIS OF N-6 AND N-3 POLYUNSATURATED FAT METABOLISM

Fat ingested is a blend of fatty acids which differs in chain length, degree of unsaturation, position of double bonds, etc. From a nutritional viewpoint, fatty acids are mainly classified as SFA (no double bonds), monounsaturated (MUFA, one double bond) and PUFA (two to six double bonds). The latter are separated into two classes (n-6 and n-3 PUFA) based on the presence of unsaturated bonds in n-6 or n-3 positions.

Most of the fatty acids present in the human tissues can be endogenously synthesized in sufficient amounts. However, linoleic acid (18:2n-6) and α-linolenic acid (18:3n-3) can not be synthesized by mammalian cells. These fatty acids are considered essential nutrients, which must be provided in the diet (Figure 31.1). The main dietary source of essential fatty acids is vegetable oil (Table 31.1). Vegetables can add double bonds in n-6 and n-3 positions of the aliphatic chain through specific desaturases.

Linoleic and α-linolenic acids are precursors of several molecules with a critical role in

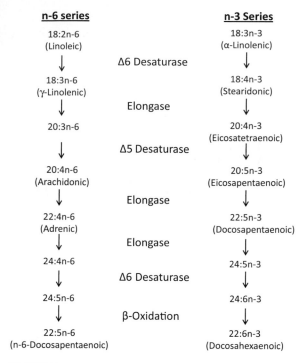

FIGURE 31.1 Cellular metabolism of n-6 and n-3 polyunsaturated fatty acids.

TABLE 31.1   Dietary Sources of Polyunsaturated Fatty Acids

Fatty acid	Source
Linoleic	Most vegetable oils (safflower oil, grape seed oil, sunflower oil, corn oil, soybean oil)
α-Linolenic	Flaxseed oil, perilla oil, canola oil, soybean oil
EPA and DHA	Fish, especially oily fish (salmon, herring, anchovy, smelt and mackerel)
AA	Animal fats, liver, egg lipids, fish

AA, araquidonic acid; EPA, eicosapentaenoic acid; DHA, docosahexaenoic acid.

cellular function. These fatty acids are converted mainly in the liver into longer and more unsaturated fatty acids through alternating desaturation and elongation reactions (Figure 31.1). The main fatty acid originated from linoleic acid is arachidonic acid (AA), while eicosapentaenoic (EPA) and docosahexaenoic (DHA) are derived from α-linolenic acid (Figure 31.1). The regulatory enzyme controlling bioconversion of linoleic and α-linolenic acids into their derivatives is Δ6 desaturase. This enzyme displays the highest affinity for α-linolenic acid, followed by linoleic, oleic, and palmitoleic acids. Since n-6 PUFA intake is several times higher than n-3 PUFA intake, and whole-body conversion from α-linolenic acid to DHA is very inefficient in humans (< 5% of α-linolenic acid is converted to DHA),[5] it remains unclear whether α-linolenic acid intake can adequately meet cellular EPA and DHA requirements. Moreover, the conversion of α-linolenic acid to its derivatives can be particularly critical in type 2 diabetes, because Δ6 desaturase activity is dependent on insulin.[6]

Newly synthesized very long-chain fatty acids are transported to extra-hepatic tissues where incorporation into cell lipids takes place. At the cellular level, very long-chain fatty acids play a structural role (as constitutive elements of cellular membranes) as well as a regulatory function through the synthesis of eicosanoids (prostaglandins, tromboxanes, leukotrienes) and recently described docosanoids (resolvins and protectins).[7] Eicosanoids can modulate insulin secretion and insulin resistance. Indeed, genetic manipulation of the ability to synthesize n-3 PUFA leads to important changes in prostaglandin production and glucose homeostasis.[8,9]

FATTY ACID QUALITY AND TYPE 2 DIABETES

The role of fatty acid quality in glucose homeostasis was first demonstrated in animals. Rats fed with high-linoleic acid oil (safflower) exhibited impaired insulin-stimulated glucose uptake. However, partial replacement of safflower oil with fish oil prevented the development of insulin resistance.[10] Recently, the gene responsible for α-linolenic acid synthesis (fat-1 omega-3 fatty acid desaturase from C. elegans) was inserted into a transgenic mouse model, and those animals were then fed an n-3 PUFA-free, high-fat diet. Interestingly, the transgenic mice showed improved glucose tolerance when compared with wild-type mice.[8] Using a similar approach, insertion of fat-1 gene into β-cells from mice increased pancreatic n-3 PUFA and decreased n-6 PUFA concentrations. This resulted in lower prostaglandin E2 synthesis (an inhibitory regulator of insulin secretion) accompanied by enhanced glucose-, amino acid-, and glucagon-like peptide-1-induced insulin secretion.[9] These studies are the basis to support the potential therapeutic role of n-3 PUFA in type 2 diabetes.

In humans, Borkman et al.[11] found that the degree of fatty acids unsaturation, especially AA content, in skeletal muscle phospholipids is inversely related to insulin resistance. Later, several epidemiological studies evaluating the relationship between PUFA intake and risk of type 2 diabetes were conducted. However, these studies are difficult to interpret and provide challenging results. For instance, a prospective study including 36,328 women found increased risk of type 2 diabetes in individuals with high long-chain n-3 PUFA intake (measured by a validated food-frequency questionnaire), particularly in individuals consuming more than two servings of fish per day.[12] It is also difficult to interpret food questionnaire-based results because of the close correlation between dietary SFA and MUFA, as animal fat is a source of both types of fat. Moreover, within SFA the effect of specific fatty acids can differ, as observed for palmitic and stearic acids. Indeed, stearic acid shows a rather neutral effect on fuel homeostasis, which is in part explained by its rapid conversion to oleic acid.[13] Furthermore, an incomplete fatty acid food composition database may result in an underestimation of actual fatty acids intake.

Measurement of fatty acid composition of plasma lipid fractions as potential improved markers of dietary exposure has been preferred. In fact, results based on objective surrogates provide more consistent and stronger results than those obtained from dietary records.[14] In this regard, increased linoleic acid content in plasma phospholipid or cholesterol ester is associated with lower incidence of type 2 diabetes, whereas individuals with higher SFA content in plasma lipid fractions have increased risk of type 2 diabetes.[14,15] Type 2 diabetes *per se* is also associated with altered plasma fatty acids composition. Pelikanova *et al.* found increased serum phospholipid AA and decreased linoleic acid content in type 2 diabetics compared to healthy subjects.[16] Taken together, longitudinal and cross-sectional data suggest that dietary fatty acid profile can play a role in the etiopathogeny of type 2 diabetes.

In contrast, reported changes in fatty acid composition between type 2 diabetic and non-diabetic subjects could well be the result of insulin deficiency through impaired Δ6 desaturase activity, which could limit conversion of n-6 and n-3 PUFA precursors into very long-chain fatty acid derivatives. This condition can be particularly critical in subjects with high n-6 and low n-3 PUFA diets, a condition often observed in Western diets.[2] Determination of the conversion rate using labeled precursors in diabetic subjects will contribute to the better understanding of the causal relationship between altered fatty acid composition and type 2 diabetes.

Controlled intervention studies evaluating the effect of fatty acid quality have also been considered. However, these interventions can not be conducted for a period long enough to detect differences in the incidence of type 2 diabetes. Alternatively, insulin resistance and insulin secretion as earlier outcomes accounting for glucose homeostasis are usually assessed in such studies.

FATTY ACID QUALITY AND INSULIN RESISTANCE

Mechanism of Fatty Acid-Mediated Insulin Resistance

A central feature of insulin resistance is increased skeletal muscle lipid accumulation. Free-fatty acid oversupply to skeletal muscle promotes formation of diglycerides and ceramides.[17] Diglycerides can activate specific serine kinases which lead to increased serine phosphorylation of IRS-1 (insulin receptor substrate 1, a key insulin signaling protein) resulting in lower IRS-1 activity. As a consequence, insulin-dependent GLUT4 translocation to the plasma membrane is reduced and muscle glucose uptake becomes impaired. Several studies have demonstrated the relevance of this mechanism in insulin resistance.[18-20]

Fatty acids could affect insulin action at different levels of cell function. Altered cell membrane composition is one of the most common mechanisms. Fatty acids can modify membrane function by changing overall membrane fluidity, affecting membrane thickness/volume, modifying lipid phase properties, inducing changes in the membrane microenvironment, or by specific protein-to-lipid interactions.[21] Alternatively, fatty acids may affect intracellular lipid balance based on its differential individual fatty acid oxidation rate[22] and ability to modify the binding of the regulatory proteins (i.e. peroxisome proliferator-activated receptors (PPARs)) to DNA response elements involved in lipid synthesis and oxidation.[3] Indeed, Pan *et al.*[23] reported differential 24-h [1-^{14}C] α-linolenic oxidation rates and ^{14}C muscle incorporation in rats fed diets enriched with lard (SFA), olive oil (MUFA), or safflower oil (n-6 PUFA) for one month. The highest 24-h $^{14}CO_2$

recovery was found in the safflower-fed group, followed by the olive oil and lard diets, whereas skeletal muscle ^{14}C incorporation followed the inverse order.

Finally, fatty acids may differentially affect inflammatory pathways, which are tightly related to insulin resistance.[24] Interestingly, palmitate added to culture media increased TLR-4-mediated cytokine generation (Toll-like receptor 4 mediates innate immune response to bacterial pathogens), whereas co-addition of DHA fully reversed this effect. At the whole-body level, TLR-4-deficient mice showed a much lower degree of lipid-dependent insulin resistance when compared to wild-type animals.[25] This mechanistic information has, however, been less consistently translated to data obtained from humans.

Intervention Studies

The effect of fatty acid quality on insulin resistance through intervention studies has been tested multiple times in type 2 diabetic subjects. However, only few of them meet the essential quality requirements to be considered.[26] Table 31.2 summarizes studies in type 2 diabetic subjects in which dietary fat quality was modified and insulin resistance determined.[27–32] Most of these studies showed no change in insulin resistance in response to manipulation of dietary fatty acid quality. However, one study found higher insulin resistance in type 2 diabetic subjects after a large fish oil dose (18 ml/day for 9 weeks) when compared with corn oil.[31] Conversely, decreased insulin resistance was reported in non-obese, obese, and type 2 diabetic subjects after a PUFA- vs SFA-enriched diet.[32] Lack of or insufficient contrast in insulin resistance among diets differing in fatty acid quality could be explained by insufficient time of exposure, insufficient amount of fatty acids supplied, or interaction with a particular genetic background.

FATTY ACID QUALITY AND INSULIN SECRETION

Mechanisms Relating Fatty Acid Quality and Insulin Secretion

Fatty acids can acutely stimulate insulin secretion when glucose is present with long-chain SFA, MUFA, or PUFA. The acute effect of fatty acids on insulin secretion is partially mediated by a G-protein-coupled receptor (GPR40) which binds long-chain fatty acids. This receptor is mostly expressed in pancreatic β-cells, although it is also found in α-cells. Activation of GPR40 by fatty acids induces intracellular calcium mobilization and subsequent stimulation of insulin secretion.[33] Indeed, mice over-expressing GPR40 in pancreatic β-cells have increased glucose-stimulated insulin secretion.[34]

Insulin secretion may also be impaired in β-cells chronically exposed to SFA. For instance, palmitate-treated pancreatic islets showed impaired glucose- and potassium-stimulated insulin secretion, whereas the inhibitory effect of palmitate was prevented after adding EPA.[35]

The contrasting effects of SFA and PUFA on insulin secretion appear to be mediated by their differential capacity to induce lipogenesis. SFA can upregulate, whereas PUFA can downregulate lipogenesis through modulation of sterol regulatory element-binding protein-1c (SREBP-1c) expression, a well-known lipogenic transcription factor.[36] SREBP-1c exerts its regulatory action on insulin secretion by controlling proteins involved in insulin secretion, such as insulin receptor substrate 2 (IRS-2), granuphilin, and uncoupling protein 2 (UCP-2).

IRS-2 participates in insulin signaling, and its expression is downregulated by SREBP-1c.[37] Over-expression of IRS-2 in isolated rat pancreatic islets increases basal and glucose-stimulated insulin secretion.[38] SREBP-1c can also increase granuphilin expression, a key component of the

TABLE 31.2   Effect of Dietary Fat Quality Intervention on Insulin Resistance in Type 2 Diabetic Subejcts

Study	Subjects (n for IR data)	Design	Time	Dietary intervention	IR method	Outcome for IR
Summers et al.[32]	Non-obese, obese and type 2 diabetic subjects[17]	Crossover, random. No washout period included	5 weeks	Fat % 42 in SFA diet and 34% in PUFA diet. Diets enriched in SFA (21%) or PUFA (9%)	Euglycemic clamp (40 mU/m^2/min)	**Higher after PUFA diet** SFA: 0.51 ± 0.08 (SD) PUFA: 0.64 ± 0.10 P = 0.02
Borkman et al.[27]	Type 2 diabetic subjects both sexes[10]	Crossover, random, double blind. Washout period for 3 weeks	3 weeks	Fat % 37. Supplementation with 10 g/day fish oil (3 g EPA+DHA) or safflower oil	Euglycemic clamp (1.1 mU/kg/min) with HGP correction	**No change** Fish: 21.5 ± 3.5 (SD) Placebo: 21.2 ± 3.8
Luo et al.[28]	Type 2 diabetic, hypertriacyl-glycerolemic men[10]	Crossover, random, double blind. Washout period for 2 months	8 weeks	Fat % 44. Supplementation with 6 g/day fish oil (1.8 g EPA+DHA) or sunflower oil	Euglycemic clamp with two insulin doses (40 and 250 mU/m^2/min) and HGP correction	**No change** Low-insulin: Fish 3.3 ± 0.2 (SD); Placebo 3.8 ± 0.5. High-insulin: Fish 8.1 ± 0.9; Placebo 8.8 ± 0.8
Boberg et al.[29]	Type 2 diabetic both sexes[14]	Crossover, random, double blind. No washout period included	8 weeks	Dietary fat % not indicated. Supplementation with 10 g/day fish oil (3 g EPA+DHA) or olive oil	Euglycemic clamp (not indicated insulin dose)	**No change** Fish 4.7; Placebo 4.9 (SD not reported)
Rivellese et al.[30]	Type 2 diabetic both sexes[16]	Parallel, random, double blind	6 months	Fat % 30. Supplementation with fish oil [first 2 months 3.2 g/day (2.6 g EPA+DHA) and last 4 months 2.1 g/day (1.7 g EPA+DHA)] or olive oil	Euglycemic clamp (2 mU/kg/min)	**No change** Fish 4.0 ± 0.5 (SD) Placebo 4.1 ± 0.5
Mostad et al.[31]	Type 2 diabetic both sexes[26]	Parallel, random, double blind	9 weeks	Fat % 38. Supplementation with 18 ml/d fish oil (5 g EPA+DHA) or corn oil	Euglycemic clamp (40 mU/m^2/min)	**Lower after fish oil** (values not reported) P = 0.049

IR, insulin resistance; SFA, saturated fatty acid; PUFA, polyunsaturated fatty acid; EPA, eicosapentaenoic acid; DHA, docosahexaenoic acid; HGP, hepatic glucose production. Insulin resistance units are different in each study and these have been not included in the table.

docking machinery of insulin-containing vesicles having a potent negative action on insulin exocytosis.[39] Indeed, mutant β-cells over-expressing granuphilin showed a dramatic decrease in insulin release.[40] In turn, SREBP-1c increases UCP-2 transcriptional activity,[41] which when over-expressed in insulin-secreting cell lines inhibits glucose-stimulated insulin secretion.[42]

In contrast, ablation of UCP-2 in leptin-deficient (Ob/Ob) mice enhances first-phase insulin secretion when compared with leptin-deficient mice.[43] Some of the mechanisms linking fatty acid quality with insulin secretion are shown in Figure 31.2.

Short-term Intervention Studies

Differential fatty acid-induced insulin secretion described in *in vitro* studies is less consistently found in clinical studies including both non-diabetic and type 2 diabetic individuals. In this regard, non-diabetic volunteers fed a MUFA-, PUFA- and SFA-enriched meal plus a heparin infusion to increase plasma FFA concentration showed higher insulin secretion after the MUFA- followed by PUFA- and then SFA-enriched meals. This differential response was accompanied by parallel changes in plasma glucagon-like peptide 1 concentration (an insulin secreting agent).[44] In contrast, overweight/obese individuals fed at regular intervals throughout the day with MUFA-, PUFA- and SFA-enriched meals showed the highest insulin secretion after the SFA- and MUFA-enriched meals, whereas the lowest insulin secretion was found after PUFA.[45] A more aggressive intervention compared insulin secretion measured by a hyperglycemic clamp in response to a simultaneous intravenous lipid infusion of soybean or fish oil in type 2 diabetic individuals. Despite dramatic changes in plasma n-3 PUFA concentration after fish oil infusion, no differences in insulin secretion were noted.[46]

Long-term Intervention Studies

Considering that the potential mechanism relating fatty acid quality and insulin secretion may require changes in cell membrane composition, it seems reasonable to assess the effect of dietary fatty acid quality on insulin secretion after a longer exposure time. To this end, a multicenter dietary intervention study compared the effect of a 3-month MUFA- *vs* SFA-enriched diet on insulin secretion in non-diabetic individuals. Additionally, within each saturated or monounsaturated diet, a second randomization including fish oil (2.4 g of EPA and DHA) or

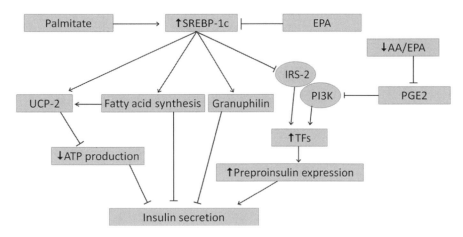

FIGURE 31.2 Mechanisms linking fatty acid quality with insulin secretion. AA, arachidonic acid; EPA, eicosapentaenoic acid; IRS-2, insulin receptor substrate-2; PGE2, prostaglandin E2; PI3K, phosphoinositide 3-kinase; SREBP-1c, sterol regulatory element-binding protein 1c; TFs: transcription factors; UCP-2, uncoupling protein-2.

olive oil capsules was conducted. None of these comparisons detected any difference in insulin secretion.[47]

Lack of differential effects after chronic exposure to different fatty acid quality has also been reported in studies including type 2 diabetic subjects, a population with frank β-cell failure. Indeed, the effect of isolated EPA and DHA for 6 weeks[48] or a large fish oil supplement (18 ml/day for 9 weeks)[31] did not modify insulin secretion. Selection of placebo oil source (e.g., olive or corn), duration of the intervention, and dose supplied add complexity to the assessment of the role of fatty acid quality in insulin secretion.

DIETARY FAT RECOMMENDATIONS IN TYPE 2 DIABETES

At present, there is not a specific dietary fat recommendation for type 2 diabetes. Indeed, an Expert Committee organized by WHO and FAO concluded that convincing evidence to support a role of dietary fat quality in type 2 diabetes is not available yet.[1] Therefore, dietary fat guidelines for type 2 diabetic subjects are mostly based on a well-established association between dietary fat quality and cardiovascular health (Table 31.3). It is believed, therefore, that such nutritional recommendations should also be beneficial for type 2 diabetic individuals. Consequently, SFA intake should be below 7% of total energy intake. In addition, participants are advised to favor edible oils with a balanced linoleic and α-linolenic acid content (canola and soybean oils) rather than highly enriched linoleic acid oils (safflower and sunflower). Since α-linolenic acid bioconversion into very long-chain n-3 PUFA is highly inefficient in humans, and it might be further impaired in type 2 diabetes, EPA plus DHA intake should be at least 670 mg/day.

TABLE 31.3 Dietary Fat Recommendations in Type 2 Diabetes

Nutrient	Recommendations
Total fat (%)[†]	25−35
Saturated fat (%)	< 7
Monounsaturated fat (%)	by difference
n-6 Polyunsaturated fat (%)	6−8
n-3 Polyunsaturated fat (%)	2−4
EPA + DHA (mg/day)*	> 670

[†]As percent of total energy.
*Achievable with two servings per week of salmon or mackerel.
EPA: eicosapentaenoic acid; DHA: docosahaxaenoic acid.

CONCLUSIONS

The role of fatty acid quality as a contributing factor to the incidence of type 2 diabetes remains unclear in humans. Evidence from epidemiological studies, particularly from studies using objective markers of dietary fatty acid intake, appears more consistent than intervention studies manipulating fatty acid quality to assess its influence on insulin resistance and insulin secretion. Indeed, epidemiological studies show a fairly consistent association between SFA and increased risk of type 2 diabetes. Conversely, PUFA, and especially n-3 PUFA, shows less well documented effects on insulin resistance and insulin secretion. Several methodological factors may explain why it has been difficult to demonstrate a more consistent role of fatty acid quality in glucose homeostasis, as reviewed elsewhere.[26] Alternatively, different results for animal vs human studies may be due to the dose used. For instance, the maximal fish oil dose used in humans is several times lower than that supplied to animals.[26] The time required to respond to the intervention may also be critical in explaining the lack of differential effects of fat quality on glucose homeostasis in humans. A relevant but not-well understood factor potentially interacting with fat quality and glucose homeostasis is genetic variability. At present, about a dozen susceptibility loci have been linked to type 2 diabetes,[49] most of which play a role in insulin secretion. It is plausible that fatty acid quality may have a more relevant role in individuals at risk of developing type 2 diabetes than in a non-susceptible population. Finally, a better understanding of n-6 and n-3 very long-chain PUFA metabolism in type 2 diabetes will allow for a more accurate estimate of adequacy between dietary supply and function.

References

1. Diet, nutrition and the prevention of chronic diseases. *World Health Organ Tech Rep Ser* 2003;**916**. i-viii, 1−149, back cover.

2. Simopoulos AP. Importance of the ratio of omega-6/omega-3 essential fatty acids: evolutionary aspects. *World Rev Nutr Diet* 2003;**92**:1−22.

3. Sampath H, Ntambi JM. Polyunsaturated fatty acid regulation of genes of lipid metabolism. *Annu Rev Nutr* 2005;**25**:317−40.

4. McGarry JD. Banting lecture 2001: dysregulation of fatty acid metabolism in the etiology of type 2 diabetes. *Diabetes* 2002;**51**:7−18.

5. Brenna JT. Efficiency of conversion of alpha-linolenic acid to long chain n-3 fatty acids in man. *Curr Opin Clin Nutr Metab Care* 2002;**5**:127−32.

6. Mimouni V, Narce M, Huang YS, Horrobin DF, Poisson JP. Adrenic acid delta 4 desaturation and fatty acid composition in liver microsomes of spontaneously diabetic Wistar BB rats. *Prostaglandins Leukot Essent Fatty Acids* 1994;**50**:43−7.

7. Ratnayake WM, Galli C. Fat and fatty acid terminology, methods of analysis and fat digestion and metabolism: a background review paper. *Ann Nutr Metab* 2009;**55**:8−43.

8. White PJ, Arita M, Taguchi R, Kang JX, Marette A. Transgenic restoration of long chain {omega}-3 fatty acids in insulin target tissues improves resolution capacity and alleviates obesity-linked inflammation and insulin resistance in high fat-fed mice. *Diabetes* 2010 Dec;**59**(12):3066−73. Epub 2010 Sep 14.

9. Wei D, Li J, Shen M, Jia W, Chen N, Chen T, Su D, Tian H, Zheng S, Dai Y, Zhao A. Cellular production of

n-3 PUFAs and reduction of n-6-to-n-3 ratios in the pancreatic beta-cells and islets enhance insulin secretion and confer protection against cytokine-induced cell death. *Diabetes* 2010;**59**:471−8.

10. Storlien LH, Kraegen EW, Chisholm DJ, Ford GL, Bruce DG, Pascoe WS. Fish oil prevents insulin resistance induced by high-fat feeding in rats. *Science* 1987;**237**:885−8.

11. Borkman M, Storlien LH, Pan DA, Jenkins AB, Chisholm DJ, Campbell LV. The relation between insulin sensitivity and the fatty-acid composition of skeletal-muscle phospholipids. *N Engl J Med* 1993;**328**:238−44.

12. Djousse L, Gaziano JM, Buring JE, Lee IM. Dietary omega-3 fatty acids and fish consumption and risk of type 2 diabetes. *Am J Clin Nutr* 2011 Jan;**93**(1):143−50. Epub 2010 Oct 27.

13. Sampath H, Ntambi JM. The fate and intermediary metabolism of stearic acid. *Lipids* 2005;**40**:1187−91.

14. Patel PS, Sharp SJ, Jansen E, Luben RN, Khaw KT, Wareham NJ, Forouhi NG. Fatty acids measured in plasma and erythrocyte-membrane phospholipids and derived by food-frequency questionnaire and the risk of new-onset type 2 diabetes: a pilot study in the European Prospective Investigation into Cancer and Nutrition (EPIC)-Norfolk cohort. *Am J Clin Nutr* 2010;**92**:1214−22.

15. Wang L, Folsom AR, Zheng ZJ, Pankow JS, Eckfeldt JH. Plasma fatty acid composition and incidence of diabetes in middle-aged adults: the Atherosclerosis Risk in Communities (ARIC) Study. *Am J Clin Nutr* 2003;**78**:91−8.

16. Pelikanova T, Kazdova L, Chvojkova S, Base J. Serum phospholipid fatty acid composition and insulin action in type 2 diabetic patients. *Metabolism* 2001;**50**:1472−8.

17. Jornayvaz FR, Samuel VT, Shulman GI. The role of muscle insulin resistance in the pathogenesis of atherogenic dyslipidemia and nonalcoholic fatty liver disease associated with the metabolic syndrome. *Annu Rev Nutr* 2010;**30**:273−90.

18. Kim JK, Gimeno RE, Higashimori T, Kim HJ, Choi H, Punreddy S, Mozell RL, Tan G, Stricker-Krongrad A, Hirsch DJ, Fillmore JJ, Liu ZX, Dong J, Cline G, Stahl A, Lodish HF, Shulman GI. Inactivation of fatty acid transport protein 1 prevents fat-induced insulin resistance in skeletal muscle. *J Clin Invest* 2004;**113**:756−63.

19. Kim JK, Fillmore JJ, Sunshine MJ, Albrecht B, Higashimori T, Kim DW, Liu ZX, Soos TJ, Cline GW, O'Brien WR, Littman DR, Shulman GI. PKC-theta knockout mice are protected from fat-induced insulin resistance. *J Clin Invest* 2004;**114**:823−7.

20. Morino K, Neschen S, Bilz S, Sono S, Tsirigotis D, Reznick RM, Moore I, Nagai Y, Samuel V, Sebastian D, White M, Philbrick W, Shulman GI. Muscle-specific

IRS-1 Ser->Ala transgenic mice are protected from fat-induced insulin resistance in skeletal muscle. *Diabetes* 2008;**57**:2644—51.

21. Salem Jr N, Shingu T, Kim HY, Hullin F, Bougnoux P, Karanian JW. Specialization in membrane structure and metabolism with respect to polyunsaturated lipids. *Prog Clin Biol Res* 1988;**282**:319—33.

22. DeLany JP, Windhauser MM, Champagne CM, Bray GA. Differential oxidation of individual dietary fatty acids in humans. *Am J Clin Nutr* 2000;**72**:905—11.

23. Pan DA, Storlien LH. Dietary lipid profile is a determinant of tissue phospholipid fatty acid composition and rate of weight gain in rats. *J Nutr* 1993;**123**:512—9.

24. Schenk S, Saberi M, Olefsky JM. Insulin sensitivity: modulation by nutrients and inflammation. *J Clin Invest* 2008;**118**:2992—3002.

25. Shi H, Kokoeva MV, Inouye K, Tzameli I, Yin H, Flier JS. TLR4 links innate immunity and fatty acid-induced insulin resistance. *J Clin Invest* 2006;**116**:3015—25.

26. Galgani JE, Uauy RD, Aguirre CA, Diaz EO. Effect of the dietary fat quality on insulin sensitivity. *Br J Nutr* 2008;**100**:471—9.

27. Borkman M, Chisholm DJ, Furler SM, Storlien LH, Kraegen EW, Simons LA, Chesterman CN. Effects of fish oil supplementation on glucose and lipid metabolism in NIDDM. *Diabetes* 1989;**38**:1314—9.

28. Luo J, Rizkalla SW, Vidal H, Oppert JM, Colas C, Boussairi A, Guerre-Millo M, Chapuis AS, Chevalier A, Durand G, Slama G. Moderate intake of n-3 fatty acids for 2 months has no detrimental effect on glucose metabolism and could ameliorate the lipid profile in type 2 diabetic men. Results of a controlled study. *Diabetes Care* 1998;**21**:717—24.

29. Boberg M, Pollare T, Siegbahn A, Vessby B. Supplementation with n-3 fatty acids reduces triglycerides but increases PAI-1 in non-insulin-dependent diabetes mellitus. *Eur J Clin Invest* 1992;**22**:645—50.

30. Rivellese AA, Maffettone A, Iovine C, Di Marino L, Annuzzi G, Mancini M, Riccardi G. Long-term effects of fish oil on insulin resistance and plasma lipoproteins in NIDDM patients with hypertriglyceridemia. *Diabetes Care* 1996;**19**:1207—13.

31. Mostad IL, Bjerve KS, Bjorgaas MR, Lydersen S, Grill V. Effects of n-3 fatty acids in subjects with type 2 diabetes: reduction of insulin sensitivity and time-dependent alteration from carbohydrate to fat oxidation. *Am J Clin Nutr* 2006;**84**:540—50.

32. Summers LK, Fielding BA, Bradshaw HA, Ilic V, Beysen C, Clark ML, Moore NR, Frayn KN. Substituting dietary saturated fat with polyunsaturated fat changes abdominal fat distribution and improves insulin sensitivity. *Diabetologia* 2002;**45**:369—77.

33. Itoh Y, Kawamata Y, Harada M, Kobayashi M, Fujii R, Fukusumi S, Ogi K, Hosoya M, Tanaka Y, Uejima H, Tanaka H, Maruyama M, Satoh R, Okubo S, Kizawa H, Komatsu H, Matsumura F, Noguchi Y, Shinohara T, Hinuma S, Fujisawa Y, Fujino M. Free fatty acids regulate insulin secretion from pancreatic beta cells through GPR40. *Nature* 2003;**422**:173—6.

34. Nagasumi K, Esaki R, Iwachidow K, Yasuhara Y, Ogi K, Tanaka H, Nakata M, Yano T, Shimakawa K, Taketomi S, Takeuchi K, Odaka H, Kaisho Y. Overexpression of GPR40 in pancreatic beta-cells augments glucose-stimulated insulin secretion and improves glucose tolerance in normal and diabetic mice. *Diabetes* 2009;**58**:1067—76.

35. Kato T, Shimano H, Yamamoto T, Ishikawa M, Kumadaki S, Matsuzaka T, Nakagawa Y, Yahagi N, Nakakuki M, Hasty AH, Takeuchi Y, Kobayashi K, Takahashi A, Yatoh S, Suzuki H, Sone H, Yamada N. Palmitate impairs and eicosapentaenoate restores insulin secretion through regulation of SREBP-1c in pancreatic islets. *Diabetes* 2008;**57**:2382—92.

36. Lin J, Yang R, Tarr PT, Wu PH, Handschin C, Li S, Yang W, Pei L, Uldry M, Tontonoz P, Newgard CB, Spiegelman BM. Hyperlipidemic effects of dietary saturated fats mediated through PGC-1beta coactivation of SREBP. *Cell* 2005;**120**:261—73.

37. Dickson LM, Rhodes CJ. Pancreatic beta-cell growth and survival in the onset of type 2 diabetes: a role for protein kinase B in the Akt? *Am J Physiol Endocrinol Metab* 2004;**287**:E192—8.

38. Mohanty S, Spinas GA, Maedler K, Zuellig RA, Lehmann R, Donath MY, Trub T, Niessen M. Overexpression of IRS2 in isolated pancreatic islets causes proliferation and protects human beta-cells from hyperglycemia-induced apoptosis. *Exp Cell Res* 2005;**303**:68—78.

39. Gomi H, Mizutani S, Kasai K, Itohara S, Izumi T. Granuphilin molecularly docks insulin granules to the fusion machinery. *J Cell Biol* 2005;**171**:99—109.

40. Plaisance V, Abderrahmani A, Perret-Menoud V, Jacquemin P, Lemaigre F, Regazzi R. MicroRNA-9 controls the expression of Granuphilin/Slp4 and the secretory response of insulin-producing cells. *J Biol Chem* 2006;**281**:26932—42.

41. Yamashita T, Eto K, Okazaki Y, Yamashita S, Yamauchi T, Sekine N, Nagai R, Noda M, Kadowaki T. Role of uncoupling protein-2 up-regulation and triglyceride accumulation in impaired glucose-stimulated insulin secretion in a beta-cell lipotoxicity model overexpressing sterol regulatory element-binding protein-1c. *Endocrinology* 2004;**145**:3566—77.

42. Hong Y, Fink BD, Dillon JS, Sivitz WI. Effects of adenoviral overexpression of uncoupling protein-2 and -3 on mitochondrial respiration in insulinoma cells. *Endocrinology* 2001;**142**:249−56.

43. Affourtit C, Brand MD. On the role of uncoupling protein-2 in pancreatic beta cells. *Biochim Biophys Acta* 2008;**1777**:973−9.

44. Beysen C, Karpe F, Fielding BA, Clark A, Levy JC, Frayn KN. Interaction between specific fatty acids, GLP-1 and insulin secretion in humans. *Diabetologia* 2002;**45**:1533−41.

45. Xiao C, Giacca A, Carpentier A, Lewis GF. Differential effects of monounsaturated, polyunsaturated and saturated fat ingestion on glucose-stimulated insulin secretion, sensitivity and clearance in overweight and obese, non-diabetic humans. *Diabetologia* 2006;**49**:1371−9.

46. Mostad IL, Bjerve KS, Basu S, Sutton P, Frayn KN, Grill V. Addition of n-3 fatty acids to a 4-hour lipid infusion does not affect insulin sensitivity, insulin secretion, or markers of oxidative stress in subjects with type 2 diabetes mellitus. *Metabolism* 2009;**58**:1753−61.

47. Vessby B, Unsitupa M, Hermansen K, Riccardi G, Rivellese AA, Tapsell LC, Nalsen C, Berglund L, Louheranta A, Rasmussen BM, Calvert GD, Maffetone A, Pedersen E, Gustafsson IB, Storlien LH. Substituting dietary saturated for monounsaturated fat impairs insulin sensitivity in healthy men and women: The KANWU Study,. *Diabetologia* 2001;**44**:312−9.

48. Woodman RJ, Mori TA, Burke V, Puddey IB, Watts GF, Beilin LJ. Effects of purified eicosapentaenoic and docosahexaenoic acids on glycemic control, blood pressure, and serum lipids in type 2 diabetic patients with treated hypertension. *Am J Clin Nutr* 2002;**76**:1007−15.

49. Voight BF, Scott LJ, Steinthorsdottir V, Morris AP, Dina C, Welch RP, Zeggini E, Huth C, Aulchenko YS, Thorleifsson G, McCulloch LJ, Ferreira T, Grallert H, Amin N, Wu G, Willer CJ, Raychaudhuri S, McCarroll SA, Langenberg C, Hofmann OM, Dupuis J, Qi L, Segre AV, van Hoek M, Navarro P, Ardlie K, Balkau B, Benediktsson R, Bennett AJ, Blagieva R, Boerwinkle E, Bonnycastle LL, Bengtsson Bostrom K, Bravenboer B, Bumpstead S, Burtt NP, Charpentier G, Chines PS, Cornelis M, Couper DJ, Crawford G, Doney AS, Elliott KS, Elliott AL, Erdos MR, Fox CS, Franklin CS, Ganser M, Gieger C, Grarup N, Green T, Griffin S, Groves CJ, Guiducci C, Hadjadj S, Hassanali N, Herder C, Isomaa B, Jackson AU, Johnson PR, Jorgensen T, Kao WH, Klopp N, Kong A, Kraft P, Kuusisto J, Lauritzen T, Li M, Lieverse A, Lindgren CM, Lyssenko V, Marre M, Meitinger T, Midthjell K, Morken MA, Narisu N, Nilsson P, Owen KR, Payne F, Perry JR, Petersen AK, Platou C, Proenca C, Prokopenko I, Rathmann W, Rayner NW, Robertson NR, Rocheleau G, Roden M, Sampson MJ, Saxena R, Shields BM, Shrader P, Sigurdsson G, Sparso T, Strassburger K, Stringham HM, Sun Q, Swift AJ, Thorand B, Tichet J, Tuomi T, van Dam RM, van Haeften TW, van Herpt T, van Vliet-Ostaptchouk JV, Walters GB, Weedon MN, Wijmenga C, Witteman J, Bergman RN, Cauchi S, Collins FS, Gloyn AL, Gyllensten U, Hansen T, Hide WA, Hitman GA, Hofman A, Hunter DJ, Hveem K, Laakso M, Mohlke KL, Morris AD, Palmer CN, Pramstaller PP, Rudan I, Sijbrands E, Stein LD, Tuomilehto J, Uitterlinden A, Walker M, Wareham NJ, Watanabe RM, Abecasis GR, Boehm BO, Campbell H, Daly MJ, Hattersley AT, Hu FB, Meigs JB, Pankow JS, Pedersen O, Wichmann HE, Barroso I, Florez JC, Frayling TM, Groop L, Sladek R, Thorsteinsdottir U, Wilson JF, Illig T, Froguel P, van Duijn CM, Stefansson K, Altshuler D, Boehnke M, McCarthy MI. Twelve type 2 diabetes susceptibility loci identified through large-scale association analysis. *Nat Genet* 2010;**42**:579−89.

Effects of Supplemental Fiber in Type 2 Diabetes Mellitus

Candis M. Morello[*,†,**], *Sarah A. Bajorek*[*]

[*] Skaggs School of Pharmacy and Pharmaceutical Sciences, University of California, San Diego, La Jolla, CA, USA [†] School of Pharmacy University of California San Francisco, San Francisco, CA, USA [**] Ambulatory Care Clinical Pharmacist Specialist, Veterans Affairs of San Diego Healthcare System, San Diego, CA, USA

INTRODUCTION

The number of Americans with type 2 diabetes mellitus (T2DM) continues to rise, currently at nearly 8% of the population, and is reaching epidemic proportions. Treatment for T2DM is multifactorial and complex, including lifestyle modifications, glycemic control, and managing common comorbidities such as hypertension and hyperlipidemia.

Randomized controlled trials have conclusively shown that intensive glycemic control reduces development or progression of microvascular complications, while effect on reducing macrovascular complications has been inconsistent.[1] Therefore, the American Diabetes Association (ADA) recommends reducing cardiovascular disease (CVD) risk factors with therapeutic lifestyle modifications (dietary and exercise), aspirin therapy, and antihypertensive and

Nutritional and Therapeutic Interventions for Diabetes and Metabolic Syndrome
DOI: 10.1016/B978-0-12-385083-6.00032-2

lipid-lowering agents.[2] One recommended dietary modification is increased consumption of soluble dietary fiber (DF) to lower cholesterol concentrations.[2,3]

DF from psyllium supplementation decreases total cholesterol and low-density lipoprotein concentrations.[4] Psyllium contains approximately 67% of natural concentrated soluble fiber.[5] In addition to lipid effects, it is postulated that psyllium and soluble fiber may slow glucose absorption in the small intestine, thereby attenuating postprandial plasma glucose (PPG) elevations.[6] Studies have suggested that increasing DF may improve insulin resistance[7,8] and the ADA now recommends individuals at high risk for developing T2DM to consume 14 g DF per 1,000 kcal daily.[2] In an 1,800–2,000-calorie daily diet, this represents consuming 24–28 g of DF each day.

Diets emphasizing foods with a low glycemic index (GI) or glycemic load have been suggested as an alternative to carbohydrate counting.[9] GI ranks foods based on the resulting increase in PPG following consumption. Lower GI foods elicit a more gradual increase in PPG and hence improve glycemic control. Low GI diets focus on increasing dietary fiber by way of consuming more whole grains, legumes, vegetables, fruit, nuts, lean protein, healthy fats, and avoiding processed foods, white bread, and rice.[10]

METHODS

Search Strategy

A literature search was conducted using the PubMed database, Cochrane Library, Natural Standard and Natural Medicines. In PubMed, literature was searched through February 2011 using the following limits: "human", "randomized controlled trial or meta-analysis", and "English". The search queries were as follows: ("Diabetes Mellitus, Type 2/diet therapy" [MeSH] AND "Dietary Fiber/therapeutic use" [MeSH]) and ("Diabetes Mellitus, Type 2" [MeSH] AND "psyllium/therapeutic use" [MeSH]). The Cochrane Library was searched with the following queries: "Diabetes Mellitus and Dietary Fiber", "Diabetes Mellitus and Psyllium" and "Diabetes Mellitus and Glycemic Index". The Natural Standard and the Natural Medicines were searched for "psyllium".

Inclusion and Exclusion Criteria

Search results were screened for the following inclusion criteria: randomized, controlled studies or meta-analyses examining the effects of dietary interventions, such as GI, fiber, or psyllium on glycemic risk factors (A1c or PPG). Eligible studies included those whose subjects had T2DM. Studies were excluded if the subjects were healthy or had type 1 diabetes mellitus, the study design was open label, dietary intervention other than psyllium, low-GI or high-fiber, or the mean A1c was below 7%.

Data Collection

Data collected included authors; publication year; study design; number of participants; intervention, including treatment, dose and duration; and primary outcomes. Primary outcomes were A1c and PPG.

RESULTS

Study Characteristics

An online literature search through February 2011 identified 80 studies, of which five met inclusion criteria. Study designs included three randomized crossover studies; one randomized parallel study; and three randomized, blinded parallel studies. Intervention study subjects were classified by authors of five original publications as having a diagnosis of T2DM) (Table 32.1). Oral hypoglycemic medication use was reported in all studies.[6,10–13] The following information was extracted from each study: authors, year of publication, design, randomization, withdrawals, losses to follow-up and primary outcome and subjects' sex, age, duration of disease, medication status, baseline fasting plasma glucose concentrations (FPG) or A1c, when reported.

Subjects with Type 2 Diabetes Mellitus

In a randomized, crossover study the effects of 6.8 g of psyllium powder *vs* placebo on PPG (N = 18) was examined.[6] Two 3.4-g packets of psyllium dissolved in 240 ml of water were given before a standardized breakfast and dinner (6.8 g per meal and 14 g of daily DF) in six men and 12 women (mean age of 54 years) with T2DM (duration of disease greater than 2 years). Six subjects were controlled on di*et alo*ne; 12 took oral hypo-glycemic medications (drug name and dosages not reported.) Baseline FPG ranged from 120 to 220 mg/dl and A1c from 8 to 12%. After the breakfast meal, change in PPG from baseline in psyllium group was 107.7 ± 11.6 mg/dl compared to 125.4 ± 11.1 mg/dl in placebo group (P = 0.08). After the dinner meal, change in PPG from baseline in the psyllium group was 53.2 ± 7.5 compared to 67.1 ± 11.1 mg/dl in the placebo group (P = 0.06). After breakfast,

TABLE 32.1 Summary of Studies Evaluating the Role of Psyllium, High-fiber Diets or Low-GI Diets in Lowering Glycemic Risk Factors in Subjects with Type 2 Diabetes

Reference	Design[a]	Treatment[b]	Daily dosage	Duration[c]	Outcomes/Conclusion
Pastors *et al.* (1991)[6]	R, CO	Psyllium	13.6 g	15 h with 7 days WO	Psyllium decreased PPG after breakfast and dinner (P = 0.08 and 0.06, respectively), and PPG 5 h after breakfast by 31% (P < 0.05)
Jenkins *et al.* (2008)[10]	R, B, P	Low GI diet High-fiber cereal diet	GI = 62, 18.7 g fiber per 1,000 kcal GI = 86, 15.7 g fiber per 1,000 kcal	6 months	After 24 weeks, the low-GI and high-fiber cereal diet decreased mean A1c (P < 0.001) and mean FPG (P < 0.05)
Frati Munari *et al.* (1998)[11]	R, CO	Acarbose Psyllium	200 mg 15 g	15 h with 3–8 d WO	Both acarbose and psyllium PPG (P < 0.05), although not statistically significant between treatments
Chandalia *et al.* (2000)[12]	R, CO	ADA diet High-fiber diet	8 g SF, 24 g TF per day[d] *25 g SF, 50 g TF per day*	6 weeks with 7 days WO	The high-fiber diet decreased APG concentrations compared to the "ADA diet" (P < 0.05), but no statistical difference in mean A1c was observed (P = 0.09)
Ma *et al.* (2008)[13]	R, P	Low GI diet ADA diet	GI < 55 CHO: 55% of daily needs, 25–35 g fiber	12 months	Both treatments significantly decreased mean A1c (P < 0.001), however the decrease was not statistically significant between treatments (P = 0.88)

[a] R, randomized; CO, crossover; B, blinded; P, parallel. CHO, carbohydrate.
[b] When only one treatment is listed, study was compared to either placebo or usual care (see text).
[c] WO, wash out period between treatments.
[d] SF, soluble fiber; TF, total fiber.

serum insulin concentrations in psyllium group were decreased ($P < 0.05$), and the area under the curve (AUC) was 17% lower ($P < 0.05$) compared to placebo. After a standardized lunch in which no psyllium was administered, residual psyllium from breakfast 5 h prior decreased PPG by 31% ($P < 0.05$) and AUC by 65% ($P < 0.05$), a phenomenon authors called "second-meal effect". Oral hypoglycemic agents did not confound results because there was no difference in PPG reduction between those using and those not using oral hypoglycemic medications. Subjects tolerated both treatments well; no adverse side effects were reported. Although standardized meals provided 14 g of DF, this should not be a confounding variable since both treatment groups consumed the same meal. Limitations of this study include small sample size, short duration of treatment, and a lack of blinding. A1c after treatment could not be assessed since study duration was too short.

A randomized, crossover study compared the effects of psyllium and the alpha-glucosidase inhibitor acarbose on GI of bread and PPG in three men and nine women (mean age 48 years) with T2DM (duration 3.6 ± 2.6 years).[11] Seven subjects were taking glibenclamide and 5 tolbutamide (dosages not reported) and all had FPG less than 200 mg/dl. Three tests were performed: 90 g of white bread [50 g of carbohydrates (CHO); control], 200 mg acarbose given immediately before 90 g of white bread and 15 g of psyllium given immediately before 90 g of white bread. GI was 26.1 ± 13.4 for acarbose plus bread and 58.9 ± 10.1 for psyllium ($P < 0.05$). Psyllium reduced peak PPG compared to control (167.9 ± 10.7 vs 207.1 ± 17.9 mg/dl; $P < 0.05$) as did acarbose (150 ± 10.7 vs 207.1 ± 17.9 mg/dl; $P < 0.05$). Although acarbose reduced PPG more than psyllium, no significant difference was observed. Neither safety data nor adverse reactions were reported. Limitations include short treatment duration (only one treatment

test was performed), use of twice-recommended doses of both psyllium and acarbose, and lack of randomization description.

A randomized, crossover study compared effects of DF as recommended by the ADA with a high fiber diet on A1c and average plasma glucose (APG) concentrations in 12 men and 1 woman (mean age of 61 years) with T2DM (duration of disease unknown).[12] Study duration was 6 weeks with a 1-week washout period. Baseline FPG were less than 200 mg/dl (no range given) and A1c ranged from 6.0 to 9.8%. While three subjects were controlled on diet alone, 10 took 2.5–20 mg/d of glyburide in conjunction with the diet. Both diets provided 55% of daily energy needs from carbohydrates, 15% from protein and 30% from fat. However, the "ADA diet" contained 8 g of soluble fiber and 16 g insoluble fiber per day while the high-fiber diet contained 25 g each of soluble and insoluble fiber per day. The high-fiber diet consisted of unfortified, fiber-rich foods (such as oats, lima beans, sweet potatoes) with no fiber supplementation. Subjects ate at least one meal daily at the research center during weekdays, while other meals were provided in packages and eaten at home. During the last study week, subjects were hospitalized for 5 days and APG concentrations were collected at 7 a.m., 11 a.m., 4 p.m., and 8 p.m. The high-fiber diet decreased APG concentrations compared to the "ADA diet" (130 ± 38 vs 142 ± 36 mg/dl; $P < 0.05$). Mean A1c was slightly lower in the high-fiber diet compared to "ADA diet" group ($6.9 \pm 1.2\%$ vs $7.2 \pm 1.3\%$; $P = 0.09$), without reaching statistical significance. Subjects tolerated the high fiber diet well, with no adverse side effects reported. All subjects completed the study. Limitations of the study include small sample size and a lack of a description of randomization or blinding. Study duration was 6 weeks, which may account for the lack of statistical significance in A1c concentrations. Authors did not report when subjects consumed test meals in relation to the plasma glucose collection, so it is unknown whether the "APG concentration" is a postprandial collection.

In a randomized, controlled, parallel study comparing effects of the "ADA diet" to a low GI diet on A1c in 19 men and 21 women (mean age 53.5 years) with T2DM (mean duration of disease 9.32 ± 9.66 years), [13] baseline A1c ranged from 7.8 to 9.0%. At the time of the study, subjects took oral hypoglycemic agents [metformin, glyburide, glipizide, pioglitazone, rosiglitazone, or repaglinide; or injectable agents (insulin or exenatide); dosages not reported]. Both diets provided 55% of daily energy needs from carbohydrates, 15% from protein and 30% from fat and recommended subjects exercise for 30 min daily most days of the week. Baseline GI for the "ADA diet" was 82 ± 1.3 compared to 79.4 ± 1.4 ($P = 0.16$) for the low GI diet. The low GI treatment diet aimed to reduce the daily GI score of carbohydrates to 55 from baseline levels. Intervention consisted of educational information regarding the treatment diet, goal setting, managing psychological influences on food choices, managing portion size, and eating out, etc. The intervention was carried out through monthly education sessions held for 6 months and then at 8 and 10 months. Fasting blood samples were measured at each session and analyzed for A1c concentrations. After 6 months of treatment, GI change from baseline was not significant between the two interventions ($P = 0.07$). A statistically significant ($P < 0.001$) decrease in mean A1c was observed in both treatment groups. However, no difference in mean A1c decrease was observed between the two groups ($P = 0.88$). PPGs were not measured. All subjects tolerated both diets well, with no adverse effects reported. Limitations of the study include baseline differences in age between treatment groups (51 ± 8.3 years in the "ADA diet" and 56.3 ± 7.9 years in the low-GI diet; $P < 0.05$) and a small sample size that is underpowered to detect the difference in A1c, the study's primary end point. Subjects

in the low GI group had a longer duration of disease (12.65 ± 11.93 years) compared to the "ADA diet" (6.62 ± 6.47 years), although the difference was not statistically significant ($P = 0.07$). The subjects received monthly dietary counseling, which may limit the applicability to real-life patients unable to receive such counseling.

A randomized, blinded, controlled, 6-month study evaluated the effects of a low-GI diet compared to a a high-fiber cereal diet on A1c in 128 men and 82 women (mean age of 61.5 years) with T2DM (duration of disease unknown). [10] Baseline glucose concentration (fasting or casual not reported) for both groups was 139.3 ± 30.4 mg/dl and baseline A1c was 7.1%. Subjects concurrently took oral hypoglycemic medications (thiazolidinedione, biguanides, sulfonylureas, meglitinides, or α-glucosidase inhibitors; drug names or dosages not reported). Subjects were stratified by sex and A1c [≤ 7.1% (54.8% of participants) and > 7.1% (45.2% of participants)] and randomized by a blinded statistician. Both diets provided 42−43% of daily energy requirements from carbohydrates. The low-GI diet emphasized foods with a GI less than 62 and provided 18.7 g of fiber per 1,000 kcal. The high-fiber cereal diet did not restrict food based on GI, although the mean GI was 86. It also provided 15.7 g of fiber per 1,000 kcal. Throughout the study, subjects completed a daily checklist of food consumed. For 7 days before each visit, subjects maintained a food journal that included actual weight or common measurements of foods consumed. After 24 weeks, there was a difference between treatment groups for daily fiber consumed ($P < 0.001$). After 24 weeks of treatment and adjusting for fiber intake, the low-GI diet significantly decreased mean A1c compared to high-fiber cereal diet (7.14−6.64% vs 7.07−6.89%, respectively; $P < 0.05$). After adjusting for fiber intake, post-treatment mean FPG decreased from baseline for both low-glycemic diet (138.8−127.7 mg/dl; $P < 0.05$)

and high-fiber cereal diet (141.2—136.8 mg/dl; $P < 0.05$). Subjects tolerated both diets well, with no adverse side effects reported. One study limitation is the narrow inclusion criteria of baseline A1c (lower range of 6.5% and upper range of 8%), which decreases the applicability to most people with T2DM. Another limitation is that the low-GI treatment group could eat All-Bran Buds®, a cereal that contained 3.5 g of psyllium fiber per 1/3 cup. It was not reported how many servings subjects consumed, which could influence the reduction in A1c in the low-GI treatment group.

DISCUSSION

Results from five randomized-controlled clinical trials suggest that psyllium fiber or a low-GI diet may improve glycemic risk factors in persons with T2DM. A daily dosage of 10.2 g of psyllium significantly decreased all-day PPG.[6] Average plasma glucose concentrations were reduced as well; however, psyllium's effect on A1c remains to be determined. The lack of statistical significance in A1c reductions could also be due to the short duration of the studies, since A1c values do not change acutely. Effect on A1c with diets emphasizing low-GI foods are inconclusive. One study was under-powered,[13] while the other study had psyllium fiber (as a cereal option for the low GI diet) as a confounding variable.[10]

In addition, one study compared the effects of acarbose or psyllium on PPG following 90 g of white bread (approximately three slices or 50 g of carbohydrate) and found no statistically significant difference between groups.[11] Double the recommended dose of both psyllium and acarbose were used. Longer studies are warranted to determine whether there is a significant treatment difference between psyllium and acarbose. If not, psyllium would be a more affordable option for treating elevated PPG following a carbohydrate-rich meal.

Dietary modifications with psyllium are generally well tolerated. The most common reported adverse effects are flatulence, cramping, cough, or rhinitis.[4] Gastric effects can be attenuated with gradual increase in DF; start with 3—5 g daily and increase by 3—5 g daily every 2—3 days). Most non-prescription psyllium powder supplements (e.g., Metamucil®) contain 3.4 g psyllium per teaspoon per dose; therefore, add one teaspoon every 2—3 days. To achieve the dosage used in studies, slowly titrate up to one dose three times a day taken 20—30 min before meals.

Individuals allergic to ingested or inhaled psyllium should avoid psyllium. Since psyllium may cause intestinal obstruction, individuals with gastrointestinal conditions such as bowel obstruction should not use psyllium. In addition, individuals requiring fluid restriction may not be candidates for psyllium therapy as each dose must be mixed with or consumed with at least 250 ml of water. While diet-related adverse events are rare with a low-glycemic diet, hypoglycemia can occur in patients taking hypoglycemic agents.[10]

Drug interactions are rare with psyllium since it does not affect CYP450 metabolizing enzymes; however, psyllium administration should be separated from other medications by at least 4 h since medications can potentially bind to psyllium, decreasing their absorption and therapeutic effects.[14]

CONCLUSION

Psyllium supplementation, specifically in the form of 10.2 g/day of psyllium fiber administered 20—30 min before meals, may be effective at reducing glycemic risk factors, such as APG and PPG concentrations. The evaluated studies showed that psyllium fiber might improve these risk factor subjects in T2DM. As evidence shows, psyllium fiber might be a beneficial adjuvant in patients with elevated PPG concentrations already receiving oral hypoglycemic medications. Further studies are necessary to determine whether psyllium supplementation is effective in decreasing PPG concentrations in people with prediabetes. Low-GI diets may decrease A1c, yet longer and larger studies with better study designs and control of confounding variables are needed.

References

1. Skyler JS, Bergenstal R, Bonow RO, Buse J, Deedwania P, Gale EA, Howard BV, Kirkman MS, Kosiborod M, Reaven P, Sherwin RS, American Diabetes Association, American College of Cardiology Foundation & American Heart Association. Intensive glycemic control and the prevention of cardiovascular events: implications of the ACCORD, ADVANCE, and VA Diabetes Trials: a position statement of the American Diabetes Association and a Scientific Statement of the American College of Cardiology Foundation and the American Heart Association. *J Am Coll Cardiol* 2009;**53**:298–304. 10.1016/j.jacc.2008.10.008.

2. American Diabetes Association. Standards of medical care in diabetes—2011. *Diabetes Care* 2011;**34**(Suppl. 1): S11–61. 10.2337/dc11-S011.

3. National Cholesterol Education Program (NCEP) Expert Panel on Detection, Evaluation, and Treatment of High Blood Cholesterol in Adults (Adult Treatment Panel III). Third Report of the National Cholesterol Education Program (NCEP) Expert Panel on Detection, Evaluation, and Treatment of High Blood Cholesterol in Adults (Adult Treatment Panel III) final report. *Circulation* 2002;**106**:3143–421.

4. Anderson JW, Allgood LD, Lawrence A, Altringer LA, Jerdack GR, Hengehold DA, Morel JG. Cholesterol-lowering effects of psyllium intake adjunctive to diet therapy in men and women with hypercholesterolemia: meta-analysis of 8 controlled trials. *Am J Clin Nutr* 2000;**71**:472–9.

5. Gelissen IC, Brodie B, Eastwood MA. Effect of Plantago ovata (psyllium) husk and seeds on sterol metabolism: studies in normal and ileostomy subjects. *Am J Clin Nutr* 1994;**59**:395–400.

6. Pastors JG, Blaisdell PW, Balm TK, Asplin CM, Pohl SL. Psyllium fiber reduces rise in postprandial glucose and insulin concentrations in patients with non-insulin-dependent diabetes. *Am J Clin Nutr* 1991;**53**: 1431–5.

7. Rave K, Roggen K, Dellweg S, Heise T, tom Dieck H. Improvement of insulin resistance after diet with a whole-grain based dietary product: results of a randomized, controlled cross-over study in obese subjects with elevated fasting blood glucose. *Br J Nutr* 2007;**98**:929–36.

8. Kim H, Stote KS, Behall KM, Spears K, Vinyard B, Conway JM. Glucose and insulin responses to whole grain breakfasts varying in soluble fiber, beta-glucan: a dose response study in obese women with increased risk for insulin resistance. *Eur J Nutr* 2009;**48**:170–5.

9. Wolever TM, Gibbs AL, Mehling C, Chiasson JL, Connelly PW, Josse RG, Leiter LA, Maheux P, Rabasa-Lhoret R, Rodger NW, Ryan EA. The Canadian Trial of Carbohydrates in Diabetes (CCD), a 1-y controlled trial of low-glycemic-index dietary carbohydrate in type 2 diabetes: no effect on glycated hemoglobin but reduction in C-reactive protein. *Am J Clin Nutr* 2008;**87**:114–25.

10. Jenkins DJ, Kendall CW, McKeown-Eyssen G, Josse RG, Silverberg J, Booth GL, Vidgen E, Josse AR, Nguyen TH, Corrigan S, Banach MS, Ares S, Mitchell S, Emam A, Augustin LS, Parker TL, Leiter LA. Effect of a low-glycemic index or a high-cereal fiber diet on type 2 diabetes: a randomized trial. *JAMA* 2008;**300**:2742–53.

11. Frati Munari AC, Benitez Pinto W, Raul Ariza Andraca C, Casarrubias M. Lowering glycemic index of food by acarbose and Plantago psyllium mucilage. *Arch Med Res* 1998;**29**:137–41.

12. Chandalia M, Garg A, Lutjohann D, von Bergmann K, Grundy SM, Brinkley LJ. Beneficial effects of high dietary fiber intake in patients with type 2 diabetes mellitus. *N Engl J Med* 2000;**342**:1392–8.

13. Ma Y, Olendzki BC, Merriam PA, Chiriboga DE, Culver AL, Li W, Hebert JR, Ockene IS, Griffith JA, Pagoto SL. A randomized clinical trial comparing low-glycemic index versus ADA dietary education among individuals with type 2 diabetes. *Nutrition* 2008;**24**:45–56.

14. Fugh-Berman A. Herb-drug interactions. *Lancet* 2000; **355**:134–8.

The Effects of Resveratrol on Diabetes and Obesity

Juan A. Sanchez, Mahesh Thirunavukkarasu, Nilanjana Maulik

Molecular Cardiology and Angiogenesis Laboratory, Department of Surgery, University of Connecticut Health Center, Farmington, CT, USA

INTRODUCTION

Diabetes mellitus currently affects approximately 5% of the population worldwide and nearly 7% of the population in the US.[1,2] As a result of the developing obesity epidemic and associated insulin resistance in the Western world and, increasingly, elsewhere, complications from diabetes are anticipated to increase considerably in the coming decades. By the year 2030, for example, the World Health Organization predicts a rise in the number of diabetics to 366 million from 171 million in 2000.[3] In the US, its prevalence is believed to increase to 12% by 2050 cutting across all slices of society including children.

While the pathophysiology of glucose homeostasis and insulin resistance is complex and the effects of longstanding diabetes on cellular and organ function incompletely understood, this condition is increasingly being characterized within the framework of oxidative

Nutritional and Therapeutic Interventions for Diabetes and Metabolic Syndrome
DOI: 10.1016/B978-0-12-385083-6.00033-4

stress biology and its operant mechanisms. It is becoming clear that adaptive and maladaptive responses to chronic free radical exposure is an important part of the organ dysfunction seen in diabetes in addition to the other inflammatory aspects of this disease. Moreover, insights obtained from other areas of investigation, including phytopharmacology, which explore oxidative cellular stress responses yield valuable data which are directly relevant to diabetes research.

RESVERATROL: A MULTIFUNCTIONAL COMPOUND

Found in the skin of red grapes and in many other plants, resveratrol (3,5,4'-trihydroxystilbene) is a bioactive polyphenol that has attracted considerable attention in recent years as a result of its antioxidant effects.[4,5] A phytoalexin, it is naturally synthesized in varying concentrations by plants ostensibly to protect against cellular injury from zoobiotic threats, radiation, and other adverse environmental conditions. Resveratrol is a derivative of stilbene and consists of an ethylene group flanked by two phenyl groups. It is found in nature in two geometric isomeric forms: trans-(E) and cis-(Z), and, in addition, as free or glucosylated forms. The two isomers have different bioactivity, trans-resveratrol being the more stable of the two.[4] It has been studied extensively as a possible therapeutic agent to reduce cardiovascular, neoplastic, and, more recently, diabetes-related morbidity and mortality.[6–9] The most abundant source of trans-resveratrol is found in the root extract of the Japanese knotweed (*Polygonum cuspidatum*), a variant of which has been used as traditional herbal tea in Japan and China for centuries.[4] In 1992, the presence of trans-resveratrol in the skin of red grapes was identified, drawing intense interest from the scientific community as well as the lay press regarding the health benefits of wine,

adding to the increasing focus on "phytoceuticals" in general.[10–14]

Caloric restriction, a strategy which extends the lifespan of many animals by up to 50%, is believed to be mediated, in part, by the actions of SIRT1, a member of the highly conserved Sir2 family of NAD(+)-dependent protein deacetylases.[15–17] Phosphorylation by cell cycle-dependent kinases appears to control the level and function of SIRT1 and the histone deacetylation of the transcriptional coactivator PGC-1 alpha is suggested as a central mechanism.[18,19] SIRT1 activation appears to have a central role in many metabolic processes and this enzyme has been implicated as a potential target for drug development in a variety of chronic metabolic, inflammatory, and age-related diseases.[9,20] A number of plant-derived compounds have been used in studies attempting to replicate this increase in the lifespan of experimental animals, both diabetic and non-diabetic, by slowing age-related degeneration.[21–23] Despite efforts to develop pharmacologic agents which mimic the effects of caloric restriction on survival, no compound has been able to replicate or even come close to this effect.[24,25] However, the considerable health effects seen with resveratrol *in vivo* mimic many of the changes found with caloric restriction, supporting the notion that analogs of resveratrol which can more vigorously stimulate SIRT1 can be developed to achieve the life extension effects of caloric restriction in the future.[22,26,27]

Streppel, in a recent study involving 1,373 men, demonstrated that wine, when taken in moderation, lowered cardiovascular-related mortality and increased life expectancy by 5 years.[28] Although grapes contain about 1.5–7.3 µg/g of trans-resveratrol and studies of wine intake in humans have shown high oral absorption via the gastrointestinal system, resveratrol is actually found in very low concentrations in plasma.[4,29,30] Its pharmacokinetics and metabolism continue to be actively investigated and synthetic analogs are under development with the goal of increasing its bioavailability and potency.[16,31–36] Sirtuin orthologs, compounds which activate SIRT1, with improved bioavailability appear to be generally safe and well-tolerated in humans and clinical trials in a variety of conditions, including the treatment of diabetes, are currently underway.[37]

One of the principal characteristics of resveratrol is its natural antioxidant properties.[38] In addition to several other cytoprotective mechanisms currently under investigation, many polyphenolic compounds exhibit antioxidant activity including the capacity to induce free radical scavenging, metal chelation, enzyme modulation, cell signaling effects, as well as the ability to regulate gene expression and protect mitochondrial function and biogenesis, thereby increasing the energy efficiency of cells under stress.[39–46] The properties of resveratrol appear to be related to its ability to increase nitric oxide synthesis and as well as its capacity to scavenge superoxide radicals.[47,48] In addition, a variety of other properties, including inhibition of tissue factor (TF) and cytokine expression as well as decreased platelet aggregation, contribute to its known anti-inflammatory and antithrombotic effects.[49] Our laboratory has shown increased expression of VEGF and its tyrosine kinase, VEGFR1 (Flt-1), in myocardial infarction models when resveratrol was given after initial injury.[50] Others have shown, in animal models, that resveratrol inhibits low-density lipoprotein (LDL) cholesterol oxidation and increases serum high-density lipoprotein (HDL) cholesterol.[11]

The molecular activities of resveratrol and related compounds are pleomorphic and ongoing investigations continue to produce surprising insights into the extraordinary variety of clinically relevant effects (Figure 33.1). Its widespread intracellular targets affect crucial processes involving cell proliferation and differentiation, programmed cell death and autophagy, and mitochondrial energy production. Findings from a large number of studies consistently show that resveratrol appears to ameliorate a number of degenerative processes that impact glucose homeostasis and the development of obesity through a variety of biochemical pathways still under investigation.[14,51]

A number of anti-inflammatory effects, both *in vitro* and in animal models, have been attributed to resveratrol.[52–54] Studies indicate significant inhibition in proliferation, antibody production, and lymphokine secretion resulting in suppression of both T- and B-cell activity and tissue macrophage function.[55] In normal human subjects, indices of oxidative and inflammatory stress were shown to be considerably and comprehensively attenuated in mononuclear cells and suppression in plasma levels of tumor necrosis factor-α (TNF-α), interleukin-6 (IL-6), and C-reactive protein compared to baseline and to placebo after a 6-week course of daily resveratrol-containing *Polygonum cuspidatum*.[52] Inhibition of chemokine-mediated inflammatory cells by resveratrol in non-obese, diabetic animals support a potent anti-inflammatory effect found for this class of compounds.[53] A number of bioactive compounds, including resveratrol, have also been demonstrated to downregulate platelet activating factor (PAF), a potent inflammatory mediator, which has been implicated in a number of conditions and diseases from cancer to diabetes.[56] In summary, the anti-inflammatory characteristics of these compounds have become abundantly clear and the metabolic syndrome/diabetes complex appears to be a fertile proving ground for their clinical effectiveness.

RESVERATROL AND DIABETES

The normal metabolic response to high-carbohydrate meals includes mechanisms which indicate oxidative stress and inflammation.[52,53,57] These indices include the expression of TLR-4, CD14, IL-1β, TNF-α, SOCS-3, along with elevated plasma concentrations of

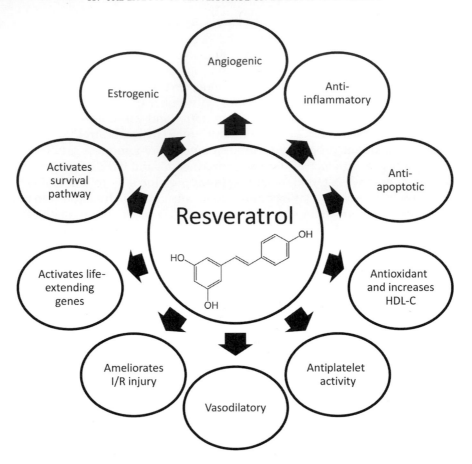

FIGURE 33.1   Biological functions of resveratrol.

lipopolysaccharide and lipoprotein binding protein among many others. Polyphenolic compounds, including resveratrol, have been shown to attenuate many of these responses and to stimulate the activity of antioxidants such as Nrf-2, a transcription factor, inducing the expression of related antioxidant genes.

The effects of dietary polyphenols on carbohydrate metabolism are attributed to a wide variety of mechanisms.[58,59] Resveratrol is known to reduce plasma glucose in both diabetic and non-diabetic animals and to normalize glucose tolerance challenges by playing a role in the intracellular transport of glucose.[60,61] The regulation of glucose uptake and its subsequent utilization is critical for the maintenance of glucose homeostasis. It is well established that glucose uptake is controlled by GLUT4 in the plasma membrane and the GLUT4 translocation to the membrane seems to be dependent on insulin-mediated signaling pathways. Adipocytes of streptozotocin-induced diabetic rats demonstrated reduction in insulin-stimulated glucose transport function and cellular glucose transporter content[62] and evidences show that the change in the glucose transporter content is more specific for GLUT4.[63] It was also reported that both GLUT4 transport and content increase after insulin treatment.[62,63] Dilated cardiomyopathy, one of the major complications during diabetes, is characterized by depletion of adenosine triphosphate (ATP) stores which is a consequence of impaired insulin-mediated glucose uptake.[64] Insulin, a major regulator of glucose metabolism, increases glucose transport by stimulating insertion of GLUT4 from the intracellular compartment into the cell surface[65] and further transition of GLUT4 to the plasma membrane fraction enriched by the caveolae.[66] Small membrane invaginations on the surface of the cells that participate in membrane signal transduction is termed as caveolae. Resveratrol increases adenosine monophosphate-activated protein kinase (AMPK) activity resulting in increased glucose uptake potentiating the sensitivity of insulin and possibly downregulating gluconeogenic enzymes in the liver.[67–69] AMPK, a serine-threonine kinase, was shown to play an important role in regulation of cellular metabolism and as a mediator of glucose metabolism.[70] Chen et al. demonstrated that activated AMPK phosphorylates eNOS both in vitro and during ischemia in rat hearts,[71] and Li et al. showed the role of nitric oxide in AMPK-mediated glucose uptake and GLUT4 translocation.[72] In the same study Li et al. also demonstrated that a relatively low concentration of nitric oxide donors stimulated GLUT4 translocation and increased glucose uptake in isolated heart muscles.[72] Thirunavukkarasu et al. demonstrated that resveratrol treatment increased myocardial function as well as reduced glucose level in diabetic rats which may be mediated through nitric oxide.[73] The resveratrol-mediated glucose uptake by modulating the Cav-1 and Cav-3 status in diabetic myocardium is mostly non-insulin related. Penumathsa et al. observed increased translocation of GLUT4 and its association with Cav-3 and dissociation of Cav-1/eNOS interaction in lipid raft fractions after resveratrol treatment. They have also documented increased phosphorylation of AMPK, eNOS and Akt on resveratrol treatment and

hypothesized that resveratrol-mediated GLUT4 translocation and glucose uptake might be AMPK/eNOS/Akt-mediated and regulated by Cav-1 and Cav-3 status which is independent of insulin signaling pathway.

SIRT1 has been shown to be downregulated in insulin-resistant cells and the addition of resveratrol in vitro appears to improve insulin sensitivity.[74,75] In vivo, the enhanced glucose uptake by many different tissues such as hepatocytes, adipocytes, and skeletal muscle, in addition to increased hepatic glycogen synthesis, does not require the presence of insulin.[8] Furthermore, its ability to activate estrogen receptors may regulate glucose metabolism through both insulin-dependent and independent mechanisms.[76] SIRT1 activation by resveratrol in a diabetic model has a considerable antihyperglycemic effect and several studies confirm the value of sirtuins in improving glucose tolerance.[77,78]

β-Cells in the pancreas are damaged through chronic exposure of supraphysiologic levels of glucose causing irreversible dysfunction resulting in further alterations in the regulation of insulin. As noted previously, oxidative stress within these cells has been confirmed by a number of investigators. Oral resveratrol has been shown to reverse this effect resulting in normalization of plasma glucose, reduce glycosylated hemoglobin (HbA1c) as well as several other indicators of antioxidation in pancreatic cells including reduced activity of superoxide dismutase (SOD), catalase, glutathione peroxidase, and glutathione-S-transferase.[79] Although the myriad effects of resveratrol on the function of islet β-cells are not completely understood, reversal of cell damage from cytokine toxicity and subsequent restoration of glucose homeostasis has been suggested.[80] Additional damage to these cells is caused by the aggregation of islet amyloid polypeptide (IAPP) into fibrils which is a hallmark of type 2 diabetes.[81–84] This process is lipid-induced and results in progressive deposition of this substance in the extracellular matrix of β-cells. By inhibiting oligomerization and amyloid formation by binding to histidine 18, resveratrol appears to reverse this deleterious effect on islet cells.

Although basal insulin secretion from islet cells is unaffected by exposure to resveratrol *in vitro*, physiologic and maximal levels of glucose appears to inhibit the insulin response.[85] This phenomenon is abrogated by blocking somatostatin receptors and by acetylcholine administration suggesting that resveratrol causes direct insulin suppression. *In vivo* experiments show that this hypoglycemic effect is not always dependent on insulin secretion and is mediated by phosphatidyl-3-kinase.[86] However, investigators have found that it can act as an insulin secretagogue through K(ATP) and K(V) channel inhibition.[87] In addition, recent evidence suggests that the improved glucose homeostasis may be also mediated via effects on the central nervous system in as well as by restoration of hepatocyte function.[88,89]

Many studies have demonstrated that advanced glycation end-products (AGEs) play a major pathogenic role in diabetes and its complications.[90] These products are the result of non-enzymatic glycation between reducing sugars and the amino groups found in a variety of molecules including proteins, lipids, and DNA. This reaction generates methylglyoxal (MGO), a reactive dicarbonyl intermediate under physiologic conditions. Stilbenes appear to be able to trap a number of adducts generated during this reaction thereby inhibiting the formation of AGEs. In addition, resveratrol prevents the impairment in lipid homeostasis, at least partially, by suppressing the AGE receptor (RAGE) via PPAR-γ activation.[91] This effect appears to be critical in the protective role played by resveratrol in diabetic atherosclerosis. Moreover, lactadherin-mediated, endothelial cell apoptosis resulting from AGE production is inhibited by resveratrol.[92]

Acceleration of protein degradation is a hallmark of the chronic diabetic state highlighting the inherent imbalance between catabolism and anabolism in this disease.[93] This effect, responsible for the observed muscle wasting in these patients, is thought to be a result of increased activity of the ubiquitin-proteasomal system mediated via nuclear factor-κB (NF-κB) transcription factor and resulting in protein oxidation.[93,94] Several studies have suggested that resveratrol and its analogs reverse muscle wasting through its antioxidant/anti-inflammatory properties.[95] For example, injection of resveratrol in rats increased microvascular blood volume in muscle and improved blood flow.[96] This effect was abolished by NO synthase inhibition indicating a nitric oxide-mediated mechanism and TNF-α prevented this microvascular recruitment. The small polyphenolic molecule, kaempferol, was able to increase skeletal muscle oxygen consumption by 30% by increasing cyclic AMP generation and protein kinase A activation, an effect which appears to be independent of esirtuin activation.[97]

RESVERATROL IN DIABETIC CARDIOMYOPATHY

The cardioprotective effects of naturally occurring polyphenols have been known for some time.[98–100] Their principal effects on the oxidative myocardial stress resulting from ischemia and reperfusion has been well documented and their unique microRNA signature in the heart recently reported.[74,101,102] Upregulation of sarcoplasmic calcium ATPase through SIRT1 activation by resveratrol has demonstrated improved cardiac function in a streptozotocin-induced diabetic animal model.[103] In addition to its beneficial effects on coronary endothelial function, it appears to improve left ventricular diastolic relaxation in type 2 diabetes, at least partially, by increasing endothelial nitric oxide synthase (eNOS) and subsequent release of nitric oxide, and by reducing both inducible nitric oxide synthase (iNOS) and nitrotyrosine expression.[104,105] As such, by inhibiting TNF-α-induced NF-κB activation and reducing oxidative and nitrative stress, resveratrol protects against cardiac dysfunction. Interestingly, insulin appears to counteract the effects of resveratrol in reducing myocardial dysfunction following acute infarction.[106] More recently, the angiogenic potential of sirtuins, particularly in a diabetic context, is receiving increasing attention.[107]

Clinical heart failure is increasing both in incidence and importance as a consequence of multiple factors including an aging population, the increasing rates of obesity and diabetes, as well as the growing number of individuals who are surviving myocardial infarction following early and aggressive medical intervention. The multiple pathways which lead to chronic impairment of ventricular performance or cardiomyopathy encompass virtually all forms of heart disease. Therapies focusing on reducing the extent of damage following an ischemic event with and without subsequent reperfusion attempt to enhance the extent to which the residual myocardium can contribute to the mechanical work of the heart. The persistent abnormalities in myocyte contractility, particularly after remodeling has occurred, continue to be fertile areas of investigation. Studies using resveratrol in experimental models of cardiomyopathy are relatively few. Some focus on reversing specific conditions such as the myopathic changes resulting from chemotherapeutic or infectious agents.[108–110]

Diabetes, in addition to increasing the risk of myocardial infarction due to its atherogenic potential, can affect cardiomyocyte contractility directly impacting both systolic and diastolic function.[111–113] One of the major pathophysiologic abnormalities found diabetic-induced cardiomyopathy involves alterations in intracellular calcium resulting from reduced expression of sarcoplasmic reticulum calcium ATPase (SERCA2a). Reduced activity of SIRT1 contributes to the inhibition of SERCA2a and SIRT1 knockout mice are highly sensitive to diabetes-induced decline in SERCA2a mRNA levels in the heart.[114]

Resveratrol, by activating SIRT1, reverses cardiac dysfunction and restores SERCA2a expression in diabetic mice. Additionally, SIRT1 activation by resveratrol is known to induce manganese-SOD (Mn-SOD) mediated resistance to oxidative stress resulting in reduced fibrosis and improved cardiomyocyte survival in a chronic heart failure model.[115] Other studies have demonstrated the ability of resveratrol to prevent pathologic cardiac hypertrophy and contractile dysfunction in spontaneously hypertensive rats.[116] Ongoing investigations focusing on the impact of oxidative stress and reactive oxygen species on mitochondrial function suggest that strategies that improve mitochondrial energetics in heart failure might be productive avenues to determine the effectiveness of a number of sirtuin analogs.[117,118]

EFFECTS OF RESVERATROL ON ENDOTHELIAL CELL FUNCTION AND VASCULAR DISEASE

Vascular oxidative stress and inflammation is a major component of the manifestations of both diabetes and metabolic syndrome.[119] The low cardiovascular morbidity attributed to the Mediterranean population, often referred to as the "French Paradox", is partially attributed to the decreased vasculopathy seen in groups of individuals with a diet consisting of antioxidant phytonutrients including the polyphenols found in grapes and other plant-based foods. As a result, endothelial cell function in response to oxidative stress and inflammation has been under intense scrutiny recently and has helped fuel an entire industry focused on alternative and complementary medicine. The combined effects of obesity, insulin resistance, and aging on the cardiovascular system have enormous implications *vis-à-vis* the anticipated increased disease burden for vascular disease in the future.

Atherosclerosis, an inflammatory disease involving medium and large blood vessels, is known to be initiated through redox signaling in a series of complex biochemical reactions involving circulating LDLs, monocytes and platelets among other factors.[120] The subsequent formation of the characteristic fibro-lipid plaque in vessel walls, in addition to reducing the cross-sectional area and increasing resistance to blood flow, impairs the ability of vessels to constrict and relax; an integral characteristic of the body's ability to regulate perfusion to organs and tissues. Ongoing oxidative stress in blood vessel walls further impairs the vasorelaxant capacity of vascular beds and the contractile response to circulating catecholamines. Resveratrol has been shown to reverse the impaired vascular response in diabetic rat aortas when stimulated to contract by noradrenaline and phenylephrine.[121,122]

The treatment of human endothelial cells with high glucose decreases SIRT1 expression and, thus, activates p53 by increasing its acetylation creating functional abnormalities and endothelial cell apoptosis.[123] Adiponectin levels in serum are elevated in response to resveratrol and are associated with a decrease in circulating endothelial cells and their fragmentation.[124] These experiments also observed a reduction in TNF-α-induced ICAM-1, VCAM-1, and caspase 3 activities in endothelial cells and suggest a mechanistic role for heme oxygenase-1 (HO-1) and increased levels of carbon monoxide. Furthermore, resveratrol and other agents can reverse the effects of glycated serum albumin on vascular smooth muscle cells by inhibiting the upregulation of IL-8 through processes involving mitogen-activated protein kinases, NF-κB and NADPH oxidase.[125]

A hallmark of vascular function is the production of nitric oxide, an important protective molecule generated by eNOS which effectively transfers electrons from NADPH via flavins using L-arginine as substrate.[126] Compounds such as trans-resveratrol, which enhance NO production by increasing eNOS expression and preventing its uncoupling, are known to have beneficial effects on endothelial cells and vascular smooth muscle. One study surprisingly found that, in smooth muscle cells cultured from diabetic and normoglycemic rat aortas, exposure to resveratrol failed to produce an anti-inflammatory response and, in fact, increased the expression of iNOS when exposed to a cytokine mixture suggesting a pro-inflammatory effect in the setting of smooth muscle cell inflammation.[127] In general, however, diabetes-induced vasculopathy appears to be alleviated by resveratrol by reducing oxidative stress and increasing NO bioavailability.[128]

In light of the inherent risk factors associated with atherosclerotic cardiovascular and cerebrovascular disease associated with diabetes and the metabolic syndrome, procoagulant pathways are of crucial concern in preventing the catastrophic complications of stroke, myocardial infarction, and other ischemic conditions. In mammals, SIRT1 inhibition is associated with enhancement of TF expression and activity, a key trigger of coagulation, by increasing NF-κB/p65 activation in human endothelial cells.[129] By reducing TF production in endothelial cells, SIRT1 activation may prevent potentially dangerous intra-arterial thrombosis and its attendant consequences. In another study, resveratrol was convincingly found to significantly modulate adenine nucleotide hydrolysis in platelets, particularly in diabetic animals, another important regulator of coagulation.[130] While a number of molecules are being developed which increase SIRT1 activity, the so-called sirtuin activators, none of these synthetic compounds have been demonstrated to achieve the wide range of constituent effects found with resveratrol.[25]

RESVERATROL AND RENAL EFFECTS OF DIABETES

End-stage renal disease and the need for chronic hemodialysis in patients with diabetes generate considerable interest given the physical and economic implications it presents for society as a whole and the truncated survival of the individual patient. The impact of direct oxidative stress on nephrocytes has, at times, been overshadowed by the microvascular effects seen in diabetes. However, diabetes is known to have adverse effects, independent of endothelial function, on the glomerular apparatus resulting in impairment of renal function. Studies examining animals with diabetes-induced nephropathy show a reduction in many of the standard stress markers of oxidation in the kidney including lipid peroxidation and the activities of key antioxidant enzymes as well as attenuation of the usual findings of renal insufficiency.[131] Studies have shown the involvement of the AMPK pathway in the pathogenesis of diabetic nephropathy and have demonstrated that resveratrol has antiproliferative and antihypertrophic effects by activating AMPK resulting in reductions in urinary albumin excretion and plasma creatinine along with a decrease in renal hypertrophy without affecting blood glucose.[132] In addition, resveratrol ameliorated renal injury and improved Mn-SOD dysfunction via an AMPK/SIRT1-independent pathway.[133] Histologic examination of glomerular basement membrane and other structures have demonstrated the effectiveness of resveratrol in alleviating glomerulosclerosis in diabetic animals and increasing nephrin expression through TGF-β/smad and ERK1/2 inhibition.[134]

RESVERATROL IN NEUROPROTECTION

Neurologic complications from diabetes are largely related to cerebrovascular disease, including stroke, and are directly attributable to the changes seen in endothelial cells, platelets, and others in the cardiovascular and coagulation systems. However, direct changes occur on nerve cells from diabetes, affecting both the central and peripheral nervous systems causing significant, albeit under-recognized, disability. The neuroprotective actions of phytocompounds are increasingly being recognized both *in vitro* and *in vivo*.[135] A study of diabetic animals found significant evidence of oxidative stress in the brain.[136] Levels of lipid peroxidation, xanthine oxidase, nitric oxide, and glutathione were considerably elevated compared to controls in the hippocampus, the cortex, the cerebellum, the brainstem, and the spinal cord. Resveratrol potently reversed all indicators of oxidative stress to normal levels after 6 weeks of administration. Antioxidant properties were seen both in the hippocampus and the striatum; however, resveratrol was unable to reverse the lower hippocampal proliferation seen in diabetes.[137] Research examining the biochemical and genetic effects of sirtuins and similar modulating compounds in neurodegenerative conditions, frequently coexisting with diabetes, including Alzheimer's disease, are under way.[138]

Resveratrol appears to also have a beneficial effect on the inherently complex mechanisms involved in the regulation of feeding behaviors resulting in obesity and is attracting considerable attention from both biomedical as well as behavioral researchers in an effort to modulate caloric intake. For example, one single intraperitoneal injection, at a dose of 100 mg/kg, was able to reduce food intake in the ensuing 48 h by as much as 20%.[139] Its effects on memory and cognition and, in particular, age-related dementia remains to be determined.[140] However, preliminary studies show that resveratrol prevents diabetes-induced increases in acetylcholinesterase (AChE) activity in the brain known to result in memory impairment.[141] In these studies, improvement in memory was related to inhibition of AChE activity in many areas of the brain including the cerebral cortex, the hippocampus, the hypothalamus, and the cerebellum. Other research shows that resveratrol may interfere with purinergic and cholinergic neurotransmission by altering NTPDase, 5'-nucleotidase, and AChE in cortical synaptosomes.[142]

Peripheral neuropathy, as with other complications of diabetes, appears to be strongly associated with oxidative stress and other mechanisms of cell injury including AGE formation and lipid peroxidation.[143,144] As such, it appears to be another potential target for antioxidative strategies. Impairment of motor nerve conduction velocity and nerve blood flow in diabetic rats was improved with resveratrol after only 2 weeks of therapy. This study also demonstrated normalization of malondialdehyde and peroxynitrite levels and a marked reduction in DNA fragmentation in sciatic nerves documenting that the neuroprotective effects seen were mediated by a reduction in oxidative stress. Chong et al. showed both early and late reductions in oxidative stress and apoptosis by resveratrol in mammalian neurons through nicotinamidase- and sirtuin-mediated pathways.[145] Neuropathic pain is also an important consideration in diabetes and is often a severely disabling complication with few effective treatments. Despite an incomplete understanding of the mechanisms involved, polyphenolic phyloalexins appear to have antinociceptive effects which suggest a role for agents such as resveratrol in attenuating the associated pain and discomfort.[146-148]

Diabetic retinopathy, a dreadful complication, appears to have a multifactorial etiology including effects on endothelial as well as neuronal cells. Retinal ganglion cell death in diabetes appears to be mediated through apoptosis and elevated calmodulin-dependent protein kinase II (CaMKII).[149] This phenomenon was completely abolished following 4 weeks of oral therapy with resveratrol. Other studies exploring the effect of diabetes on retinal pigment epithelial cells have demonstrated the inhibition of connexin downregulation and improved gap junction intercellular communication with resveratrol in a dose-dependent fashion.[150]

RESVERATROL AND FAT METABOLISM

The constellation of abnormalities associated with the metabolic syndrome resulting in insulin resistance and elevated cardiovascular risk, poses a significant public health threat as a consequence of the obesity epidemic. The low-level, chronic inflammatory state found in obese individuals adds credence to the theory that oxidative stress is a major component of the metabolic syndrome.[151] Polyphenols appear to mitigate the cardio-metabolic consequences of this syndrome predominantly via its anti-inflammatory mechanisms.[152-154] Insulin resistance in adipose tissue is associated with the production of reactive oxygen species and a proinflammatory adipokine pattern that can be induced by protracted exposure to high concentrations of fatty acids.[155] This pattern is characterized by a decrease in adiponectin and increases in IL-6, IL-1B, COX-2, plasminogen activator inhibitor-1, and monocyte chemotactic protein-1 mRNA expression.[151] Exposure to resveratrol reverses these responses and reduces the generation of reactive oxygen species, at least partially, by increasing Fox01 protein levels and translocating FOX01 to the nucleus. Macrophage accumulation in adipose tissue is prevalent in obesity-induced diabetes and is induced by monocyte chemoattractant protein (MCP-1) as a result of certain cytokine profiles dominated by TNF-α.[156] Resveratrol inhibits the DNA binding activity of the NF-κB complex suppressing its transcriptional activity in adipocytes stimulated by TNF-α.[156,157]

The lipemia and accelerated atherosclerosis seen in diabetes is exacerbated by the dysregulation of lipid metabolism in the liver.[158] Resveratrol, by activating SIRT1 and AMPK, prevents the expression of fatty acid synthase and lipid accumulation in hepatocytes exposed to high glucose concentrations.[158–160] Moreover, in a model of hepatic steatosis, it inhibits TNF-α production, lipid peroxidation, and other signs of reduced oxidative stress.[161] In addition, resveratrol induces fatty acid oxidation in fibroblasts from patients with inherited disorders in mitochondrial fatty acid oxidation.[162]

These results suggest that polyphenols such as resveratrol can potentially impact the course of the metabolic syndrome significantly. However, while considerable interest exists in the use of an agent which can reduce the inflammatory nature of the metabolic syndrome, normalize the distorted lipid metabolism, and restore insulin resistance, no large-scale trials on humans have yet been carried out demonstrating the safety and efficacy of this strategy.[163,164]

OTHER BENEFICIAL EFFECTS

Studies involving the impact of diabetes on embryopathy and the physiology of the maternal–fetal interface in diabetes continue to explore mechanisms of impaired organogenesis and fetal injury resulting from oxidative stress and apoptosis. In one such study, diabetic rodents were shown to have reduced glutathione levels, increased thiol and lipid peroxidation as well as nearly three-fold rates of embryonic apoptosis compared to control.[165] Resveratrol reduced the incidence of embryonic maldevelopment and improved the metabolic profile of the dams with reduced serum glucose, cholesterol, and triglyceride levels. Some investigators have hypothesized a role for resveratrol and other SIRT1 activators in inducing immune tolerance at the maternal–fetal interface and other autoimmune conditions via their anti-inflammatory effects targeting NAD-dependent proteins.[166] In addition, numerous studies exist suggesting a role for resveratrol and related compounds in the treatment of a variety of neoplastic diseases both via mechanisms which accelerate cellular responses to DNA damage and which preserve genome integrity.[167–169] Other potential effects are beginning to be examined including the role of resveratrol in the prophylaxis and treatment of infectious diseases and other conditions.[170]

CONCLUSIONS

Polyphenolic compounds such as resveratrol possess a wide variety of biologic activity addressing many of the deleterious consequences of oxidative stress and inflammation found in diabetes mellitus and the metabolic syndrome. Many, but not all, of these effects are related to the ability of these agents to activate SIRT1 as well as the synergistic effects of insulin. Unfortunately, naturally occurring forms of these agents may not be sufficiently bioavailable to impact human disease. With increasing attention to this group of potential therapeutic agents, it is probable that synthetic analogs with improved pharmacokinetics and increased potency can result in the development of new ways to clinically treat this highly morbid and dangerous set of pathologic conditions.

References

1. WHO Expert Committee on Diabetes Mellitus: Second Report, World Health Organ. *Tech Rep Ser* 1980;**646**:1–80.
2. Zunino S. Type 2 diabetes and glycemic response to grapes or grape products. *J Nutr* 2009 Sep;**139**(9): 1794S–800S.
3. Narayan KM, Boyle JP, Geiss LS, Saaddine JB, Thompson TJ. Impact of recent increase in incidence on future diabetes burden: US, 2005-2050. *Diabetes Care* 2006;**29**(9):2114–6.
4. Burns J, Yokota T, Ashihara H, Lean MEJ, Crozier A. Plants foods and herbal sources of resveratrol. *J Agric Food Chem* 2002;**50**(11):3337–40.
5. Marques FZ, Markus MA, Morris BJ. Resveratrol: cellular actions of a potent natural chemical that

confers a diversity of health benefits. *Int J Biochem Cell Biol* 2009 Nov;**41**(11):2125–8.

6. Wu JM, Hsieh T. Resveratrol: A cardioprotective substance. *Ann N Y Acad Sci* 2011;**1215**:16–21.

7. Atten MJ, Attar BM, Milson T, Holian O. Resveratrol-induced inactivation of human gastric adenocarcinoma cells through a protein kinase C-mediated mechanism. *Biochem Pharmacol* 2001;**62**(10):1423–32.

8. Su HC, Hung LM, Chen JK. Resveratrol, a red wine antioxidant, possesses an insulin-like effect in streptozotocin-induced diabetic rats. *Am J Physiol Endocrinol Metab* 2006 Jun;**290**(6):E1339–46.

9. Balcerczyk A, Pirola L. Therapeutic potential of activators and inhibitors of sirtuins. *Biofactors* 2010 Sep;**36**(5):383–93.

10. Siemann EH, Creasy LL. Concentration of the phytoalexin resveratrol in wine. *Am J Enol Vitic* 1992;**43**:49–52.

11. Soleas GJ, Diamondis EP, Goldberg DM. Resveratrol: A molecule whose time has come? And gone? *Clinical Biochemistry* 1997;**30**(2):91–113.

12. Frémont L. Biological effects of resveratrol. *Life Sciences* 2000;**66**(8):663–73.

13. Lim CG, Fowler ZL, Hueller T, Schaffer S, Koffas MA. High-yield resveratrol production in engineered escherichia coli. *Appl Environ Microbiol* 2011 May;**77**(10):3451–60.

14. Kawaguchi K, Matsumoto T, Kumazawa Y. Effects of antioxidant polyphenols on TNF-alpha-related diseases. *Curr Top Med Chem* 2011;**11**(14):1767–79.

15. Zarse K, Schmeisser S, Birringer M, Falk E, Schmoll D, Ristow M. Differential effects of resveratrol and SRT1720 on lifespan of adult Caenorhabditis elegans. *Horm Metab Res* 2010 Nov;**42**(12):837–9.

16. Milne JC, Lambert PD, Schenk S, Carney DP, Smith JJ, Gagne DJ, Jin L, Boss O, Perni RB, Vu CB, Bemis JE, Xie R, Disch JS, Ng PY, Nunes JJ, Lynch AV, Yang H, Galonek H, Israelian K, Choy W, Iffland A, Lavu S, Medvedik O, Sinclair DA, Olefsky JM, Jirousek MR, Elliott PJ, Westphal CH. Small molecule activators of SIRT1 as therapeutics for the treatment of type 2 diabetes. *Nature* 2007 Nov 29;**450**(7170):712–6.

17. Jiang WJ. Sirtuins: novel targets for metabolic disease in drug development. *Biochem Biophys Res Commun* 2008 Aug 29;**373**(3):341–4.

18. Sasaki T, Maier B, Koclega KD, Chruszcz M, Gluba W, Stukenberg PT, Minor W, Scrable H. Phosphorylation regulates SIRT1 function. *PLoS One* 2008;**3**(12):e4020.

19. Koo SH, Montminy M. In vino veritas: a tale of two sirt1s? *Cell* 2006 Dec 15;**127**(6):1091–3.

20. Dittenhafer-Reed KE, Feldman JL, Denu JM. Catalysis and mechanistic insights into sirtuin activation. *Chembiochem* 2011 Jan 24;**12**(2):281–9.

21. Yang H, Baur JA, Chen A, Miller C, Adams JK, Kisielewski A, Howitz KT, Zipkin RE, Sinclair DA. Design and synthesis of compounds that extend yeast replicative lifespan. *Aging Cell* 2007 Feb;**6**(1):35–43. Erratum in: Aging Cell. 2007 Aug;**6**(4):593.

22. Ingram DK, Zhu M, Mamczarz J, Zou S, Lane MA, Roth GS, et al. Calorie restriction mimetics: an emerging research field. *Aging Cell* 2006;**5**(2):97–108.

23. Wenzel U. Nutrition, sirtuins and aging. *Genes Nutr* 2006 Jun;**1**(2):85–93.

24. Markus MA, Morris BJ. Resveratrol in prevention and treatment of common clinical conditions of aging. *Clin Interv Aging* 2008;**3**(2):331–9.

25. Camins A, Sureda FX, Junyent F, Verdaguer E, Folch J, Pelegri C, Vilaplana J, Beas-Zarate C, Pallàs M. Sirtuin activators: designing molecules to extend life span. *Biochim Biophys Acta* 2010 Oct-Dec;**1799**(10-12):740–9.

26. Mayers JR, Iliff BW, Swoap SJ. Resveratrol treatment in mice does not elicit the bradycardia and hypothermia associated with calorie restriction. *FASEB J* 2009 Apr;**23**(4):1032–40.

27. Baur JA. Resveratrol, sirtuins, and the promise of a DR mimetic. *Mech Ageing Dev* 2010 Apr;**131**(4):261–9.

28. Streppel MT, Ocke MC, Boshuizen HC, Kok FJ, Kromhout D. Long-term wine consumption is related to cardiovascular mortality and life expectancy independently of moderate alcohol intake: the Zutphen Study. *J Epidemiol Community Health* 2009;**63**:534–40.

29. Goldberg DM, Yan J, Soleas GJ. Absorption of three wine-related polyphenols in three different matrices by healthy subjects. *Clin Biochem* 2003;**36**(1):79–87.

30. Walle T, Hsieh F, DeLegge MH, Oatis Jr JE, Walle UK. *Drug Metab Dispos* 2004;**32**(12):1377–82.

31. Knutson MD, Leeuwenburgh C. Resveratrol and novel potent activators of SIRT1: effects on aging and age-related diseases. *Nutr Rev* 2008 Oct;**66**(10):591–6.

32. Sivakumar G, Medina-Bolivar F, Lay Jr JO, Dolan MC, Condori J, Grubbs SK, Wright SM, Baque MA, Lee EJ, Paek KY. Bioprocess and bioreactor: next generation technology for production of potential plant-based antidiabetic and antioxidant molecules. *Curr Med Chem* 2011;**18**(1):79–90.

33. Fröjdö S, Durand C, Pirola L. Metabolic effects of resveratrol in mammals—a link between improved insulin action and aging. *Curr Aging Sci* 2008 Dec;**1**(3):145–51.

34. Mattoo AK, Shukla V, Fatima T, Handa AK, Yachha SK. Genetic engineering to enhance

crop-based phytonutrients (nutraceuticals) to alleviate diet-related diseases. *Adv Exp Med Biol* 2010; **698**:122−43.

35. Pacholec M, Bleasdale JE, Chrunyk B, Cunningham D, Flynn D, Garofalo RS, Griffith D, Griffor M, Loulakis P, Pabst B, Qiu X, Stockman B, Thanabal V, Varghese A, Ward J, Withka J, Ahn K. SRT1720, SRT2183, SRT1460, and resveratrol are not direct activators of SIRT1. *J Biol Chem* 2010 Mar 12;**285**(11):8340−51.

36. Malik R, Kashyap A, Bansal K, Sharma P, Rayasam GV, Davis JA, Bora RS, Ray A, Saini KS. Comparative deacetylase activity of wild type and mutants of SIRT1. *Biochem Biophys Res Commun* 2010 Jan 1;**391**(1):739−43.

37. Elliott PJ, Jirousek M. Sirtuins: novel targets for metabolic disease. *Curr Opin Investig Drugs* 2008 Apr;**9**(4):371−8.

38. Rodrigo R, Miranda A, Vergara L. Modulation of endogenous antioxidant system by wine polyphenols in human disease. *Clin Chim Acta* 2011 Feb 20;**412**(5-6):410−24.

39. Harikumar KB, Aggarwal BB. Resveratrol: a multi-targeted agent for age-associated chronic diseases. *Cell Cycle* 2008 Apr 15;**7**(8):1020−35.

40. Urquiaga I, Leighton F. Plant polyphenol antioxidants and oxidative stress. *Biological Research* 2000;**33**(2):55−64.

41. Aribal-Kocatürk P, Kavas GO. Büyükkağnici DI. Pretreatment effect of resveratrol on streptozotocin-induced diabetes in rats. *Biol Trace Elem Res* 2007 Sep;**118**(3):244−9.

42. Ungvari Z, Sonntag WE, de Cabo R, Baur JA, Csiszar A. Mitochondrial protection by resveratrol. *Exerc Sport Sci Rev* 2011 Jul;**39**(3):128−32.

43. James JS. Resveratrol: why it matters in HIV. *AIDS Treat News* 2006 Oct;(420):3−5.

44. Roy M, Sinha D, Mukherjee S, Paul S, Bhattacharya RK. Protective effect of dietary phyto-chemicals against arsenite induced genotoxicity in mammalian V79 cells. *Indian J Exp Biol* 2008 Oct;**46**(10):690−7.

45. Csiszar A, Labinskyy N, Pinto JT, Ballabh P, Zhang H, Losonczy G, Pearson K, de Cabo R, Pacher P, Zhang C, Ungvari Z. Resveratrol induces mitochondrial biogenesis in endothelial cells. *Am J Physiol Heart Circ Physiol* 2009 Jul;**297**(1):H13−20.

46. Banks AS, Kon N, Knight C, Matsumoto M, Gutiér-rez-Juárez R, Rossetti L, Gu W, Accili D. SirT1 gain of function increases energy efficiency and prevents diabetes in mice. *Cell Metab* 2008 Oct;**8**(4):333−41.

47. Tsai SH, Lin Shiau SY, Lin JK. Suppression of nitric oxide synthase and the down regulation of the

activation of NF B in macrophages by resveratrol. *British Journal of Pharmacology* 1999;**126**(3):673−80.

48. Kavas GO, Aribal-Kocatürk P. Büyükkağnici DI. Resveratrol: is there any effect on healthy subject? *Biol Trace Elem Res* 2007 Sep;**118**(3):250−4.

49. Pendurthi UR, Williams T, Rao VM. Resveratrol, a polyphenolic compound found in wine, inhibits tissue factor expression in vascular cells. *Arterioscler Thromb Vasc Biol* 1999;**19**(2):419−26.

50. Fukuda S, Kaga S, Zhan L, Bagchi D, Das DK, Bertelli A, Maulik N. Resveratrol ameliorates myocardial damage by inducing vascular endothelial growth factor-angiogenesis and tyrosine kinase receptor Flk-1. *Cell Biochem Biophys* 2006;**44**(1):43−9.

51. Chaudhary N, Pfluger PT. Metabolic benefits from Sirt1 and Sirt1 activators. *Curr Opin Clin Nutr Metab Care* 2009 Jul;**12**(4):431−7.

52. Ghanim H, Sia CL, Abuaysheh S, Korzeniewski K, Patnaik P, Marumganti A, Chaudhuri A, Dandona P. An antiinflammatory and reactive oxygen species suppressive effects of an extract of Polygonum cuspidatum containing resveratrol. *J Clin Endocrinol Metab* 2010 Sep;**95**(9):E1−8.

53. Lee SM, Yang H, Tartar DM, Gao B, Luo X, Ye SQ, Zaghouani H, Fang D. Prevention and treatment of diabetes with resveratrol in a non-obese mouse model of type 1 diabetes. *Diabetologia* 2011 May;**54**(5): 1136−46.

54. Xie W, Du L. Diabetes is an inflammatory disease: evidence from traditional Chinese medicines. *Diabetes Obes Metab* 2011 Apr;**13**(4):289−301.

55. Sharma S, Chopra K, Kulkarni SK, Agrewala JN. Resveratrol and curcumin suppress immune response through CD28/CTLA-4 and CD80 co-stimulatory pathway. *Clin Exp Immunol* 2007 Jan;**147**(1):155−63.

56. Tsoupras AB, Fragopoulou E, Nomikos T, Iatrou C, Antonopoulou S, Demopoulos CA. Characterization of the de novo biosynthetic enzyme of platelet activating factor, DDT-insensitive cholinephospho-transferase, of human mesangial cells. *Mediators Inflamm* 2007;**2007**:27683.

57. Chan WH. Effect of resveratrol on high glucose-induced stress in human leukemia K562 cells. *J Cell Biochem* 2005 Apr 15;**94**(6):1267−79.

58. Hanhineva K, Törrönen R, Bondia-Pons I, Pekkinen J, Kolehmainen M, Mykkänen H, Poutanen K. Impact of dietary polyphenols on carbohydrate metabolism. *Int J Mol Sci* 2010 Mar 31;**11**(4):1365−402.

59. Szkudelski T, Szkudelska K. Anti-diabetic effects of resveratrol. *Ann N Y Acad Sci* 2011 Jan;**1215**:34−9.

60. Szkudelski T. Resveratrol-induced inhibition of insulin secretion from rat pancreatic islets: evidence

for pivotal role of metabolic disturbances. *Am J Physiol Endocrinol Metab* 2007 Oct;**293**(4):E901—7.

61. Youl E, Bardy G, Magous R, Cros G, Sejalon F, Virsolvy A, Richard S, Quignard JF, Gross R, Petit P, Bataille D, Oiry C. Quercetin potentiates insulin secretion and protects INS-1 pancreatic β-cells against oxidative damage via the ERK1/2 pathway. *Br J Pharmacol* 2010 Oct;**161**(4):799—814.

62. Berger J, Biswas C, Vicario PP, Strout HV, Saperstein R, Pilch PF. Decreased expression of the insulin-responsive glucose transporter in diabetes and fasting. *Nature* 1989 Jul 6;**340**(6228):70—2.

63. Garvey WT, Huecksteadt TP, Birnbaum MJ. Pre-translational suppression of an insulin-responsive glucose transporter in rats with diabetes mellitus. *Science* 1989 Jul 7;**245**(4913):60—3.

64. Nikolaidis LA, Sturzu A, Stolarski C, Elahi D, Shen YT, Shannon RP. The development of myocardial insulin resistance in conscious dogs with advanced dilated cardiomyopathy. *Cardiovasc Res* 2004 Feb 1;**61**(2):297—306.

65. Bryant NJ, Govers R, James DE. Regulated transport of the glucose transporter GLUT4. *Nat Rev Mol Cell Biol* 2002 Apr;**3**(4):267—77.

66. Gustavsson J, Parpal S, Stralfors P. Insulin-stimulated glucose uptake involves the transition of glucose transporters to a caveolae-rich fraction within the plasma membrane: implications for type II diabetes. *Mol Med* 1996 May;**2**(3):367—72.

67. Park CE, Kim MJ, Lee JH, Min BI, Bae H, Choe W, Kim SS, Ha J. Resveratrol stimulates glucose transport in C2C12 myotubes by activating AMP-activated protein kinase. *Exp Mol Med* 2007 Apr 30;**39**(2):222—9.

68. Zhang F, Sun C, Wu J, He C, Ge X, Huang W, Zou Y, Chen X, Qi W, Zhai Q. Combretastatin A-4 activates AMP-activated protein kinase and improves glucose metabolism in db/db mice. *Pharmacol Res* 2008 Apr;**57**(4):318—23.

69. Um JH, Park SJ, Kang H, Yang S, Foretz M, McBurney MW, Kim MK, Viollet B, Chung JH. AMP-activated protein kinase-deficient mice are resistant to the metabolic effects of resveratrol. *Diabetes* 2010 Mar;**59**(3):554—63.

70. Rutter GA. Da Silva Xavier G, Leclerc I. Roles of 5'-AMP-activated protein kinase (AMPK) in mammalian glucose homoeostasis. *Biochem J* 2003 Oct 1;**375**(Pt 1):1—16.

71. Chen ZP, Mitchelhill KI, Michell BJ, Stapleton D, Rodriguez-Crespo I, Witters LA, et al. AMP-activated protein kinase phosphorylation of endothelial NO synthase. *FEBS Lett* 1999 Jan 29;**443**(3):285—9.

72. Li J, Hu X, Selvakumar P, Russell 3rd RR, Cushman SW, Holman GD, et al. Role of the nitric oxide pathway in AMPK-mediated glucose uptake and GLUT4 translocation in heart muscle. *Am J Physiol Endocrinol Metab* 2004 Nov;**287**(5):E834—41.

73. Thirunavukkarasu M, Penumathsa SV, Koneru S, Juhasz B, Zhan L, Otani H, et al. Resveratrol alleviates cardiac dysfunction in streptozotocin-induced diabetes: Role of nitric oxide, thioredoxin, and heme oxygenase. *Free Radic Biol Med* 2007 Sep 1;**43**(5):720—9.

74. Sun C, Zhang F, Ge X, Yan T, Chen X, Shi X, Zhai Q. SIRT1 improves insulin sensitivity under insulin-resistant conditions by repressing PTP1B. *Cell Metab* 2007 Oct;**6**(4):307—19.

75. de Kreutzenberg SV, Ceolotto G, Papparella I, Bortoluzzi A, Semplicini A, Dalla Man C, Cobelli C, Fadini GP, Avogaro A. Downregulation of the longevity-associated protein sirtuin 1 in insulin resistance and metabolic syndrome: potential biochemical mechanisms. *Diabetes* 2010 Apr;**59**(4):1006—15.

76. Deng JY, Hsieh PS, Huang JP, Lu LS, Hung LM. Activation of estrogen receptor is crucial for resveratrol-stimulating muscular glucose uptake via both insulin-dependent and -independent pathways. *Diabetes* 2008 Jul;**57**(7):1814—23.

77. Sharma S, Misra CS, Arumugam S, Roy S, Shah V, Davis JA, Shirumalla RK, Ray A. Antidiabetic activity of resveratrol, a known SIRT1 activator in a genetic model for type-2 diabetes. *Phytother Res* 2011 Jan;**25**(1):67—73.

78. Nakae J, Cao Y, Daitoku H, Fukamizu A, Ogawa W, Yano Y, Hayashi Y. The LXXLL motif of murine forkhead transcription factor FoxO1 mediates Sirt1-dependent transcriptional activity. *J Clin Invest* 2006 Sep;**116**(9):2473—83.

79. Palsamy P, Subramanian S. Resveratrol, a natural phytoalexin, normalizes hyperglycemia in streptozotocin-nicotinamide induced experimental diabetic rats. *Biomed Pharmacother* 2008 Nov;**62**(9):598—605.

80. Lee JH, Song MY, Song EK, Kim EK, Moon WS, Han MK, Park JW, Kwon KB, Park BH. Overexpression of SIRT1 protects pancreatic beta-cells against cytokine toxicity by suppressing the nuclear factor-kappaB signaling pathway. *Diabetes* 2009 Feb;**58**(2):344—51.

81. Wei L, Jiang P, Xu W, Li H, Zhang H, Yan L, Chan-Park MB, Liu XW, Tang K, Mu Y, Pervushin K. The molecular basis of distinct aggregation pathways of islet amyloid polypeptide. *J Biol Chem* 2011 Feb 25;**286**(8):6291—300.

82. Radovan D, Opitz N, Winter R. Fluorescence microscopy studies on islet amyloid polypeptide fibrillation at heterogeneous and cellular membrane

interfaces and its inhibition by resveratrol. *FEBS Lett* 2009 May 6;**583**(9):1439—45.

83. Evers F, Jeworrek C, Tiemeyer S, Weise K, Sellin D, Paulus M, Struth B, Tolan M, Winter R. Elucidating the mechanism of lipid membrane-induced IAPP fibrillogenesis and its inhibition by the red wine compound resveratrol: a synchrotron X-ray reflectivity study. *J Am Chem Soc* 2009 Jul 15;**131**(27): 9516—21.

84. Mishra R, Sellin D, Radovan D, Gohlke A, Winter R. Inhibiting islet amyloid polypeptide fibril formation by the red wine compound resveratrol. *Chembiochem* 2009 Feb 13;**10**(3):445—9.

85. Szkudelski T. The insulin-suppressive effect of resveratrol — an in vitro and in vivo phenomenon. *Life Sci* 2008 Feb 13;**82**(7-8):430—5.

86. Chi TC, Chen WP, Chi TL, Kuo TF, Lee SS, Cheng JT, Su MJ. Phosphatidylinositol-3-kinase is involved in the antihyperglycemic effect induced by resveratrol in streptozotocin-induced diabetic rats. *Life Sci* 2007 Apr 10;**80**(18):1713—20.

87. Chen WP, Chi TC, Chuang LM, Su MJ. Resveratrol enhances insulin secretion by blocking K(ATP) and K(V) channels of beta cells. *Eur J Pharmacol* 2007 Jul 30;**568**(1-3):269—77.

88. Ramadori G, Gautron L, Fujikawa T, Vianna CR, Elmquist JK, Coppari R. Central administration of resveratrol improves diet-induced diabetes. *Endocrinology* 2009 Dec;**150**(12):5326—33.

89. Palsamy P, Sivakumar S, Subramanian S. Resveratrol attenuates hyperglycemia-mediated oxidative stress, proinflammatory cytokines and protects hepatocytes ultrastructure in streptozotocin-nicotinamide-induced experimental diabetic rats. *Chem Biol Interact* 2010 Jul 30;**186**(2):200—10.

90. Lv L, Shao X, Wang L, Huang D, Ho CT, Sang S. Stilbene glucoside from Polygonum multiflorum Thunb.: a novel natural inhibitor of advanced glycation end product formation by trapping of methylglyoxal. *J Agric Food Chem* 2010 Feb 24;**58**(4):2239—45.

91. Zhang Y, Luo Z, Ma L, Xu Q, Yang Q, Si L. Resveratrol prevents the impairment of advanced glycosylation end products (AGE) on macrophage lipid homeostasis by suppressing the receptor for AGE via peroxisome proliferator-activated receptor gamma activation. *Int J Mol Med* 2010 May;**25**(5): 729—34.

92. Li BY, Li XL, Cai Q, Gao HQ, Cheng M, Zhang JH, Wang JF, Yu F, Zhou RH. Induction of lactadherin mediates the apoptosis of endothelial cells in response to advanced glycation end products and protective effects of grape seed procyanidin B2 and resveratrol. *Apoptosis* 2011 Jul;**16**(7):732—45.

93. Resmi H. The combination of bortezomib and resveratrol may prevent muscle wasting in diabetes. *Med Hypotheses* 2011 Feb;**76**(2):291—2.

94. Tisdale MJ. The ubiquitin-proteasome pathway as a therapeutic target for muscle wasting. *J Support Oncol* 2005 May-Jun;**3**(3):209—17.

95. Dirks Naylor AJ. Cellular effects of resveratrol in skeletal muscle. *Life Sci* 2009 May 8;**84**(19-20):637—40.

96. Wang N, Ko SH, Chai W, Li G, Barrett EJ, Tao L, Cao W, Liu Z. Resveratrol recruits rat muscle microvasculature via a nitric oxide-dependent mechanism that is blocked by TNFα. *Am J Physiol Endocrinol Metab* 2011 Jan;**300**(1):E195—201.

97. da-Silva WS, Harney JW, Kim BW, Li J, Bianco SD, Crescenzi A, Christoffolete MA, Huang SA, Bianco AC. The small polyphenolic molecule kaempferol increases cellular energy expenditure and thyroid hormone activation. *Diabetes* 2007 Mar;**56**(3): 767—76.

98. Kroon PA, Iyer A, Chunduri P, Chan V, Brown L. The cardiovascular nutrapharmacology of resveratrol: pharmacokinetics, molecular mechanisms and therapeutic potential. *Curr Med Chem* 2010;**17**(23):2442—55.

99. Bravo L. Polyphenols: chemistry, dietary sources, metabolism, and nutritional significance. *Nutrition reviews* 1998;**56**(11):317—33.

100. Zhang C. Cardiovascular physiology at the bench for application in the clinic. *World J Cardiol* 2011 Feb 26;**3**(2):59—64.

101. Penumathsa SV, Maulik N. Resveratrol: a promising agent in promoting cardioprotection against coronary heart disease. *Can J Physiol Pharmacol* 2009 Apr;**87**(4):275—86.

102. Penumathsa SV, Thirunavukkarasu M, Zhan L, Maulik G, Menon VP, Bagchi D, Maulik N. Resveratrol enhances GLUT-4 translocation to the caveolar lipid raft fractions through AMPK/Akt/eNOS signalling pathway in diabetic myocardium. *J Cell Mol Med* 2008 Dec;**12**(6A):2350—61. Erratum in: J Cell Mol Med. 2010 Oct;**14**(10):2539.

103. Sulaiman M, Matta MJ, Sunderesan NR, Gupta MP, Periasamy M, Gupta M. Resveratrol, an activator of SIRT1, upregulates sarcoplasmic calcium ATPase and improves cardiac function in diabetic cardiomyopathy. *Am J Physiol Heart Circ Physiol* 2010 Mar;**298**(3): H833—43.

104. Ungvari Z, Bagi Z, Feher A, Recchia FA, Sonntag WE, Pearson K, de Cabo R, Csiszar A. Resveratrol confers endothelial protection via activation of the antioxidant transcription factor Nrf2. *Am J Physiol Heart Circ Physiol* 2010 Jul;**299**(1):H18—24.

105. Zhang H, Morgan B, Potter BJ, Ma L, Dellsperger KC, Ungvari Z, Zhang C. Resveratrol improves left

ventricular diastolic relaxation in type 2 diabetes by inhibiting oxidative/nitrative stress: in vivo demonstration with magnetic resonance imaging. *Am J Physiol Heart Circ Physiol* 2010 Oct;**299**(4):H985–94.

106. Huang JP, Huang SS, Deng JY, Chang CC, Day YJ, Hung LM. Insulin and resveratrol act synergistically, preventing cardiac dysfunction in diabetes, but the advantage of resveratrol in diabetics with acute heart attack is antagonized by insulin. *Free Radic Biol Med* 2010 Dec 1;**49**(11):1710–21.

107. Wykrzykowska JJ, Bianchi C, Sellke FW. Impact of aging on the angiogenic potential of the myocardium: implications for angiogenic therapies with emphasis on sirtuin agonists. *Recent Pat Cardiovasc Drug Discov* 2009 Jun;**4**(2):119–32.

108. Yoshida Y, Shioi T, Izumi T. Resveratrol ameliorates experimental autoimmune myocarditis. *Circ J* 2007 Mar;**71**(3):397–404.

109. Tatlidede E, Sehirli O, Velioğlu-Oğünc A, Cetinel S, Yeğen BC, Yarat A, Süleymanoğlu S, Sener G. Resveratrol treatment protects against doxorubicin-induced cardiotoxicity by alleviating oxidative damage. *Free Radic Res* 2009 Mar;**43**(3):195–205.

110. Wang ZP, Hua YM, Zhang X, Wang YB, Shi XQ, Li MY. [Effect of resveratrol on myocardial fibrosis in mice with chronic viral myocarditis]. *Zhongguo Dang Dai Er Ke Za Zhi* 2009 Apr;**11**(4):291–5. Chinese.

111. Galderisi M, Anderson KM, Wilson PW, Levy D. Echocardiographic evidence for the existence of a distinct diabetic cardiomyopathy (the Framingham Heart Study). *Am J Cardiol* 1991 Jul 1;**68**(1):85–9.

112. Mizushige K, Yao L, Noma T, Kiyomoto H, Yu Y, Hosomi N, Ohmori K, Matsuo H. Alteration in left ventricular diastolic filling and accumulation of myocardial collagen at insulin-resistant prediabetic stage of a type II diabetic rat model. *Circulation* 2000 Feb 29;**101**(8):899–907.

113 Regan TJ, Lyons MM, Ahmed SS, GE Levinson, Oldewurtel HA, Ahmad MR, Haider B. Evidence for cardiomyopathy in familial diabetes mellitus. *J Clin Invest* 1997 oct;**60**(4):884–99.

114. Sulaiman M, Matta MJ, Sunderesan NR, Gupta MP, Periasamy M, Gupta M. Resveratrol, an activator of SIRT1, upregulates sarcoplasmic calcium ATPase and improves cardiac function in diabetic cardiomyopathy. *Am J Physiol Heart Circ Physiol* 2010 Mar;**298**(3):H833–43.

115. Tanno M, Kuno A, Yano T, Miura T, Hisahara S, Ishikawa S, Shimamoto K, Horio Y. Induction of manganese superoxide dismutase by nuclear translocation and activation of SIRT1 promotes cell survival in chronic heart failure. *J Biol Chem* 2010 Mar 12;**285**(11):8375–82.

116. Thandapilly SJ, Wojciechowski P, Behbahani J, Louis XL, Yu L, Juric D, Kopilas MA, Anderson HD, Netticadan T. Resveratrol prevents the development of pathological cardiac hypertrophy and contractile dysfunction in the SHR without lowering blood pressure. *Am J Hypertens* 2010 Feb;**23**(2):192–6.

117. Schwartz DR, Sack MN. Targeting the mitochondria to augment myocardial protection. *Curr Opin Pharmacol* 2008 Apr;**8**(2):160–5.

118. Addabbo F, Montagnani M, Goligorsky MS. Mitochondria and reactive oxygen species. *Hypertension* 2009 Jun;**53**(6):885–92.

119. Labinskyy N, Csiszar A, Veress G, Stef G, Pacher P, Oroszi G, Wu J, Ungvari Z. Vascular dysfunction in aging: potential effects of resveratrol, an anti-inflammatory phytoestrogen. *Curr Med Chem* 2006;**13**(9): 989–96.

120. Schwartz CJ, Valente AJ, Sprague EA, Kelley JL, Cayatte AJ, Mowery J. Atherosclerosis. Potential targets for stabilization and regression. *Circulation* Dec 1992;**86**(Suppl. 6):III117–23.

121. Silan C. The effects of chronic resveratrol treatment on vascular responsiveness of streptozotocin-induced diabetic rats. *Biol Pharm Bull* 2008 May;**31**(5):897–902.

122. Roghani M, Baluchnejadmojarad T. Mechanisms underlying vascular effect of chronic resveratrol in streptozotocin-diabetic rats. *Phytother Res* 2010 Jun;**24**(Suppl. 2):S148–54. Erratum in: Phytother Res. 2010 Jun;24 Suppl. 2:S233–4.

123. Orimo M, Minamino T, Miyauchi H, Tateno K, Okada S, Moriya J, Komuro I. Protective role of SIRT1 in diabetic vascular dysfunction. *Arterioscler Thromb Vasc Biol* 2009 Jun;**29**(6):889–94.

124. Rodella LF, Vanella L, Peterson SJ, Drummond G, Rezzani R, Falck JR, Abraham NG. Heme oxygenase-derived carbon monoxide restores vascular function in type 1 diabetes. *Drug Metab Lett* 2008 Dec;**2**(4):290–300.

125. Choi KH, Park JW, Kim HY, Kim YH, Kim SM, Son YH, Park YC, Eo SK, Kim K. Cellular factors involved in CXCL8 expression induced by glycated serum albumin in vascular smooth muscle cells. *Atherosclerosis* 2010 Mar;**209**(1):58–65.

126. Förstermann U, Li H. Therapeutic effect of enhancing endothelial nitric oxide synthase (eNOS) expression and preventing eNOS uncoupling. *Br J Pharmacol* 2011 Sep;**164**(2):213–23.

127. Cignarella A, Minici C, Bolego C, Pinna C, Sanvito P, Gaion RM, Puglisi L. Potential pro-inflammatory action of resveratrol in vascular smooth muscle cells from normal and diabetic rats. *Nutr Metab Cardiovasc Dis* 2006 Jul;**16**(5):322–9.

128. Akar F, Pektas MB, Tufan C, Soylemez S, Sepici A, Ulus AT, Gokalp B, Ozturk K, Surucu HS. Resveratrol shows vasoprotective effect reducing oxidative stress without affecting metabolic disturbances in insulin-dependent diabetes of rabbits. *Cardiovasc Drugs Ther* 2011 Apr;**25**(2):119−31.

129. Breitenstein A, Stein S, Holy EW, Camici GG, Lohmann C, Akhmedov A, Spescha R, Elliott PJ, Westphal CH, Matter CM, Lüscher TF, Tanner FC. Sirt1 inhibition promotes in vivo arterial thrombosis and tissue factor expression in stimulated cells. *Cardiovasc Res* 2011 Feb 1;**89**(2):464−72.

130. Schmatz R, Schetinger MR, Spanevello RM, Mazzanti CM, Stefanello N, Maldonado PA, Gutierres J, Corrêa Mde C, Girotto E, Moretto MB, Morsch VM. Effects of resveratrol on nucleotide degrading enzymes in streptozotocin-induced diabetic rats. *Life Sci* 2009 Mar 13;**84**(11-12):345−50.

131. Sharma S, Anjaneyulu M, Kulkarni SK, Chopra K. Resveratrol, a polyphenolic phytoalexin, attenuates diabetic nephropathy in rats. *Pharmacology* 2006;**76**(2):69−75.

132. Ding DF, You N, Wu XM, Xu JR, Hu AP, Ye XL, Zhu Q, Jiang XQ, Miao H, Liu C, Lu YB. Resveratrol attenuates renal hypertrophy in early-stage diabetes by activating AMPK. *Am J Nephrol* 2010;**31**(4): 363−74.

133. Kitada M, Kume S, Imaizumi N, Koya D. Resveratrol improves oxidative stress and protects against diabetic nephropathy through normalization of Mn-SOD dysfunction in AMPK/SIRT1-independent pathway. *Diabetes* 2011 Feb;**60**(2):634−43.

134. Chen KH, Hung CC, Hsu HH, Jing YH, Yang CW, Chen JK. Resveratrol ameliorates early diabetic nephropathy associated with suppression of augmented TGF-β/smad and ERK1/2 signaling in streptozotocin-induced diabetic rats. *Chem Biol Interact* 2011 Mar 15;**190**(1):45−53.

135. Albani D, Polito L, Forloni G. Sirtuins as novel targets for Alzheimer's disease and other neurodegenerative disorders: experimental and genetic evidence. *J Alzheimers Dis* 2010;**19**(1):11−26.

136. Ates O, Cayli SR, Yucel N, Altinoz E, Kocak A, Durak MA, Turkoz Y, Yologlu S. Central nervous system protection by resveratrol in streptozotocin-induced diabetic rats. *J Clin Neurosci* 2007 Mar;**14**(3): 256−60.

137. Venturini CD, Merlo S, Souto AA, Fernandes Mda C, Gomez R, Rhoden CR. Resveratrol and red wine function as antioxidants in the nervous system without cellular proliferative effects during experimental diabetes. *Oxid Med Cell Longev* 2010 Nov-Dec; **3**(6):434−41.

138. Albani D, Polito L, Signorini A, Forloni G. Neuroprotective properties of resveratrol in different neurodegenerative disorders. *Biofactors* 2010 Sep;**36**(5):370−6.

139. Kim SJ, Lee YH, Han MD, Mar W, Kim WK, Nam KW. Resveratrol, purified from the stem of Vitis coignetiae Pulliat, inhibits food intake in C57BL/6J Mice. *Arch Pharm Res* 2010 May;**33**(5):775−80.

140. Daffner KR. Promoting successful cognitive aging: a comprehensive review. *J Alzheimers Dis* 2010;**19**(4): 1101−22.

141. Schmatz R, Mazzanti CM, Spanevello R, Stefanello N, Gutierres J, Corrêa M, da Rosa MM, Rubin MA, Chitolina Schetinger MR, Morsch VM. Resveratrol prevents memory deficits and the increase in acetylcholinesterase activity in streptozotocin-induced diabetic rats. *Eur J Pharmacol* 2009 May 21;**610**(1-3):42−8.

142. Schmatz R, Mazzanti CM, Spanevello R, Stefanello N, Gutierres J, Maldonado PA, Corrêa M, da Rosa CS, Becker L, Bagatini M, Gonçalves JF, Jaques Jdos S, Schetinger MR, Morsch VM. Ectonucleotidase and acetylcholinesterase activities in synaptosomes from the cerebral cortex of streptozotocin-induced diabetic rats and treated with resveratrol. *Brain Res Bull* 2009 Dec 16;**80**(6):371−6.

143. Kumar A, Sharma SS. NF-kappaB inhibitory action of resveratrol: a probable mechanism of neuroprotection in experimental diabetic neuropathy. *Biochem Biophys Res Commun* 2010 Apr 2;**394**(2):360−5.

144. Kumar A, Kaundal RK, Iyer S, Sharma SS. Effects of resveratrol on nerve functions, oxidative stress and DNA fragmentation in experimental diabetic neuropathy. *Life Sci* 2007 Mar 6;**80**(13):1236−44.

145. Chong ZZ, Maiese K. Enhanced tolerance against early and late apoptotic oxidative stress in mammalian neurons through nicotinamidase and sirtuin mediated pathways. *Curr Neurovasc Res* 2008 Aug;**5**(3):159−70.

146. Sharma SS, Kumar A, Arora M, Kaundal RK. Neuroprotective potential of combination of resveratrol and 4-amino 1,8 naphthalimide in experimental diabetic neuropathy: focus on functional, sensorimotor and biochemical changes. *Free Radic Res* 2009 Apr;**43**(4):400−8.

147. Sharma S, Kulkarni SK, Chopra K. Effect of resveratrol, a polyphenolic phytoalexin, on thermal hyperalgesia in a mouse model of diabetic neuropathic pain. *Fundam Clin Pharmacol* 2007 Feb;**21**(1):89−94.

148. Sharma S, Chopra K, Kulkarni SK. Effect of insulin and its combination with resveratrol or curcumin in attenuation of diabetic neuropathic pain: participation of nitric oxide and TNF-alpha. *Phytother Res* 2007 Mar;**21**(3):278−83.

149. Kim YH, Kim YS, Kang SS, Cho GJ, Choi WS. Resveratrol inhibits neuronal apoptosis and elevated Ca2+/calmodulin-dependent protein kinase II activity in diabetic mouse retina. *Diabetes* 2010 Jul;**59**(7):1825−35.

150. Losso JN, Truax RE, Richard G. Trans-resveratrol inhibits hyperglycemia-induced inflammation and connexin downregulation in retinal pigment epithelial cells. *J Agric Food Chem* 2010 Jul 28;**58**(14):8246−52.

151. Gonzales AM, Orlando RA. Curcumin and resveratrol inhibit nuclear factor-kappaB-mediated cytokine expression in adipocytes. *Nutr Metab (Lond)* 2008 Jun 12;**5**:17.

152. Sadruddin S, Arora R. Resveratrol: biologic and therapeutic implications. *J Cardiometab Syndr* 2009; **4**(2):102−6. Spring.

153. Beaudeux JL, Nivet-Antoine V, Giral P. Resveratrol: a relevant pharmacological approach for the treatment of metabolic syndrome? *Curr Opin Clin Nutr Metab Care* 2010 Nov;**13**(6):729−36.

154. Kang L, Heng W, Yuan A, Baolin L, Fang H. Resveratrol modulates adipokine expression and improves insulin sensitivity in adipocytes: Relative to inhibition of inflammatory responses. *Biochimie* 2010 Jul;**92**(7):789−96.

155. Subauste AR, Burant CF. Role of FoxO1 in FFA-induced oxidative stress in adipocytes. *Am J Physiol Endocrinol Metab* 2007 Jul;**293**(1):E159−64.

156. Zhu J, Yong W, Wu X, Yu Y, Lv J, Liu C, Mao X, Zhu Y, Xu K, Han X, Liu C. Anti-inflammatory effect of resveratrol on TNF-alpha-induced MCP-1 expression in adipocytes. *Biochem Biophys Res Commun* 2008 May 2;**369**(2):471−7.

157. McCarty MF. Potential utility of natural polyphenols for reversing fat-induced insulin resistance. *Med Hypotheses* 2005;**64**(3):628−35.

158. Hou X, Xu S, Maitland-Toolan KA, Sato K, Jiang B, Ido Y, Lan F, Walsh K, Wierzbicki M, Verbeuren TJ, Cohen RA, Zang M. SIRT1 regulates hepatocyte lipid metabolism through activating AMP-activated protein kinase. *J Biol Chem* 2008 Jul 18;**283**(29): 20015−26.

159. Ponugoti B, Kim DH, Xiao Z, Smith Z, Miao J, Zang M, Wu SY, Chiang CM, Veenstra TD, Kemper JK. SIRT1 deacetylates and inhibits SREBP-1C activity in regulation of hepatic lipid metabolism. *J Biol Chem* 2010 Oct 29;**285**(44):33959−70.

160. Colak Y, Ozturk O, Senates E, Tuncer I, Yorulmaz E, Adali G, Doganay L, Enc FY. SIRT1 as a potential therapeutic target for treatment of nonalcoholic fatty liver disease. *Med Sci Monit* 2011 May 2;(5):17. HY5-9.

161. Bujanda L, Hijona E, Larzabal M, Beraza M, Aldazabal P, García-Urkia N, Sarasqueta C, Cosme A, Irastorza B, González A, Arenas Jr JI. Resveratrol inhibits nonalcoholic fatty liver disease in rats. *BMC Gastroenterol* 2008 Sep 9;**8**:40.

162. Bastin J, Lopes-Costa A, Djouadi F. Exposure to resveratrol triggers pharmacological correction of fatty acid utilization in human fatty acid oxidation-deficient fibroblasts. *Hum Mol Genet* 2011 May 15;**20**(10):2048−57.

163. Sonnett TE, Levien TL, Gates BJ, Robinson JD, Campbell RK. Diabetes mellitus, inflammation, obesity: proposed treatment pathways for current and future therapies. *Ann Pharmacother* 2010 Apr;**44**(4):701−11.

164. Szkudelska K, Szkudelski T. Resveratrol, obesity and diabetes. *Eur J Pharmacol* 2010 Jun 10;**635**(1-3):1−8. Epub 2010 Mar 19. Review.

165. Singh CK, Kumar A, Hitchcock DB, Fan D, Goodwin R, Lavoie HA, Nagarkatti P, Dipette DJ, Singh US. Resveratrol prevents embryonic oxidative stress and apoptosis associated with diabetic embryopathy and improves glucose and lipid profile of diabetic dam. *Mol Nutr Food Res*; 2011 Jan 20. doi:10.1002/mnfr.201000457.

166. Penberthy WT. Pharmacological targeting of IDO-mediated tolerance for treating autoimmune disease. *Curr Drug Metab* 2007 Apr;**8**(3):245−66.

167. Wang RH, Sengupta K, Li C, Kim HS, Cao L, Xiao C, Kim S, Xu X, Zheng Y, Chilton B, Jia R, Zheng ZM, Appella E, Wang XW, Ried T, Deng CX. Impaired DNA damage response, genome instability, and tumorigenesis in SIRT1 mutant mice. *Cancer Cell* 2008 Oct 7;**14**(4):312−23.

168. Wang RH, Zheng Y, Kim HS, Xu X, Cao L, Luhasen T, Lee MH, Xiao C, Vassilopoulos A, Chen W, Gardner K, Man YG, Hung MC, Finkel T, Deng CX. Interplay among BRCA1, SIRT1, and Survivin during BRCA1-associated tumorigenesis. *Mol Cell* 2008 Oct 10;**32**(1):11−20.

169. Shankar S, Singh G, Srivastava RK. Chemoprevention by resveratrol: molecular mechanisms and therapeutic potential. *Front Biosci* 2007 Sep 1; **12**:4839−54.

170. Lu CC, Lai HC, Hsieh SC, Chen JK. Resveratrol ameliorates Serratia Apr;**83**(4):1028−37.

CHAPTER

34

Meal Plans for Diabetics: Caloric Intake, Calorie Counting, and Glycemic Index

Paulin Moszczynski*, Jan A. Rutowski†

*Malopolska University, Brzesko, Poland †E. Szczeklic's Specialistic Hospital, Tarnow, Poland, and Scientific Committee of the EAHP in Brussels, Belgium

INTRODUCTION

Major causes of morbidity and mortality in the world are related to poor diet and a sedentary lifestyle. Many of the cancers common in the Western world, including colon, prostate, and breast cancers, are thought to relate to dietary habits.[1] This process is very complex, genetically determined by the production of various hormones, neurotransmitters, the development of sensory organs, the influence of environmental factors, culture, and knowledge about the value of such food. A child in the selection of food is primarily guided by its flavor, aroma, color, and appearance, rather than

nutritional value. That is why it is so important for the nutritional value of food products to be associated with subjective values experienced by the consumer, which ensures the quality of life. Profound secular changes in the food environment and eating habits may play an important role in consumer health. In particular, consumption of foods prepared outside the home has greatly increased. The data from the prospective Black Women's Health Study revealed that among 44,072 participants aged 30–69 years and free of diabetes at baseline, 2,873 incident cases of type 2 diabetes occurred during 10 years of follow-up. Consumption of restaurant meals such as hamburgers, fried

Nutritional and Therapeutic Interventions for Diabetes and Metabolic Syndrome
DOI: 10.1016/B978-0-12-385083-6.00034-6

431

chicken, fried fish, and Chinese food were independently associated with an increased risk of type 2 diabetes. Control for body mass index (BMI) greatly reduced the estimates, which suggests that the associations are mediated through weight gain and obesity.[2]

Recommendations for energy intake include consideration of the physical activity level of each individual, and strong evidence indicates that the current level of calorie intake is too high, given physical activity levels in the US.[3] The Recommended Dietary Allowance (RDA) for carbohydrate is set at 130 g/d for adults and children based on the average minimum amount of glucose utilized by the brain. The median intake of carbohydrates is approximately 220–330 g/d for men and 180–230 g/d for women. Thus, the types of carbohydrates supplied and source of their origin play a key role. These are the factors affecting the rate of absorption and glycemic response of the organism to the ingested carbohydrates. The importance of these elements is reflected in the concept of glycemic index (GI) foods.[4–6] The consumption of 5 energy % from protein at the expense of 5 energy % from carbohydrate or fat increased diabetes risk by about 30%.[7]

CALORIE INTAKE AND ENERGY BALANCE

Energy balance refers to the balance between calories consumed through eating and drinking and those calories expended through physical activity and metabolic processes.[8] Energy consumed must equal energy expended for a person to remain at the same body weight.[2] Overweight and obesity will result from excess calorie intake and/or inadequate physical activity. Weight loss is associated with calorie deficit, which can be achieved by eating less, being more physically active, or a combination of the two.[9] The diabetes research focused on the causal relationship between obesity and

insulin resistance, a major characteristic of type 2 diabetes.[10] It is only within the past 20 years that the notion of inflammation as a cause of insulin resistance has begun to surface. In obesity, inflammation develops when macrophages infiltrate adipose tissue and stimulate adipocyte secretion of inflammatory cytokines that in turn affect energy balance, glucose and lipid metabolism, leading to insulin resistance.[11] The inflammatory component in obesity and diabetes is now firmly established with the discovery of causal links between inflammatory mediators and insulin receptor signaling and the elucidation of the underlying molecular mechanisms, such as c-Jun NH_2-terminal kinase (JNK), an inhibitor of nuclear factor-κB kinase, -mediated transcriptional and post-translational modifications that inhibit insulin action. More recently, obesity-induced endoplasmic reticulum stress (chronic high-fat diet) has been demonstrated to underlie the initiation of obesity-induced JNK activation, inflammatory responses, and generation of peripheral insulin resistance. The three members of the JNK group of serine/threonine kinases, JNK-1, -2, and -3, belong to the mitogen-activated protein kinase family. Many studies have demonstrated that JNK is a central player in the modulation of insulin action and a critical component of the pathogenesis of obesity, fatty liver disease, and type 2 diabetes.[12,13] From a conceptual understanding to molecular discoveries, a century-old story of inflammation and insulin resistance is re-born with new ideas.[14]

In recent years, several alternative dietary approaches, including high-protein and low-glycemic-load (GL) diets, have produced faster rates of weight loss than traditional low-fat, high-carbohydrate diets.[15] These diets share an under-recognized unifying mechanism: the reduction of postprandial glycemia and insulinemia. Similarly, some food patterns and specific foods (potatoes, white bread, soft drinks) characterized by hyperglycemia are associated with higher risk of adiposity and type 2 diabetes.[11,16–18] Profound compensatory hyperinsulinemia, exacerbated by overweight, occurs during critical periods of physiological insulin resistance such as pregnancy and puberty. The dramatic rise in gestational diabetes and type 2 diabetes in the young may therefore be traced to food patterns that exaggerate postprandial glycemia and insulinemia.[19,20] The dietary strategy with the strongest evidence of being able to prevent type 2 diabetes is not the accepted low-fat, high-carbohydrate diet, but alternative dietary approaches that reduce postprandial glycemia and insulinemia without adversely affecting other risk factors.[21–25] Diabetes is the most common and important metabolic dysfunction in pregnancy. Dietary advice throughout pregnancy recommends frequent small meals which contain carbohydrates that are not highly processed, rich with slowly absorbed starches and non-soluble polysaccharides and with a low GI. The recommended daily caloric intake is individually suited to every woman. The main goals of nutritional management are to maintain balanced glucose levels and to provide enough energy and nutrients for all pregnant women, while avoiding ketosis, and minimizing the risk of hypoglycemia (in women treated with insulin). Healthcare providers should use the window of opportunity of pregnancy to change dietary patterns and to replace them with a healthy lifestyle for both the mother and her family.[26] Overweight and increased energy intake before conception are powerful risk factors in the development of gestational diabetes mellitus (GDM) and may also represent important determinants of the so-called fetal (mal-)programming, which may have long-term consequences for the health of the newborn. Thus, an adequate intake of energy and nutrients is of fundamental significance in the treatment of GDM, along with regular self-monitoring of blood glucose. This concept suffices in most cases to achieve the strict therapeutic goal of normoglycemia. However, because of a lack of data from interventional studies, there is uncertainty about the optimal macronutrient composition of the diet (carbohydrates, fat, and protein) and meal distribution, as well as of the mode of calorie restriction in overweight and obese women with GDM. Varying the carbohydrate intake between 40 and 55% of total energy intake appears to be acceptable and may be distributed across main meals and snacks. Thus, individualized nutritional treatment together with other specific lifestyle interventions are the principal components in the management of GDM.[26–28]

CALORIC INTAKE AND HEALTH CONSEQUENCES

The Report of the DGAC on the Dietary Guidelines for Americans includes consideration of the physical activity level of each individual, and strong evidence indicates that the current level of calorie intake is too high, given physical activity levels in the US.[3] Recent literature has tried to quantify the energy gap that has led to the current obesity epidemic, with estimations ranging from 100 to 400 extra calories per day. Although the magnitude of this energy imbalance has been debated, there is consensus that weight gain occurs as a result of a positive energy balance—consuming more calories than are expended. As illustrated by the increase in the prevalence of overweight and obesity in the US, energy intakes are exceeding energy expenditure for many Americans. Moreover, recent data from the National Health and Nutrition Examination Survey (NHANES) 2005–2006 indicates that many of the top food sources of calories among the US population are energy-dense and are not in nutrient-dense forms.[3] For example, 1 g of pure ethyl alcohol = 7 kcal.[29] Several factors increase the risk of diabetes, including being overweight, lack of physical activity, and family history of diabetes. There is growing consensus that alcohol consumption is an influencing factor.

The biological mechanism is uncertain, but there are several factors that may explain the relationship, including increases in insulin sensitivity after moderate alcohol consumption, changes in levels of alcohol metabolites and increases in high-density lipoprotein (HDL) cholesterol concentrations, or via the anti-inflammatory effect of alcohol.[30] Moderate daily alcohol intake is associated with lower insulin secretion—an effect that warrants further investigation.[31] The meta-analysis of 20 cohort studies has confirmed the U-shaped relationships between average amount of alcohol consumed per day and the relative risk incident for type 2 diabetes type 2 among men and women. Compared with lifetime abstainers, the relative risk for type 2 diabetes among men was most protective when consuming 22 g/day and became deleterious at just over 60 g/day alcohol. Among women, consumption of 24 g/day alcohol was most protective and became deleterious at about 50 g/day alcohol. Moderate alcohol consumption among apparently healthy Japanese men was associated with reduced risk for development of elevated fasting plasma glucose concentration or type 2 diabetes. Amount of calorie adopted is adjusted by organism by a number of external and internal factors.[32]

The changes which took place in recent years in the dietary treatment of diabetes were designed to precisely meet these requirements.[33–35] The FDA allows companies to make three types of health-related claims on food packages: Nutrient-content claims, Health claims, Qualified health claims. Diet in diabetes should be well balanced in terms of biochemical energy and should indicate the percentage of basic food ingredients in the diet. A typical day's meals and snacks would provide about 1,500 to 2,000 calories with about 50% of the calories from carbohydrate, about 20% from protein, and about 30% from fat. If a patient's nutritional needs are more or less than provided by these meal plans, individualized adjustments may be required. Patients who may require adjustments include children,

adolescents, metabolically stressed patients, pregnant women, and geriatric patients.[36] The Mayo Clinic Healthy Weight Pyramid is a tool designed to help you eat a balanced, nutritious diet while achieving a healthy weight.[37] It illustrates the types and amounts of food from each of the five represented food groups that need to be eaten every day. The sample menu shows how the Mayo Clinic Healthy Weight Pyramid can help to plan daily meals and snacks. Recommendations for energy requirements for basic food ingredients for diabetic diet flared anew after the publication of the recommendations of the prestigious American Diabetes Center, Joslin Diabetes Center (Clinical nutrition guideline for overweight and obese adults with type 2 diabetes, prediabetes or at high risk for developing type 2 diabetes).[38] Joslin's approach to diabetes management has always been to focus on the individual, and not dictate a "one size fits all" strategy. At a time when the diet advice waters are muddied with thousands claiming the answer to the battle of the bulge, Joslin offers evidence-based clinical nutrition guidelines for overweight and obese people with type 2 diabetes, prediabetes or at high risk for developing type 2 diabetes. The ultimate goal is to help these populations improve cardiovascular health, reduce body fat and increase sensitivity to insulin. The biggest difference between the USDA's guidelines and Joslin's is the recommendation of fewer carbohydrates and more protein in the diet, as recent studies have shown that this helps people eat less and lose weight. The following are Joslin's guideline essentials (shown as approximate percentages of daily calories): Carbohydrate: 40% from carbohydrates, including at least 20–35 g of fiber. Best carbohydrate/high-fiber sources: fresh vegetables, fruits, beans and wholegrain foods. Eat less of these carbohydrates: pasta, white bread, white potatoes and sugary cereals. Protein: 20–30% from protein (unless you have kidney disease). Best protein sources: fish, skinless chicken or turkey, non-fat or low-fat dairy products, tofu and legumes (beans and peas). Fat: 30–35%

from fat (mostly mono- and polyunsaturated fats). Best fat sources: olive oil, canola oil, nuts, seeds, and fatty fish like salmon.[39] With the aim of developing a rational diet for diabetics, researchers at the Mayo Clinic developed the Healthy Weight Pyramid, which shows the number of calories per serving of the food. On the first level there are vegetables (one serving = 25 calories) and fruit (one serving = 60 calories); at least four servings per day should be consumed. The second level involves carbohydrates: cereals, grains, and seeds, and wholegrain bread (four to eight servings recommended, one serving = 70 calories). The third level of the pyramid is reserved for skimmed milk products (three to seven servings with a portion of protein = 70 calories). The fourth level involves fats: olive oil, vegetable oils such as canola oil, or rich in omega-3 fatty acids canola oil (oil from the seeds of Brassica campestris), nuts, and avocados (three to five servings recommended per day, one serving = 45 calories (Table 34.1).[40,41]

An important element of diabetic diet is a daily meal plan. Patients with type 1 diabetes who have a history of recurrent hypoglycemia or hypoglycemia unawareness or who are poorly controlled are at very high risk for developing severe hypoglycemia. Hypo- and hyperglycemia may also occur in patients with type 2 diabetes, but is generally less frequent and has less severe consequences than in patients with type 1 diabetes.[42] The first main meal in diabetics should be breakfast. In health, the rise in plasma glucose after lunch is less if breakfast is eaten. In obese type 2 diabetic subjects, the rise in plasma glucose was 95% less after lunch when the lunch had been preceded by breakfast, confirming the occurrence of the second-meal metabolic effect. Postprandial glucose metabolism in type 2 diabetes is facilitated by suppression of plasma free fatty acid concentration after a previous meal. The plasma free fatty acid concentration at lunchtime directly related to plasma glucose rise after lunch (r = 0.67, P = 0.0005). The standard breakfast consisted of 50 g muesli, 100 g milk, two slices of toast (56 g), 20 g marmalade, 20 g margarine, and 200 ml orange juice (106 g carbohydrate, 18 g fat, 15 g protein, 646 kcal). The standard lunch comprised a cheese sandwich, 200 ml orange juice, 170 g yogurt, and 150 g jelly (103 g carbohydrate, 30 g fat, 44 g protein, 858 kcal).[43] Here's what forms the core of a healthy breakfast (Nutrition and healthy eating www.mayoclinic.com/health/healthy-weight-pyramid) [41]: (1) Whole grains. Options include wholegrain rolls, bagels, hot or cold whole-grain cereals, low-fat bran muffins, crackers, or melba toast. (2). Low-fat protein. Options include hard-boiled eggs, peanut butter, lean slices of meat and poultry, or fish, such as water-packed tuna or slices of salmon. (3) Low-fat dairy. Options include skim milk, low-fat yogurt and

TABLE 34.1 Recommendations of the Main Diabetes Associations

Main source of calories	Main diabetes associations	Joslin Diabetes Center
Carbohydrates	40–65% of calories	40% of calories
Proteins	10–20% of calories	30% of calories
Fats	30–35% of calories	30% of calories

Recommendations of the main diabetes associations (ADA, EASD, CAD, AACE, Diabetes UK) and Joslin Diabetes Center regarding the percentage of calories from carbohydrates, proteins and fats in the diet of diabetics, recommended by the main diabetes associations [ADA (American Diabetes Association), EASD (European Association for the Study of Diabetes), CAD (Canadian Diabetes Association), Diabetes UK, JDC (Joslin Diabetes Center)].

low-fat cheeses, such as cottage and natural cheeses. (4). Fruits and vegetables. Options include fresh fruits and vegetables or 100% juice beverages without added sugar.

GLYCEMIC INDEX: DEFINITION AND GENERAL CHARACTERISTICS

The GI is a physiological assessment of a food's carbohydrate content through its effect on postprandial blood glucose concentrations. It measures the glycemia-raising potential of a single food by expressing the rise in glycemia in response to a 50-g available carbohydrate portion of that food as a percentage of the rise in glycemia in response to a 50-g available carbohydrate portion of a reference food (white bread or glucose).[43] Low GI is a value ≤ 55, the average 56–69, and high ≥ 70.[44] The aim of the GI classification of foods was therefore to assist in the physiological classification of carbohydrate foods which, it was hoped, would be of relevance in the prevention and treatment of chronic diseases such as diabetes. The merits and limitation of the GI concept have been debated since its introduction in 1981 by Jenkins and coworkers as an alternative system for classifying carbohydrate-containing food. Since then, several hundred scientific articles and numerous popular diet books have been published on the topic.[45,46] However, the clinical significance of the GI remains the subject of debate. Although variability in GI can be high, mean GI values for single foods are largely unaffected by age, sex, BMI, ethnicity, and glucose tolerance of subjects; blood compartment sampled, glucose assay, and reference food.

The results of many investigations clearly show that the GI is an important element in differentiating metabolic effects of food carbohydrates and in evaluating the relationship between dietary carbohydrates and the risk of diabetes, atherosclerosis, and certain cancers.[47]

The studies indicate, among others, a connection between diet with high GI and risk of colorectal cancer or cancers of the breast. It is also important for researchers to consider factors such as ethnicity, family income, and alcohol intake as potential confounders when investigating the associations of dietary GL and GI with disease.[48] One found that modifying GI in a single meal (i.e. at breakfast) alone resulted in lower fasting blood glucose levels and induced satiety until lunch. The American Diabetes Association (ADA) in their evidence-based guidelines maintained their position that carbohydrate quantity is a more important consideration than quality, dismissing the value of the GI in diabetes therapy. In contrast, most other major international diabetes organizations have interpreted the available data differently, supporting the application of the GI concept in the management of diabetes in their most recent guidelines. These organizations include the Canadian Diabetes Association (CDA) Diabetes Australia (DA), Diabetes UK and the European Association for the Study of Diabetes (EASD). Proponents of giving priority to carbohydrate quality argue that GI is a robust measurement, predicts the relative glycemic response to mixed meals, is easy to implement and follow, results in consistent improvements in glycemic control when applied in people with diabetes, and shows consistency for a benefit of low GI in the prevention and treatment of diabetes across the three main levels of evidence: epidemiology, clinical interventions, and basic science.[49] In contrast, the opponents that favor giving priority to carbohydrate quantity argue that GI is highly variable, not physiological, can not reliably predict mixed meal responses, is difficult to learn and follow, and has inconsistent effects on markers of glycemic control and other aspects of metabolic control in people with diabetes.[50] The GI classification of foods has been used as a tool to assess potential prevention and treatment strategies for diseases where glycemic control is of importance, such as diabetes (Table 34.2). Low GI diets

TABLE 34.2 List of Food Products According to GI[53]

The average GI of 62 common foods derived from multiple studies by different laboratories					
Breakfast cereals		**Vegetables**		**Dairy products and alternatives**	
Cornflakes	81 ± 6	Potato, boiled	78 ± 4	Milk, full fat	39 ± 3
Wheat flake biscuits	69 ± 2	Potato, instant mash	67 ± 3	Milk, skim	37 ± 4
Porridge, rolled oats	55 ± 2	Potato, french fries	63 ± 5	Ice cream	51 ± 3
Instant oat porridge	79 ± 3	Carrots, boiled	39 ± 4	Yogurt, fruit	41 ± 2
Rice porridge/congee	78 ± 9	Sweet potato, boiled	63 ± 6	Soy milk	34 ± 4
Millet porridge	67 ± 5	Pumpkin, boiled	64 ± 7	Rice milk	86 ± 7
Muesli	57 ± 2	Plantain/green banana	55 ± 6		
		Taro, boiled	53 ± 2		
		Vegetable soup	48 ± 5		
Legumes		**Snack products**		**Sugar**	
Chickpeas	28 ± 9	Chocolate	40 ± 3	Fructose	15 ± 4
Kidney beans	24 ± 4	Popcorn	65 ± 5	Sucrose	65 ± 4
Lentils	32 ± 5	Potato crisps	56 ± 3	Glucose	103 ± 3
Soya beans	16 ± 1	Soft drink/soda	59 ± 3	Honey	61 ± 3
		Rice crackers/crisps	87 ± 2		
High-carbohydrate foods		**Fruit and fruit products**			
White wheat bread*	75 ± 2	Apple, raw[†]	36 ± 2		
Whole wheat/whole meal bread	74 ± 2	Orange, raw[†]	43 ± 3		
Specialty grain bread	53 ± 2	Banana, raw[†]	51 ± 3		
Unleavened wheat bread	70 ± 5	Pineapple, raw	59 ± 8		
Wheat roti	62 ± 3	Mango, raw[†]	51 ± 5		
Chapatti	52 ± 4	Watermelon, raw			
Corn tortilla	46 ± 4	Dates, raw	76 ± 4		
White rice, boiled*	73 ± 4	Peaches, canned[†]	42 ± 4		
Brown rice, boiled	68 ± 4	Strawberry jam/jelly	43 ± 5		
Barley	28 ± 2	Apple juice	49 ± 3		

* *Low-GI varieties were also identified.*
[†] *Average of all available data.*
Data are ± SEM.
Source: Fiona S. Atkinson, Kaye Foster-Powell, Jennie C. Brand-Miller (2008) International tables of glycemic index and glycemic load values. Diab. Care *31: 2281–2283.*

have also been reported to improve the serum lipid profile, reduce C-reactive protein (CRP) concentrations, and aid in weight control. In cross-sectional studies, low GI or GL diets (mean GI multiplied by total carbohydrate) have been associated with higher levels of HDL cholesterol (HDL-C), with reduced CRP concentrations, and, in cohort studies, with decreased risk of developing diabetes and cardiovascular disease (CVD).[51] In addition, some case-control and cohort studies have found positive associations between dietary GI and risk of various cancers, including those of the colon, breast, and prostate. Although inconsistencies in the current findings still need to be resolved, sufficient positive evidence, especially with respect to renewed interest in postprandial events, suggests that the GI may have a role to play in the treatment and prevention of chronic diseases associated with overconsumption and inactivity leading to central obesity and insulin resistance.[52,53]

METABOLIC, BIOCHEMICAL, AND HEALTH EFFECTS

A meta-analysis conducted has shown that low-GI diet was associated with a reduction in HbA1c by 0.43%. It is worth noting that this effect is greater than other dietary interventions, such as reducing the total amount of carbohydrates and increasing the fibrin content in the diet.[33] In 210 participants with type 2 diabetes, 6-month treatment with a low-GI diet resulted in moderately lower HbA1c levels compared with a high-cereal fiber diet. Continuous blood glucose monitoring in youths with type 1 diabetes revealed that the consumption of low GI meals may reduce glucose excursions, improving glycemic control.[53,54] The GI provides a good summary of postprandial glycemia. It predicts the peak (or near peak) response, the maximum glucose fluctuation, and other attributes of the response curve.

Chronic insulin resistance contributes to subclinical inflammation, thrombosis/impaired fibrinolysis, and dyslipidemia. A diet characterized by low-GI starchy foods lowers the glucose and insulin responses throughout the day and improves the lipid profile and capacity for fibrinolysis, suggesting a therapeutic potential in diabetes. The study suggests that altering the GI of high-carbohydrate energy-restricted diets does not impact on the improvement in glycemic control that is observed normally during energy restriction. However, a low-GI diet including low-GI cereal and fruits, wholegrain bread, pasta and wheat-meal biscuits may be slightly better at improving glycemic control and lipoprotein metabolism in overweight subjects previously diagnosed with type 2 diabetes with variable glucose tolerance.[55] In subjects with type 2 diabetes managed by diet alone with optimal glycemic control, long-term HbA1c was not affected by altering the GI or the amount of dietary carbohydrate. Differences in total HDL cholesterol among diets had disappeared by 6 months. However, because of sustained reductions in postprandial glucose and CRP, a low-GI diet may be preferred for the dietary management of type 2 diabetes. The consumption of a meal with a high GI results in a postprandial surge of counterregulatory hormones and free fatty acids that "resembles a state of fasting normally reached only after many hours without food". In contrast to insulin, which is vasodilatory, all the counterregulatory hormones (glucocorticoids, catecholamines, glucagon, and growth hormone) increase cardiovascular tone. There is recent evidence that fatty acids do so as well.[56] The high-glycemic index/glycemic load (high-GI/GL) diet resulted in significant, but unexpected, reductions in total and low-density lipoprotein (LDL) cholesterol, whereas HDL cholesterol concentration was significantly reduced on the high-GI/GL diet compared with the low-GI/GL diet.[57] Overall, high- and low-GI/GL diets of 4 weeks' duration had no consistent effects on coronary heart disease (CHD) risk factors in this group of overweight/obese men.[57] Hyperglycemia and insulin resistance are independent risk factors for CVD. Postprandial glycemic "spikes" adversely affect vascular structure and function via multiple mechanisms including oxidative stress, inflammation, LDL oxidation, protein glycation, and procoagulant activity.[58]

Glycemic responses can be reliably predicted by considering both the quantity and quality of carbohydrate. The GI, a measure of carbohydrate quality, has provided insights that knowledge of the sugar or starch content has not. In prospective observational studies, dietary GI and/or GL (the product of the amount of carbohydrate and GI) independently predict CVD, with relative risk ratios of 1.2−1.9 comparing highest and lowest quartiles. In randomized controlled trials in overweight subjects, diets based on low-GI carbohydrates have decreased plasminogen activator inhibitor-1 activity and other CVD risk factors over and above that of conventional low-fat diets. Taken together, the findings suggest that clinicians may be able to improve CVD outcomes by recommending the judicious use of low GI/GL foods. In the Italian cohort, high dietary GL and carbohydrate intake from high-GI foods increase the overall risk of CHD in women but not men. Among 36,019 women 48−83 years old without baseline heart failure, diabetes, or myocardial infarction, dietary GI did not appear to be associated with incident heart failure events. Authors have determined whether altering dietary GI in addition to healthy eating and weight loss advice affects arterial compliance and 24-h blood pressure (BP), and CHD risk factors.[59] Middle-aged men with at least one CHD risk factor were randomized to a 6-month low-GI (LGI) or high-GI (HGI) diet. All subjects were advised on healthy eating and weight loss. They were seen monthly to assess dietary compliance and anthropometrics. Carotid-femoral pulse wave velocity (PWV), fasting blood lipid profile, and glucose and insulin concentrations were measured at baseline and at months 3 and 6. Six-hour postprandial glucose and insulin responses and 24-h ambulatory BP were also assessed at baseline and month 6. Thirty-eight subjects completed the study. At month 6, groups differed significantly in dietary GI, GL, and carbohydrate intake. Fasting insulin concentration and insulin resistance (calculated by homeostatic model assessment) were lower in the LGI than the HGI group (P < 0.01). The reduction in total cholesterol and 24-h BP was more pronounced in the LGI than the HGI group (P < 0.05); and only the LGI group exhibited significant reductions in PWV, LDL cholesterol, and triacylglycerol concentration. There were no differences in postprandial glucose or insulin responses between the groups.

The other results suggest that an LGI diet may be more beneficial in reducing CHD risk, including carotid-femoral pulse wave velocity and 24-h blood pressure even in the setting of healthy eating and weight loss; and thus, further study is warranted. While a low-GI diet was seen to be beneficial for some outcomes for both mother and child, results from the review were inconclusive. Further trials with large sample sizes and longer follow-up are required to make more definitive conclusions. High dietary GI and GL may promote tumorigenesis by increasing endogenous concentrations of insulin-like growth factor I (IGF-I) or the bioavailability of estradiol. *In vitro* studies have shown that uterine leiomyoma (UL) cells proliferate in response to IGF-I and display increased IGF-I gene expression and protein synthesis. Previous epidemiologic studies suggest that a high GL is a risk factor for endometrial and ovarian cancers, which, like UL, are hormone-responsive tumors. The study has suggested that high dietary GI and GL may be associated with an increased UL risk in some women.[60] Women with polycystic ovarian syndrome (PCOS) are intrinsically insulin resistant and have a high risk of cardiovascular disease and type 2 diabetes. Authors compared changes in insulin sensitivity and clinical outcomes after similar weight losses after consumption of a low-GI diet compared with a conventional healthy diet in women with PCOS. The study provides the objective evidence to justify the use of low-GI diets in the management of PCOS. There was a significant diet—metformin interaction, with greater improvement in oral-glucose-tolerance test among women prescribed both metformin and the low-GI diet. Compared with women who consumed the conventional healthy diet, more women who consumed the low-GI diet showed improved menstrual cyclicity. Among the biochemical measures, only serum fibrinogen concentrations showed significant differences between diets.[61] A meta-analysis was performed to explore the association between GI and GL and cancer risk from 39 published studies. Overall, both GL and GI were significantly associated with a greater risk of colorectal and endometrial cancers, whereas no association was found for pancreatic cancer.

The GI classification of foods has been used as a tool to assess potential prevention and treatment strategies for diseases where glycemic control is of importance, such as diabetes. Low GI diets have also been reported to improve the serum lipid profile, reduce CRP concentrations, and aid in weight control. In cross-sectional studies, low-GI or -GL diets (mean GI multiplied by total carbohydrate) have been associated with higher levels of HDL-C, with reduced CRP concentrations, and in cohort studies, with decreased risk of developing diabetes and cardiovascular disease. In addition, some case-control and cohort studies have found positive associations between dietary GI and risk of various cancers, including those of the colon, breast, and prostate. Although inconsistencies in the current findings still need to be resolved, sufficient positive evidence, especially with respect to renewed interest in postprandial

events, suggests that the GI may have a role to play in the treatment and prevention of chronic diseases. Carbohydrates and dietary GI influence the secretion of insulin and insulin-related growth factors and may play a role in the development of diabetes and obesity, both of which have been related to pancreatic cancer risk. The positive association with high GI, in the absence of an association with dietary GL, fruit, or total carbohydrates, likely reflects the positive association between sweets or refined carbohydrates and pancreatic cancer. The Netherlands Cohort Study which consisted of 120,852 men and women failed to support the notion that GL, GI, or intake of carbohydrates and mono- and disaccharides were positively associated with esophageal adenocarcinoma and pancreatic cancer risk.[62] Although inconsistencies in the current findings still need to be resolved, sufficient positive evidence, especially with respect to renewed interest in postprandial events, suggests that the GI may have a role to play in the treatment and prevention of chronic diseases.

References

1. Erber E, Hopping BN, Grandinetti S, Park S-Y, Kolonel LN, Maskarinec G. Dietary patterns and risk for diabetes: The Multiethnic Cohort. *Diabetes Care* 2010;**33**:532–8.
2. Drewnowski A, Bellisle F. Liquid calories, sugar, and body weight. *Am J Clin Nutr* 2007;**85**:651–61.
3. Report of the DGAC on the Dietary Guidelines for Americans. *D1–2. Recommendations for energy intake include consideration of the physical activity level of each individual, and strong evidence indicates that the current level of calorie intake is too high, given physical activity levels in the United States (US)*, http://www.cnpp.usda.gov/Publications/DietaryGuide; 2010.
4. Willett W, Manson J, Lin S. Glycemic index, glycemic load and risk of type 2 diabetes. *Am J Clin Nutr* 2002;**76**(Suppl.):274S–80S.
5. Jakobsen MU, Dethlesten C, Joensen AM, Stegger J, Tjonneland A, Schmidt EB, Overvad K. Intake of carbohydrates compared with intake of satured fatty acids and risk of myocardial infarction: importance of the glycemic index. *Am J Clin Nutr* 2010;**91**:1764–8.

6. Garg A. High-monounsaturated-fat diets for patients with diabetes mellitus: a meta-analysis. *Am J Clin Nutr* 1998;**67**(Suppl. 3):S577–82.

7. Ivonne S, Beulens JWJ, van der Daphne AL, Annemieke SMW, van der Schouw GDE, Yvonne T. Dietary intake of total animal, and vegetable protein and risk of type 2 diabetes in the European Prospective Investigation into Cancer and Nutrition (EPIC)-NL study. *Diabetes Care* 2010;**33**:43–8.

8. Poppitt S, Swann D, Black A, Prentice A. Assessment of selective under-reporting of food intake by both obese and non-obese women in a metabolic facility. *Int J Obes Relat Metab Disord* 1998;**22**:303–11.

9. White JS. Straight talk about high-fructose corn syrup: what it is and what it ain't. *Am J Clin Nutr* 2008;**88**: 1716–21.

10. Bray G. How bad is fructose? *Am J Clin Nutr* 2007;**86**: 895–6.

11. Parks EJ, Skokan LE, Timlin MT, Dingfelder CS. Dietary sugars stimulate fatty acid synthesis in adults. *J Nutr* 2008;**138**:1039–46.

12. Hotamisligil GS. Role of endoplasmic reticulum stress and c-Jun NH$_2$-terminal kinase pathways in inflammation and origin of obesity and diabetes. *Diabetes* 2005;**54**(Suppl. 2):S73–8.

13. Gregor MF, Yang L, Fabbrini E, Mohammed BS, Eagon JC, Hotamisligil GS, Klein S. Endoplasmic reticulum stress is reduced in tissues of obese subjects after weight loss. *Diabetes* 2009;**58**:693–700.

14. Kim JK. Inflammation and insulin resistance: an old story with new ideas. *Korean Diabetes J* 2010;**34**:137–45.

15. Willett W. *Nutritional Epidemiology*. 2 ed. USA: Oxford University Press; 1998.

16. Akhavan T, Anderson GH. Effects of glucose-to-fructose ratios in solutions on subjective satiety, food intake, and satiety hormones in young men. *Am J Clin Nutr* 2007;**86**:1354–63.

17. Rodin J, Reed D, Jamner L. Metabolic effects of fructose and glucose: implications for food intake. *Am J Clin Nutr* 1988;**47**:683–9.

18. Hoekstra JH, van den Aker JH. Facilitating effect of amino acids on fructose and sorbitol absorption in children. *J Pediatr Gastroenterol Nutr* 1996;**23**:118–24.

19. Mukherjee S, Thakur G, Kumar BD, Mitra A, Chakraborty C. Long-term effects of a carbohydrate-rich diet on fasting blood sugar, lipid profile, and serum insulin values in rural Bengalis. *J Diabetes* 2009;**1**:288–95.

20. Rodin J. Comparative effects of fructose, aspartame, glucose, and water preloads on calorie and macronutrient intake. *Am J Clin Nutr* 1990;**51**:428–35.

21. American Diabetes Association (ADA). Nutrition recommendations and principles for people with diabetes mellitus. *Diabetes Care* 2000;**23**(Suppl. 1):S1–116.

22. American Diabetes Association (ADA). Postprandial blood glucose. *Diabetes Care* 2001;**24**:775–8.

23. American Diabetes Association (ADA). Evidence-based nutrition principles and recommendations for the treatment and prevention of diabetes and related complications. *Diabetes Care* 2002;**25**:202–12.

24. Commission of the European Communities. *Reports of the Scientific Committee for Food (thirty-first series): Nutrient and energy intakes for the European Community*. GT-29-98-003-EN-C (accessed 11 December 1992), http://europa.eu.int/comm/food/fs/sc/scf/reports/scf_reports_43.pdf; 1992.

25. Buyken AE, Mitchell P, Ceriello A, Brand-Miller J. Optimal dietary approaches for prevention of type 2 diabetes: a life-course perspective. *Diabetologia* 2010;**53**: 406–18.

26. Shimron-Nachmias L, Frishman S, Hod M. Dietary management of diabetic pregnancy. *Harefuah* 2006;**145**: 768–72.

27. Amann-Gassner U, Hauner H. Nutrition therapy for gestational diabetes. *Dtsch Med Wochenschr* 2008;**133**: 893–8 (in German).

28. *What We Eat in America, National Health and Nutrition Examination Survey (WWEIA, NHANES), 2005–2006, individuals*. USDA, http://www.ars.usda.gov/ba/bhnrc/fsrg; 2008.

29. Drzewiecki J. *Diabetes Quick Lexicon*. Poland: Delta Publishing Advertising Agency; 2005. pp.68–68 (in Polish).

30. Hendriks HF. Moderate alcohol consumption and insulin sensitivity: observations and possible mechanisms. *Ann Epidemiol* 2007;**17**(Suppl. 5):S40–2.

31. Cortez-Pinto H, Chatham J, Chacko VP, Arnold C, Rashid. A, Diehl AM. Alterations in liver ATP homeostasis in human nonalcoholic steatohepatitis: a pilot study. *JAMA* 1999;**282**:1659–64.

32. Daniluk U, Kaczmarski M, Wasilewska J, Matuszewska E, Krasnow A, Skiba E. Physiological and pathological mechanisms regulating of human appetite. *Terapia* 2002;**116**:34–7 (in Polish).

33. Klupa T. Diet in diabetes – current opinions. *Terapia* 2007;**103**:17–20 (in Polish).

34. Moszczynski P. Diabetes. Part.I. Pathogenesis, classification, metabolic disorders. *Drug in Poland* 2002;**12**:73–84 (in Polish).

35. Watts SA, Anselmo J. Nutrition for diabetes – all in a day's work. *Nursing* 2006;**36**:46–8.

36. American Diabetes Association. Evidence based nutrition principles and recommendations. *Diabetes Care* 2004;**27**(Suppl. 1):S36–46.

37. Reedy J, Krebs-Smith SM. Dietary sources of energy, solid fats, and added sugars among children and adolescents in the United States. *J Am Diet Assoc* 2010;**110**:1477–84.

38. American Diabetes Center, Joslin Diabetes Center. *Clinical nutrition guideline for overweight and obese adults with type 2 diabetes, prediabetes or at high risk for developing type 2 diabetes*, http://www.joslin.org; 2007.

39. Hamdy O, Campbell A. *Joslin Diabetes Center*, http://www.joslin.org; 2005.

40. Mayo Clinic Healthy Weight Pyramid. *A sample menu. Example of a 1,200-calorie menu*, http://www.mayoclinic.com/health/healthy-weight-pyramid; 2008.

41. Mayo Clinic Healthy Weight Pyramid servings. *Vegetables, Fruits, Carbohydrates, Protein and Dairy Fats*, http://www.healthierus.gov/dietaryguidelines; 2008.

42. Jovanovic S, Gerrard J, Taylor R. The second-meal phenomenon in type 2 diabetes. *Diabetes Care* 2009;**32**:1199−201.

43. Venn BJ, Green TJ. Glycemic index and glycemic load: measurement issues and their effect on diet−disease relationships. *Eur J Clin Nutr* 2007;**61**(Suppl. 1): S122−31.

44. Moszczynski P. The plant foods are the important ingredients of Mediterranean diet. *Drug in Poland* 2007;**17**:94−104 (in Polish).

45. Wolever TM, Jenkins DJ, Jenkins AL, Josse RG. The glycemic index: methodology and clinical implications. *Am J Clin Nutr* 1991;**54**:846−54.

46. Jenkins DJ, Wolever TM, Jenkins AL, Josse RG, Wong GS. The glycaemic response to carbohydrate foods. *Lancet* 1984;**324**:388−91.

47. Bessesen DH. The role of carbohydrates in insulin resistance. *J Nutr* 2001;**131**:2782−6.

48. Puchau BM, Zulet Á, de Echávarri AG, Hermsdorff HHM, Martínez AJ. Study of Women's Health Across the Nation (SWAN). Dietary total antioxidant capacity: A novel indicator of diet quality in healthy young adults. *J Am Coll Nutr* 2009;**28**: 648−56.

49. Greenwood JLJ, Stanford JB. Preventing or improving obesity by addressing specific eating patterns. *J Am Board Fam Med* 2008;**21**:135−40.

50. Miller JC. Importance of glycemic index in diabetes. *Am J Clin Nutr* 1994;**59**:747S−52S.

51. Choi HK, Curhan G. Soft drinks, fructose consumption, and the risk of gout in men: prospective cohort study. *Brit Med J* 2008;**336**:309−12.

52. Jeppesen J, Schaaf P, Jones C, Zhou MY, Chen YD, Reaven GM. Effects of low-fat, high-carbohydrate diets on risk factors for ischemic heart disease in postmenopausal women. *Am J Clin Nutr* 1997;**65**:1027−33.

53. Atkinson FS, Foster-Powell K, Brand-Miller JC. International Tables of Glycemic Index and Glycemic Load Values. *Diabetes Care* 2008;**31**:2281−3.

54. Nansel TR, Gellar L, McGill A. Effect of varying glycemic index meals on blood glucose control assessed with continuous glucose monitoring in youth with type 1 diabetes on basal-bolus insulin regimens. *Diabetes Care* 2008;**31**:695−7.

55. Burton-Freeman BM, Keim NL. Glycemic index, cholecystokinin, satiety and disinhibition: is there an unappreciated paradox for overweight women? *Int J Obes (Lond)* 2008;**32**:1647−54.

56. Ludwig DS. The Glycemic Index: Physiological mechanisms relating to obesity, diabetes, and cardiovascular disease. *JAMA* 2002;**287**:2414−23.

57. Shikany JM, Phadke RP, Redden DT, Gower BA. Effects of low- and high-glycemic index/glycemic load diets on coronary heart disease risk factors in overweight/obese men. *Metabolism* 2009;**58**:1793−801.

58. Hollenbeck C. Dietary fructose effects on lipoprotein metabolism and risk for coronary artery disease. *Am J Clin Nutr* 1993;**58**(Suppl. 5):800S−9S.

59. Sieri S, Krogh V, Berrino F, Evangelista A, Agnoli C, Brighenti F, Pellegrini N, Palli D, Masala G, Sacerdote C, Veglia F, Tumino R, Frasca G, Grioni S, Pala V, Mattiello A, Chiodini P, Panico S. Dietary glycemic load and index and risk of coronary heart disease in a large italian cohort: The EPICOR Study. *Arch Intern Med* 2010;**170**:640−7.

60. Janket SJ, Manson JE, Sesso H, Buring JE, Liu S. A prospective study of sugar intake and risk of type 2 diabetes in women. *Diabetes Care* 2003;**26**:1008−15.

61. Marsh KA, Steinbe-Lamarcheck KS, Atkinson FS, Petocz P, Brand-Miller JC. Effect of a low glycemic index compared with a conventional healthy diet on polycystic ovary syndrome. *Am J Clin Nutr* 2010;**92**:83−92.

62. Thompson CL, Khiani V, Chak A, Berger NA, Li L. Carbohydrate consumption and esophageal cancer: an ecological assessment. *Am J Gastroenterol* 2008;**103**: 555−61.

CHAPTER

35

Ayurveda and Metabolic Diseases: The Whole is Greater than the Sum of the Parts

Amrutesh Puranik*, Bhushan Patwardhan[†]

*Department of Integrative Biology and Stress Physiology, University of Minnesota, Minneapolis, MN, USA [†]Bio-medical Research Cluster, Symbiosis International University, Lavale, Pune, India

INTRODUCTION

The World Health Organization (WHO) estimates that non-communicable metabolic diseases are contributing significantly to increasing morbidity and mortality.[1] There is an explosion of literature citing the rising prevalence and incidence of metabolic diseases that have insulin resistance (IR) as their underlying pathology. The International Diabetes Federation

Nutritional and Therapeutic Interventions for Diabetes and Metabolic Syndrome
DOI: 10.1016/B978-0-12-385083-6.00035-8

443

(IDF) states that every 10 s, a person dies of diabetes or a related cause. Within same 10 s another two people develop the disease. Today 230 million people live with diabetes. Eighty percent of diabetics live in low- and middle-income countries.[2] Realizing the complex pathology of metabolic diseases, an alliance of four international federations (International Diabetes Federation, Union for International Cancer Control, International Union Against Tuberculosis and Lung Disease, and the World Heart Federation), representing the four main non-communicable diseases (NCDs), have contributed to the World Health Organization's 2008−2013 Action Plan for NCDs.

IR and inflammation were postulated as two pathways that play causal roles in the cluster of metabolic diseases.[3] There is ample evidence suggesting cross-communication between IR and inflammation. Thus inflammation and IR are the primary targets in the therapy of all metabolic disorders.[4] The ominous octet—liver, muscle, β-cells, adipose tissue, gastrointestinal tissue, pancreatic α-cells, kidney, and brain—are the target organs involved.[5] Thus, to address multiple target organs there is a need for multiple drugs. The therapeutic strategy for glucose control includes drugs like insulin (long, intermediate and short acting), metformin (biguanide), pioglitazone (thiazolidinedione), exenatide (glucagon-like peptide analogs), repaglinide, glipizide (insulin secretogogues), sitagliptin (dipeptidyl peptidase inhibitors), SIRT1 activators[6] and sodium-glucose co-transporter 2 (SGLT) inhibitors.[7] However, the above-mentioned, newer, single-target modulators either have limited information on safety or are known to have cardiovascular risks. Indeed, metformin coupled with lifestyle modification forms the first line of treatment of type 2 diabetes (T2DM).[4] However, arresting the complications of T2DM still remains a challenge. Drug discovery programs using single target-based approaches have met with limited success and there is a need for a systems approach which

will positively modulate multiple targets in metabolic diseases.

Herbal(s) (also referred to as herbal formulations, herbal drugs, herbal medicine, herbal extracts, or dietary supplements in this chapter) can be considered important in multimodal therapeutics. Herbals, often administered as powders or extracts, are mixtures of interacting compounds that can modulate multiple pharmacological targets and provide clinical efficacy beyond the reach of single-compound-based drugs.[8,9] Rationally designed, carefully standardized, synergistic traditional herbals with robust scientific evidence can also be used as alternatives in chronic diseases.[10] Herbals have been used for glucose homeostasis inflammation, and to arrest diabetic complications.[11−15] While the herbal market is growing, the need for more rigorous clinical and scientific research is strongly advocated for greater acceptance and visibility.[16] Herbals are often adapted from *Ayurveda* and/or Traditional Chinese Medicine (TCM) and directly subjected to modern medicine's double-blind randomized trials or reductionist biology. However, the wisdom of the ancient literature is lost in such transitions. There is a need to study Systems *Ayurveda* and then to adopt novel strategies for herbal drug research based on *Ayurveda* and TCM.

T2DM AND CLUSTER OF METABOLIC DISEASES

T2DM is a progressive disease in which the risks of myocardial infarction, stroke, microvascular events, and mortality are all strongly associated with hyperglycemia. The disease course is characterized by increase in inflammatory mediators, worsening of IR and consequently a decline in the pancreatic β-cell function. T2DM coexists with chronic conditions like obesity, hypertriglyceridemia, hypertension, cardiovascular diseases, polycystic ovarian disease, osteoarthritis, Alzheimer's disease, and cancer. National Center for Biotechnology Information (NCBI) classifies all of the above diseases as metabolic disease. Simultaneous existence of any of the above three conditions is also refererred to as Metabolic Syndrome (MS) or Syndrome X. It is now well-established that IR and inflammation leads to MS.[3]

EPIDEMIOLOGY, MORTALITY, MORBIDITY, AND GLOBAL ECONOMIC BURDEN

The IDF Atlas, 2009, reports global prevalence of T2DM as 6.6% in 2010, which is projected to increase up to 7.8% by 2030. More worrying is the 7.9% prevalence of patients with impaired glucose tolerance (IGT)—a prediabetic stage that is projected to increase up to 8.4% by 2030 (http://www.idf.org/Facts_and_Figures). T2DM, once thought to be a disease of rich (developed) countries, is more prevalent in developing countries like India and China. India is the diabetes capital of the world with 12% prevalence of T2DM.[17] Today (2010) India has around 50.8 million diabetics, and this number is predicted to increase to 87 million by 2030. The prevalence of T2DM in urban Indian adults has increased from < 3% in the 1970s to > 12% in 2010. The rising prevalence of metabolic diseases has a direct correlation with related comorbidity like cardiovascular diseases (CVDs). The IDF estimates that there were close to 4,000,000 deaths due to diabetes in the 20–79 age groups in 2010, accounting for 6.8% of global all-cause mortality in this age group. This estimated number of premature deaths is similar in magnitude to deaths in this age group from several infectious diseases. The highest number of deaths due to diabetes is expected to occur in countries with large populations as they have the largest numbers of people with diabetes. Metabolic diseases impose a large economic burden on the individual, on the national healthcare system,

and on the economy. Healthcare expenditures on diabetes are expected to account for 11.6% of the total healthcare expenditure in the world in 2010. About 80% of countries are predicted to spend between 5% and 13% of their total healthcare dollars on diabetes. The US is projected to spend US$198 billion or 52.7% of global expenditure in 2010, while India, the country with the largest population of people living with diabetes, is expected to spend an estimated US$2.8 billion (http://www.idf.org/Facts_and_Figures.)[18] Traditional drug discovery programs have limited potential to arrest the complications of metabolic diseases. There is a need to undertake holistic and safe approaches like *Ayurveda* to manage metabolic diseases.

AYURVEDA UNDERSTANDING OF METABOLIC DISEASES

Ayurveda is a comprehensive, personalized and sustainable health system based on logical principles. The nature of logic in *Ayurveda* differs from the modern medicine's reductionist approach. Unlike ethnopharmacology, *Ayurveda* is the "science of life" (*Ayusho veda*) and hence differs principally and fundamentally from modern medicine. *Ayurveda* defines health as "the equilibrium of the three biological humors or the *doshas* (*Vata, pitta* and *kapha*), seven *dhatus*, *agni* and a state of pleasure or happiness of the soul, senses and the mind". Ayurvedic understanding of metabolic diseases involves a multifaceted approach. *Prameha* has been described in most of the available classics of *Ayurveda*. According to *Ayurveda*, *Prameha* is the disease which affects several systems; it depends on genetic and environmental factors and leads to complications if not managed in the proper way. *Prameha* is a metabolic disease and not just localized to urinary tract pathology. However, the environment of urinary tract is associated frequently in this disease almost in every case in the advanced stage. Thus, the manifestation of the metabolic abnormality as well as the urinary tract pathology is included in two symptoms: *Prabhuta mutrata*, excess urination both in terms of quantity and frequency; and "*Avila mutrata*", urine turbidity. *Ayurveda* has a systemic diagnosis, treatment principles, and clinical insights for managing certain stages of *Prameha* and their complications. It affirms that certain conditions of *Prameha* are curable (*Sadhya*), some are just manageable (*Yapya*) and a few others are incurable (*Asadhya*).[19,20] Detailed information on *Prameha* is available in the mentioned references or NCBI book database, or in recent reviews by Nanda *et al.* and Sharma *et al.*[21–23] There is a need to create evidence base to *Ayurveda* so that it could be accepted freely by modern medicine. Integrated approaches of ethnopharmacology and modern medicine are being undertaken to generate mechanistic understanding of *Ayurveda*.[24–26]

PATHOGENESIS OF T2DM

IR in muscle and liver, and pancreatic β-cell failure represent the core pathophysiologic defects in T2DM. DeFronzo in his Banting Memorial Lecture considers eight body organs, namely muscle, liver, β-cell, adipose tissue (accelerated lipolysis), gastrointestinal tract (incretin deficiency/resistance), α-cell (hyperglucagonemia), kidney (increased glucose reabsorption), and brain (insulin resistance) in the development of glucose intolerance in T2DM.[5] Collectively, these eight players comprise the ominous octet. IR has been linked to an increase in adiposity. Secondary mediators that participate in the pathogenic mechanisms of metabolic disease like homocysteine, nitric oxide (NO), AMPKinase, peroxisome proliferated activated receptors (PPAR), nuclear factor kappa B (NF-κB), insulin receptor substrates (IRS), sirtuins (SIRT), glucagon-like peptide (GLIPs) and other related adipocytokines are mentioned in the reviewed text; however, their individual discussion is out of the scope of this review.

Increased Adiposity

Increased adiposity is accumulation of more body fat than the lean mass. Czech *et al.* describe this as a disorienting outcome of modern-day human behavior in relation to feeding and physical activity or a resolute adaption to a sedentary lifestyle.[27] Adipose tissue is a master endocrine regulatory tissue that controls body lipid flux. Adipose tissue secretes adipokines—bioactive factors that participate in regulation of IR and energy homeostasis. Among them, relevant adipokines for this thesis are discussed below. Leptin is an adipose tissue-derived signal to brain and other tissues, and acts as a negative feedback loop for maintenance of energy homeostasis. Leptin is also considered as a marker for whole-body adiposity. Deficiency or resistance to action of leptin causes lipoatrophy and diabetes with clinical features such as non-alcohol steatohepatitis (NASH), hyperglycemia, hyperinsulinemia, elevated free fatty acids (FFA) and triglycerides (TG).[28] Adiponectin is a beneficial adipokine. Plasma concentration of adiponectin is associated with a lower risk of T2DM. Adiponectin also has anti-inflammatory and anti-atherosclerotic effects. Mechanistically, adiponectin stimulates AMP-activated protein kinase (AMPK)—a mediator that regulates the mitochondrial biogenesis and function, thus preventing IR.[29] Thus, conserving and improving adiponectin is considered a potentially important therapeutic strategy. TG droplets stored in an adipocyte define its insulin sensitivity. Smaller droplets make adipocytes more insulin sensitive. In early phases of overnutrition, adipocytes expand because of increased TG deposition within the cells. Hypertrophied adipocytes trigger secretion of monocyte chemoattractant protein (MCP-1) and TNF-α, adipokines that are pro-inflammatory in nature. These effects are discussed in next section.

Chronic Inflammation

Chronic inflammation is marked by presence of elevated pro-inflammatory adipokines. The Insulin Resistance Atherosclerosis Study (IRAS) in non-diabetics, the Atherosclerosis Risk in Communities (ARIC) in chronic diabetics show relation of white blood cell count (WBC), C-reactive protein (CRP), and fibrinogen with T2DM.[30] Hypertrophied adipocytes in overnourished individuals secrete MCP-1 which promotes macrophage infiltration in to adipocytes. Macrophage in turn secretes large amounts of chemoattractants and cytokines like TNF-α, IL-1β and IL-6. Independently these cytokines are known to precipitate IR. The production of TNF-α requires both IKKβ-NF-κB and the JNK-MAP4K4-AP1 (Jun N−terminal kinase-4-activator protein-1) signaling pathways. Cytokines also trigger increased lipolysis and inhibit peroxisome proliferator-activated receptor-γ (PPAR-γ)-mediated synthesis of TG. This results in an increase in circulating FFA that are taken up by skeletal muscles, liver and pancreatic β-cells. These FFA attenuate expression of genes that are involved in mitochondrial function such as PPAR-γ co-activator-1 (PGC-1). Thus arresting inflammation by decreasing adiposity can be a target of intervention. Chronic inflammation also triggers increased platelet aggregation which increases the risk of CVD.[31]

Insulin Resistance

In normal physiology, intake of glucose (food) stimulates the pancreatic β-cells residing in the Islets of Langerhans to secrete insulin. Insulin in turn promotes glucose uptake and utilization in the cells via insulin receptors located on the cell membrane. Insulin binds to insulin receptor at the cell surface, which activates the intracellular domains of the receptor to trans-autophosphorylate at specific tyrosine residues. The receptor can then transduce the insulin signal into the cell and to its various effectuating

systems, such as glucose uptake via glucose transporters (GLUT). Downstream signal-mediating proteins are members of the insulin receptor substrate (IRS) family, in particular IRS-1, which is rapidly phosphorylated at specific tyrosine residues by the activated receptor. Insulin regulates glucose homeostasis primarily by suppression of hepatic glucose production and stimulation of peripheral glucose uptake. Glucose stimulates insulin release and released insulin, in turn, stimulates glucose disposal. This appears to be a robust closed feedback loop. Resistance to this anabolic action is called IR. It impairs glucose disposal action of insulin. This in turn signals pancreatic β-cells to produce more insulin. Insulin secretion increases progressively with IR in a hyperbolic pattern and failure of β-cells to compensate for IR sets up a self-promoting pathology characterized by impaired glucose tolerance, impaired fasting glucose. This, if untreated, progresses to T2DM.[32] When reviewing IR, it is important to distinguish what is responsible for the IR in the fasting state and what is responsible for the insulin resistance in the insulin-stimulated state. Both the liver and muscle are severely resistant to insulin in individuals with T2DM. The brain has an obligate need for glucose and is responsible for ~ 50% of glucose utilization under basal or fasting conditions. This glucose demand is met primarily by glucose production by the liver and kidneys. In T2DM basal hepatic glucose production (HGP) is greater than in healthy individuals. This overproduction of glucose by the liver occurs in the presence of fasting plasma insulin which is increased 2.5- to 3-fold, indicating severe resistance to the suppressive effect of insulin on HGP. In addition to hepatic IR, multiple other factors contribute to the accelerated rate of HGP including: (i) increased circulating glucagon levels and enhanced hepatic sensitivity to glucagon; (ii) lipotoxicity leading to increased expression and activity of phosphoenolpyruvate carboxykinase and pyruvate carboxylase, the rate-limiting enzymes for gluconeogenesis; and (iii) glucotoxicity, leading to increased expression and activity of glucose-6-phosphatase, the rate-limiting enzyme for glucose escape from the liver. Defronzo *et al.* demonstrated that muscle insulin resistance could account for over 85–90% of the impairment in total body glucose disposal in T2DMs.[33] In these patients there is presence of multiple intramyocellular defects in insulin action including impaired glucose transport and phosphorylation, reduced glycogen synthesis and decreased glucose oxidation.

Lipotoxicity

IR is known to be precipitated by excess deposition of fat in liver and muscle, i.e. lipotoxicity, deposition of long-chain (LC)-fatty acyl CoAs, diacylglycerol, and ceramide in the β-cell leads to impaired insulin secretion and β-cell failure. FFA play a causal role in IR. FFA modulate insulin-stimulated glucose disposal, hepatic gluconeogenesis, and glycogenolysis. Physiologically excess circulating glucose is stored as TG in adipose tissue. TG are broken down to FFA and glycerol and are released into the circulation in fasting stages. In overnutrition FFA play a crucial role in stimulating the liver to produce TG-rich lipoproteins (LC-CoA). In normal physiology LC-CoA are taken up by mitochondria where they undergo β-oxidation to release energy. Overnutrition induces an increase in malonyl CoA which in turn inhibits carnitine palmitoyltransferase-1, a rate-limiting enzyme in import of LC-CoA in mitochondria. Thus LC-CoA accumulate in endoplasmic reticulum (ER) exerting a stress on ER leading to protein misfolding. The physiological function of insulin is to inhibit β-oxidation. This function is fairly retained even in IR. Thus overnutrition triggers IR, lipid synthesis, inhibits β-oxidation, and impedes insulin-mediated suppression of hepatic gluconeogenesis. Together these events set up a stage for the development of hepatic steatosis during a sustained period of overnutrition. Increased TG in circulating blood shifts the TG/HDL ratio towards TG, thus accelerating cardiovascular risk. FFA promote recruitment of macrophage to adipose tissue. Macrophages secrete TNF-α through activation of IKKβ-NF-κB (inhibitor of nuclear factor (NF)–κB (IκB) kinase–β-NF-κB) triggering an inflammatory flux. FFA also alter the ratio of pro-inflammatory (leptin, TNF-α, IL-6, IL-1β) and anti-inflammatory (adiponectin) adipokines. The cumulative effect of this low-grade chronic inflammation is a CVD risk.[34] Recently the ProActive UK Research Group highlighted positive association between moderate intensity activity, improvement in insulin sensitivity and the prevention of T2DM.[35] A chronic unhealthy diet coupled with a sedentary lifestyle initiates IR which plays a causal role by gluco- and lipotoxicity steadily shifting the balance from normal physiology to obesity, T2DM, and MS.[36] Other factors like glucotoxicity, hypersecretion of islet amyloid polypeptide (IAPP), which is co-secreted in a one-to-one ratio with insulin and abnormalities in the incretin axis can lead to progressive β-cell failure.[5]

Mitochondrial Dysfunction

The mitochondrion plays a central role in fuel utilization. It is the site for oxidation of fat, carbohydrates, and fatty acids, and formation of adenosine-5′-triphosphate (ATP) which is the "molecular currency" of a cell. ATP formation involves two major steps: (i) the oxidation of reducing equivalents (NADH or FADH2) that are produced by enzymatic pathways involved in the metabolism of substrates; and (ii) the phosphorylation of adenosine diphosphate (ADP) to ATP, also known as oxidative phosphorylation (OP). OP is known to be reduced in prediabetic stages.[36] The detailed physiology of mitochondria is not in the scope of this review. Here we will discuss the pathogenesis of mitochondrial dysfunction due to overproduction of

substrates—a pre- prediabetic situation that stems from overfeeding. Lowell *et al.* in their review have described mitochondrial function. The cellular metabolism of substrates generates electrons in the form of the reduced hydrogen carriers NADH and FADH2. They donate electrons to the electron-transport chain (ETC), which comprises protein complexes that are located in the mitochondrial inner membrane. As electrons are transferred in ETC, protons (H+) are pumped from the mitochondrial matrix into the mitochondrial intermembrane space. This establishes a proton gradient across the mitochondrial inner membrane. The energy that is conserved in this proton gradient drives the synthesis of ATP from ADP and inorganic phosphate (Pi) by ATP synthase as protons are transported back from the intermembrane space into the mitochondrial matrix. Proton leak is mediated by the uncoupling proteins (UCPs), which uncouple the processes of electron transport/proton-gradient generation on the one hand, and ATP synthesis on the other. By dissipating the proton gradient, the energy that is derived from the oxidized substrates is released as heat. Superoxide production is dependent on the proton gradient and is controlled by UCPs by an autoregulatory feedback loop.[37] This means that when there is high caloric intake of substrates, there will be an increase in mitochondrial membrane potential (MMP) and thus an increase in the production of superoxides. These superoxides will activate the UCP causing the proton leak and this decreasing the MMP. Sustained overfeeding will increase the amount of substrates undergoing oxidation thus initiating stress on mitochondria. Conversely, caloric restriction (CR) will increase the ratio of AMP:ATP in mitochondria in turn stimulating AMPK which triggers PGC-1. CR also stimulates sirtuins (SIRT1), a nutrient deprivation sensor that contributes in activating the PGC-1. Sirtuins are an attractive therapeutic target since they can be found in all organs and their modulation can be achieved through caloric restriction. Acute stressors like exercise, exposure

to cold, caloric restriction, and macrophage activation, all contribute in modulating AMPK-PGC group bringing robustness to the biological function and regulating IR. These data suggest a causal role of mitochondria in IR.[6]

β-Cell Dysfunction

Pancreatic β-cell dysfunction means either loss of function or decrease in the cell mass or apoptosis. Initially β-cell mass was thought to be genetically predetermined; however, now we know that β-cells interact with nutrients and other environmental stressors. Pancreatic β-cells respond to various secretogogues like pyruvate, FFA, amino acids, catecholamines, or the incretin regulator-like glucagon-like peptide (GLP-1). However, all of them require some threshold stimulatory concentration of glucose in the bloodstream for their effects. However, glucose is a direct stimulus for β-cells. Overnutrition increases metabolism of glucose and other substrates in mitochondria resulting in an increased donation of electrons to the ETC. This will result in an increase in the amount of protons that are pumped out of the mitochondrial matrix, thus generating a high MMP. As a consequence, large amounts of superoxide will be produced in the mitochondrial matrix owing to an increase in 'random' single-electron transfer reactions from components of the ETC to molecular oxygen. Furthermore, UCP2 expression is increased. These independent events lead to a deleterious activation of the superoxide–UCP2 pathway, which causes decreased ATP production from glucose by ATP synthase and, subsequently, loss of glucose-stimulated insulin secretion.[37,38] ER-stress because of gluco-lipotoxicity also plays an important role in β-cell dysfunction. IR stimulates β-cells to secrete insulin. This increases demand for insulin biosynthesis leading to ER stress and increased protein misfolding. ER stress is initially relieved by unfolded protein response (UPR), but sustained stress makes UPR ineffective. Deleterious effects of ER stress thus lead to cell death mediated by inositol-requiring-kinase-1 (IRE1). Insulin hypersecretion is accompanied by amylin secretion, which in humans can form amyloid fibrils that accumulate at the surface of β-cells inducing dysfunction and apoptosis.[39]

OXIDATIVE STRESS AND ADVANCED GLYCATED END PRODUCTS (AGE)

Chronic hyperglycemia has longstanding effects like generation of reactive oxygen species (ROS) that mediate the micro- and macro-vascular complications representing a substantial cause of morbidity and mortality. Diabetic patients without known vascular complications display enhanced platelet activation and decreased antioxidant status. Organ damage can be triggered by both extracellular and intracellular increases in glucose. Increased extracellular glucose leads to non-enzymatic glycosylation of proteins and subsequent formation of AGE. Chemically AGE are formed when there is interaction between the highly reactive aldehyde group of glucose with any free amino group on proteins. This creates a Schiff's base, which spontaneously rearranges itself into an Amadori's product. A stable Amadori product ultimately leads to the formation of AGEs. These in turn interact with their respective receptor (RAGE) on the cell membrane and promote the production of ROS. Increased intracellular glucose generates ROS through mitochondria promoting the polyol pathway. Together increased ROS and AGE target tissues causing diabetic retinopathy, diabetic nephropathy, atherosclerosis, and diabetic neuropathy.[40]

Significance of Stress in T2DM

Stress has central as well as peripheral effects. Central effects deal with alertness, arousal, aggression, inhibiting vegetative functions and activating counter-regulatory feedback loops mediated via hypothalamic hormones arginine vasopressin (AVP), cortico-tropin-releasing hormone (CRH)-cortisol, the pro-opiomelanocortin-derived peptides, norepinephrine, and many other hormone intermediates present in brainstem and midbrain. Peripheral effects are oxygenation, increase in nutrition of brain, heart, muscles, increased cardiovascular tone and increased catabolism mediated via hypothalamic-pituitary-adrenal (HPA) axis. Undernutrition or overnutrition also activates NF-κB and JNK pathways via the ER stress. In case of chronic stress the normal equilibrium of the body witnesses a sustained disequilibrated state resulting from hypersecretion of stressor mediators. For example, chronic ER stress activates IkkB/NF-κB pathways in the hypothalamus which in turn inhibits physiological actions of insulin and leptin. Also, chronic increase in cortisol or catecholamines will trigger release of FFA from the adipocyte. Recent studies have also demonstrated that stress-induced increases in neuropeptide Y contribute to increases in obesity. Taken together these findings suggest a strong correlation of stress in metabolic disease.[41] Peripheral upregulation of NPY receptor-2 (Y2) is implicated in obesity.[42] Efforts to study Y2 inhibitors for treatment of obesity are ongoing.[43,44]

From the above review it is evident that the body is a robust, dynamic and complex system. Like stimulus has a response, the body tries to cope with every challenge. The response to a stimulus is memorized, evaluated, and replicated with necessary corrections by the brain. This robustness allows the body to keep itself in a constant state of equilibrium. However, sustained abnormal stimulus cripples the robustness of the system and this disequilibrium is stress. Chronic diseases do not develop overnight, but they are a result of a loss of robustness of the system. Modern medicine should try to restore the lost balance in metabolic disease with the help of medical and nutritional therapy. Thus modern medicine should target metabolic disease as a whole, rather than as a sum of its parts.

APPROACHES FOR STUDYING HERBALS

Herbal drug development requires novel approaches like reverse pharmacology that can fast-track drug development.[10] This is because reverse pharmacology selects herbs that are already used in *Ayurveda*. These drugs are then evaluated during exploratory clinical studies. Experimental studies can be carried simultaneously to conclude mechanistic explanations for the clinical activity.[45] Ayurvedic therapeutics follows the systems approach and, therefore, has more promise in the treatment of multi-target disease. For chronic diseases including diabetes and cardiovascular conditions where long-term treatment is needed, co-administration of herbals and modern medicines may pose higher risk of adverse events and hence sufficient evidence of safety is necessary. Approaches such as Safety Pharmacology (SP) should be undertaken for herbals.[46,47] The aim of SP is to characterize the pharmacodynamic/pharmacokinetic relationship of a drug's adverse effects using continuously evolving methodology at therapeutic dose. Unlike toxicology, SP includes a regulatory requirement to predict the risk of rare lethal events. This gives SP its unique character. SP could be used as an important tool for adverse event liability and clinical safety monitoring for herbals.

Approaches for studying the effect of herbals should include first, the whole system, and second, mechanistic studies elucidating the multiple targets. It is observed that in India, PhD students take multiple plants and observe the effects of multiple plants on a particular disease. Such observations remain unexplored for their mechanisms of action. Without mechanism of action it is difficult for modern medicine to accept such formulations in mainstream therapeutics. Therefore, it is time to take a next step and study the mechanism of action of these formulations. It is easier to file a patent on such observations but such patents remain on-shelf forever. A recent review extensively covers the number and quality of patents filed from India that are based on herbals.[48] However, there are very few patents that succeed in market.

HERBAL MARKET: EXPECTATIONS AND CONFUSION FROM THE KNOWN

In India, China, Egypt, and Sudan, around 70% of the rural population uses traditional medicine. Similar situations exist in a large number of developing countries. It is estimated that 17.7% of Americans use herbals, and in 2007 they spent US$33.9 billion on complementary and alternative medicine (CAM).[49] Out of that, US$14.8 billion was spent on herbals (dietary supplements). This detailed survey was conducted by National Institutes of Health's (NIH), National Center for Complementary and Alternative Medicine (NCCAM)—National Health Interview Survey (NHIS), http://nccam. nih.gov/news/2008/nhsr12.pdf. However, data on safety are sparse when compared to the use. Patients have reported many adverse herbal reactions, unexpected herb—drug interactions, and inefficacy of treatment. Grant *et al.* 2009, examined 16 trials lasting 4 weeks to 2 years involving 1,391 participants receiving 15 different Chinese herbal medicines in eight different comparisons. No trial reported on mortality, morbidity, or costs. No serious adverse events like severe hypoglycemia were observed. Meta-analysis of the eight trials showed that those receiving Chinese herbal medicines combined with lifestyle modification were more than twice as likely to have their fasting plasma glucose levels return to normal levels compared to lifestyle modification alone. Thus subjects/patients receiving the Chinese herbs were less likely to progress to T2DM over the duration of the trial. However, authors conclude that all trials had a considerable risk of bias and none of the specific herbal medicines comparison data was available from more than one study. Moreover, results could have been confounded by rates of natural reversion to normal glucose levels.[50]

Efforts to address these inadequacies are being undertaken by respective authorities. Recently CAM researchers from China developed and validated a tool to assess the quality of the case series studies in herbal medicine.[51] Similarly Narahari et al.[52] and Tillu et al.[53,54] discuss the problem of evaluating multimodal integrative medicine treatments for complex pathological conditions. Both the articles are recognized by the Consolidated Standards of Reporting Trials (CONSORT) guidelines. Vaidya et al. argue that TCM and Ayurveda require a different kind of evidence which might not fit in the domains of modern medicine. Hence there may be a need to develop newer assessment tools and different evaluating models. Bhaishajyaratnavali, an ancient Ayurvedic text, enlists 164 formulations for Prameha and Madhumeha (biomedical approximation of Prameha and Madhumeha can be "Metabolic Diseases"). Ayurvedic practitioners regularly use most of these in the treatment of metabolic diseases using Ayurvedic wisdom. However, there is a need for focused research that will help to establish the use of herbals in pathological conditions like T2DM, obesity, hypertension, hypertriglyceridemia, and CVDs.[55] TCM is way ahead of Ayurveda in terms of its herbal exports, market share, research, development of new tools for TCM validation, and patents. This is covered by Patwardhan et al.[56]

Marketed herbs for diabetes in and around Mumbai, India were surveyed by Nabar et al. (Personal discussion). We searched for published manuscripts elucidating mechanistic aspects of these herbs (Table 35.1). To our surprise, there is sparse literature available that can elucidate the mechanisms of action of the herbs that are consumed by diabetic patients. Independently isolated compounds like curcuminoids, polyphenols from different sources, have been studied extensively. However, integrated approaches towards drug development from Ayurveda and other Indian systems of medicines need more time.[57]

NEW STRATEGIES FOR INTEGRATED RESEARCH ON METABOLIC DISEASES BASED ON AYURVEDA

Modern medicine recognizes an individual either in health or disease. However, it is known that there is a slow, yet progressive conversion from a healthy state to diseased state. Ayurveda elaborates on a six-stage process of disease manifestation as Shatkriyakaal.[58,23] These Shatkriyakaal or six stages permit the recognition and management of disease much before it progresses into evidently differentiated clinical symptoms. Patwardhan et al. are in the process of developing a multi-institutional molecular epidemiology project that would aim to understand the steps involved in progression from health to Prameha using Shatkriyakaal. Prameha is considered as a biomedical approximation to metabolic diseases. This project targets metabolic diseases in which insulin resistance is the underlying pathology. Ayurveda defines symptomatic factors for Poorvaroopa (pre-stages) of Prameha. These anthropometric, biochemical, psychological, genetic, epigenetic, and metabolomic variables would be considered as biomarkers of Prameha pathogenesis. Presently the project is in the process of conceptualizing a scale or instrument, called "Prameha Proclivity Factors" (PPF). PPF would be generated, which could predict

TABLE 35.1 List of Top 10 Herbs Used in the Indian Market for Diabetes, as Obtained from the Pharmacoepidemiology Survey by Nabar *et al.*

Sr. No	Top 10 herbs used in the Indian market for diabetes	Published articles				Articles discussing molecular mechanisms	Possible targets suggested for diabetes
		Total[#]	Reviews	Original studies			
				Clinical	Experimental		
1	*Syzygium cumini* (Jambhul)	(58) 17	4	4	14*	—	Adenosine deaminase
2	*Gymnema sylvestre* (Gudmar)	(137) 43	15	4	21	2	↑ Calcium flux in pancreatic β-cells
3	*Azadirachta indica* (Neem)	(488) 19	3	1	14	—	—
4	*Momordica charantia* (Karela)	(451) 107	25	9	60	8	↑ AMPK, PPARα, insulin, ↓apoB, triacylglycerol, insulino-mimetic
5	*Curcuma longa* (Haridra)	(642) 32	9	—	17	9	↑ PPAR-γ, glucose uptake, cholesterol-7a-hydroxylase; ↓ ROS, adipogenesis (Wnt signaling)
6	*Emblica officinalis* (Amalki)	(142) 7	—	—	7	—	
7	*Trigonella foenum-graecum* (Methi)	(192) 60	6	2	40	7	↑ HDL, LDL receptor, glucose uptake, GLUT4 translocation, phosphoenol pyruvate kinase and pyruvate kinase
8	*Tinospora cordifolia* (Guduchi)	(123) 23	4	—	16	—	
9	*Aegle marmelos* (Bilva)	(105) 21	2	—	16	1	Normalizing membrane-bound ATPases by umbelliferone
10	*Enicostemma littorale* (Mamejwa)	(16) 12	—	2	8	2	↑ HDL and glucose-induced insulin release through K(+)-ATP channel dependent pathway independent of Ca influx
11**	*Cassia auriculata* (Avartaki)	(44) 13	—	—	12	1	↓ α-Glucosidase activity

[#] *Number in parentheses is total number of articles published on that plant up to 29-05-2010.*
* *Published manuscript covered clinical + experimental study; the classification is based on the abstract and/or full text; if full text or abstract was not available the article is not listed in the table.*
** *Cassia auriculata is not a member in the top 10 marketed herbs, but is included only for comparison.*
The table shows a Pubmed search of 10 herbs and classification of the same in to Reviews, Clinical, Experimental and Mechanisms elucidating studies. Keywords searched only in Pubmed are 'botanical name of the plant' AND diabetes using Endnote software (demo version).

FIGURE 35.1 Complex of metabolic diseases elucidating inflammation and IR are causal to T2DM, obesity, hypertension, hypertriglyceridemia, polycystic ovarian disease, CVD, cancer, and Alzheimer's Disease. This cluster of metabolic diseases stems from inflammation triggering IR and targets almost all the organs of the body and therefore cause increase in risk of morbidity and mortality. *(Adapted from PhD Thesis of Dr Amrutesh Puranik.)*

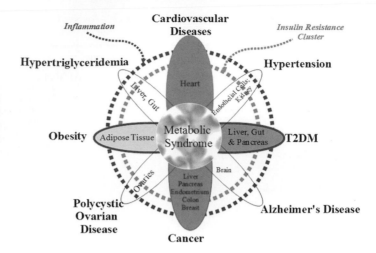

susceptibility of an individual for *Prameha* or metabolic disease. Such projects based on integrated approaches would bring a scientific rigor to *Ayurveda*[59] and contribute to preventing the progression of metabolic diseases.

Acknowledgment

ASP acknowledges support of Dr Zofia Zukowska, Professor, Integrative Biology and Stress Physiology, University of Minnesota.

References

1. Zarocostas J. Need to increase focus on non-communicable diseases in global health, says WHO. *BMJ* 2010;**341**:c7065.
2. Dans A, Ng N, Varghese C, Tai ES, Firestone R, Bonita R. The rise of chronic non-communicable diseases in southeast Asia: time for action. *Lancet* 2011;**377**:680–9.
3. Taubes G. Insulin resistance. Prosperity's plague. *Science* 2009;**325**:256–60.
4. Nathan DM, Buse JB, Davidson MB, Ferrannini E, Holman RR, Sherwin R, Zinman B. Medical management of hyperglycaemia in type 2 diabetes mellitus: a consensus algorithm for the initiation and adjustment of therapy: a consensus statement from the American Diabetes Association and the European Association for the Study of Diabetes. *Diabetologia* 2009;**52**:17–30.
5. Defronzo RA. Banting Lecture. From the triumvirate to the ominous octet: a new paradigm for the treatment of type 2 diabetes mellitus. *Diabetes* 2009;**58**:773–95.
6. Milne JC, Lambert PD, Schenk S, Carney DP, Smith JJ, Gagne DJ, Jin L, Boss O, Perni RB, Vu CB, Bemis JE, Xie R, Disch JS, Ng PY, Nunes JJ, Lynch AV, Yang H, Galonek H, Israelian K, Choy W, Iffland A, Lavu S, Medvedik O, Sinclair DA, Olefsky JM, Jirousek MR, Elliott PJ, Westphal CH. Small molecule activators of SIRT1 as therapeutics for the treatment of type 2 diabetes. *Nature* 2007;**450**:712–6.
7. DeSouza C, Fonseca V. Therapeutic targets to reduce cardiovascular disease in type 2 diabetes. Nature reviews. *Drug Discovery* 2009;**8**:361–7.
8. Schmidt BM, Ribnicky DM, Lipsky PE, Raskin I. Revisiting the ancient concept of botanical therapeutics. *Nature Chemical Biology* 2007;**3**:360–6.
9. Bent S. Herbal medicine in the United States: review of efficacy, safety, and regulation: grand rounds at University of California, San Francisco Medical Center. *Journal of General Internal Medicine* 2008;**23**:854–9.
10. Patwardhan B, Mashelkar RA. Traditional medicine-inspired approaches to drug discovery: can *Ayurveda* show the way forward? *Drug Discovery Today* 2009;**14**:804–11.
11. Kelly GS. Insulin resistance: lifestyle and nutritional interventions. *Alternative Medicine Review: A Journal of Clinical Therapeutics* 2000;**5**:109–32.

12. Babu PA, Suneetha G, Boddepalli R, Lakshmi VV, Rani TS, Rambabu Y, Srinivas K. A database of 389 medicinal plants for diabetes. *Bioinformation* 2006;**1**:130−1.

13. Shane-McWhorter L. Botanical dietary supplements and the treatment of diabetes: what is the evidence? *Current Diabetes Reports* 2005;**5**:391−8.

14. Sharma H, Chandola HM, Singh G, Basisht G. Utilization of *Ayurveda* in health care: an approach for prevention, health promotion, and treatment of disease. Part 2 − *Ayurveda* in primary health care. *Journal of Alternative and Complementary Medicine* 2007;**13**:1135−50.

15. Shekelle PG, Hardy M, Morton SC, Coulter I, Venuturupalli S, Favreau J, Hilton LK. Are Ayurvedic herbs for diabetes effective? *The Journal of Family Practice* 2005;**54**:876−86.

16. Liu Y, Wang MW. Botanical drugs: challenges and opportunities: contribution to Linnaeus Memorial Symposium 2007. *Life Sciences* 2008;**82**:445−9.

17. Mohan V, Venkatraman JV, Pradeepa R. Epidemiology of cardiovascular disease in type 2 diabetes: the Indian scenario. *Journal of Diabetes Science and Technology* 2010;**4**:158−70.

18. Bagchi D, Preuss HG, editors. *Obesity: Epidemiology, Pathophysiology, and Prevention*, Vol. 1. CRC Press; 2007.

19. Baruah D, Gupta OP. A comparative study of *Prameha Roga* from the Brihatrayee. *Bulletin of the Indian Institute of History of Medicine* 2002;**32**:93−107.

20. Nanda GC, Padhi MM, Pathak NN, Choppra KK. Screening of Madhumehaghna (anti diabetic) plants in Vrihattrayee. *Bulletin of the Indian Institute of History of Medicine* 2000;**30**:15−26.

21. Sharma H, Chandola HM. *Prameha* in *Ayurveda*: Correlation with obesity, metabolic syndrome, and diabetes mellitus. Part 2 − Management of *Prameha*. *Journal of Alternative and Complementary Medicine* 2011;**17**(7):589−99.

22. Sharma H, Chandola HM. *Prameha* in *Ayurveda*: Correlation with obesity, metabolic syndrome, and diabetes mellitus. Part 1 − Etiology, classification, and pathogenesis. *Journal of Alternative and Complementary Medicine* 2011;**17**:491−6.

23. Morandi A, Tosto C, Sartori G, Roberti di Sarsina P. Advent of a link between *Ayurveda* and modern health science: The Proceedings of the First International Congress on *Ayurveda*, "*Ayurveda*: The Meaning of Life-Awareness, Environment, and Health" March 21-22, 2009, Milan, Italy. *Evidence-based Complementary and Alternative Medicine: eCAM* 2011;**2011**. 929083.

24. Mukherjee PK, V. P., Ponnusankar S. Ethnopharmacology and integrative medicine − Let the history tell the future. *J Ayurveda Integr Med* 2010;**1**:9.

25. Raut AA. Integrative endeavor for renaissance in *Ayurveda*. *J Ayurveda Integr Med* 2011;**2**:3.

26. Patwardhan B. *Ayurveda* for all: 11 action points for 2011. *J Ayurveda Integr Med* 2010;**1**:3.

27. Spiegelman BM, Enerback S. The adipocyte: a multifunctional cell. *Cell Metabolism* 2006;**4**:425−7.

28. Waki H, Tontonoz P. Endocrine functions of adipose tissue. *Annual Review of Pathology* 2007;**2**:31−56.

29. Hock MB, Kralli A. Transcriptional control of mitochondrial biogenesis and function. *Annual Review of Physiology* 2009;**71**:177−203.

30. Gnasso A, Carallo C, Irace C, Spagnuolo V, De Novara G, Mattioli PL, Pujia A. Association between intima-media thickness and wall shear stress in common carotid arteries in healthy male subjects. *Circulation* 1996;**94**:3257−62.

31. Schmidt MI, Duncan BB, Sharrett AR, Lindberg G, Savage PJ, Offenbacher S, Azambuja MI, Tracy RP, Heiss G. Markers of inflammation and prediction of diabetes mellitus in adults (Atherosclerosis Risk in Communities study): a cohort study. *Lancet* 1999;**353**:1649−52.

32. Nathan DM, Davidson MB, DeFronzo RA, Heine RJ, Henry RR, Pratley R, Zinman B. Impaired fasting glucose and impaired glucose tolerance: implications for care. *Diabetes Care* 2007;**30**:753−9.

33. Pendergrass M, Bertoldo A, Bonadonna R, Nucci G, Mandarino L, Cobelli C, Defronzo RA. Muscle glucose transport and phosphorylation in type 2 diabetic, obese nondiabetic, and genetically predisposed individuals. American Journal of Physiology. *Endocrinology and Metabolism* 2007;**292**:E92−100.

34. de Rooij SR, Nijpels G, Nilsson PM, Nolan JJ, Gabriel R, Bobbioni-Harsch E, Mingrone G, Dekker JM. Low-grade chronic inflammation in the relationship between insulin sensitivity and cardiovascular disease (RISC) population: associations with insulin resistance and cardiometabolic risk profile. *Diabetes Care* 2009;**32**:1295−301.

35. Helmerhorst HJ, Wijndaele K, Brage S, Wareham NJ, Ekelund U. Objectively measured sedentary time may predict insulin resistance independent of moderate- and vigorous-intensity physical activity. *Diabetes* 2009;**58**:1776−9.

36. Kahn SE, Hull RL, Utzschneider KM. Mechanisms linking obesity to insulin resistance and type 2 diabetes. *Nature* 2006;**444**:840−6.

37. Lowell BB, Shulman GI. Mitochondrial dysfunction and type 2 diabetes. *Science* 2005;**307**:384−7.

38. Robertson RP, Harmon J, Tran PO, Poitout V. Beta-cell glucose toxicity, lipotoxicity, and chronic oxidative stress in type 2 diabetes. *Diabetes* 2004;**53**(Suppl. 1): S119−24.

39. Muoio DM, Newgard CB. Mechanisms of disease: molecular and metabolic mechanisms of insulin resistance and beta-cell failure in type 2 diabetes. Nature reviews. *Molecular Cell Biology* 2008;**9**:193–205.

40. Vericel E, Januel C, Carreras M, Moulin P, Lagarde M. Diabetic patients without vascular complications display enhanced basal platelet activation and decreased antioxidant status. *Diabetes* 2004;**53**:1046–51.

41. Kuo LE, Kitlinska JB, Tilan JU, Li L, Baker SB, Johnson MD, Lee EW, Burnett MS, Fricke ST, Kvetnansky R, Herzog H, Zukowska Z. Neuropeptide Y acts directly in the periphery on fat tissue and mediates stress-induced obesity and metabolic syndrome. *Nature Medicine* 2007;**13**:803–11.

42. Shi YC, Lin S, Castillo L, Aljanova A, Enriquez RF, Nguyen AD, Baldock PA, Zhang L, Bijker MS, Macia L, Yulyaningsih E, Zhang H, Lau J, Sainsbury A, Herzog H. Peripheral-specific Y2 receptor knockdown protects mice from high-fat diet-induced obesity. *Obesity (silver spring)*; 2011 May. Ahead of print.

43. Yulyaningsih E, Zhang L, Herzog H, Sainsbury A. NPY receptors as potential targets for anti-obesity drug development. *British Journal of Pharmacology* 2011 July;**163**(6):1170–202.

44. Zhang L, Bijker MS, Herzog H. The neuropeptide Y system: Pathophysiological and therapeutic implications in obesity and cancer. *Pharmacology & Therapeutics* 2011;**131**:91–113.

45. Vaidya AD, Vaidya RA, Nagral SI. *Ayurveda* and a different kind of evidence: from Lord Macaulay to Lord Walton (1835 to 2001 AD). *The Journal of the Association of Physicians of India* 2001;**49**:534–7.

46. Puranik AS, Halade G, Kumar S, Mogre R, Apte K, Vaidya ADB, Patwardhan B. Cassia auriculata: Aspects of safety pharmacology and drug interaction. Evidence-based complementary and alternative medicine. *eCAM* 2011;**8**.

47. MacKenzie I. Safety pharmacology for the non-clinical assessment of medicinal products. *Drug Discovery Today* 2002;**7**:232–4.

48. Sahoo N, Manchikanti P, Dey SH. Herbal drug patenting in India: IP potential. *Ethnopharmacol* 2011 Sep;**137**(1):289–97.

49. Nahin RL, Barnes PM, Stussman BJ, Bloom B. Costs of complementary and alternative medicine (CAM) and frequency of visits to CAM practitioners: United States, 2007. *National Health Statistics Reports* 2009;**18**:1–14.

50. Grant SJ, Bensoussan A, Chang D, Kiat H, Klupp NL, Liu JP, Li X. Chinese herbal medicines for people with impaired glucose tolerance or impaired fasting blood glucose. *Cochrane Database of Systematic Reviews*; 2009:CD006690.

51. Yang AW, Li CG, Da Costa C, Allan G, Reece J, Xue CC. Assessing quality of case series studies: development and validation of an instrument by herbal medicine CAM researchers. *Journal of Alternative and Complementary Medicine* 2009;**15**:513–22.

52. Narahari SR, Ryan TJ, Aggithaya MG, Bose KS, Prasanna KS. Evidence-based approaches for the Ayurvedic traditional herbal formulations: toward an Ayurvedic CONSORT model. *Journal of Alternative and Complementary Medicine* 2008;**14**:769–76.

53. Chopra A, Saluja M, Tillu G. *Ayurveda*-modern medicine interface: A critical appraisal of studies of Ayurvedic medicines to treat osteoarthritis and rheumatoid arthritis. *Journal of* Ayurveda *and Integrative Medicine* 2010;**1**:190–8.

54. Sarmukaddam S, Chopra A, Tillu G. Efficacy and safety of Ayurvedic medicines: Recommending equivalence trial design and proposing safety index. *International Journal of* Ayurveda *Research* 2010;**1**:175–80.

55. Vaidya AD, Devasagayam TP. Current status of herbal drugs in India: an overview. *Journal of Clinical Biochemistry and Nutrition* 2007;**41**:1–11.

56. Patwardhan B, Warude D, Pushpangadan P, Bhatt N. *Ayurveda* and traditional Chinese medicine: a comparative overview. Evidence-based complementary and alternative medicine: *eCAM* 2005;**2**:465–73.

57. Mukherjee PK, Wahile A. Integrated approaches towards drug development from *Ayurveda* and other Indian system of medicines. *Journal of Ethnopharmacology* 2006;**103**:25–35.

58. Singh RH. An assessment of the ayurvedic concept of cancer and a new paradigm of anticancer treatment in *Ayurveda*. *Journal of Alternative and Complementary Medicine* 2002;**8**:609–14.

59. Patwardhan B. *Ayurveda*, evidence-base and scientific rigor. *Journal of* Ayurveda *and Integrative Medicine* 2010;**1**:169–70.

PREVENTION AND TREATMENT 2: DRUGS AND PHARMACEUTICALS

The Evolution of Glucose-Lowering Drugs for Type 2 Diabetes

Andrew J. Krentz, Alan J. Sinclair

Institute of Diabetes for Older People (IDOP), Bedfordshire and Hertfordshire Postgraduate Medical School, University of Bedfordshire, Luton, UK

OUTLINE

INTRODUCTION

After many years of stagnation, some new classes of glucose-lowering drugs have entered the market; still more are currently being evaluated in clinical trials. Novel drugs for type 2 diabetes are currently being positioned within treatment algorithms alongside more established agents. These new drugs avoid some of the adverse effects and limitations of older drugs such as biguanides and sulfonylureas. However, no diabetes drugs are devoid of unwanted effects. By definition, clinical experience of newer drugs is limited and their long-term efficacy and safety have yet to be quantified. Unanticipated safety issues that have emerged after many years

Nutritional and Therapeutic Interventions for Diabetes and Metabolic Syndrome
DOI: 10.1016/B978-0-12-385083-6.00036-X

of use—most notably with the thiazolidine-diones (glitazones)—have altered the perceptions of risks and benefits of glucose-lowering agents.[1,2] The rosiglitazone controversy has prompted regulators to insist on more rigorous assessment of cardiovascular outcomes in patients with type 2 diabetes. This is of enormous importance because the risk of athero-thrombotic events (macrovascular disease), primarily ischemic heart disease and stroke, are greatly increased in type 2 diabetes.[3,4] The fact that these complications are the leading cause of death among patients with diabetes makes exclusion of adverse cardiovascular effects of new drugs imperative. However, separating the intrinsic risk of ischemic events from toxic effects of new drugs can be problematic.

On a more positive note, the place of metformin as foundation therapy has been cemented by the results of the United Kingdom Prospective Diabetes Study (UKPDS)[5] and the subsequent 10-year follow-up of the participants.[6] Sulfonylureas are still used extensively although the advantages of new drugs, notably avoidance of weight gain and freedom from hypoglycemia, are increasingly being considered by physicians. These attributes, especially freedom from hypoglycemia, have led the American Association of Clinical Endocrinologists/American College of Endocrinology (AACE/ACE)[7] to recommend their use as first-line therapy. Other expert groups such as the American Diabetes Association/European Association for the Study of Diabetes (ADA/EASD) consensus group[8] have taken a more cautious approach.

A detailed exposition of the aims and approaches of managing type 2 diabetes is outside the scope of this chapter. However, a few guiding principles are warranted. The management of type 2 diabetes centers on attaining glycemic control to relieve acute osmotic symptoms and preventing, or at least retarding, the development of long-term microvascular and macrovascular complications. More often than not, lifestyle measures have to be supplemented with pharmacological therapy. In general, oral glucose-lowering agents are used first as long as hyperglycemia is not too extreme, particularly if osmotic symptoms are marked and major insulin deficiency is likely. Metabolic decompensation requires immediate insulin treatment and intensive supportive measures. Balancing the risk—benefit profile of glucose-lowering drugs and setting and maintaining glycemic targets appropriate to the individual patient are major tenets of therapy. Special care must be taken in highly vulnerable groups such as the older patients and those with comorbidities such as renal or hepatic impairment, or a history of cardiovascular disease. Great care is also needed in women of childbearing age because of the risk of pregnancy. Diabetes in pregnancy requires specialist care.

Sufficient residual pancreatic β-cell function is necessary for most of these drugs to exert their maximal glucose-lowering effects. Combinations of drugs from different agents, e.g., insulin sensitizers + insulin secretagogues, are often required as endogenous insulin production wanes. Ultimately, insulin replacement therapy is required by many patients after failure to maintain glycemic control with two to three oral agents. Various options are available when transitioning to insulin and often one, less commonly more than one, oral agents are continued in combination with insulin.

Glucose-lowering therapy must be complemented by measures directed at reducing the risk of athero-thrombotic (macrovascular) complications: these are the leading cause of premature mortality in type 2 diabetes. Non-glucose-dependent effects of drugs for diabetes, such as improvements in lipid profiles and reductions in blood pressure, are therefore of considerable relevance. However, positive effects on these risk factors can not be assumed to translate into better clinical outcomes in the long term. This lesson has been brought home by the aforementioned storm of controversy that led to major regulatory restrictions on the use of rosiglitazone.

In this chapter we briefly review the more established classes of glucose-lowering drugs that are used for type 2 diabetes, although some are more more popular than others. This section includes biguanides, sulfonylureas, α-glucosidase inhibitors, the thiazolidinediones, and amylin agonists. We then consider the range of newer agents acting on the incretin axis and discuss their roles within the pharmacological armamentarium. Finally, we look ahead to some novel agents that are currently in development.

WELL-ESTABLISHED DRUGS

Biguanides

Metformin

Metformin (dimethylbiguanide) is the only member of this class available in many countries. Phenformin was withdrawn from the UK and other markers in the l970s because of its association with lactic acidosis.[9] Worldwide, metformin is the most extensively used oral agent for type 2 diabetes. The drug, which has been in use since the 1950s, is widely regarded as first-line monotherapy for type 2 diabetes inadequately controlled by lifestyle measures. In the UKPDS, metformin not only provided protection against microvascular complications of diabetes but also reduced the incidence of athero-thrombotic events compared with diet therapy.[5] In contrast to sulfonylureas or insulin, metformin also reduced diabetes-related deaths and all-cause mortality in the overweight and obese participants who were initially randomized to the drug. Metformin has been credited with vasoprotective effects not shared by other classes of glucose-lowering agents.[10] These include increased rates of fibrinolysis and reduced levels of plasminogen activator inhibitor-1. However, attributing the relative contributions of these actions and the glucose-lowering effects of

metformin has been problematic.[11] An additional issue is that some studies, notably the UKPDS, have suggested that combination therapy using metformin with a sulfonylurea may be detrimental.[5,12] More recently, a putative role for metformin as an anticancer agent has emerged.[13]

Metformin acts mainly by improving insulin action, i.e. by reducing insulin resistance.[14] Blood glucose is lowered without any appreciable risk of hypoglycemia at therapeutic dosages. However, hypoglycemia may become an issue when metformin is used in combination with an insulin-releasing agent, e.g., a sulfonylurea, or insulin. The full efficacy of metformin requires the presence of islet β-cell function that is adequate to provide the necessary levels of circulating insulin. At the cellular level, metformin improves insulin signaling thereby activating the cellular energy regulating enzyme adenosine 5′-monophosphate-activated protein kinase (AMPK).[15]

The predominant action of metformin is to reduce the inappropriately elevated levels of hepatic glucose production that drive fasting hyperglycemia in type 2 diabetes.[16] This is achieved predominantly through decreased gluconeogenesis. Metformin also reduces hepatic glycogenolysis. Insulin-stimulated glucose uptake and glycogen formation in skeletal muscle are also enhanced. Reduced fatty acid oxidation also contributes to improvements in intermediary metabolism.

Metformin is the drug of choice for overweight or obese patients because it does not cause weight gain and may aid weight reduction. Metformin can be used in combination with any other class of oral glucose-lowering agent as well as with insulin. In the UK, it is recommended that the dose of metformin be reviewed if estimated glomerular filtration rate (eGFR) falls below 45 ml/min. At eGFR rates < 30 ml/min metformin should be avoided. This caution reflects concerns about the most feared, if uncommon, adverse event— lactic acidosis. Use of the drug in patients with cardiac or respiratory insufficiency and during major intercurrent illnesses such as severe infection, dehydration, recent myocardial infarction, or shock that predispose to tissue hypoxia and hyperlactatemia must also be avoided. Liver disease, alcohol abuse, or a history of metabolic acidosis are additional contraindications. Metformin may cause resumption in women with polycystic ovary syndrome (PCOS). Optimally titrated metformin monotherapy can generally be expected to reduce fasting plasma glucose by approximately 2–4 mmol/l and decreases hemoglobin A1c (HbA1c) by 1–2%. However, as with all drugs for diabetes, responses are variable between patients and depend on factors such as the pretreatment HbA1c and the degree of insulin deficiency in the individual. As a broad generalization, however, it is reasonable to say that no particular class of oral glucose-lowering drugs can be regarded as being clearly the most efficacious.[17]

Tolerability issues are well recognized with metformin.[18] These are mainly related to the gastrointestinal tract and include abdominal discomfort and diarrhea. Low doses of the drug may be tolerated but approximately 5–10%, perhaps more, of patients find that gastrointestinal symptoms preclude long-term therapy. Metformin can reduce absorption of vitamin B_{12}.

Sulfonylureas

The first generation of sulfonylureas have largely been replaced by potent second-generation sulfonylureas, including glibenclamide (also known as glyburide in the US and Canada), gliclazide, glipizide, and glimepiride.[19]

The liver metabolizes all sulfonylureas although metabolite activity and routes of elimination vary. It has long been recognized that sulfonylureas with a longer duration of action carry a higher risk of hypoglycemia.

Sulfonylureas stimulate insulin secretion from β-cells. The drugs bind to the sulfonylurea receptor (SUR1), a component of the transmembrane complex that includes the ATP-sensitive Kir 6.2 potassium channels (K-ATP channels). Binding closes the K-ATP channels, leading to intracellular events that culminate in the release of insulin from preformed granules. Cardiac and vascular smooth muscle cells express different isoforms of the SUR.[20] Concerns about potential cardiotoxicity of sulfonylureas date back to the 1970s and have not been satisfactorily resolved.[21]

Avoidance of asymptomatic or symptomatic hypoglycemia is an important objective in managing diabetes. All sulfonylureas have the capacity to cause hypoglycemia because they will stimulate insulin release even at low blood glucose concentrations. Cardiac and vascular smooth muscle cells express various isoforms of the SUR.

Sulfonylureas are preferred for patients who are not overweight since they often cause some weight gain. Starting doses should always be at the lower end of the dose range. The efficacy of sulfonylureas is similar to that of metformin. Irreversible deterioration of glycemic control during sulfonylurea therapy occurs in perhaps 5–10% of patients per year is held to be a consequence of the progressive β-cell failure that characterizes type 2 diabetes.

Alpha-Glucosidase Inhibitors

Alpha-glucosidase inhibitors retard carbohydrate digestion via competitive inhibition of the activity of α-glucosidase enzymes located in the brush border of the enterocytes that line the intestinal villi.[22] The inhibitors bind to these enzymes preventing breakdown of disaccharide and oligosaccharide substrates into absorbable monosaccharides. Glucose absorption is completed over a longer period and postprandial hyperglycemia is reduced. The secretion of gastric inhibitory polypeptide (GIP) may be reduced whereas secretion of glucagon-like peptide-1 (7-36 amide) (GLP-1) is increased.[19]

When used as monotherapy in patients complying with dietary advice, an α-alpha-glucosidase inhibitor can be expected to reduce peak postprandial glucose concentrations by approximately 1–3 mmol/l. Furthermore, there is often a reduction in fasting hyperglycemia of up to 1 mmol/l. The improvement in HbA1c is generally less pronounced than with sulfonyl-ureas or metformin, i.e. ~0.5%, but sometimes exceeding 1% if a high dose of the drug is tolerated and dietary modifications are maintained. Alpha-glucosidase inhibitors do not cause weight gain. The fermentation of unabsorbed carbohydrates in the large bowel is responsible for the common problems of flatulence, abdominal discomfort, and diarrhea.

Acarbose has never been popular in the UK but is widely used in some countries such as China. Low rates of use of the drug in the UK mainly reflect the aforementioned poor tolerability of acarbose. Two other α-glucosidase inhibitors, miglitol and voglibose, are available in some countries.

Thiazolidinediones

The thiazolidinediones were introduced into clinical practice at the end of the 20th century. High hopes surrounded this novel class of glucose-lowering drugs which seemed to offer a means of countering insulin resistance, present in the great majority of patients with type 2 diabetes.[23] The drugs improve insulin sensitivity by stimulating a widely distributed nuclear receptor known as the peroxisome proliferator-activated receptor-γ (PPAR-γ).[24] This promotes adipocyte differentiation and lipogenesis mainly in subcutaneous depots. Stimulation of lipogenesis reduces circulating non-esterified fatty acids thereby facilitating glucose uptake by muscle and insulin-sensitive adipocytes; hepatic gluconeogenesis is reduced.

The first thiazolidinedione, troglitazone, was withdrawn because of severe hepatotoxicity. Two others, rosiglitazone and pioglitazone, subsequently became available, neither of which was associated with adverse hepatic effects. However, rosiglitazone was withdrawn from the European market in 2010 and use of the drug was restricted in the US. As detailed below, these actions were the culmination of a highly charged debate that revolved around concerns that rosiglitazone might be associated with an increased risk of myocardial ischemic events.

Thiazolidinedione monotherapy can reduce fasting plasma glucose by 2–3 mmol/l and HbA1c by approximately 1.5%.[19] All thiazolidinediones have the propensity to cause fluid retention with increased plasma volume, reduced hematocrit and a decrease in hemoglobin. The drugs should be avoided in patients with heart failure. Precise exclusions on the basis of cardiac status vary between Europe and the US. Fluid retention accounts for some of the weight gain that is commonly encountered with these drugs. Visceral adipose depots may be reduced while subcutaneous adipose depots increase. Used as monotherapy or in combination with drugs such as metformin, thiazolidinediones do not cause hypoglycemia. Rosiglitazone causes a small rise in total cholesterol levels, accounted for by a rise in both low-density lipoprotein (LDL) cholesterol and high-density lipoprotein[25] (HDL) cholesterol. Elevations of triglyceride levels are a well-recognized consequence of rosiglitazone therapy. Pioglitazone has little effect on total cholesterol, raises HDL cholesterol and reduces fasting triglycerides. More recent safety concerns have centered on (i) the impact of the drugs on cardiovascular outcomes, and (ii) adverse effects of bone metabolism.

The European Medicines Agency (EMA) approved the use of pioglitazone and rosiglitazone in 2000, but demanded post-marketing cardiovascular outcome studies, there being no long-term safety and efficacy data.[26] This deficiency notwithstanding, the thiazolidinediones enjoyed a growth in use as other drugs, notably sulfonylureas in the UK market, declined. The class attained so-called blockbuster status until worrying data about cardiovascular events associated with rosiglitazone came to light.[2] In 2007, rosiglitazone came under intense scrutiny with the publication of a controversial meta-analysis.[27] This suggested a statistically significant 43% increase in risk of myocardial infarction and a 64% rise in cardiovascular death risk among patients taking rosiglitazone compared with placebo or other classes of glucose-lowering drugs. A series of subsequent meta-analyses were unable to confirm or refute the concern that rosiglitazone increased the risk of myocardial infarction.[28]

The results of the Rosiglitazone Evaluated for Cardiovascular Outcomes (RECORD) study were reassuring,[29] although critics pointed to methodological issues that in their opinion may have precluded firm conclusions. Current evidence for pioglitazone suggests protection against athero-thrombotic vascular events, albeit at the cost of an increased incidence of heart failure.[30–33]

Both rosiglitazone and pioglitazone increase the risk of distal bone fractures in women. Thiazolidinediones contribute to bone loss, the effect being most prominent in postmenopausal women.[34] This unwanted effect was not anticipated and emerged only after the drugs had been in clinical use for a decade. Macular edema has been reported with thiazolidinediones.

Amylin Analogs

Islet amyloid polypeptide, or amylin, is a peptide hormone co-secreted with insulin from islet β-cells. The hormone activates central neural pathways that decrease glucagon release from pancreatic α-cells, retard gastric emptying, and promote satiety.

Pramlintide is a soluble synthetic amylin analog.[35] In the US pramlintide is approved for use in patients with type 2 diabetes as add-on therapy to certain orally active glucose-lowering agents or insulin. The drug can promote weight loss in addition to improving glycemic control. The principal adverse effects of the drug are nausea and hypoglycemia.[36]

NEW DRUGS FOR TYPE 2 DIABETES

The latest classes of glucose-lowering drugs increase insulin secretion through the so-called incretin axis. This approach circumvents some of the unwanted effects of the sulfonylureas—principally weight gain and hypoglycemia. These new agents also provide an alternative to thiazolidinediones, thereby avoiding weight gain, fluid retention, heart failure, and increased risk of fractures.

The incretin effect is held to account for up to 70% of postprandial insulin secretion in healthy subjects. The most important incretin hormones are glucagon-like peptide-1 (GLP-1) and glucose-dependent insulinotropic peptide (GIP).[37] These are secreted by the L cells of the distal ileum and colon, and the K cells of the duodenum and upper jejunum, respectively. Plasma levels of the incretin hormones rise within minutes of eating. GLP-1 and GIP act on β-cell G-protein-coupled receptors to enhance glucose—stimulated insulin secretion. Acute release of insulin is followed by insulin biosynthesis and insulin gene transcription. The acute effect of GLP-1 serves to potentiate glucose-dependent insulin release of preformed insulin; importantly, this only occurs when circulating glucose concentrations are raised. Thus, as glucose levels return to normal the incretin-induced release of insulin is switched off and insulin levels rapidly decline.

GLP-1, but not GIP, slows gastric emptying and suppresses appetite via central effects (Table 36.1). The incretin effect is deficient in

TABLE 36.1   Major Effects of the Incretin Hormones GLP-1 (Glucagon-like Peptide-1) and GIP (Glucose-Dependent Insulinotropic Polypeptide) on Factors Influencing Glucose Homeostasis

	GLP-1	GIP
Effects on pancreatic islets		
Increase nutrient-induced insulin secretion	Y	Y
Suppress glucagon secretion	Y	-
Extra-pancreatic effects		
Slow gastric emptying	Y	-
Promote satiety and weight reduction	Y	-

patients with type 2 diabetes.[38] Thus, postprandial GLP-1 secretion from the gut is reduced and the insulinotropic action of GIP is attenuated. The secretion of glucagon—a potent stimulus to hepatic glucose production—is reduced by GLP-1. In type 2 diabetes glucagon levels from the islet α-cells are not adequately suppressed by hyperglycemia. This has been a somewhat neglected aspect of the pathophysiology of type 2 diabetes that, in part, reflects the limited scope for therapeutic manipulation. GLP-1 and GIP are rapidly degraded, principally by a widely distributed proteolytic cell surface enzyme, dipeptidyl peptidase-4 (DPP-4).

As a consequence, the half-life of GLP-1 in the circulation is less than 2 min.

Novel glucose-lowering therapies exploiting the defective incretin effect in type 2 diabetes have been developed, based on the pathophysiology of the incretin hormone axis.[39] Include the orally active DPP-4 inhibitors which increase the endogenous levels of the incretin hormones (Figure 36.1). The injectable GLP mimetics include: (i) derivatives of GLP-1 that have been modified to resist proteolysis; and (ii) novel peptides that have metabolic actions similar to GLP-1 and are intrinsically resistant to proteolysis.[40]

Dipeptidyl Peptidase-4 Inhibitors

Members of this new class of orally active glucose-lowering drugs are also known as gliptins. The first three DPP-4 inhibitors to be marketed were sitagliptin, vildagliptin, and saxagliptin (Figure 36.2). Clinically relevant differences in metabolism and safety profiles are evident between the three drugs (Table 36.2). The Food and Drug Administration (FDA) deferred approval of vildagliptin. because of skin lesions in a primate model and issues of safety in patients with renal impairment. Linagliptin, which is non-renally eliminated, was approved in 2011. Others are in development. DPP-4 inhibitors can raise the

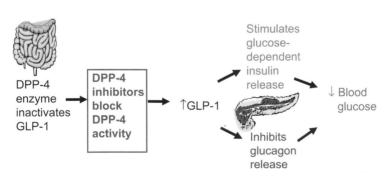

FIGURE 36.1   Effect of DPP-4 inhibitors on GLP-1 (glucagon-like peptide-1) metabolism and its physiological actions. Note that GLP-1 receptor agonists also exert effects on satiety and gastric emptying that are not observed with DPP-4 inhibitors.

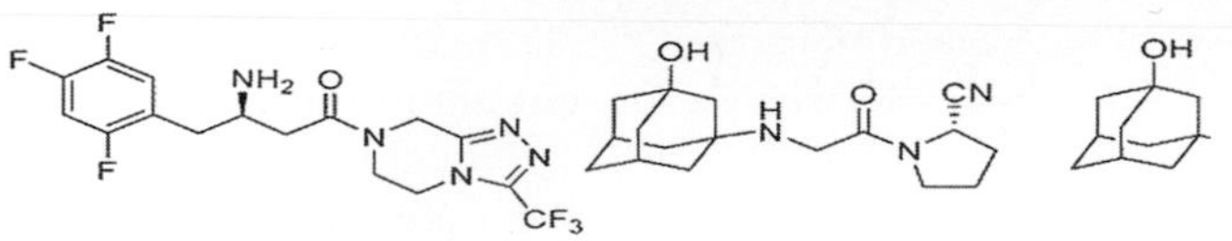

FIGURE 36.2   Chemical structure of sitagliptin, vildagliptin, and saxagliptin.

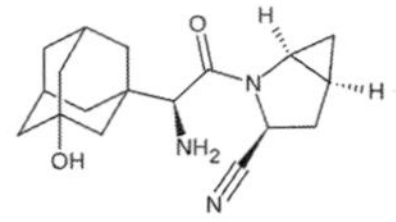

levels of active incretin hormone concentrations two- to three-fold.

Sitagliptin is a competitive inhibitor of DPP-4 that has high bioavailability (~90%) with a plasma half-life of 8–14 h; t-max is 1–4 h. Plasma protein binding is approximately 40%. A small proportion of the drug is metabolized by CYP3A4 and CYP2C6 with about 80% of sitagliptin being eliminated unchanged in the urine through renal tubular secretion. In a single dose, 100 mg sitagliptin achieves near complete

inhibition of DPP-4 activity for about 12 h with around 80% inhibition up to 24 h.

Vildagliptin forms a reversible covalent complex with DPP-4. The drug has a plasma half-life of approximately 1.5–4.5 h; t-max is less than 2 h. Bioavailability of the drug is around 85%. More than two-thirds of vildagliptin is metabolized, predominantly through renal metabolism, to inactive metabolites. There is a negligible contribution from CYP 450 isoforms with 85% being eliminated in the urine. A dose

TABLE 36.2   Dosages and Precautions of DPP-4 Inhibitors

	Usual dose	Liver disease	Renal disease	Other comments
Sitagliptin	100 mg o.d.	May be used in mild-to-moderate liver disease, i.e. Child–Pugh score 7–9 (a composite of biochemical and clinical criteria)	Creatinine clearance ≥ 30 to < 50 ml/min, use 50 mg daily If < 30 ml/min, use 25 mg daily	
Vildagliptin	50 mg b.d.	Avoid if serum transaminase levels elevated ×3 or more before or during therapy	Not recommended if creatinine clearance < 50 ml/min	Check liver function before initiation, every 3 months during first year of treatment, and periodically thereafter
Saxagliptin	5 mg o.d.	No dose reduction required	Use 2.5 mg daily if creatinine clearance < 50 ml/min	

DPP-4 dipeptidyl peptidase-4.

of 50–100 mg vildagliptin provides almost complete inhibition of DPP-4 for about 12 h with 40% inhibition at 24 h. Plasma protein binding is low at approximately 10%.

Saxagliptin provides maximal inhibition of DPP-4 for approximately 2–3 h through reversible covalent complex formation; DPP-4 inhibition extends to approximately 24 h. As for sitagliptin and vildagliptin, saxagliptin has greater specificity for DPP-4 than for either cytosolic DPP-8 or DPP-9, members of the same gene family as DPP-4. Saxagliptin is eliminated by renal and hepatic pathways. Kidney metabolism generates a hydroxylated metabolite that has 50% of the activity of the parent compound. There is some evidence of active renal excretion of the parent compound and blood levels of drug and metabolite are increased by renal impairment. *In vitro*, serum protein binding of saxagliptin is $\leq 30\%$.

The indications for use of these drugs differ between countries. In theory, they can be used as monotherapy, in combination with metformin, a sulfonylurea, or a thiazolidinedione. Combining a DPP-4 inhibitor with insulin can also be advantageous. Full efficacy of DPP-4 inhibitors requires the presence of adequate β-cell function. While the class is regarded as being weight-neutral, some studies have shown modest degrees of weight loss. The latter property contrasts with sulfonylurea or thiazolidinediones making DPP-4 inhibitors an attractive option for overweight and obese patients. Because insulin secretion is closely linked to blood glucose concentration DPP-4 inhibitors carry a low risk of hypoglycemia. This is the case when they are used as monotherapy, or in conjunction with agents such as metformin or thiazolidinediones. If hypoglycemia occurs when a DPP-4 inhibitor is combined with a sulfonylurea, reducing the dose of the sulfonylurea or withdrawal of the DPP-4 inhibitor is recommended. A reduced dose of sitagliptin, i.e. 50 mg once daily, is recommended in moderate renal insufficiency, i.e. creatinine clearance ≥ 30 to

< 50 ml/min. With more severe renal insufficiency or end-stage renal disease, a dose of 25 mg once daily should be considered. Sitagliptin can be used in patients with minor to moderate impairment of liver function. Circulating levels of saxagliptin and its metabolite are reduced if liver function is impaired. Vildagliptin use is not recommended in patients with either moderate or severe renal impairment. A reduced dose, i.e. 2.5 mg daily, is recommended if creatinine clearance is less than 50 ml/min. Reversible elevations in hepatic transaminase concentrations have been observed in association with vildagliptin. Liver function should be assessed before starting treatment, at 3-month intervals during the first year, and periodically thereafter. A marked rise in liver enzymes, > 3 times the upper limit of the normal range, or other evidence of hepatic impairment, are contraindications to vildagliptin. All DPP-4 inhibitors should be avoided in pregnancy and in women planning or at risk of conception.

In clinical trials, administration of 100 mg/day sitagliptin as monotherapy or add-on therapy to other agents reduces HbA1c from a baseline of ~8% by ~0.7 percentage points after 24–52 weeks. At higher baseline HbA1c levels reductions in HbA1c $> 1\%$ have been reported. Fasting blood glucose is reduced by 1.0–1.5 mmol/l. Postprandial glucose levels after a standard mixed meal are reduced by approximately 3 mmol/l. A single daily dose of 50–100 mg/day vildagliptin shows similar efficacy and tolerability to sitagliptin when used as monotherapy, or as add-on therapy to metformin or a thiazolidinedione. A daily dose of 5 mg saxagliptin either as monotherapy, or in combination with metformin, a sulfonylurea, or a thiazolidinedione produces mean placebo-subtracted reductions in HbA1c of 0.60–0.65%.

No serious adverse effects have been reported to date with DPP-4 inhibitors. In phase 3 trials tolerability has generally been good with a low frequency of adverse events. Compared with placebo and comparator drugs, a slightly higher incidence of upper respiratory tract infections has been reported. Theoretical concerns about interference with innate immunity have been raised because DPP-4 also functions as the lymphocyte CD36 protein. However, neither CD26 knockout mice nor the DPP-4 inhibitors used in humans have shown any significant untoward effects on immune function. These reassuring observations notwithstanding, minor decreases in blood lymphocyte count have been observed in association with sitagliptin and saxagliptin in human studies.

In 2009 the FDA revised the prescribing information for sitagliptin following reports of acute pancreatitis. Patients should be monitored for the development of clinical features of pancreatitis after initiating a DPP-4 inhibitor initiation and when dosages are increased. Until a clearer picture emerges, DPP-4 inhibitors should be used cautiously in patients with a history of pancreatitis.

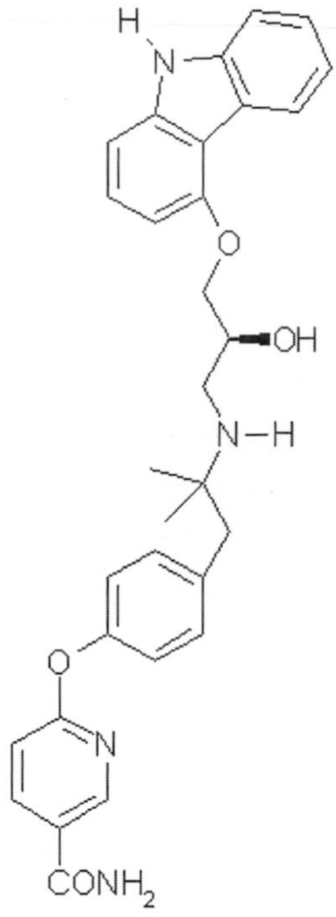

Glucagon-Like Peptide-1 Receptor Agonists

GLP-1 mimetics mimic the actions of native GLP-1. Agents in this class, all of which require subcutaneous administration, are designed to be resistant to the actions of DPP-4.[40] Compared with DPP-4 inhibitors, use of GLP-1 agonists is generally associated with greater reductions in blood glucose that is often accompanied by loss of body weight (Table 36.1). Islet β-cell function is improved by GLP-receptor agonists, but no evidence has emerged that this is sustained beyond the duration of treatment. Thus, to date, no drugs used for glucose control in type 2 diabetes can be said to be disease-modifying.

The long-term impact of GLP-1 agonists on clinical outcomes remains to be determined.

Exenatide

Synthetic exendin-4, or exenatide (Figure 36.3), was approved for use in the US in 2005; the drug

FIGURE 36.3   Chemical structure of exenatide.

has been available in the UK since 2007. Exendin-4 is an agonist for the GLP-1 receptor present in the venom of *Heloderma suspectum*, the Gila monster of the Southwestern US. The intrinsic resistance of exendin-4 to inactivation by DDP-4 provided the development of exenatide.[40] In 2009, liraglutide entered clinical practice. The main attributes of GLP-1 agonists are reduction of hyperglycemia in concert with the potential for simultaneous weight loss and an intrinsically low risk of hypoglycemia. GLP-1 mimetics lower glycated hemoglobin by approximately 1% compared with placebo. Moreover, GLP-1 receptor agonists can produce weight loss of between 1.5 kg and 4.5–5.0 kg *vs* placebo and insulin therapy, respectively. This contrasts with the weight gain observed in some oral agents and insulin.[41] Open label extension studies show that reductions in glycemic control are sustained and progressive reductions in body weight may be achieved in some patients. Improvements in vascular risk factors including blood pressure and lipid profiles have been reported. Reductions in hepatic transaminase levels have also been observed.

Exenatide has approximately 50% sequence homology with human GLP-1. However, the drug has a 20- to 30-fold longer half-life and much greater potency than GLP-1 in its effects on blood glucose. Resistance to DDP-4 is achieved through substitution of Gly2 for Ala2 at the inactivation site of the molecule. Exenatide is rapidly absorbed, and is detectable in the circulation within 15 min after subcutaneous injection. Maximum drug concentrations are achieved at 2–3 h. The formation of antibodies to exenatide can reportedly increase the C_{max} and may extend the half-life of the drug. Effects on blood glucose are evident for 6–8 h after injection. Thus, twice-daily administration is required. Elimination half-life is 3–4 h. Clearance of the drug is reduced in patients with severe renal impairment. The clinical significance of exenatide antibodies, which have been observed in approximately 40% of patients in some studies, is uncertain. There is evidence that the metabolic effects of exenatide may be impaired by high antibody titers in a minority (< 5%) of patients.

In the US, exenatide is licensed as adjunctive therapy for patients with inadequate glycemic control on metformin, a sulfonylurea, a thiazolidinedione, a combination of metformin and a sulfonylurea, or a combination of metformin and a thiazolidinedione.

Exenatide is administered using a pre-filled pen device in the thigh, abdomen, or upper arm. The starting dose is 5 µg given any time within the 60-min period before the main morning and evening meals, or before the two main meals of the day about 6 h apart or longer. If tolerated, the dose is increased to 10 µg twice daily after 4 weeks if the therapeutic response demands a higher dose. If gastrointestinal side effects pose difficulties, dose escalation can be deferred another 4–6 weeks. Because insulin secretion is coupled to blood glucose levels no reduction in dose is necessary for meal size or physical activity levels. There is a small risk of hypoglycemia when exenatide is used in conjunction with a sulfonylurea and the dose of the latter drug may need to be reduced. If added to metformin, no dose adjustment of either drug is required.

In older people exenatide should be used with caution; dose escalation from 5 µg to 10 µg should proceed with care in patients > 70 years. Clinical experience in patients > 75 years is limited. No dosage adjustment is required for patients with mild renal impairment, defined as a creatinine clearance of 50–80 ml/min. If creatinine clearance is 30–50 ml/min dose escalation should proceed cautiously. Exenatide is not recommended in patients if creatinine clearance is < 30 ml/min. No dosage adjustment is necessary if hepatic function is impaired.

Nausea is the most common side effect; this is usually relatively mild and tends to dissipate with time but affects 30–50% of recipients.[42] Vomiting may be troublesome and preclude long-term therapy. There are no adequate studies of exenatide in pregnancy and the drug should be avoided in lactation. Post-marketing reports of acute pancreatitis in patients taking exenatide have generated some concern. Most of the patients affected had pre-existing risk factors for acute pancreatitis such as gallstones, severe hypertriglyceridemia or excessive alcohol consumption. None the less, the FDA requested a change to the package insert that warns about pancreatitis. Patients should be informed of the symptoms of pancreatitis and the need to seek prompt medical attention should they develop. Exenatide should be discontinued if pancreatitis is suspected.

Exenatide LAR was approved for clinical use in 2011. This is a sustained release formulation of injectable microspheres of exenatide and poly(D,L lactic-co-glycolic acid) which is a biodegradable medical polymer. Gradual drug delivery at a controlled rate enables once-weekly injection. Other GLP-1 receptor agonists that require less frequent administration are in development, including taspoglutide and albuglitide.

Liraglutide

Liraglutide is a GLP-1 mimetic that is resistant to DPP-4. The drug has a 97% sequence identify to native GLP-1 that comprises a modified GLP-1 peptide sequence that is attached to a palmitoyl chain (Figure 36.4).[43] This enables non-covalent binding to albumin after subcutaneous injection. Islet β-cell function is improved with enhanced potentiation of meal-associated insulin secretion. Postprandial blood glucagon levels are decreased, in line with the aforementioned actions of GLP-1.

Binding to albumin retards renal elimination, giving liraglutide a half-life of approximately 12 h. The slow absorption of liraglutide from subcutaneous tissues produces a maximum blood concentration after 8–12 h, thereby permitting once-daily injection. It is postulated that avoiding peaks of the drug helps to reduce the characteristic gastrointestinal side effects.

In the UK, liraglutide is approved for the treatment of adults with type 2 diabetes in combination with metformin or a sulfonylurea, in combination with metformin and a sulfonylurea, or added to metformin and a thiazolidinedione.

Liraglutide is formulated as a solution for subcutaneous injection in pre-filled pens delivering 0.6, 1.2 or 1.8 mg per dose. The suggested starting dose is 0.6 mg daily, increasing after not less than a week to the maintenance dose of 1.2 mg daily. After at least another week, the dose can be increased to 1.8 mg if required, although this dose is not recommended by the UK's National Institute of Health and Clinical Excellence (NICE).[42] The agency has also specified criteria that should prompt abandonment of therapy based on a combination of weight reduction and glycemic effects; these restrictions also apply to exenatide in the UK. If an inadequate response is observed after 6 months of treatment, alternative glucose-lowering drugs should be considered. Use of liraglutide is not recommended in patients with moderate degrees of renal impairment, i.e. where creatinine clearance is 30–60 ml/min. Liraglutide has not been studied in patients with severely impaired renal function, and data in patients with hepatic impairment are limited.

In patients with type 2 diabetes liraglutide can significantly lower HbA1c with concomitant improvements in fasting and postprandial blood glucose levels. Body weight is dose-dependently reduced by approximately 1–3 kg. The main adverse events are nausea and diarrhea, although the frequency of gastrointestinal side

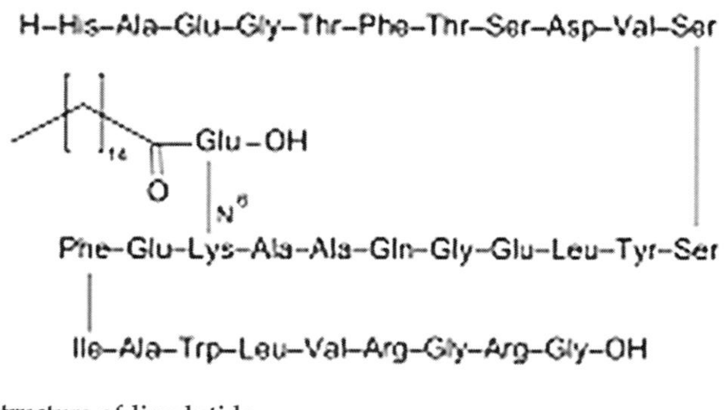

FIGURE 36.4   Chemical structure of liraglutide.

effects will often decrease over time. Lowering of triglycerides and reductions in blood pressure have also been observed.

In preclinical studies C-cell thyroid tumors were observed in rodent models. In clinical use, increased rates of clinical thyroid-related adverse events including neoplasms, elevated blood calcitonin levels and goiter have been observed in ≤ 1% of liraglutide-treated patients. Antibody formation has been reported in < 10% of patients but their presence does not appear to have a significant impact on the efficacy of the drug. A small number of cases of acute pancreatitis have been reported. However, no evidence of causality has been established. The utility of liraglutide as a weight-reducing drug in nondiabetic obesity is under investigation.

DRUGS CURRENTLY IN DEVELOPMENT FOR TYPE 2 DIABETES

Several classes of orally active new drugs for type 2 diabetes are being investigated (Table 36.3). In addition, new insulin analogs that might also be used in type 2 diabetes are

TABLE 36.3 Examples of Novel Glucose-Lowering Drugs Reported to be in Development for the Treatment of Type 2 Diabetes

SGLT2 inhibitors

PPAR-modulators

SPPARMs

Sulfonylurea receptor modulators

Glucokinase activators

GPR119 agonists

Glucocorticoid pathway modulators

SGLT2, sodium-glucose co-transporter type 2 diabetes; PPAR, peroxisome-proliferator activated receptor; SPPARM, selective peroxisome proliferator-activated receptor-γ modulators; GPR119, G protein-coupled receptor 119.

in development, as are more GLP-1 receptor agonists and DPP-4 inhibitors. We will briefly review three classes of oral glucose-lowering agents.

Sodium—Glucose Co-Transporter Type 2 Inhibitors

Approximately 160—180 g of glucose is filtered daily via the kidney into the urine in healthy adults. Reabsorption of glucose is proportional to the filtered glucose load until the transport maximum is exceeded. Glucose requires carrier proteins to move across cell membranes. Sodium-glucose co-transporter-2 (SGLT2) and SGLT1 reabsorb 90% and 10%, respectively, of filtered glucose.[44] SGLT2 is expressed almost entirely on proximal renal tubule cell membranes. This low-affinity, high-capacity transporter couples reabsorption of each glucose molecule to a sodium ion.

A new class of glucose-lowering agents, the SGLT2 inhibitors, are in the late stages of development.[45] These drugs, e.g., dapagliflozin, promote renal glucose excretion thereby reducing blood glucose concentrations.[46] They are predicted to carry a low risk of hypoglycemia. Urinary calorie loss, which can reach 200—300 kcal/day, promotes weight reduction. An increased frequency of uro-genital infections has consistantly been reported in clinical trials of SGLT2 inhibitors.

Peroxisome-Proliferator Activated Receptor Agonists

The efficacy and safety of pairing the metabolic benefits of thiazolidinediones with the lipid-modifying effects of fibric acid derivatives has led to the creation of a new class of drugs: combined PPAR-α and -γ agonists, or glitazars. Improvements in glucose and lipid metabolism have raised hopes of beneficial effects on cardiovascular disease.[47] However, the development of several agents has been discontinued because of a range of toxicity problems. Of note, muraglitazar was found to be associated with an increased risk of serious adverse cardiovascular effects, underscoring the need for careful clinical evaluation of all new drugs for type 2 diabetes.[48]

Glucokinase Activators

Glucokinase is a member of hexokinase family of enzymes that are responsible for the phosphorylation of glucose to glucose-6-phosphate. The enzyme has a key role in maintaining glucose homeostasis in islet β-cells and hepatocytes. Drugs that activate glucokinase have entered clinical studies.[49,50] Theoretical concerns include the risk of inducing hypoglycemia.

CONCLUSIONS

All drugs for lowering blood glucose in patients with type 2 diabetes have limitations in terms of long-term efficacy and the potential for adverse, potentially fatal in some circumstances, effects. The arrival of drugs with novel modes of action that can be used alongside more established agents is welcome. However, caution is required until the risk–benefit profiles of these new agents are fully evaluated. The recent lessons from the rosiglitazone controversy have strengthened regulatory requirements for new glucose-lowering drugs. However, the potential for the emergence of unanticipated serious adverse effects after many years of clinical use underlines the need for circumspection.

References

1. Cohen D. Rosiglitazone: what went wrong? BMJ (Clinical research ed 341:c4848).
2. Krentz AJ. Rosiglitazone: trials, tribulations and termination. *Drugs* **71**(2):123–30.
3. Woodcock J, Sharfstein JM, Hamburg M. Regulatory action on rosiglitazone by the U.S. Food and Drug Administration. *The New England Journal of Medicine* **363**(16):1489–91.
4. Blind E, Dunder K, de Graeff PA, Abadie E. Rosiglitazone: a European regulatory perspective. *Diabetologia* **54**(2):213–8.
5. Effect of intensive blood-glucose control with metformin on complications in overweight patients with type 2 diabetes (UKPDS 34). UK Prospective Diabetes Study (UKPDS) Group. *Lancet* 1998;**352**(9131):854–65.
6. Holman RR, Paul SK, Bethel MA, Matthews DR, Neil HA. 10-year follow-up of intensive glucose control in type 2 diabetes. *The New England Journal of Medicine* 2008;**359**(15):1577–89.
7. Rodbard HW, Jellinger PS, Davidson JA, et al. Statement by an American Association of Clinical Endocrinologists/American College of Endocrinology consensus panel on type 2 diabetes mellitus: an algorithm for glycemic control. *Endocr Pract* 2009;**15**(6):540–59.
8. Nathan DM, Buse JB, Davidson MB, et al. Medical management of hyperglycaemia in type 2 diabetes mellitus: a consensus algorithm for the initiation and adjustment of therapy: a consensus statement from the American Diabetes Association and the European Association for the Study of Diabetes. *Diabetologia* 2009;**52**(1):17–30.
9. Nattrass M, Alberti KG. Biguanides. *Diabetologia* 1978;**14**(2):71–4.
10. Nagi DK, Yudkin JS. Effects of metformin on insulin resistance, risk factors for cardiovascular disease, and plasminogen activator inhibitor in NIDDM subjects. A study of two ethnic groups. *Diabetes Care* 1993;**16**(4):621–9.
11. Lamanna C, Monami M, Marchionni N, Mannucci E. Effect of metformin on cardiovascular events and mortality: a meta-analysis of randomized clinical trials. *Diabetes, Obesity & Metabolism* **13**(3):221–8.
12. Olsson J, Lindberg G, Gottsater M, et al. Increased mortality in Type II diabetic patients using sulphonylurea and metformin in combination: a population-based observational study. *Diabetologia* 2000;**43**(5):558–60.
13. Ben Sahra I, Le Marchand-Brustel Y, Tanti JF, Bost F. Metformin in cancer therapy: a new perspective for an old antidiabetic drug? *Molecular Cancer Therapeutics* **9**(5):1092–99.
14. Bailey CJ, Turner RC. Metformin. *The New England Journal of Medicine* 1996;**334**(9):574–9.
15. Boyle JG, Salt IP, McKay GA. Metformin action on AMP-activated protein kinase: a translational research approach to understanding a potential new therapeutic target. *Diabet Med* **27**(10):1097–106.

16. Natali A, Ferrannini E. Effects of metformin and thiazolidinediones on suppression of hepatic glucose production and stimulation of glucose uptake in type 2 diabetes: a systematic review. *Diabetologia* 2006;**49**(3): 434–41.

17. Inzucchi SE. Oral antihyperglycemic therapy for type 2 diabetes: scientific review. *Jama* 2002;**287**(3):360–72.

18. Krentz AJ, Ferner RE, Bailey CJ. Comparative tolerability profiles of oral antidiabetic agents. *Drug Saf* 1994;**11**(4):223–41.

19. Krentz AJ, Bailey CJ. Oral antidiabetic agents: current role in type 2 diabetes mellitus. *Drugs* 2005;**65**(3): 385–411.

20. Gribble FM, Reimann F. Pharmacological modulation of K(ATP) channels. *Biochem Soc Trans* 2002;**30**(2): 333–9.

21. Krentz AJ. Sulfonylureas in the prevention of vascular complications: from UKPDS to the ADVANCE study. In: Crepaldi GTA, Avogaro A, editors. *The metabolic syndrome: diabetes, obesity, hyperlipidemia and hypertension*. Amsterdam: Excertpa Medical International Conference Series; 2002. p. 261–77.

22. Balfour JA, McTavish D, Acarbose. An update of its pharmacology and therapeutic use in diabetes mellitus. *Drugs* 1993;**46**(6):1025–54.

23. Reaven GM. Banting Lecture 1988. Role of insulin resistance in human disease. *Diabetes* 1988;**37**(12): 1595–607.

24. Yki-Jarvinen H. Thiazolidinediones. *The New England Journal of Medicine* 2004;**351**(11):1106–18.

25. Goldberg RB, Kendall DM, Deeg MA, et al. A comparison of lipid and glycemic effects of pioglitazone and rosiglitazone in patients with type 2 diabetes and dyslipidemia. *Diabetes Care* 2005;**28**(7):1547–54.

26. Krentz AJ, Bailey CJ, Melander A. Thiazolidinediones for type 2 diabetes. New agents reduce insulin resistance but need long term clinical trials. *BMJ* 2000;**321**(7256):252–3 (Clinical research ed).

27. Nissen SE, Wolski K. Effect of rosiglitazone on the risk of myocardial infarction and death from cardiovascular causes. *The New England Journal of Medicine* 2007;**356**(24):2457–71.

28. Schernthaner G, Chilton RJ. Cardiovascular risk and thiazolidinediones—what do meta-analyses really tell us? *Diabetes, Obesity & Metabolism* **12**(12):1023–35.

29. Home PD, Pocock SJ, Beck-Nielsen H, et al. Rosiglitazone evaluated for cardiovascular outcomes in oral agent combination therapy for type 2 diabetes (RECORD): a multicentre, randomised, open-label trial. *Lancet* 2009;**373**(9681):2125–35.

30. Dormandy JA, Charbonnel B, Eckland DJ, et al. Secondary prevention of macrovascular events in patients with type 2 diabetes in the PROactive Study (PROspective pioglitAzone Clinical Trial In macroVascular Events): a randomised controlled trial. *Lancet* 2005;**366**(9493):1279–89.

31. Krentz A. Thiazolidinediones: effects on the development and progression of type 2 diabetes and associated vascular complications. *Diabetes/Metabolism Research and Reviews* 2009;**25**(2):112–26.

32. Lincoff AM, Wolski K, Nicholls SJ, Nissen SE. Pioglitazone and risk of cardiovascular events in patients with type 2 diabetes mellitus: a meta-analysis of randomized trials. *JAMA* 2007;**298**(10):1180–8.

33. Graham DJ, Ouellet-Hellstrom R, MaCurdy TE, et al. Risk of acute myocardial infarction, stroke, heart failure, and death in elderly Medicare patients treated with rosiglitazone or pioglitazone. *JAMA*;**304**(4):411–8.

34. Tolman KG. The safety of thiazolidinediones. *Expert Opin Drug Saf* 2011 may;**10**(3):419–28. Epub 2011 mar 3.

35. Edelman S, Blashki G. Managing anxious patients: cognitive behaviour therapy in general practice. *Australian Family Physician* 2007;**36**(4):212–4;7-20.

36. Dunican KC, Adams NM, Desilets AR. The role of pramlintide for weight loss. *The Annals of Pharmacotherapy* **44**(3):538–45.

37. Vilsboll T, Holst JJ. Incretins, insulin secretion and Type 2 diabetes mellitus. *Diabetologia* 2004;**47**(3):357–66.

38. Drucker DJ. Enhancing incretin action for the treatment of type 2 diabetes. *Diabetes Care* 2003;**26**(10): 2929–40.

39. Meier JJ, Gallwitz B, Nauck MA. Glucagon-like peptide 1 and gastric inhibitory polypeptide: potential applications in type 2 diabetes mellitus. *BioDrugs* 2003;**17**(2):93–102.

40. Drucker DJ, Nauck MA. The incretin system: glucagon-like peptide-1 receptor agonists and dipeptidyl peptidase-4 inhibitors in type 2 diabetes. *Lancet* 2006;**368**(9548):1696–705.

41. Gentilella R, Bianchi C, Rossi A, Rotella CM. Exenatide: a review from pharmacology to clinical practice. *Diabetes, Obesity & Metabolism* 2009;**11**(6):544–56.

42. Wilding JP, Hardy K. Glucagon-like peptide-1 analogues for type 2 diabetes. *BMJ* 2011;**342**:d410 (Clinical research ed).

43. Davies MJ, Kela R, Khunti K. Liraglutide – overview of the preclinical and clinical data and its role in the treatment of type 2 diabetes. *Diabetes, Obesity & Metabolism* **13**(3):207–20.

44. Gerich JE. Role of the kidney in normal glucose homeostasis and in the hyperglycaemia of diabetes mellitus: therapeutic implications. *Diabet Med* **27**(2): 136–42.

45. Idris I, Donnelly R. Sodium-glucose co-transporter-2 inhibitors: an emerging new class of oral antidiabetic drug. *Diabetes, Obesity & Metabolism* 2009;**11**(2):79–88.

46. List JF, Woo V, Morales E, Tang W, Fiedorek FT. Sodium-glucose cotransport inhibition with dapagliflozin in type 2 diabetes. *Diabetes Care* 2009;**32**(4):650–7.

47. Cavender MA, Lincoff AM. Therapeutic potential of aleglitazar, a new dual PPAR-alpha/gamma agonist: implications for cardiovascular disease in patients with diabetes mellitus. *Am J Cardiovasc Drugs* **10**(4):209–16.

48. Nissen SE, Wolski K, Topol EJ. Effect of muraglitazar on death and major adverse cardiovascular events in patients with type 2 diabetes mellitus. *JAMA* 2005;**294**(20):2581–6.

49. Agius L. New hepatic targets for glycaemic control in diabetes. *Best Practice & Research* 2007;**21**(4):587–605.

50. Piya MK, Tahrani AA, Barnett AH. Emerging treatment options for type 2 diabetes. *British Journal of Clinical Pharmacology*.

37

Antidiabetic Drugs for Elderly Population

Raffaele Marfella, Giuseppe Paolisso

Department of Geriatric Medicine and Metabolic Diseases, Second University of Naples, Naples, Italy

INTRODUCTION

The management of type 2 diabetes in the elderly poses unique challenges.[1] A multitude of factors complicate the management of diabetes in this age group. Patients' overall health status, coexisting illnesses, social environment, psychological well-being and the degree of cognitive function must be assessed prior to initiating antihyperglycemic therapy in elderly diabetic patients.[2] Therefore, treatment of diabetes, although not substantially different from the type 2 diabetes therapy in adults, requires a different approach that must take into account all these variables, and above all it must be targeted to have a multidisciplinary approach.[3] Thus, an individualized approach in managing elderly persons with diabetes is appropriate, acknowledging the variability and complexity of this population. Although we can not find a disease clinically defined as "senile diabetes", we must make a distinction between people with diabetes who become older and older people who become diabetic. The first group requires a continuous review of therapeutic goals according to the gradual advancement of age and the consequent clinical conditions. In the second group, the characteristics typical of their age significantly affect the therapeutic aspects and management of diabetes.

Thus, it is important to know the history of the disease and the patient's clinical condition. The clinical evaluation must be integrated with assessments such as fasting blood glucose, glycosylated hemoglobin, lipid profile, creatinine, urinalysis, and cardiovascular assessment.[3] In general, the metabolic target of elderly diabetic patients is not different from that of the adult diabetic patient. However, many studies emphasize that the geriatric patients with diabetes often exhibit non-optimal metabolic control. Interestingly, it was also proposed to change the therapeutic target in relation to the health of the elderly. Particularly in diabetic patients in good health it would be desirable to achieve values of fasting of approximately 7 mmol/l (130 mg/dl) and 11 mmol/l (200 mg/dl) 2 h after the meal with values of glycosylated hemoglobin <7%. On the contrary, in elderly patients with diabetes not in good health ("frail elderly") it would be desirable to achieve blood glucose values of fasting of approximately 10 mmol/l (180 mg/dl), 14 mmol/l (250 mg/dl) 2 h after the meal and glycosylated hemoglobin values <8%. In the elderly it is important to approach the antidiabetic therapy in steps:

(i) change the therapy in relation to life expectancy, cognitive deficits, the patient's physical performance (including the quantification of disability), and social support which the patient has access to (living alone or not? lives in the community or in a protected environment? etc.);

(ii) use simple therapeutic regimens in both their implementation and the management;

(iii) encourage the decision-making autonomy in the therapeutic field with an appropriate education;

(iv) attempt to maintain glycosylated hemoglobin to <7% whereas higher values may also be accepted in relation to

life expectancy, the severity of diabetes, degree of disability, and finally to avoid hypoglycemia;

(v) schedule an eye examination every 2 years (except in cases with documented diabetic or hypertensive retinopathy) and an examination of the feet to evaluate neuropathy in diabetic foot each year;

(vi) screening for depression, cognitive deficits, and major geriatric syndromes that can make the elderly diabetic patient even more "fragile";

(vii) assessment of possible drug interference, such as those caused by the use of antiplatelet agents and/or antithrombotic, antihypertensive, anti-dyslipidemic, and drugs acting on the central nervous system such as hypno-inducing and/or anxiolytics.

In particular, the therapy aims to improve metabolic control (avoiding hypoglycemia) and to prevent the development and progression of complications, both macro- and microangiopathy. Age-related changes in physiology, diabetes-associated morbidities and other comorbidities, and polypharmacy make standard oral antihyperglycemic therapy and insulin use problematic in many cases. Avoidance of hypoglycemia is important in elderly subjects with diabetes, and many commonly-used antidiabetic medications are associated with substantial risk of hypoglycemia. Any antihyperglycemic medication that can be used in younger patients can also be used in older patients. However, many of these medications have adverse effects that are of particular concern in the elderly as elderly patients have age-related decreases in renal function, higher frequency of polypharmacy, and higher rates of comorbidity, including diabetes-related conditions that increase their risk for adverse effects. As noted, hypoglycemia is a primary concern in the elderly population, because it can have such a profound impact on patient health, function and quality of life. Avoiding hypoglycemia can significantly improve quality of life and patient compliance with anti-diabetic treatment. Therefore, the target of anti-diabetic therapy in elderly patients is the optimization of metabolic control by means of a procedure "stepwise" or "progressive" that includes both non-pharmacological therapy (diet and exercise, consistent with the physical conditions of the elderly patient) and drug therapy.[4]

NON-PHARMACOLOGICAL THERAPY

Diet and exercise play a central role in non-pharmacological therapy. In addition, elderly patients may have disorders of taste, salivation, and difficulties with dentition, all phenomena which may further reduce the compliance of diabetic patients to diet therapy. In general, the diet is important to maintain the ideal body weight, and should be high in complex carbohydrates and fiber. These aspects of the diet may play a dual role beneficial both for the delayed absorption of carbohydrates and may also help to stabilize the intestinal function. The American Diabetes Association (ADA) recommends a diet consisting of 50–60% of calories as carbohydrates, 10–20% as monounsaturated fats, 10–20% protein and less than 30% of calories from fat with keeping saturated fat less than 7% and polyunsaturated fat less than 10%.[5] The diet type that would result in high glycemic control is still unknown. Overall, the amount of carbohydrate may be more important than the source of carbohydrate ingested.[5] Studies looking at the glycemic index of particular food products have been controversial. It is more practical to emphasize the need for control of carbohydrate intake rather than eliminate specific sources of carbohydrates.[5] The amount of protein prescribed to an elderly diabetic patient depends on several factors.

The recommended dietary allowance of 0.8 g/kg may be sufficient for most healthy elderly patients, in chronic disease or catabolic states.[5] The ADA does not recommend routine supplementation of vitamins and mineral unless a specific deficiency is present.[5,6] A dietary regimen must be individualized, based on the patient's eating habits, motivation, and metabolic goals. Age-related physiologic changes such as alteration in taste and smell must be taken into consideration. Causes of malabsorption, renal status, polypharmacy, and depression must be carefully evaluated. The latter may all result in anorexia in which case prescribing more calories becomes a priority in order to prevent malnutrition. A modest reduction in body weight results in significant improvement of glycemic control in overweight elderly diabetic patients.[7] A physical exercise program appropriate for the patient's fitness and mobility is an important aspect of the management. However, the role of exercise in the elderly diabetic patient is extremely limited by comorbidity and disability. Physical activity in the elderly is particularly beneficial: increasing insulin sensitivity; lowering of plasma lipids; reducing blood pressure; increasing bone mineral density; decreasing the risk of hypercoagulability.[8] More importantly, physical exercise has a positive impact on the patient's ability to ambulate, reduces risk of falls, and improves psychological well-being and quality of life. However, a careful medical history and physical examination must be performed prior to prescribing an exercise regimen. It is necessary to assess the presence of heart and cerebrovascular diseases by performing a test of tolerance to cardiovascular stress, the assessment of the osteoarticular and muscular integrity, and the presence of diabetic neuropathy. Finally, exercise can be associated with an increased incidence of hypoglycemic episodes especially if the patient is being treated with oral antidiabetic medications of long duration.

DRUG THERAPY

Five classes of drugs are currently used to control blood glucose. The different mechanisms of action are reported in Figure 37.1. When considering an appropriate agent in elderly patients with diabetes, it is important to consider the efficacy, half-life, duration of action, metabolic pathway, drug interactions, adverse reactions, safety profile, ease of use, and costs.[9] In the geriatric population sulfonylureas and metformin are the most widely used oral antidiabetic agents. Clinical experience related to alpha-glucosidase inhibitors, the glinides, the glytazones, and incretin hormones are limited.

Sulfonylureas

The sulfonylureas (SFU) should be used with extreme caution in the elderly population to avoid the risk of hypoglycemia. SFU promote insulin secretion by direct stimulation of pancreatic β-cells. SFU bind to ATP-sensitive potassium channels and inhibit the efflux of potassium. The resulting depolarization promotes calcium influx through voltage-dependent calcium channels. Insulin release is triggered by the accumulation of intracytosolic calcium.[10] The secondary failure due to β-cell "depletion" occurs in approximately 10% of patients per year.[10] After 10 years of treatment, about 50% of patients treated with SFU become non-responders.[10] In elderly patients the most appropriate

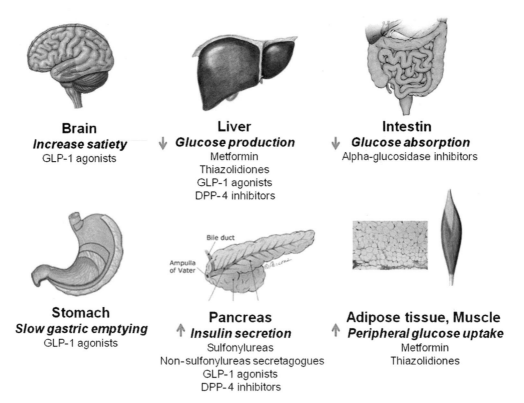

Brain
Increase satiety
GLP-1 agonists

Liver
↓ *Glucose production*
Metformin
Thiazolidiones
GLP-1 agonists
DPP-4 inhibitors

Intestin
↓ *Glucose absorption*
Alpha-glucosidase inhibitors

Stomach
Slow gastric emptying
GLP-1 agonists

Pancreas
↑ *Insulin secretion*
Sulfonylureas
Non-sulfonylureas secretagogues
GLP-1 agonists
DPP-4 inhibitors

Adipose tissue, Muscle
↑ *Peripheral glucose uptake*
Metformin
Thiazolidiones

FIGURE 37.1 Mechanism of action of the currently available oral agents for type 2 diabetes. (*See the color plate section at the back of the book.*)

therapeutic approach is to start therapy with antidiabetic sulfonylureas at low doses, which should be increased gradually over a period of days or weeks to obtain better values for glycated hemoglobin between 7 and 8%. Sulfonylureas, which are currently most widely used, are those of the second generation, which differ from previous ones in order to have greater pharmacological potency, a longer duration of action and can be administered 1 or 2 times a day. These drugs are mainly metabolized in the liver, and therefore can be administered in patients who have mild to moderate renal insufficiency (serum creatinine levels between 1.8 and 2.0 mg/dl). Unfortunately most of these drugs have the disadvantage of having pharmacokinetic profiles that do not allow an appropriate reduction of the postprandial hyperglycemic peaks, and frequently lead to hypoglycemia. A new molecule of this class, glimepiride, has some interesting characteristics. It also binds to receptors of sulfonylurea, but acts through a subunit (65 kDa) different from that (140 kDa) which binds other sulfonylureas, and perhaps this is why it does not interact with the ATP-dependent potassium channels of the cardiovascular system. In addition, the binding of glimepiride with the receptor for sulfonylureas occurs at a rate two- to three-times higher and the dissociation with a speed eight-times higher compared to glibenclamide. This leads to a more rapid onset of its secretory effect followed by a phase of slow release. Hepatic excretion makes it safer for diabetics in older age who frequently have diminished renal function. The lower frequency of hypoglycemic events and the ability to administer a single dose in the morning allow greater safety and better compliance in the elderly.

Meglitinides

These agents are non-sulfonylureas secretagogues, with sulfonylurea-like mechanisms of action. They target a different binding site on pancreatic β-cells, leading to a similar cascade of events triggering insulin release.[11] Repaglinide and nateglinide are examples of this class of agents. Their pharmacokinetic profile is favorable in terms of targeting postprandial hyperglycemia.[11] Repaglinide is metabolized by cytochrome P450 and transformed into active metabolites that are eliminated via bile. The pharmacokinetics of repaglinide was determined by therapeutic trials in groups of elderly patients fewer than 70 years. The results showed no differences in the elderly population in relation to adults, and especially there was a lower rate of hypoglycemia in elderly patients treated with repaglinide.[11] Since there are no specific studies for patients above 75 years, it is not recommended to use these drugs in this class of patients. Repaglinide has a very short duration of action and it results in an immediate release of insulin, mimicking the physiological release, and therefore is an ideal drug for patients who have irregular eating habits, or those who exhibit frequent hypoglycemia when treated with SFU.

Biguanides

Metformin is the biguanide prescribed most worldwide. It is much safer than earlier biguanides, phenformin, and buformin. Its principal action is to reduce hepatic gluconeogenesis. To a lesser degree, possibly an indirect effect, metformin increases insulin-mediated glucose uptake and glucose utilization in peripheral tissues. Therefore, the use of metformin as an antihyperglycemic agent may be an attractive option in the obese and overweight elderly patients with insulin resistance.[12] There are no significant studies that have analyzed the effects of biguanides in the geriatric population. The larger part of the cases are mostly of studies in small cohorts of patients, made with the inclusion criteria limiting and non-randomized.[12] In any case, it was noted that the metformin is effective and safe as monotherapy in elderly obese patients.[13] As for side effects, gastrointestinal pain and diarrhea are the most frequent (30%), but the most severe is lactic acidosis. Lactic acidosis is favored by conditions which are not specific but is more frequently associated with renal failure and tissue hypoxia. Biguanides however do not expose the patient to the risk of hypoglycemia. In obese patients, biguanides could be considered the drug of first use as monotherapy because they enhance insulin sensitivity, reduce lipid levels, promote weight loss and, very importantly as stated above, do not induce hypoglycemia.

Thiazolidinediones

Thiazolidinediones (TZDs) enhance glucose uptake and utilization in peripheral tissues, mainly skeletal muscle tissue. TZDs bind to specific nuclear receptors called peroxisome proliferator activated receptor gamma (PPAR-γ) that induce gene expression of proteins involved in the action at the post-insulin receptor level. Nuclear receptors are most highly expressed in adipose tissue, skeletal muscle, liver, intestine, kidney, vascular smooth muscle, heart and macrophages. Once activated, PPAR-γ receptors bind to DNA leading to transcriptional modulation of genes involved in lipid and carbohydrate metabolism.[14] TZDs decrease insulin resistance in peripheral tissues with a minor effect on hepatic glucose production at high doses.[14] In particular, they increase insulin sensitivity in adipose tissue, muscle and to a lesser extent in the liver. Due to their mechanism of action, glitazones have a hypoglycemic effect, reduce lipolysis, increase lipid synthesis in adipose tissue, lower levels of FFA in the circulation, increase HDL and appear to reduce microalbuminuria, levels of PAI-1 and fibrinogen. The glitazones induce a general improvement in all the main events that are associated with the metabolic syndrome and diabetes. Moreover, the glitazones cause an increase in adipocyte numbers and thus an increase in body weight, but the increase of fat is limited to the subcutaneous tissue, and visceral fat. However, TZDs reduce the content of fat in liver and in muscle fibers. Since TZDs are insulin-sensitizing drugs and not insulin-secretory agents, they do not cause hypoglycemia. However, they can cause a degree of fluid retention, which can be dangerous in patients with impaired cardiac function (heart failure) in which their use is contraindicated. The currently available agent is pioglitazone; rosiglitazone was withdrawn from the market because of its association with increased incidence of heart mortality.[15] Pioglitazone has hypoglycemic efficacy superior to that of troglitazone and does not cause acute liver failure or liver dysfunction. However, the use of pioglitazone should be avoided in patients with increased alanine transaminase (ALT) levels. In addition, the FDA recommends monitoring liver function in patients treated with pioglitazone every 2 months during the first year of treatment and less frequently thereafter.

TZDs may be an attractive antidiabetic agent in elderly diabetic patients. However, TZDs cause weight gain secondary to fluid retention and stimulation of adipogenesis.[15] Plasma expansion may lead to decompensation of congestive heart failure. Therefore, TZDs are contraindicated in heart failure (New York Heart Association classes 3 and 4). These agents may be used in elderly diabetic patients without heart failure and hepatic impairment.

α-Glucosidase Inhibitors

Over half of patients with type 2 diabetes have postprandial hyperglycemia.[16] Postprandial hyperglycemia has been linked with cardiovascular mortality.[16] Alpha-glucosidase inhibitors target postprandial hyperglycemia. Their action on fasting blood sugar is minimal.[16] There are three agents in this category that are currently marketed worldwide. These include acarbose, miglitol, and voglibose. These agents competitively inhibit alphaglucosidases, the brush border enzymes of the proximal small intestinal epithelium. This reversible inhibition delays hydrolysis of polysaccharides into absorbable monosaccharides (e.g., glucose). Carbohydrate absorption occurs over a greater portion of the small intestine, blunting post-prandial glucose excursions.[16] The non-systemic mode of action, lack of association with hypoglycemia, and minimal drug interaction make this class of agents an attractive anti-diabetic drug option in the elderly.[16] However, the administration of these drugs is associated with a number of side effects in the intestines (flatulence and diarrhea) that dramatically reduce the degree of compliance that the elderly patient has towards these drugs.

Incretins

A new class of drugs is represented by incretins.[17] The importance of incretin therapy comes from the observation that glucose given orally produces a better insulin response to that induced by the same amount of glucose given intravenously, suggesting that the intestinal hormones (incretins) may increase the secretion insulin. The intestinal hormone more active in this regard is the glucagon-like peptide-1 (GLP-1). GLP-1 has functional effects on Langerhans cells modulating the secretion of both α- and β-cells. In particular, the GLP-1 is able to enhance the secretion of β-cells and inhibit α-cells. The GLP-1 has extra-pancreatic effects such as increasing the feeling of satiety and delayed gastric emptying. The increase in satiety and slow gastric emptying (with consequent delay in the absorption of carbohydrates) are useful effects in the treatment of obese subjects.

In addition, several studies have shown that GLP-1 plays an important role in improving the survival of β-cells. In fact, many animal studies have shown that GLP-1 increases β-cell mass by stimulating neogenesis of β-cells and their growth and proliferation, while *in vitro*

studies with GLP-1 were associated with a significant apoptosis reduction in the preparations. These effects of GLP-1 are of particular interest in the treatment of type 2 diabetes, as the gradual reduction and β-cell dysfunction is a major pathophysiological mechanism of the disease.[18]

In addition, we must consider that patients with type 2 diabetes show a reduced "incretin effect" compared to non-diabetic patients regardless of age or degree of obesity. Moreover, administration of GLP-1 in patients with type 2 diabetes has been shown to increase insulin secretion and normalize both fasting and the postprandial glucose. However, even if treatment with subcutaneous GLP-1 appears to be reasonably effective and beneficial, the effect of treatment with GLP-1 on blood glucose and insulin secretion is disappointing in patients with type 2 diabetes. This is because plasma half-life of this incretin is extremely short. In fact, the GLP-1 is metabolized within minutes by dipeptidyl peptidase-4 (DDP-4), a membrane enzyme present in many tissues (kidney, intestine, endothelium, capillary, etc.). Based on this, drugs have been produced to exploit essentially two options: (i) the use of GLP-1 from synthetic (exanetide) or its analogs resistant to enzymatic degradation of DDP-4 (liraglutide); (ii) the use of the DDP-4 inhibitors (vildagliptin, sitagliptin, saxagliptin, SYR-322) able to prevent the degradation of GLP-1 and then to increase its circulating levels intact or biologically active.

Sitagliptin (Januvia: MSD) and vildagliptin (GalvusR: Novartis), both approved by FDA and EMEA, are both available. Januvia is a molecule that is used once-daily (100 mg). Treatment with sitagliptin 100 mg/day was effective in the treatment of type 2 diabetes because it can reduce the average glycosylated hemoglobin by about 1 percentage point, and also with the same degree of metabolic control as seen with other drugs, and with smaller numbers of hypoglycemia (whether serious or minor that night). Finally, sitagliptin was not associated with weight gain which is the case with treatment with sulfonylureas, glitazones, and insulin. Vildagliptin has a shorter duration of action and is administered at least twice daily at a dose of 50 mg. The drug is generally well tolerated with few adverse events (such as itching and pharyngitis). The paucity of the side effects and the low proportion of severe hypoglycemic reactions after its administration make these drugs particularly suitable for the treatment of diabetes in geriatric patients.[17]

Insulin

Age should not be an excuse to deny insulin therapy to elderly diabetic patients. However, insulin therapy in the elderly should be individualized. These patients may have other comorbid conditions, diminished eyesight, difficulty of motility, and cognitive impairment. The types of insulin regimen adopted for geriatric patients are not based on comparative studies. The choice of treatment depends on the therapeutic target, the risk of hypoglycemia, and particularly the possibility of handling.[19] Insulin treatment is usually adopted when the oral hypoglycemic agents are not sufficient to ensure adequate glycemic control even in higher doses.[19] In patients starting insulin therapy who have a good quality of life and who are able to manage blood sugar symptoms, the therapeutic target would be the maintenance of HbA1c below 7%. This target clearly can not be attained by frail patients, who are socially isolated and have low expectations of life, so in these cases, insulin therapy may be useful to prevent osmotic complications and infections. Finally, elderly patients with poor glycemic control and weight loss may benefit from insulin treatment.[19]

The main problem with insulin therapy is hypoglycemia. The use of insulin analogs with short half-life significantly reduces the hypoglycemic events. In fact, compared to conventional regular insulin, the analogs have a faster absorption. Currently there are two analogs on the market: insulin lispro, achieved after conversion of the amino acids proline and lysine, insulin aspart, obtained by replacing a proline with aspartic acid.[20] In addition, there is also availability of slow insulins (glargine and detemir), which last about 24 h. Unlike classical ultralente, glargine and detemir do not show peaks that may result in hypoglycemia. Prolonged action of detemir is mediated by the strong self-association of detemir molecules at the injection site and albumin binding via fatty acid side chains.[21] Detemir has a slower, more prolonged absorption over 24 h and a flatter time–action profile as compared with Neutral Protamine Hagedorn (NPH).[22]

Age-related changes in functional ability, cognitive functions, eyesight, and impaired manual dexterity may affect the patient's ability to administer insulin, monitor blood glucose, and manage hypoglycemia, which is a consideration in starting insulin therapy in the elderly population. The benefits and disadvantages of insulin therapy, including hypoglycemia, must be explained to and understood by the patients and family.[23] The conventional insulin therapy is simpler insulin regimens, including a single daily injection of slow insulins, or two injections per day of combined regular and NPH insulin given in fixed amounts before breakfast and dinner. Intensive insulin therapies utilize basal insulin with multiple premeal injections of a rapidly acting insulin to provide a tighter glycemic control. The time to peak and the duration of action of human insulin preparations (NPH and regular insulin) do not replicate endogenous basal and postprandial insulin secretion. However, insulin analogs (lispro, aspart, glulisine, glargine, detemir) were developed with the goal of more nearly replicating endogenous insulin secretion.[19]

Regimens for elderly type 2 diabetic patients include the following:

1. Glargine insulin once a day.
2. Detemir insulin twice a day.

3. Intermediate-acting premixed twice daily.
4. Insulin basal/bolus lispro or aspart before meals.
5. Combination glargine or detemir before going to bed and oral medications.

The prescribed insulin therapy should be as simple as possible to ensure compliance and prevent errors. Home capillary blood glucose monitoring should be thoroughly explained and encouraged. Its frequency can vary depending on the goal of therapy. Accurate recording of the finger stick capillary blood glucose value on a logbook or data sheet is essential to the physician for appropriate recommendations. In elderly diabetic patients with insulin secretory capacity, a single daily injection of detemir or glargine may be sufficient. The injection is best given at bedtime to control fasting hyperglycemia. Insulin glargine and detemir, unlike NPH insulin, can not be mixed with short- or ultra-rapid-acting insulins. The use of premixed insulin such as 70/30 insulin or 75/25 lispro insulin offers a convenient alternative for elderly patients who have difficulty in mixing insulins. However, the evening (pre-dinner) administration of these pre-mixed insulins often causes midnight hypoglycemia. To initiate insulin therapy, a dose between 0.2 and 0.5 units/kg of body weight can be used. Two-thirds of the dose could be given in the morning and one-third in the evening.

CONCLUSIONS

The control of hyperglycemia (with either oral agents, insulin or a combination) not only provides beneficial metabolic effects, but also a better quality of life in elderly diabetic patients. Glycosuria and the resulting osmotic diuresis may lead to fatigue and dehydration. Furthermore, several studies have shown that adequate glycemic control may provide improvement in well-being and in cognitive function in elderly diabetic patients. In general, the management of diabetes mellitus in the elderly is challenging and must be highly individualized.

References

1. Oiknine R, Mooradian AD. Drug therapy of diabetes in the elderly. *Biomed Pharmacother* 2003;**57**:231−9.
2. Gregg EW, Brown A. Cognitive and physical disabilities and aging-related complications of diabetes. *Clinical Diabetes* 2003;**21**:113−8.
3. Olson DE, Norris SL. Diabetes in older adults. Overview of Ags guidelines for the treatment of diabetes mellitus in geriatric population. *Geriatrics* 2004;**59**:18−24.
4. Brown AF. Guideline for improving the care of the older person with diabetes mellitus. *JAGS* 2003;**51**: S265−80.
5. Franz MJ, Bantle JP, Beebe CA, Brunzell JD, Chiasson JL, Garg A. Technical review: evidence-based nutrition principles and recommendations for the treatment and prevention of diabetes and related complications. *Diabetes Care* 2002;**25**:148−98.
6. Thurman J, Mooradianm AD. Vitamin supplementation therapy in the elderly. *Drugs Aging* 1997;**11**:433−49.
7. Horani MH, Mooradian AD. Management of obesity in the elderly. Special considerations. *Treat Endocrinol* 2002;**1**:387−98.
8. American Diabetes Association. Physical activity/exercise and diabetes mellitus. *Diabetes Care* 2003;**26**(Suppl. 1):S73−7.
9. Chehade JM, Mooradian AD. Drug therapy: current and emerging agents. In: Sinclair AJ, Finucane P, editors. *Diabetes in old age*. 2nd ed. Chichester, UK: John Wiley and Sons; 2001. p. 199−214.
10. Chehade J, Mooradian AD. A rational approach to drug therapy of type 2 diabetes mellitus. *Drugs* 2000;**60**:95−113.
11. Jovanovic L, Daily G, Huang WC, Strange P, Goldstein BJ. Repaglinide in type 2 diabetes: 24-week fixed dose efficacy and safety study. *J Clin Pharmacol* 2000;**40**:49−57.
12. Prospective Diabetes Study (UKPDS) Group UK. Effect of intensive blood-glucose control with metformin on complications in overweight patients with type 2 diabetes (UKPDS 34). *Lancet* 1998;**352**:854−65.
13. Abbatecola AM, Paolisso G, Corsonello A, Bustacchini S, Lattanzio F. Antidiabetic oral treatment in older people: does frailty matter? *Drugs Aging* 2009;**1**:53−62.
14. Silverberg AB, Ligaray KP. Oral diabetic medications and the geriatric patient. *Clin Geriatr Med* 2008;**24**:541−9.

15. Graham DJ, Ouellet-Hellstrom R, Mac Curdy TE, Ali F, Sholley C, Worral C, Kelman JA. Risk of acute myocardial infarction, stroke, heart failure, and death in elderly Medicare patients treated with rosiglitazone or pioglitazone. *JAMA* 2010;**304**:411−8.

16. Rabasa-Lhoret R, Chiaisson JL. Potential of alpha-glucosidase inhibitors in elderly patients with diabetes mellitus and impaired glucose tolerance. *Drugs Aging* 1998;**13**:131−43.

17. Mathieu C, Bollaerts K. Antihyperglycaemic therapy in elderly patients with type 2 diabetes: potential role of incretin mimetics and DPP-4 inhibitors. *Intern J Clin Pract* 2007;**61**(Suppl. 154):29−37.

18. Inzucchi SE, Darren K. New drugs for the treatment of diabetes: part II: incretin-based therapy and beyond. *Circulation* 2008;**117**:574−84.

19. Ober SK, Watts S, Lawrence RH. Insulin use in elderly diabetic patients. *Clin Interv Aging* 2006;**1**: 107−13.

20. Owens DR, Zinman B, Bolli GB. Insulins today and beyond. *Lancet* 2001;**358**(9283):739−46.

21. Owens DR, Bolli GB. Beyond the era of NPH insulin—Long-acting insulin analogs: Chemistry, comparative pharmacology, and clinical application. *Diabetes Technol Ther* 2008;**10**:333−49.

22. Heinemann L, Linkeschova R, Rave K. Time-action profile of the long-acting insulin analog insulin glargine (HOE901) in comparison with those of NPH insulin and placebo. *Diabetes Care* 2000;**23**: 644−9.

23. Hendra TJ. Starting insulin therapy in elderly patients. *J R Soc Med* 2002;**95**:453−5.

DIABETES IN ANIMALS AND TREATMENT

38

Diabetes Mellitus in Animals: Diagnosis and Treatment of Diabetes Mellitus in Dogs and Cats

Deborah S. Greco

Nestle Purina PetCare, St Louis, MO, USA

OUTLINE

INTRODUCTION

The field of companion animal diabetology is in its infancy but new discoveries are being made every day. The overlap between human and companion animal medicine and research grows larger with each new discovery. This chapter covers the diagnosis and treatment of diabetes mellitus in companion animals, such as the dog and cat. Dogs develop insulin-dependent diabetes mellitus and most dogs require insulin therapy; however, cats develop type 2 diabetes and can be managed with diet alone or diet combined with insulin or oral hypoglycemic

Nutritional and Therapeutic Interventions for Diabetes and Metabolic Syndrome
DOI: 10.1016/B978-0-12-385083-6.00038-3

therapy. The etiology, clinical signs, clinical pathology and diagnostic tests for diabetes in dogs and cats will be covered along with treatment modalities such as diet, oral hypoglycemics, and insulin. Finally, a discussion of monitoring options for small animal diabetics is included.

DIABETES IN DOGS AND CATS

Insulin-dependent diabetes mellitus (IDDM) is a diabetic state in which endogenous insulin secretion is never sufficient to prevent ketone production. Type 1 diabetes mellitus is a diabetic state in which insulin secretion may be reduced or absent and which is readily corrected by exogenous insulin. Most dogs suffer from type 1 diabetes or IDDM which is thought to have an autoimmune basis in both dogs and man.[1] Dogs suffering from diabetes mellitus range in age from 4 to 14 years with a peak incidence at 7–9 years.[1] In dogs, females are twice as likely to develop diabetes than males. A genetic basis for diabetes mellitus is suspected in the keeshonden and golden retriever.[1] Other commonly affected breeds include poodles, dachshunds, miniature schnauzers, beagles, puliks, Cairn terriers, and miniature pinschers.[1]

Etiology: Feline Diabetes Mellitus

Diabetes mellitus is a commonly occurring feline endocrinopathy. In cats, neutered males are 1.5 times more likely than females to develop diabetes mellitus. Risk factors for the development of diabetes mellitus in cats include increased body weight (> 6.8 kg), older age (>10 years) and neutering.[1,2]

Historically, feline diabetics were suspected to be insulinopenic; however, recent research indicates that most cats develop diabetes similar to type 2 diabetes mellitus (DM) in humans.[3,4] Obesity and amyloidosis is involved in the pathogenesis of type 2 DM in cats. It is now

recognized that the classic metabolic abnormalities found in type 2 DM, decreased insulin secretion and peripheral insulin resistance, are both consequences of abnormal amyloid production by pancreatic β-cells. In 1986, a previously unidentified protein called islet-amyloid polypeptide (IAPP or amylin) was identified as the main component of amyloid deposits in a human insulinoma. This novel protein was also found to be the main component of islet amyloid (IA) isolated from pancreatic islets in cats with type 2 DM.[3]

Another major distinguishing feature of type 2 diabetes is peripheral insulin resistance. Obesity plays a significant role in the insulin resistance seen in feline diabetics. The resistance is due to internalization of the insulin receptors in membranes of muscle and fat cells. Obesity also decreases receptor affinity for the insulin molecule. Both the amount and distribution of adipose tissue plays a role in insulin resistance and other obesity-related disorders.[4] Obese cats have low GLUT4 (insulin sensitive glucose transporter) expression in both muscle and adipose tissue; however, the expression of GLUT1 (insulin insensitive glucose transporter) is not different in lean *vs* obese cats.[5] The glucose transporter in pancreatic β-cells is actually GLUT2 and a decreased expression of these receptors causes a loss of the first phase of insulin secretion but normal second phase of insulin secretion similar to that seen in later stages of obesity in the cat. Insulin secretion is affected early on in the course of type 2 diabetes mellitus; particularly glucose-mediated insulin secretion. Insulin resistance in β-cells may lead to a decrease in insulin secretion. In some forms of diabetes in humans, a mutation of the glucokinase enzyme may lead to impaired insulin secretion. The feline liver exhibits normal hexokinase activity but glucokinase activity is virtually absent.[7] Glucokinase converts glucose to glycogen for storage in the liver and is important in "mopping" up excess postprandial glucose. Normal cats are in fact similar to human beings with type 2 diabetes mellitus whose glucokinase levels drop precipitously with persistent hyperglycemia.

To summarize the current hypothesis of the pathogenesis of type 2 DM, peripheral insulin resistance (due to obesity, elevated plasma IAPP, or both) causes chronic stimulation of insulin production in the pancreatic β-cells.[3–7] Amylin is co-synthesized with the insulin; therefore, impaired insulin secretion causes insulin and IAPP to accumulate in the β-cells.[3] The high local concentration of IAPP causes polymerization of IAPP to form insular amyloid. Deposition of insular amyloid further impairs glucorecognition and diffusion of nutritive substances into the β-cells. Eventually, insular amyloidosis leads to necrosis of the β-cells and release of amyloid into the extracellular space.[3,4]

Pathogenesis of Clinical Signs: IDDM

Hyperglycemia, caused by insulin deficiency, results primarily from impaired glucose utilization; however, increased hepatic gluconeogenesis and glycogenolysis by the liver contributes to hyperglycemia. Decreased peripheral utilization of glucose leads to accumulation of glucose in the serum; as the renal threshold for glucose is exceeded, osmotic diuresis ensues. Progressive dehydration results in the classic clinical signs of diabetes such as polyuria with compensatory polydipsia. Impaired glucose utilization by the hypothalamic satiety center combined with loss of calories in the form of glycosuria causes polyphagia and weight loss, respectively. Insulin is anabolic; therefore, insulin deficiency leads to protein catabolism and contributes to the clinical signs of weight loss and muscle atrophy. With insulin deficiency, the *hormone-sensitive lipase* system which is normally suppressed by insulin, becomes activated. As a consequence of this increased lipase activity, adipose tissue is broken down at an accelerated rate into nonesterified fatty acids. The unrestrained lipolytic activity of *hormone sensitive lipase* results in the clinical signs of weight loss in a previously obese or overweight animal.

Pathogenesis of Clinical Signs: NIDDM

In cats with type 2 DM, the initial abnormality is insulin resistance. Cats, like human beings with type 2 diabetes, may show very few or no signs of "classic" diabetes until progressive amyloid deposition and glucose toxicity impair insulin secretion to the point that hyperglycemia exceeds the renal threshold (about 15 mmol/l in cats which is higher than in dogs). At this point, the diabetes mellitus has become insulin dependent, at least temporarily. Lowering of blood glucose via exogenous insulin or oral hypoglycemic agents may be sufficient to reverse glucose toxicity and result in resolution of the clinical signs of polydipsia and polyuria. However, it should be emphasized that cats with resolved IDDM still have the underlying pathophysiology of type 2 DM, i.e. insulin resistance and impaired insulin secretory capacity.

Clinical signs of type 2 diabetes mellitus are subtle and progressive over a period of months to years. In the author's experience, obesity combined with fasting or postprandial hyperglycemia may be the only clinical "sign" of early type 2 DM. Prior to the onset of polydipsia and polyuria, a constellation of gastrointestinal abnormalities and signs of diabetic neuropathy may also be observed. In diabetic cats, the first signs of diabetes mellitus may be periodic vomiting, anorexia, and less frequently diarrhea. These gastrointestinal signs may originate as a result of autonomic diabetic neuropathy or possibly as a result of concurrent pancreatitis, cholangiohepatitis or inflammatory bowel disease. Another observation, in the author's experience, is that owners of diabetic cats will report gait abnormalities, weakness, and problems with jumping prior to the onset of polydipsia and polyuria. There is often a history of administration of diabetogenic medications, such as glucocorticoids or progestins, in cats presenting for type 2 DM.

Clinical Signs of Non-Ketotic Diabetes Mellitus

Most diabetic dogs and cats present with the classic clinical signs of polyuria and polydipsia. Polydipsia was the most common clinical sign of diabetes mellitus in dogs (93%).[2] Polyuria, however, was observed in only 77% of dogs. In cats, polydipsia (77%) and polyuria (72%) occur with equal frequency.[2] Dramatic and rapid weight loss in an animal with a good or even ravenous appetite will often alert the owner to seek veterinary advice. Weight loss is observed more commonly in dogs (62%) compared with cats (44%).[2] Only 12% of cats and 19% of dogs exhibited polyphagia as a clinical sign of diabetes mellitus.[2]

In dogs, progressive polyuria, polydipsia, and weight loss develop relatively rapidly usually over a period of several weeks. Another common presenting complaint of diabetes mellitus in dogs is acute onset of blindness caused by bilateral cataract formation. Cats will present with chronic complications of diabetes, such as gait abnormalities (13%) resulting from diabetic neuropathy, or with chronic gastrointestinal signs such as vomiting, diarrhea, and anorexia.[2] There is often a history of inappropriate elimination or house soiling as a result of muscle weakness caused by neuropathy (inability to climb stairs or get into or out of the litter pan) and polyuria.

Physical Examination Findings

Physical examination findings of non-ketotic diabetes mellitus in cats and dogs are typically non-specific. The most common physical examination findings in cats are lethargy and depression (70%), dehydration (63%), unkempt haircoat (35%) and muscle wasting (47%).[2] Cats may present with "frosty paws" or accumulation of cat litter on the hind legs and paws as a result of diabetic neuropathy and sticky urine caused by glucosuria. Cats often have concurrent gastrointestinal disease such as pancreatitis, inflammatory bowel disease, and cholangiohepatitis.[8]

Plantigrade rear limb stance resulting from diabetic neuropathy is observed in approximately 8% of diabetic cats in previous studies. However, recent evidence suggests that diabetic cats can have a variety of clinical signs suggestive of diabetic neuropathy including pain on palpation of distal extremities, hypersensitivity, gait abnormalities, and palmagrade stance. Based on EMG, nerve biopsy and nerve conduction studies, all diabetic cats have some degree of diabetic neuropathy at the time of presentation.[9]

In dogs, the most common physical examination findings are dehydration (48%) and muscle wasting or thin body condition (44%). About 35% of cats and 20% of dogs are obese upon initial examination; obese diabetic animals are more likely to suffer from non-insulin dependent diabetes mellitus. Hepatomegaly is observed in both diabetic cats (30%) and dogs (17%). Cataracts are observed in approximately 40% of diabetic dogs.

Ketoacidotic, Hyperosmolar or Complicated Diabetes Mellitus: Pathophysiology and Clinical Signs

Lipid metabolism in the liver becomes deranged with insulin deficiency and non-esterified fatty acids are converted to acetyl-CoA rather than being incorporated into triglycerides. Acetyl-CoA accumulates in the liver and is converted into acetoacetyl-CoA and then ultimately to acetoacetic acid. Finally, the liver starts to generate large amounts of ketones including acetoacetic acid, beta-hydroxybutyrate and acetone. As insulin deficiency culminates in DKA, accumulation of ketones and lactic acid in the blood and loss of electrolytes and water in the urine results in profound dehydration, hypovolemia, metabolic acidosis, and shock. Ketonuria and osmotic diuresis caused by glycosuria result in urinary sodium and potassium loss which exacerbates hypovolemia and dehydration. Nausea, anorexia and vomiting, caused by stimulation of the chemoreceptor trigger zone via ketonemia and hyperglycemia, contribute to the dehydration caused by osmotic diuresis. Dehydration and shock lead to prerenal azotemia and a decline in glomerular filtration rate (GFR). Declining GFR leads to further accumulation of glucose and ketones in the blood. Stress hormones such as cortisol and epinephrine contribute to the hyperglycemia in a vicious cycle. Eventually severe dehydration may result in hyperviscosity, thromboembolism, severe metabolic acidosis, renal failure, and finally death.

The most common historical findings in cats and dogs with diabetic ketoacidosis are anorexia (61%), weakness, depression, and vomiting.[2] Physical examination findings may include shock, depression, tachypnea, dehydration, weakness, vomiting, and occasionally, a strong acetone odor on the breath. Cats can present recumbent or comatose; this may be a manifestation of mixed ketotic hyperosmolar syndrome. In cats, 33% exhibited clinical icterus at presentation.[2]

Clinical Pathology of Diabetes Mellitus in Animals

In dogs, a diagnosis of diabetes mellitus should be based on the presence of clinical signs compatible with diabetes mellitus and evidence of fasting hyperglycemia and glycosuria. Common clinicopathologic features of diabetes mellitus in dogs and cats include: fasting hyperglycemia, hypercholesterolemia, increased liver enzymes (ALP, ALT), neutrophilic leukocytosis, proteinuria, increased urine specific gravity, and glycosuria. Common clinicopathologic findings in diabetic ketoacidosis include all of the above plus azotemia, hyponatremia, hyperkalemia, hyperlipasemia, hyperamylasemia, ketonemia, regenerative or degenerative left shifts, hyperosmolality, ketonuria, bacteriuria, hematuria, and pyuria.

Many cats are susceptible to "stress-induced" hyperglycemia in which the serum glucose concentrations may approach 300−400 mg/dl. In addition, renal glycosuria may be found in animals with renal tubular disease and occasionally with stress-induced hyperglycemia. It may be difficult to differentiate early type 2 diabetes in cats from stress-induced hyperglycemia, because cats with early NIDDM are often asymptomatic.

Glycosylated proteins, such as glycosylated hemoglobin and fructosamine may aid in the diagnosis of early type 2 DM in cats.[10] Glycosylated hemoglobin is formed by an irreversible, non-enzymatic binding of glucose to hemoglobin. As plasma glucose concentrations increase, hemoglobin glycosylation increases proportionately. Normal glycosylated hemoglobin (mean $\pm$ SD) values are: $2.95 \pm 0.15\%$ in dogs and $1.6 \pm 0.5\%$ in cats.[10]

Serum fructosamine is formed by glycosylation of serum protein such as albumin. The concentration of fructosamine in serum is directly related to blood glucose concentration. However, due to the shorter lifespan of albumin compared with hemoglobin, fructosamine concentrations reflect more recent (1−3 weeks) changes in serum glucose concentrations. Serum fructosamine measurement may be beneficial in differentiating early or subclinical diabetes mellitus in the cat from stress-induced hyperglycemia.[11−13] One study in 17 normal cats showed that transient glucose administration (1 g/kg 50% glucose solution, intravenously) did not cause increased serum fructosamine concentrations.[13] Furthermore, hyperglycemic serum samples from sick cats were analyzed for serum fructosamine content; approximately 40% exhibited normal fructosamine concentrations consistent with transient hyperglycemia. In the same study, it was noted that the 50% of sick cats showed mold increases in serum fructosamine concentrations consistent with subclinical or mildly clinical diabetes mellitus even when the serum glucose concentrations were in the normal or near normal range.[13] This finding suggests that subclinical type 2 diabetes mellitus is probably much more common than previously believed and that obese cats with increased serum fructosamine should be followed carefully for evidence of developing diabetes mellitus. Normal fructosamine concentrations in dogs are 254 ± 42 µmol/l and in cats normal fructosamine concentrations are 283 ± 32 µmol/l.[11–13]

TREATMENT OF DIABETES MELLITUS IN CATS AND DOGS

The Role of Diet

The goals of dietary therapy in diabetes mellitus for both cats and dogs are to provide sufficient calories to maintain ideal body weight and correct obesity or emaciation, to minimize postprandial hyperglycemia, and to facilitate ideal absorption of glucose by timing meals to coincide with insulin administration. Caloric intake should be 60–70 kcal/kg per day for smaller dogs and 50–60 kcal/kg per day for larger dogs. Most cats will consume between 200 and 250 kcal/day. Obese animals should have their body weight reduced gradually over a period of 2–4 months by feeding 60–70% of the calculated caloric requirements for ideal body weight. The feeding schedule should be adjusted to the insulin therapy and most patients are fed twice daily.

One approach to managing diabetes mellitus in dogs uses nutritional components such as starch blends, carboymethyl cellulose and fermentable fiber blends. Barley and sorghum are used to blunt the postprandial rise in blood glucose, adjust postprandial insulin to appropriate levels, and to help blunt glucose surge.

Fermentable fibers, such as FOS, beet pulp, and gum arabic, increase short-chain fatty acids from the large intestine which in turn increases glucagon-like peptide-1 (GLP-1) secretion and activity. GLP-1 is necessary for normal insulin secretion and for normal timing of insulin secretion after eating. Another approach is to limit carbohydrate in the diet to less than 30% of metabolizable energy.

The cat is an obligate carnivore; therefore, amino acids, rather than glucose, are the signal for insulin release in cats.[14] Another unusual aspect of feline metabolism is the increase in hepatic gluconeogenesis seen after a normal meal. Normal cats maintain essential glucose requirements from gluconeogenic precursors (i.e. amino acids) rather than from dietary carbohydrates. As a result, cats can maintain normal blood glucose concentrations even when deprived of food for over 72 h.[15] When type 2 diabetes occurs in cats, the metabolic adaptations to a carnivorous diet become even more deleterious leading to severe protein catabolism; feeding a diet rich in carbohydrates may exacerbate hyperglycemia and protein wasting in these diabetic cats. A low-carbohydrate (< 15% of dry matter) or ultra-low (< 10% of dry matter), high-protein diet, which is similar in fact to a cat's natural diet (mice), may ameliorate some of the abnormalities associated with diabetes mellitus in the cat. Initial studies using a canned high-protein/low-carbohydrate diet and the starch blocker acarbose have shown that 58% of cats discontinue insulin injections and those with continued insulin requirements could be regulated on a much lower dosage (1 U BID).[16] Comparison of canned high-fiber *vs* low-carbohydrate diets showed that cats fed low-carbohydrate diets were twice as likely to discontinue insulin injections.[17]

Oral Hypoglycemic Therapy

Oral hypoglycemic agents are used in cats only to attenuate the physiologic abnormalities of type 2 diabetes by decreasing hepatic glucose output and glucose absorption from the intestine, increasing peripheral insulin sensitivity, and increasing insulin secretion from the pancreas. In cats, the clinician must rely on the *response* to oral hypoglycemic agents as a guide to whether the cat has sufficient β-cell function to be managed with oral hypoglycemic agents. Oral hypoglycemic agents used in cats include the sulfonylureas (glipizide) and α-glucosidase inhibitors (acarbose).[16,18] Indications for oral hypoglycemic therapy in cats include normal or increased body weight, lack of ketones, probable type 2 diabetes with no underlying disease (pancreatitis, pancreatic tumor), history of diabetogenic medications, and owners' willingness to administer oral medication rather than an injection. Diet should consist of low-carbohydrate/high-protein foods only.

The mechanism of action of the sulfonylureas is to increase insulin secretion and improve insulin resistance. Sulfonylureas, because of provocation of insulin release, may promote progression of pancreatic amyloidosis. In cats, glipizide has been used to successfully treat diabetes mellitus at a dosage of 2.5 mg BID when combined with a high-protein, low-carbohydrate diet. The patient is evaluated weekly or every 2 weeks for a period of 2–3 months. Cats with early type 2 diabetes are most likely to respond to any oral hypoglycemic agent. Gastrointestinal side effects, which occur in about 15% of cats treated with glipizide, resolve when the drug is administered with food.[18]

The α-glucosidase inhibitors impair glucose absorption from the intestine by decreasing fiber digestion and hence glucose production from food sources. Acarbose is used as initial therapy in obese prediabetic patients suffering from insulin resistance or as adjunct therapy with sulfonylureas to enhance the hypoglycemic effect in patients with diabetes mellitus. Side effects include flatulence, loose stools, and diarrhea at high dosages. One advantage of these medications is that they are not absorbed systemically and may be used in conjunction with other oral hypoglycemics or insulin. The author has had experience with acarbose at a dosage of 12.5 mg/cat BID with meals; side effects, although rare if diet is adjusted, include semi-formed stool or in some cases overt diarrhea.[16] The glucose-lowering effect of acarbose alone is mild with blood glucose concentrations decreasing only into the 250–300 mg/dl range. However, acarbose is an excellent agent when combined with insulin to improve glycemic control.

Insulin Therapy

Recombinant human and synthetic insulin including neutral protamine Hagedom insulin (NPH), lente, glargine, protamine zinc, and detemir have been used in animals.[19–22] Preliminary studies on glargine have shown that it has some advantages over other types of insulin in cats. In fact, early studies showed that combination of glargine with a low-carbohydrate, high-protein diet resulted in 100% remission of insulin dependence in cats. Detemir insulin is rapidly becoming the insulin of choice in dogs due to greater efficacy and longer half-life. Detemir is unusual in that it is "stored" on protein binding sites on albumin in the blood and slowly dissociates throughout the day which leads to a long half-life. Because of differences in albumin binding in dogs and cats *vs* humans, animals require one-quarter the dose of detemir compared with humans.

The primary difference between insulin designed for use in animals (PZI, lente) and for humans (glargine, NPH, detemir) is the insulin concentration; U-40 insulin is available for PZI and lente insulin, however, NPH, glargine and detemir are only available as U-100 insulin.[20] Care should be taken when using insulin syringes; U-100 syringes for U-100 insulin and U-40 syringes for U-40 insulin to prevent accidental overdose. In dogs, with conventional insulin therapy (NPH, lente,

PZI, glargine), a starting dose of 0.5 U/kg is recommended; however, detemir is dosed at 0.1–0.2 U/kg because of the aforementioned albumin binding. Most cats are readily managed on 2 units twice daily as a starting dose. If intermediate-acting insulin is used, it must be administered twice daily because of the short duration of action in cats. If PZI insulin is used, a dosage of 1–3 units per cat is often recommended as once-daily therapy. Glargine (Lantus insulin) should be used cautiously in the cat to avoid hypoglycemia. A dosage of 1–2 units twice daily is recommended along with careful blood or urine monitoring to avoid hypoglycemic episodes.

The site of insulin injection should be discussed with the pet owner. Absorption of insulin from various injection sites in the body may differ. In animals, the back of the neck or scruff has commonly been used as a site for insulin injection. However, this site has several disadvantages because of lack of blood flow and increased fibrosis caused by repeated injections at this site. The author recommends administration of insulin at sites along the lateral abdomen and thorax. The owner should rotate the site of injection each day.

Treatment of Diabetic Ketoacidosis in Animals

Treatment of diabetic ketoacidosis (DKA) includes the following steps in order of importance: (i) fluid therapy initially using shock doses of 0.9% saline; (ii) short-acting insulin therapy (low-dose intramuscular or intravenous); (iii) electrolyte supplementation (potassium chloride and/or potassium phosphate); (iv) reversal of metabolic acidosis.[25,26]

Fluid therapy should consist of 0.9% NaCl supplemented with potassium when insulin therapy is initiated. Normal saline is the fluid of choice initially and when the blood glucose decreases to below 250 mg/dl, fluid therapy is changed to 5% or 2.5% dextrose in water and 0.45% saline

when the blood glucose falls below 250 mg/dl.[24] A large central venous catheter should be used to administer fluid therapy as animals in DKA are severely dehydrated and require rapid fluid administration. Use of hypotonic solutions is controversial in that hyperosmolality often causes idiogenic osmoles in the brain which are "trapped" when serum osmolality is decreased rapidly resulting in cerebral edema.

Insulin therapy should be initiated as soon as possible and the author prefers intravenous insulin therapy as previously described.[23] Regular insulin is mixed in a 250-ml saline bag at a dosage of 2.2 units of regular insulin/kg of body weight for dogs and 1.1 U/kg for cats. Approximately 50 ml of fluid and insulin is allowed to run through the intravenous drip set and is discarded because insulin binds to the plastic tubing. The species of regular insulin (beef, pork, or human) used does not affect response; however, the type of insulin given is very important. Regular insulin must be used; lente, ultralente, and NPH *should never be given intravenously*.

The diluted regular insulin is administered initially at a rate of 10 ml/h via an infusion pump and decreased according to the drop in serum glucose. As serum glucose decreases, the insulin fluid rate is decreased from 10 ml/h to 7 ml/h to 5 ml/h and finally shut off as blood glucose approaches the normal range (100 mg/dl). Concurrently with the decrease in serum glucose, fluid therapy is changed from normal saline to saline dextrose mixtures. When blood glucose decreases below 250 mg/dl, the fluid is changed to 2.5% dextrose and 0.45% NaCl. When the blood glucose falls below 150 mg/dl, the fluids are changed to 5% dextrose and 0.45% NaCl. Using this method, blood glucose decreases to below 250 mg/dl in approximately 10 h in dogs and in cats after about 16 h. Insulin is administered through a separate catheter than the fluids to allow for more flexible insulin administration. Once euglycemia has been achieved, the animal is maintained on subcutaneous regular insulin (0.1 U/kg, SQ q 4–6 h) until it starts to eat and/or the ketosis has resolved. Another protocol is to use low-dose intramuscular insulin at an initial dosage of 0.2 U/kg followed by hourly IM injections of 0.1 U/kg until the blood glucose concentration is < 250 mg/dl. After the blood glucose drops to < 250 mg/dl, regular insulin is administered subcutaneously every 6–8 h. The disadvantage of this protocol is that blood glucose levels may drop precipitously as depots of intramuscular insulin are absorbed from previously poorly perfused muscle tissue.

Electrolyte, specifically potassium, balance may be difficult to manage during a ketoacidotic crisis. Potassium should be supplemented as soon as insulin therapy is initiated. While serum potassium may be normal or elevated in DKA, the animal actually suffers from total body depletion of potassium. Furthermore, correction of the metabolic acidosis tends to drive potassium intracellularly in exchange for hydrogen ions. Insulin facilitates this exchange and the net effect is a dramatic decrease in serum potassium which must be attenuated with appropriate potassium supplementation in fluids. General guidelines list 40–80 meq/l as appropriate supplementation; however, as much as 100 meq/l may be required to maintain serum potassium within the normal range in some diabetic cats. Monitoring serum potassium frequently during the course of treatment of DKA is essential to avoid under- or over-supplementation of potassium and other electrolytes.

Serum and tissue phosphorus may also be depleted during a ketoacidotic crisis and some of the potassium supplementation should consist of potassium phosphate (0.01–0.03 mmol phosphate/kg h), particularly in small dogs and cats who are most susceptible to hemolysis caused by hypophosphatemia. Another cause of hemolysis in cats with DKA is Heinz body anemia. While Heinz body anemia usually does not result in overt hemolysis by itself, it probably shortens the lifespan of red blood cells and when coupled with low phosphorus levels may precipitate a hemolytic crisis.

Finally, serum pH should be addressed after administration of fluids, insulin, and potassium. Often, the first three steps will result in normalization of serum acid–base status; however, bicarbonate therapy may be necessary in some patients. Caution with bicarbonate therapy is recommended as metabolic alkalosis may be difficult to reverse.

MONITORING DIABETIC ANIMALS

Although often overlooked, clinical signs, such as polydipsia or polyuria, are the best indicators of adequate diabetic regulation.[27] Under-regulation is often manifested as continued or worsening polydipsia, polyuria, weight loss, vomiting, diarrhea, anorexia, neuropathy in cats and cataracts in dogs. Over-regulation can be detected by weight gain (as a result of the anabolic effects of insulin), progression of diabetic neuropathy or nephropathy, progression of cataracts, and signs of hypoglycemia such as weakness or coma. Body weight should remain stable or normalize with underweight animals gaining and overweight animals losing weight. Irritability or changes in personality (aggressiveness, biting) should alert the clinician to a worsening diabetic situation in a cat. Signs of ketosis include vomiting, diarrhea, weakness, and acetone odor to the breath in both dogs and cats. Hyperosmolar or mixed ketotic-hyperosmolar syndrome in cats may manifest as weakness, severe dehydration, bradycardia, hypotension, and eventually coma.

Urine glucose is a measure of trends in blood glucose, and should not be used alone to increase insulin dosage. Urine glucose monitoring may be performed at home by the owner, is not affected by stress, and may indicate insulin-induced hyperglycemia (Somogyi effect).[28] Urine glucose should decrease to trace or one plus with appropriate therapy. Consistently high urine glucose indicates the need for blood glucose evaluation.

Glucose monitors designed for home monitoring in human beings and animals are inexpensive, accurate, rapid, and require only a drop of blood.[29,30] Although reasonably accurate in the blood glucose range of 60–120 mg/dl (4–12.5 mmol/l), these glucose monitors are designed to read lower than the actual value as glucose approaches the hypoglycemic range. Factors that affect accuracy of these monitors include altitude, oxygen therapy, patient hematocrit, shock, dehydration, severe infection, and out of date or improperly stored test strips. Whole blood glucose concentrations are lower than serum glucose and the manufacturer should be consulted about the suitability of these monitors for canine patients. Recently, a veterinary glucose monitor has been developed and marketed as the Abbott AlphaTRAK. AlphaTRAK has the highest correlation to clinical laboratory sample analysis of glucose. The Bayer Ascensia Contour and the Roche Accu-Chek Advantage are both excellent human monitors, but fall short of the accuracy of the Abbott product in cats.

The ideal glucose curve has a glucose nadir (lowest blood glucose concentration on the curve) between 100 and 150 mg/dl (4–6 mmol/l). The time of the glucose nadir indicates peak insulin action. The nadir should occur approximately halfway through the dosing interval. For example, if insulin is being given every 12 h, the nadir should fall 5–6 h after the dose. The glucose differential is the difference between the glucose nadir and the blood glucose concentration prior to the next insulin dose. The glucose differential should be less than 100–150 mg/dl (5–7 mmol/l) in dogs to prevent cataract formation and between 150 and 200 mg/dl (7.5 mmol/l) in cats. The duration of insulin action is related to both the time of the glucose nadir and the absolute concentration of the glucose nadir. One can not make a determination of insulin duration unless the target glucose nadir concentration (80–120 mg/dl) has been achieved. If the glucose nadir occurs approximately halfway through the dosing interval, the duration of action of insulin should be adequate. Unfortunately, blood glucose curves are highly variable in cats and dogs and since cats are susceptible to stress-induced hyperglycemia, the response to therapy may be masked.[31] The best use of blood glucose curves in cats is to determine whether insulin is being absorbed adequately and if the insulin is lasting throughout the day (short duration of action).

Glycosylated blood proteins are indicative of mean glucose concentrations in serum over an extended period of time.[32,33] Glycated blood proteins may be used to monitor long-term insulin therapy; these proteins are particularly useful in monitoring diabetic cats that may be stressed by hospitalization and serial blood glucose curves. As plasma glucose concentrations increase, hemoglobin glycosylation increases proportionately. Serum fructosamine is formed by glycosylation of serum protein such as albumin. The concentration of fructosamine in serum is directly related to blood glucose concentration.[33] However, due to the shorter lifespan of albumin compared with hemoglobin, fructosamine concentrations reflect more recent (1–3 weeks) changes in serum glucose concentrations. Fructosamine concentrations less than 350–450 μmol/l are associated with good to excellent diabetic control, whereas serum fructosamine of 450–500 μmol/l indicates fair to good control, serum fructosamine greater than 500 μmol/l indicates poor glycemic control. Relative changes in serum fructosamine may be more helpful than absolute values in some cases.

References

1. Nelson RW. Diabetes mellitus. In: Ettinger SJ, Feldman EC, editors. *Textbook of Veterinary Internal Medicine*. 4th ed. Philadelphia: WB Saunders; 1995.
2. Greco DS. Diagnosis of diabetes mellitus in dogs and cats. In: Behrend EN, Kemppainen RJ, editors. *Vet Clin North Am*, vol. 31. Philadelphia: WB Saunders; 2001. p. 845–53.

3. O'Brien TD, Butler PC, Westermark P, Johnson KH. Islet amyloid polypeptide: A review of its biology and potential roles in the pathogenesis of diabetes mellitus. *Vet Pathol* 1993;**30**:317−32.

4. Lutz TA, Rand JS. A review of new developments in type 2 diabetes mellitus in human beings and cats. *Brit Vet J* 1993;**149**:527−36.

5. Brennan CL, Hoenig M, Ferguson DC. GLUT4 but not GLUT1 expression decreases early in the development of feline obesity. *Dom Anim Endocrin* 2004;**26**(4): 291−301.

6. Rand Jacquie S. Canine and feline diabetes mellitus: Nature or nurture? *Journal of Nutrition* 2004;**134**: 2072S−80S.

7. Ballard FJ. Glucose utilization in mammalian liver. *Comp Biochem and Physiol* 1965;**14**:437−43.

8. Diehl KJ. Long-term complications of diabetes mellitus, Part II: Gastrointestinal and Infectious. In: Greco DS, Peterson ME, editors. *Vet Clin N Amer* 1995;**25**. p. 731−40.

9. Munana KR. Long-term complications of diabetes mellitus, Part I: Retinopathy, nephropathy, neuropathy. In: Greco DS, Peterson ME, editors. *Vet Clin N Amer* 1995;**25**. p. 715−30.

10. Haberer B, Reusch CE. Glycated haemoglobin in various pathological conditions: investigations based on a new, fully automated method. *J Sm Anim Pract* 1998;**39**:510−7.

11. Reusch CE, Liehs MR, Hoyer M, Vochezer R. Fructosamine. A new parameter for diagnosis and metabolic control in diabetic dogs and cats. *JVIM* 1993;**7**:177−82.

12. Thoresen SI, Bredal WP. Clinical usefulness of fructosamine measurements in diagnosing and monitoring feline diabetes mellitus. *J Sm Anim Pract* 1996;**37**:64−8.

13. Lutz TA, Rand JS. Fructosamine concentrations in hyperglycemic cats. *Can Vet J March* 1995;**36**(3):155−9.

14. Kitamura T, Yasuda J, Hashimoto A. Acute insulin response to intravenous arginine in nonobese healthy cats. *J Vet Intern Med* 1999;**13**(6):549−56.

15. Kettlehut IC, Foss MC, Migliorini RH. Glucose homeostasis in a carnivorous animal (cat) and in rats fed a high-protein diet. *Amer J Physiol* 1978;**239**:R115−21.

16. Mazzaferro EM, Greco DS, Turner AS, Fettman MJ. Treatment of feline diabetes mellitus with a high protein diet and acarbose. *J Fel Med Surg* 2003;**5**:183−9.

17. Bennett N, Greco DS, Peterson ME, Kirk CE, Mathes M, Fettman ME. Comparison of a low carbohydrate vs high fiber canned diet for the treatment of diabetes mellitus in cats. *J Fel Med Surg* 2006;**8**(2):73−84. Apr.

18. Ford S. NIDDM in the cat: treatment with the oral hypoglycemic medication, glipizide. Greco DS, Peterson ME, editors. *Vet Clin N Amer* 1995;**25**(3):599.

19. Nelson RW, Lynn RC, Wagner-Mann CC, Michels GM. Efficacy of protamine zinc insulin for treatment of diabetes mellitus in cats. *J Amer Vet Med Assoc* 2001;**218**:38−42.

20. Greco DS, Broussard JD, Peterson ME. Insulin therapy. *Vet Clinics of N Amer Sm Anim Pract* 1995;**25**(3):677.

21. Gilor C, Ridge TK, Attermeier KJ, Graves TK. Pharmacodynamics of insulin detemir and insulin glargine assessed by an isoglycemic clamp method in healthy cats. *J Vet Int Med* 2010;**24**(4):870−4.

22. Graham PA, Nash AS, McKellar QA. Pharmacokinetics of a porcine insulin zinc suspension in diabetic dogs. *J Sm Anim Pract* 1997;**38**:434−8.

23. Fleeman LM, Rand JS. Management of canine diabetes. In: Behrend EN, Kemppainen RJ, editors. *Vet Clin North Am*, vol. 31. Philadelphia: WB Saunders Co; 2001. p. 855−80.

24. Rand JS, Martin GJ. Management of feline diabetes mellitus. In: Behrend EN, Kemppainen RJ, editors. *Vet Clin North Am*, vol. 31. Philadelphia: WB Saunders Co; 2001. p. 881−913.

25. Macintire DK. Treatment of diabetic ketoacidosis in dogs by continuous low-dose intravenous infusion of insulin. *J Amer Vet Med Assoc* 1993;**202**:1266−72.

26. MacIntyre, DK. Emergency therapy of diabetic crises: insulin overdose, diabetic ketoacidosis and hyperosmolar coma. Greco DS, Peterson ME, editors. *Vet Clin N Amer* 1995;**25**(3)639−50.

27. Briggs CE, Nelson RW, Feldman EC, Elliott DA, Neal LA. Reliability of history and physical examination findings for assessing control of glycemia in dogs with diabetes mellitus: 53 cases (1995−1998). *J Amer Vet Med Assoc* 2000;**217**:48−53.

28. Schaer M. A justification for urine glucose monitoring in the diabetic dog and cat. *J Amer Anim Hosp Assoc* 2001;**37**:311−2.

29. Wess G, Reusch C. Capillary blood sampling from the ear of dogs and cats and use of portable meters to measure glucose concentration. *J Sm Anim Pract* 2000;**41**:60−6.

30. Reusch CE, Wess G, Casella M. Home monitoring of blood glucose concentration in the management of diabetes mellitus. *Comp Cont Ed* 2001;**23**:544−56.

31. Fleeman LM, Rand JS. Evaluation of day-to-day variability in serial blood glucose concentrations in diabetic dogs. *J Amer Vet Med Assoc* 2003;**222**:317−21.

32. Elliott DA, Nelson RW, Feldman EC, Neal LA. Glycosylated hemoglobin concentration for assessment of glycemic control in diabetic cats. *J Vet Int Med* 1997;**11**:161−5.

33. Elliott DA, Nelson RW, Reusch CE, Feldman EC, Neal LA. Comparison of serum fructosamine and blood glycosylated hemoglobin concentrations for assessment of glycemic control in cats with diabetes mellitus. *J Vet Int Med* 1998;**12**:1794−8.

VII. DIABETES IN ANIMALS AND TREATMENT

CHAPTER

39

Overview of Diabetes Treatment in Animals

Erica L. Reineke

Department of Clinical Studies—Philadelphia, University of Pennsylvania School of Veterinary Medicine, Philadelphia, PA, USA

OUTLINE

INTRODUCTION

Diabetes mellitus is the most commonly encountered spontaneously occurring endocrine disease in veterinary medicine affecting many species including dogs, cats, horses, cattle, and ferrets. Historically, dogs have played a major role in our understanding of the pathophysiology and treatment of diabetes mellitus in people. The first animal model of diabetes was created in 1889 when the scientists Joseph von Mering and Oskar Minkowski realized that polyuria and polydipsia resulted when the pancreas was removed from healthy dogs. These scientists correctly concluded that the pancreas secreted an "antidiabetogenic" factor that enables the body to utilize glucose.[1] Approximately 30 years later, it was also the dog that was the first recipient of exogenous insulin, paving the way for the treatment of diabetes mellitus.[2]

Today, the incidence of spontaneously occurring diabetes mellitus in dogs is estimated to be

Nutritional and Therapeutic Interventions for Diabetes and Metabolic Syndrome
DOI: 10.1016/B978-0-12-385083-6.00039-5

499

0.0005–1.5%.[3,4] In a population of insured dogs from Sweden, the reported incidence of diabetes mellitus was 13 cases per 10,000 dog years at risk. In other words, one of 100 dogs reaching 12 years of age would develop diabetes mellitus in this country.[5] In cats, diabetes mellitus has been reported to affect about 1 in 400 cats in the US. Additionally in the US, the hospital prevalence rate of diabetes in both cats and dogs appears to be increasing over the past 30 years. This may be due in part to improvements in diagnosis and management of diabetes in addition to a rise in risk factors such as obesity and physical inactivity.[6–8]

The prevalence of diabetes mellitus in other domesticated species is unknown with only sporadic reports of its occurrence in the veterinary literature. Recently there has been increased interest in diabetes mellitus in horses which is likely due to both an increased awareness of the disease as well as an increasing population of elderly horses.[9]

TYPES OF DIABETES

In veterinary medicine, the classification of diabetes mellitus generally follows the model used in human medicine with animals classified into type 1 (insulin-dependent) and type 2 (non-insulin dependent) diabetes mellitus based on the underlying etiology. Type 1 diabetes mellitus is characterized by an absolute deficiency of insulin secretion due to T-cell mediated autoimmune destruction of pancreatic β-cells whereas type 2 diabetes is characterized by insulin resistance and progressive β-cell dysfunction.

Recently, a group of canine diabetic researchers from the UK have suggested a slightly different classification scheme based on disease pathogenesis, rather than clinical response to insulin therapy. In this system, diabetic dogs are classified into two groups: primary insulin deficiency diabetes (IDD) and primary insulin resistance diabetes (IRD). In dogs with IDD,

hyperglycemia is secondary to hypoinsulinemia whereas in IRD hyperglycemia coexists with hyperinsulinemia.[10]

The development of IDD in dogs is most commonly thought to occur secondary to T-cell-mediated autoimmune destruction of β-cells in the pancreas, a similar feature of type 1 diabetes in people. This is supported by the finding of antibodies against β-cells in 50% of newly diagnosed diabetic dogs.[11] There is also recent evidence for the presence of glutamic acid decarboxylase (GAD65) and islet antigen auto-antibodies in diabetic dogs providing additional evidence for an auto-immune etiology.[10] In contrast to people with type 1 diabetes, lymphocytic infiltration of islets is infrequently detected in dogs.[12] An extreme form of diabetes may occur in which there is a congenital absolute deficiency of β-cells and pancreatic islet hypoplasia or aplasia leading to the onset of diabetes in dogs less than 12 months of age.[13] Finally chronic pancreatitis, reported in 28–40% of diabetic dogs, may give rise to diabetes in dogs.[14] It has been proposed that the inflammatory response associated with pancreatitis may initiate β-cell damage and the subsequent release of antigens may stimulate an immune response that exacerbates islet destruction leading to diabetes mellitus.[12]

IRD, similar to type 2 diabetes mellitus in people, is uncommon to rare in the dog and is usually associated with concurrent insulin antagonistic diseases or drugs. Most commonly, IRD in the dog occurs during the diestrus phase of the reproductive cycle in female dogs and resembles gestational diabetes in people.[10] This phase of the reproductive cycle is characterized by a high concentration of circulating progesterone which antagonizes insulin function resulting in impaired glucose tolerance. Recently, gestational diabetes mellitus was reported in 13 dogs. Following parturition, diabetes resolved in nine dogs; however, four dogs continued to require long-term insulin therapy to maintain glycemic control.[15] In other reports, diabetes mellitus has resolved following ovario-hysterectomy or following discontinuation of diabetogenic drugs.[16–18] Hyperadrenocorticism, a common concurrent condition recognized in diabetic dogs, may also lead to insulin resistance and, if left untreated, cause progression to diabetes mellitus.[14] Although cause and effect has yet to be definitely established, hyperadrenocorticism was diagnosed concurrently in 22% of diabetic ketoacidotic dogs at one veterinary teaching institution.[19]

Unlike dogs, type 1 diabetes mellitus or IDD in cats appears to be rare. In a study of 26 newly diagnosed diabetic cats, none of the cats was found to have antibodies directed against β-cells or endogenous insulin.[20] In addition, lymphocytic infiltration as a marker of immune-mediated destruction has only been described in a very small number of diabetic cats.[21] Therefore, it is generally assumed that the majority of diabetic cats suffer from a form of diabetes that most closely resembles type 2 in people. This is supported by the presence of islet amyloidosis with significant loss of β-cells in the pancreatic islets, a characteristic of type 2 diabetes mellitus in people. In fact, over 90% of cats with diabetes mellitus have histologic evidence of islet amyloidosis, a similar proportion to that seen in people with type 2 diabetes mellitus.[22–24]

CLINICAL FEATURES

Diabetes typically occurs in middle-aged to older dogs with the highest prevalence between 10 and 15 years.[8,25] Certain breeds of dog appear to be predisposed to diabetes with the Miniature Schnauzer, Bichon Frise, Miniature Poodle, Samoyed, and Cairn Terrier as having an increased risk of disease suggesting a genetic component.[8] Similar to the dog, diabetic cats tend to be middle-aged to older when diagnosed with diabetes mellitus. In one recent epidemiological study, cats ≥ 7 years of age were found

to have the highest risk of developing diabetes and this risk increases with age.[6] A genetic component to diabetes mellitus has also been demonstrated in the cat in two separate studies; one out of Australia and the second out of the UK. In both of these studies, the rate of diabetes in Burmese cats was four times higher compared with domestic cats.[26–28] A similar breed predilection has not been seen in Burmese cats in the US and other breeds at risk have not been reported. Major risk factors identified for the development of diabetes mellitus in cats include: male gender, neuter status, physical inactivity, glucocorticoid and progestin administration, and obesity.[27,29] Obesity is of particular importance in the cat as obese cats are 3.9 times more likely to develop diabetes mellitus compared with cats of an optimal weight.[30]

Diabetic dogs and cats are typically presented to a veterinarian for the classical symptoms of diabetes mellitus including polyuria, polydipsia, polyphagia, and weight loss. In addition to these classic signs, a diabetic dog may be brought to a veterinarian for an inability to make it through the night without having to be let outside or having urinary accidents in the house. Sudden blindness in a dog due to cataract formation may be another reason for an owner seeking veterinary care for their diabetic pet. Although cataracts do occur in cats with diabetes mellitus they are much less severe than in dogs and typically do not cause blindness.[31]

In cats, in addition to the classic signs associated with diabetes mellitus, there may also be overt signs of diabetic neuropathy including hindlimb weakness, a decreased ability to jump, and a plantigrade posture while standing or walking. These signs are generally restricted to the pelvic limbs but can also affect the thoracic limbs. Although diabetic dogs also develop histologic nerve lesions similar to those seen in human diabetics and cats, it is rare for dogs to develop overt clinical signs of diabetic neuropathy.[32,33]

If the owner does not recognize the clinical signs associated with uncomplicated diabetes mellitus, the pet is at risk for developing life-threatening diabetic ketoacidosis (DKA) from progressive ketonemia. Clinical signs associated with DKA include lethargy, anorexia, vomiting, weakness, depression, dehydration, tachypnea, and weight loss. The risk of diabetic mellitus progressing to life-threatening DKA in companion animals is high. In the largest study to date of 127 dogs diagnosed with DKA at a veterinary teaching hospital, 65% were newly diagnosed with diabetes mellitus.[19]

DIAGNOSIS

A diagnosis of diabetes mellitus requires documentation of appropriate clinical signs (i.e. polyuria, polydipsia, polyphagia, weight loss) in addition to persistent fasting hyperglycemia and glucosuria. The blood glucose concentration can be measured in the veterinary hospital using a cage-side portable blood glucose monitoring device (PBGM) on venous or capillary blood. A urine sample (free catch voided sample or via cystocentesis) should be obtained to check for the presence of glucosuria. Urine reagent test strips (e.g., KetoDiastix; Ames Division, Miles Laboratories, Inc, Elkhart, Ind.) can also be used cage-side in the veterinary hospital allowing for rapid confirmation of diabetes mellitus in addition to evaluating for the presence or absence of ketonuria.

Normal blood glucose concentrations vary from 53 to 117 mg/dl (2.9—6.5 mmol/l) in the resting state in dogs and from 57 to 131 mg/dl (3.1—7.2 mmol/l) in cats.[34] Hyperglycemia is considered to be present when the blood glucose concentration exceeds 117 mg/dl in dogs. In cats, hyperglycemia is less well defined but is usually considered to be present when the blood glucose concentration exceeds 130 mg/dl. There is no set cut-off value established for blood glucose concentration above which the

animal is considered to be diabetic. However, mild to moderate hyperglycemia is unlikely to cause recognizable clinical signs and therefore veterinary care will not be sought by the owner until the blood glucose concentration exceeds the renal capacity for glucose reabsorption (approximately 300 mg/dl in cats, 180 mg/dl in dogs). In addition, *persistent* hyperglycemia as well as glucosuria must be documented before a diagnosis of diabetes mellitus can be established as other factors may be contributing. Documented causes of hyperglycemia and/or glucosuria in small animal patients in addition to diabetes mellitus include stress, critical illness (such as heart failure and sepsis), administration of drugs, and renal defects. In cats, stress hyperglycemia is a well-documented and frequent cause of mild to severe elevations in blood glucose. In one study of healthy cats, blood glucose measurements as high as 613 mg/dl, with and without glucosuria, were associated with struggling during venipuncture.[35] Typically, stress hyperglycemia should resolve within 90—120 min although in some hospitalized sick cats moderate hyperglycemia may be persistent. It is this author's recommendation to repeat a blood glucose measurement in 3 h to monitor for resolution or persistence of hyperglycemia when stress hyperglycemia is suspected.

Fructosamine, a product of an irreversible reaction between glucose and the amino groups of plasma proteins, reflects the mean blood glucose concentration over the preceding 1—2 weeks (*vs* 2—3 weeks in people). In a cat experimental study, fructosamine levels have been demonstrated to increase above the reference range within 3—7 days and to reach a steady state within 8—20 days depending on the degree of hyperglycemia.[36] When the serum fructosamine levels are well above the normal range (> 400 mmol/l) in a dog or cat, this test provides additional supportive evidence for the diagnosis of diabetes. Additionally, since serum fructosamine levels are not affected by sudden changes in blood glucose concentration, it can be a used to differentiate between transient stress-induced hyperglycemia and diabetes in cats.[36–39] However, it should be noted that a normal fructosamine level does not rule out a diagnosis of diabetes in an animal since normal values may be obtained when the onset of diabetes is recent or when only mild to moderate increases in blood glucose are occurring. In addition, fructosamine may also be influenced by hypoalbuminemia (< 2.5 g/dl), hyperlipidemia (triglycerides > 150 mg/dl), and concurrent hyperthyroidism (likely due to increased plasma protein turnover).[40–42] Therefore, fructosamine levels should be interpreted cautiously in animals with these concurrent conditions. Despite these limitations, fructosamine can still provide additional supporting evidence for a diagnosis of diabetes mellitus and is frequently used for evaluation of glycemic control in the longer-term management of this disease.

Measurements of plasma insulin concentrations are not routinely done to diagnose diabetes mellitus in dogs and cats. Generally, insulin concentrations are low at the time of diagnosis and are not predictive of whether diabetic remission (in cats) will be possible.

Once a diagnosis of diabetes mellitus has been established, a thorough clinicopathologic evaluation is recommended to evaluate for other concurrent conditions. Concurrent diseases, such as pancreatitis, may be present which may worsen insulin resistance and hinder successful disease treatment. The minimum laboratory evaluation that is recommended for the newly diagnosed diabetic animal includes a complete blood count, serum biochemical panel, and urinalysis with bacterial culture. A bacterial culture of the urine is recommended even in animals with an unremarkable urine sediment. Additionally, a blood measurement of pancreatic lipase immunoreactivity (PLI) in both dogs and cats should be considered as pancreatitis is a common concurrent

disease in diabetic animals.[14] If available, abdominal ultrasonography can be used to further evaluate the abdominal organs for presence of disease.

THERAPY

The administration of exogenous insulin remains the mainstay of therapy for treatment of diabetes mellitus and should be initiated as soon as possible after a diagnosis is established. In people, there is a large body of evidence confirming that tight glycemic control is essential in preventing long-term complications of diabetes.[43–45] In contrast, there is no similar established benefit of tight glycemic control in veterinary patients. Therefore the goal of insulin therapy in veterinary patients is to alleviate the clinical signs of diabetes (polyuria, polydipsia) while minimizing adverse effects such as hypoglycemia rather than achieving sustained euglycemia.

Insulin

There are many different insulin products, both human (recombinant human and synthetic insulin analogs) as well as veterinary insulin preparations that are available to treat diabetes mellitus in animals. Unfortunately, no specific canine or feline insulin products are available but the development of anti-insulin antibodies appears to be low in both dogs and cats.[46,47] The one exception to this is beef-sourced insulin where approximately 50% of dogs will develop serum insulin antibodies leading to poor glycemic control. Therefore, beef-source insulin preparations are not recommended for the treatment of diabetic dogs.[48,49]

The insulin preparations available are classified according to their duration of action as short-acting, intermediate-acting, and long-acting. Short-acting insulin (100% regular crystalline insulin and the newer synthetic insulin analogs, aspart and lispro) products are generally reserved for the treatment of diabetic ketoacidosis, hyperglycemic hyperosmolar diabetes, or anorexic, ill diabetic animals. Intermediate- and long-acting insulin preparations are prescribed for the long-term management of stable diabetic animals. Insulin preparations commonly used in dogs and cats include neutral protamine Hagedorn (NPH), purified porcine zinc lente insulin (Vetsulin®/Caninsulin®, Intervet/ Schering Plough Animal Health), protamine zinc insulin (PZI) and glargine (Lantus®; Aventis Pharmaceuticals, Bridgewater, New Jersey). Mixtures of NPH with regular insulin in fixed ratios (from 10/90 to 50/50) are not currently recommended for treatment of diabetic animals.

Vetsulin® is the only FDA-approved insulin for use in both dogs and cats. This porcine-derived insulin product is identical to canine insulin and differs from feline insulin by only three amino acids. Recent studies evaluating the use of this insulin in diabetic dogs and cats have shown that it is safe and effective.[47,49–52] However, due to recent issues with quality and possible bacterial contamination, it is no longer being manufactured or sold.

PZI has been extensively used in the treatment of feline diabetes due to its longer duration of action compared with NPH. For a period of time, the use of PZI was limited due to its withdrawal from the human market and a lack of veterinary products. However, a human recombinant protamine zinc insulin product (PROZINC®, Boehringer Ingelheim Vetmedica, St Joseph, MO) was recently introduced and approved for use in feline diabetes. This insulin was evaluated in a large multicenter study of 133 diabetic cats. The results of this study indicated that 60% of cats receiving twice-daily PZI exhibited good glycemic control based on blood glucose measurements and improvement in clinical signs.[53]

Glargine, a genetically engineered insulin analog, is being increasingly used in the management of diabetic cats. In healthy cats, glargine was shown to have a long duration of action, which ranged from 12 to > 24 h and a glucose nadir occurring between 10 and 24 h.[54,55] In dogs, there is currently only one study evaluating the pharmacodynamics of glargine compared to the more commonly used insulin NPH. Glargine's duration of action was much longer at 18–24 h with a pronounced peak at 7 h compared with a 12-h duration of activity for NPH and a peak at 5 h.[56] There is limited information on the clinical use of glargine in diabetic dogs at this time and it is not typically recommended for initial therapy. See Table 39.1 for insulin types and dosing recommendations for dogs and cats.

Insulin therapy is typically initiated at 0.25 U/kg subcutaneously in both dogs and cats twice daily. In dogs, the duration of action of both lente and NPH insulin has been found to be between 10 and 14 h and twice-a-day insulin therapy is effective in controlling blood glucose concentrations.[57,58] Ideally, insulin is administered concurrently with meals. However, since most cats are fed *ad libitum*, insulin is given every 12 h at times that are suitable to the owner's schedule.

During initiation of insulin therapy, hospitalization to monitor blood glucose concentrations every 3–4 h is typically recommended to monitor for the development of hypoglycemia. If hypoglycemia is detected, the insulin dose should be lowered. Conversely, the insulin dose should not be adjusted if blood glucose concentration remains high because it can take several days for full insulin action to develop. Initiation of insulin therapy may also be done on an outpatient basis with the owner educated to monitor for signs of hypoglycemia at home.

Oral Hypoglycemic Agents

Oral hypoglycemic agents are primarily used in the treatment of type 2 diabetes (non-insulin dependent) and therefore have limited use in the treatment of diabetic dogs. In contrast, oral

TABLE 39.1   Insulin Types and Initial Dose Recommendations

Insulin	Concentration	Recommended initial dose	
		Dog	Cat
NPH	100 units/ml	0.25–0.5 U/kg every 12 h	1 unit/cat every 12 h
Porcine Zinc (Lente)*	40 units/ml	0.5 U/kg every 12 h	1–2 U/cat or 0.25–0.5 U/kg every 12 h**
PZIR	40 units/ml	Not recommended	0.22–0.66 U/kg every 12 h or 1–3 U/cat every 12 h
Glargine	100 units/ml	Not currently recommended***	0.25–0.5 U/kg every 12–24 h

*Currently unavailable.

**A recommended starting dose is 0.25 U/kg twice daily if the blood glucose concentration is between 216 and 342 mg/dl, and 0.5 U/kg twice daily if the blood glucose concentration is > 360 mg/dl. Alternatively, a dose of 1 U/cat twice daily for cats weighing less than 4 kg and 1.5–2.0 U/cat twice daily for cats weighing > 4 kg can be used to initiate therapy.

***Only one study evaluating the effect of glargine in diabetic dogs currently exists in the veterinary literature. These dogs were given glargine (0.05–0.1 U/kg) concurrently with NPH insulin.[56]

hypoglycemic agents should be theoretically useful in the treatment of cats with diabetes since most cats suffer from type 2 diabetes mellitus. These drugs work by stimulating pancreatic insulin secretion, enhancing tissue sensitivity to insulin, or slowing postprandial intestinal glucose absorption.

Glipizide, in the sulfonylurea class of drugs, stimulates insulin secretion from β-cells and is the most commonly used oral hypoglycemic agent in diabetic cats. This drug is only successful in about 30% of diabetic cats and may have the unfortunate complication of accelerating β-cell loss.[59] Therefore, glipizide is not generally recommended in the standard treatment of diabetic cats. Its use may be considered in a situation where insulin administration is not possible (i.e. an aggressive cat or owner unwillingness to administer insulin) if the cat is otherwise healthy and only exhibiting mild clinical signs of diabetes mellitus. Other hypoglycemic medications, such as metformin, α-glucosidase inhibitors, and chromium, have only been evaluated in a very small number of diabetic cats and therefore their routine use cannot be recommended at this time.

Dietary Management

Dietary therapy is an important component in the management of diabetes mellitus. The goal of dietary therapy should be to provide a diet that is readily consumed by the animal ensuring predictable food intake, that either corrects or prevents obesity, and that helps to minimize postprandial increases in blood glucose concentration.

In dogs, diets containing increased fiber content have the potential benefit of improving glycemic control by slowing intestinal glucose absorption.[60–62] In cats, utilization of a low-carbohydrate, high-protein diet results in better clinical control and possibly diabetic remission.[63,64] This is likely secondary to the cat's unique metabolism that is highly adapted to protein and fat with a more limited ability to metabolize carbohydrates. Unfortunately, most commercially available dry food diets contain a high percentage of carbohydrates. Prescription veterinary diets specifically with a high protein concentration have been marketed and are available for use in diabetic cats. Alternatively, commercially available canned kitten food containing higher concentrations of protein compared with adult dry food formulations can be fed to the diabetic cat.

Treatment of Concurrent Disease

Identification and treatment of concurrent disease and discontinuation of insulin antagonistic drugs (if possible) is vital to the successful treatment of a diabetic animal.[14,65] Both concurrent disease and diabetogenic drugs, such as glucocorticoids, can decrease tissue responsiveness to insulin (either through decreased number of insulin receptors, alterations in insulin binding, or impaired insulin action) resulting in insulin resistance. Any concurrent disease in the diabetic animal can contribute to insulin resistance and the animal should be evaluated for infectious, inflammatory, neoplastic, and cardiac disorders. Therefore, it is essential that a full medical history, physical examination, and a complete diagnostic evaluation be completed on all newly diagnosed diabetic dogs and cats.

DIABETIC REMISSION

Diabetic remission (or transient diabetes), which is defined as the maintenance of normoglycemia without exogenous insulin therapy, has been reported in the veterinary literature in 41—84% of cats affected with diabetes mellitus.[51,66,67] This term is generally used in cats when insulin administration can be withdrawn for at least four consecutive weeks. During this time period, normoglycemia should be achieved as well as resolution of the clinical signs of diabetes mellitus.[68] Even in cats with previous episodes of diabetic ketoacidosis suggesting

a more severe form of type 2 diabetes mellitus, diabetic remission is possible.[68,69] The reason why remission occurs in some cats is uncertain but the current hypothesis is that glycemic control with insulin may reverse glucose toxicity in the endocrine pancreas.[51,66,67]

A recent study evaluating clinical predictors of diabetic remission in 90 newly diagnosed diabetic cats found that older, obese cats were more likely to achieve diabetic remission compared with younger cats. In this study, the diabetic remission rate was 50%. However, insulin therapy had to be later resumed in 29% of cats that had achieved diabetic remission. The median length of the diabetic remission in this study was 114—151 days.[68] In a much smaller study of 24 newly diagnosed diabetic cats, blood glucose concentration at day 17 was predictive of diabetic remission. In this study, the mean blood glucose concentration was lower in cats treated with the insulin glargine compared with PZI or lente insulin and all eight cats treated with glargine achieved remission. Although small, this study suggests that better initial glycemic control with insulin glargine is more likely to result in diabetic remission.[51]

Diabetic remission in dogs is uncommon due to the underlying etiology more closely resembling type 1 diabetes mellitus in people. However, transient diabetes when reported in dogs is usually associated with progestins (intact females) and administration of diabetogenic drugs, such as glucocorticoids. Diabetes in these cases has resolved following ovariohysterectomy or cessation of drug therapy.[16–18] As previously mentioned, resolution of gestational diabetes has also been reported in dogs.[15,70]

MONITORING OF GLYCEMIC CONTROL

The goal of insulin therapy is to maintain a blood glucose concentration between 80 mg/dl and 250 mg/dl (in cats, up to

300 mg/dl is also considered acceptable). At this time, the benefit of intensive insulin therapy to maintain euglycemia has not been evaluated in dogs, although there is some evidence (as stated above) that better initial glycemic control in cats may improve the chance for diabetic remission.[51] However, the risk of hypoglycemia must be carefully considered when managing diabetic pets, as most owners are not capable or willing to monitor blood glucose concentrations at home. The assessment of adequate glycemic control can be made by owner observation of improvement in clinical signs in addition to periodic evaluations by a veterinarian for blood glucose monitoring and serum fructosamine concentrations.

A normal physical examination, stable body weight and owner reports of improvement of clinical signs are generally supportive of adequate glycemic control. A serum fructosamine concentration can provide additional evidence of glycemic control over the preceding 2–3 weeks. A fructosamine level that is significantly below the lower end of normal should alert the veterinarian to possible episodes of hypoglycemia while fructosamine levels that are significantly high (> 600 μmol/l) may indicate a serious lack of glycemic control. Fructosamine levels are always evaluated concurrently with physical exam findings and clinical signs and should not be used as the sole test of glycemic control.

Urine glucose and ketone monitoring at home are recommended for diabetic pets, especially in animals with recurrent ketosis or hypoglycemia. A daily adjustment of insulin by the owner based on urine glucose measurements is not recommended by this author. However, urine glucose monitoring can be helpful to screen for life-threatening hypoglycemia, especially when the urine is persistently negative for glucose.

Blood glucose curves are recommended whenever an adjustment to insulin is being made and may need to be done frequently during the initial regulation of the diabetic patient. Blood glucose curves are generated over a 12- or 24-h period. Generally, the dog or cat is dropped off at the hospital 1 h after insulin is administered by the owner. Blood glucose concentrations are measured every 1–2 h throughout the day allowing for the identification of a peak and nadir insulin effect as well as the duration of action. Blood glucose curves can also help to identify whether severe fluctuations in blood glucose concentrations are occurring. Continuous glucose monitoring devices that allow for non-invasive interstitial glucose measurements are also being used with increasing frequency in veterinary patients to assess glycemic control both in the hospital setting and at home.[71–75]

PROGNOSIS

Treatment of companion animals with diabetes mellitus requires commitment by the pet owner (financial as well as emotional) and complications are possible. Reported complications of diabetes mellitus include blindness from cataract formation (uncommon in cats), pancreatitis, recurring infections, hypoglycemia, and ketoacidosis. In one study of diabetic dogs, it was found that most do not live beyond 5 years from the time of diagnosis with a mean survival time of 2–3 years.[5] In a study of 104 diabetic cats, 50% were dead within 17 months of diagnosis of diabetes mellitus.[76] However, reporting actual survival times is problematic in veterinary medicine as euthanasia (rather than natural death) may be chosen by the pet owner for reasons that may be related or unrelated to diabetes mellitus.

DIABETES IN HORSES

Diabetes in horses, resulting from primary insulin deficiency, is reported infrequently in the veterinary literature.[77,78] Type 2 diabetes, or non-insulin dependent diabetes is considered to be the more common form and is reported most commonly in elderly horses in association with pituitary pars intermedia dysfunction (PPID) or due to a slow and insidious pathogenesis.[9] Based only on 14 cases of diabetes mellitus in the literature, the mean age was 19 years (range 7–30 years) with five geldings and four mares affected.[77–90]

In a recent report of three horses, type 2 diabetes mellitus with pancreatic failure was identified in all horses based on low insulin sensitivity and low to no discernible pancreatic β-cell response to exogenous glucose. One horse was found to have concurrent PPID, based on an increased plasma concentration of ACTH, and this was likely the underlying reason for the insulin resistance. In the other two horses, no concurrent disease was identified.[9]

Horses, just like other species, exhibit the classic clinical signs of diabetes including weight loss, polyuria, and polydipsia, with occasional reports of polyphagia, depression, and exercise intolerance. Currently, there is no recommended standard treatment of diabetes in horses. In the most recent report of the three diabetic horses mentioned previously, the two horses without concurrent PPID were initially treated with the oral hypoglycemic agent, metformin (15 mg/kg PO every 12 h). Following 22 days of this therapy, there was no improvement in clinical signs, hyperglycemia, or serum insulin concentrations in one horse. Therefore, oral glibenclamide therapy (0.3 mg/kg PO every 12 h) was initiated in this horse along with a strict cereal-free diet. The second horse receiving metformin in this report developed clinical signs consistent with hypoglycemia 10 days after initiation of therapy. The metformin was discontinued and hyperglycemia recurred 5 days later. Metformin was re-instituted in this horse at a lower dose (7.5–9.5 mg/kg PO every 12 h) and euglycemia was achieved. This horse was also fed a high-fiber diet,

low-carbohydrate diet, and supplemented with oil or copra meal following diagnosis of diabetes mellitus.[9] In summary, when concurrent disease is present, such as PPID, treatment for diabetes in horses is directed at the underlying disorder responsible for insulin resistance. In cases where no underlying disorder is identified, oral hypoglycemic medications, dietary modifications, and exercise should be considered. However, caution should be used when prescribing oral hypoglycemic medications as pharmacokinetic and bioavailability studies have yet to be performed in the horse.[91]

References

1. Von Mering J, Minkowski O. Diabetes mellitus nach pancreas extirpation. *Arch Exp Pathol Pharmakol* 1890;**26**:371–81.
2. Banting FG, Best CH, Collip JP, Campbell WR, Fletcher AA. Pancreatic extracts in the treatment of diabetes mellitus. *Can Med Assoc J* 1922;**12**:141–6.
3. Wilkinson JS. Spontaneous diabetes mellitus. *Vet Rec* 1960;**72**:548–53.
4. Mattheeuws D, Rottiers R, Kaneko JJ, Vermeulen A. Diabetes mellitus in dogs: relationship of obesity to glucose tolerance and insulin response. *Am J Vet Res* 1984;**45**:98–103.
5. Fall T, Hamlin HH, Hedhammar A, Kampe O, Egenvall A. Diabetes mellitus in a population of 180,000 insured dogs: incidence, survival, and breed distribution. *J Vet Intern Med* 2007 Nov-Dec;**21**(6):1209–16.
6. Prahl A, Guptill L, Glickman NW, Tetrick M, Glickman LT. Time trends and risk factors for diabetes mellitus in cats presented to veterinary teaching hospitals. *J Feline Med Surg* 2007 Oct;**9**(5):351–8.
7. Panciera DL, Thomas CB, Eicker SW, Atkins CE. Epizootiologic patterns of diabetes mellitus in cats: 333 cases (1980–1986). *J Am Vet Med Assoc* 1990 Dec 1;**197**(11):1504–8.
8. Guptill L, Glickman L, Glickman N. Time trends and risk factors for diabetes mellitus in dogs: analysis of veterinary medical data base records (1970–1999). *Vet J* 2003 May;**165**(3):240–7.
9. Durham AE, Hughes KJ, Cottle HJ, Rendle DI, Boston RC. Type 2 diabetes mellitus with pancreatic beta cell dysfunction in 3 horses confirmed with minimal model analysis. *Equine Vet J* 2009 Dec;**41**(9):924–9.

10. Catchpole B, Ristic JM, Fleeman LM, Davison LJ. Canine diabetes mellitus: can old dogs teach us new tricks? *Diabetologia* 2005 Oct;**48**(10):1948—56.

11. Hoenig M, Dawe DL. A qualitative assay for beta cell antibodies. Preliminary results in dogs with diabetes mellitus. *Vet Immunol Immunopathol* 1992 May;**32**(3—4):195—203.

12. Hoenig M. Comparative aspects of diabetes mellitus in dogs and cats. *Mol Cell Endocrinol* 2002 Nov 29;**197**(1-2):221—9.

13. Brenner K, Harkin KR, Andrews GA, Kennedy G. Juvenile pancreatic atrophy in Greyhounds: 12 cases (1995-2000). *J Vet Intern Med* 2009 Jan-Feb;**23**(1):67—71.

14. Hess RS, Saunders HM, Van Winkle TJ, Ward CR. Concurrent disorders in dogs with diabetes mellitus: 221 cases (1993—1998). *J Am Vet Med Assoc* 2000 Oct 15;**217**(8):1166—73.

15. Fall T, Johansson Kreuger S, Juberget A, Bergstrom A, Hedhammar A. Gestational diabetes mellitus in 13 dogs. *J Vet Intern Med* 2008 Nov-Dec;**22**(6):1296—300.

16. Edwards DF. Transient diabetes mellitus and ketoacidosis in a dog. *J Am Vet Med Assoc* 1982 Jan 1;**180**(1):68—70.

17. Campbell KL, Latimer KS. Transient diabetes mellitus associated with prednisone therapy in a dog. *J Am Vet Med Assoc* 1984 Aug 1;**185**(3):299—301.

18. Hess RS, Ilan I. Renal abscess in a dog with transient diabetes mellitus. *J Small Anim Pract* 2003 Jan;**44**(1):13—6.

19. Hume DZ, Drobatz KJ, Hess RS. Outcome of dogs with diabetic ketoacidosis: 127 dogs (1993—2003). *J Vet Intern Med* 2006 May-Jun;**20**(3):547—55.

20. Hoenig M, Reusch C, Peterson ME. Beta cell and insulin antibodies in treated and untreated diabetic cats. *Vet Immunol Immunopathol* 2000 Nov 23;**77**(1—2):93—102.

21. Hall DG, Kelley LC, Gray ML, Glaus TM. Lymphocytic inflammation of pancreatic islets in a diabetic cat. *J Vet Diagn Invest* 1997 Jan;**9**(1):98—100.

22. Johnson KH, Hayden DW, O'Brien TD, WP. Spontaneous diabetes mellitus-islet amyloid complex in adult cats. *Am J Pathol* 1986;**125**(5):416—9.

23. Yano BL, Hayden DW, Johnson KH. Feline insular amyloid: association with diabetes mellitus. *Vet Pathol* 1981 Sep;**18**(5):621—7.

24. O'Brien TD, Butler PC, Westermark P, Johnson KH. Islet amyloid polypeptide: a review of its biology and potential roles in the pathogenesis of diabetes mellitus. *Vet Pathol* 1993 Jul;**30**(4):317—32.

25. Marmor M, Willeberg P, Glickman LT, Priester WA, Cypess RH, Hurvitz AI. Epizootiologic patterns of diabetes mellitus in dogs. *Am J Vet Res* 1982 Mar;**43**(3):465—70.

26. Rand JS, Bobbermien LM, Hendrikz JK, Copland M. Over representation of Burmese cats with diabetes mellitus. *Aust Vet J* 1997 Jun;**75**(6):402—5.

27. McCann TM, Simpson KE, Shaw DJ, Butt JA, Gunn-Moore DA. Feline diabetes mellitus in the UK: the prevalence within an insured cat population and a questionnaire-based putative risk factor analysis. *J Feline Med Surg* 2007 Aug;**9**(4):289—99.

28. Lederer R, Rand JS, Jonsson NN, Hughes IP, Morton JM. Frequency of feline diabetes mellitus and breed predisposition in domestic cats in Australia. *Vet J* 2009 Feb;**179**(2):254—8.

29. Slingerland LI, Fazilova VV, Plantinga EA, Kooistra HS, Beynen AC. Indoor confinement and physical inactivity rather than the proportion of dry food are risk factors in the development of feline type 2 diabetes mellitus. *Vet J* 2009 Feb;**179**(2):247—53.

30. Scarlett JM, Donoghue S. Associations between body condition and disease in cats. *J Am Vet Med Assoc* 1998 Jun 1;**212**(11):1725—31.

31. Williams DL, Heath MF. Prevalence of feline cataract: results of a cross-sectional study of 2000 normal animals, 50 cats with diabetes and one hundred cats following dehydrational crises. *Vet Ophthalmol* 2006 Sep-Oct;**9**(5):341—9.

32. Mizisin AP, Nelson RW, Sturges BK, Vernau KM, Lecouteur RA, Williams DC, et al. Comparable myelinated nerve pathology in feline and human diabetes mellitus. *Acta Neuropathol* 2007 Apr;**113**(4):431—42.

33. Estrella JS, Nelson RN, Sturges BK, Vernau KM, Williams DC, LeCouteur RA, et al. Endoneurial microvascular pathology in feline diabetic neuropathy. *Microvasc Res* 2008 Apr;**75**(3):403—10.

34. Willard MD, Tvedten H, Turnwald GH. *Small animal clinical diagnosis by laboratory methods*. 3rd ed. Philadelphia, PA: W.B. Saunders; 1999.

35. Rand JS, Kinnaird E, Baglioni A, Blackshaw J, Priest J. Acute stress hyperglycemia in cats is associated with struggling and increased concentrations of lactate and norepinephrine. *J Vet Intern Med* 2002 Mar-Apr;**16**(2):123—32.

36. Link KR, Rand JS. Changes in blood glucose concentration are associated with relatively rapid changes in circulating fructosamine concentrations in cats. *J Feline Med Surg* 2008 Dec;**10**(6):583—92.

37. Reusch CE, Liehs MR, Hoyer M, Vochezer R. Fructosamine. A new parameter for diagnosis and metabolic control in diabetic dogs and cats. *J Vet Intern Med* 1993 May-Jun;**7**(3):177—82.

38. Plier ML, Grindem CB, MacWilliams PS, Stevens JB. Serum fructosamine concentration in nondiabetic and diabetic cats. *Vet Clin Pathol* 1998;**27**(2):34—9.

39. Lutz TA, Rand JS, Ryan E. Fructosamine concentrations in hyperglycemic cats. *Can Vet J* 1995 Mar;**36**(3):155–9.

40. Reusch CE, Tomsa K. Serum fructosamine concentration in cats with overt hyperthyroidism. *J Am Vet Med Assoc* 1999 Nov 1;**215**(9):1297–300.

41. Reusch CE, Haberer B. Evaluation of fructosamine in dogs and cats with hypo- or hyperproteinaemia, azotaemia, hyperlipidaemia and hyperbilirubinaemia. *Vet Rec* 2001 Mar 24;**148**(12):370–6.

42. Graham PA, Mooney CT, Murray M. Serum fructosamine concentrations in hyperthyroid cats. *Res Vet Sci* 1999 Oct;**67**(2):171–5.

43. Nathan DM, Cleary PA, Backlund JY, et al. Intensive diabetes treatment and cardiovascular disease in patients with type 1 diabetes. *N Engl J Med* 2005;**353**:2643–53.

44. Tkac I. Effect of intensive glycemic control on cardiovascular outcomes and all-cause mortality in type 2 diabetes: Overview and metaanalysis of five trials. *Diabetes Res Clin Pract* 2009 Dec;**86**(Suppl. 1):S57–62.

45. Akalin S, Berntorp K, Ceriello A, Das AK, Kilpatrick ES, Koblik T, et al. Intensive glucose therapy and clinical implications of recent data: a consensus statement from the Global Task Force on Glycaemic Control. *Int J Clin Pract* 2009 Oct;**63**(10):1421–5.

46. Davison LJ, Ristic JM, Herrtage ME, Ramsey IK, Catchpole B. Anti-insulin antibodies in dogs with naturally occurring diabetes mellitus. *Vet Immunol Immunopathol* 2003 Jan 10;**91**(1):53–60.

47. Martin GJ, Rand JS. Pharmacology of a 40 IU/ml porcine lente insulin preparation in diabetic cats: findings during the first week and after 5 or 9 weeks of therapy. *J Feline Med Surg* 2001 Mar;**3**(1):23–30.

48. Haines DM. A re-examination of islet cell cytoplasmic antibodies in diabetic dogs. *Vet Immunol Immunopathol* 1986 Mar;**11**(3):225–33.

49. Davison LJ, Walding B, Herrtage ME, Catchpole B. Anti-insulin antibodies in diabetic dogs before and after treatment with different insulin preparations. *J Vet Intern Med* 2008 Nov-Dec;**22**(6):1317–25.

50. Martin GJ, Rand JS. Control of diabetes mellitus in cats with porcine insulin zinc suspension. *Vet Rec* 2007 Jul 21;**161**(3):88–94.

51. Marshall RD, Rand JS, Morton JM. Treatment of newly diagnosed diabetic cats with glargine insulin improves glycaemic control and results in higher probability of remission than protamine zinc and lente insulins. *J Feline Med Surg* 2009 Aug;**11**(8):683–91.

52. Fleeman LM, Rand JS, Morton JM. Pharmacokinetics and pharmacodynamics of porcine insulin zinc suspension in eight diabetic dogs. *Vet Rec* 2009 Feb 21;**164**(8):232–7.

53. Nelson RW, Henley K, Cole C. PZIR Clinical Study Group. Field safety and efficacy of protamine zinc recombinant human insulin for treatment of diabetes mellitus in cats. *J Vet Intern Med* 2009 Jul-Aug;**23**(4):787–93.

54. Gilor C, Ridge TK, Attermeier KJ, Graves TK. Pharmacodynamics of insulin detemir and insulin glargine assessed by an isoglycemic clamp method in healthy cats. *J Vet Intern Med* 2010 Jul-Aug;**24**(4):870–4.

55. Marshall RD, Rand JS, Morton JM. Insulin glargine has a long duration of effect following administration either once daily or twice daily in divided doses in healthy cats. *J Feline Med Surg* 2008 Oct;**10**(5):488–94.

56. Mori A, Sako T, Lee P, Motoike T, Iwase K, Kanaya Y, et al. Comparison of time-action profiles of insulin glargine and NPH insulin in normal and diabetic dogs. *Vet Res Commun* 2008 Oct;**32**(7):563–73.

57. Monroe WE, Laxton D, Fallin EA, Richter KP, Santen DR, Panciera DL, et al. Efficacy and safety of a purified porcine insulin zinc suspension for managing diabetes mellitus in dogs. *J Vet Intern Med* 2005 Sep-Oct;**19**(5):675–82.

58. Hess RS, Ward CR. Effect of insulin dosage on glycemic response in dogs with diabetes mellitus: 221 cases (1993–1998). *J Am Vet Med Assoc* 2000 Jan 15;**216**(2):217–21.

59. Feldman EC, Nelson RW, Feldman MS. Intensive 50-week evaluation of glipizide administration in 50 cats with previously untreated diabetes mellitus. *J Am Vet Med Assoc* 1997 Mar 15;**210**(6):772–7.

60. Nelson RW, Duesberg CA, Ford SL, Feldman EC, Davenport DJ, Kiernan C, et al. Effect of dietary insoluble fiber on control of glycemia in dogs with naturally acquired diabetes mellitus. *J Am Vet Med Assoc* 1998 Feb 1;**212**(3):380–6.

61. Graham PA, Maskell IE, Nash AS. Canned high fiber diet and postprandial glycemia in dogs with naturally occurring diabetes mellitus. *J Nutr* 1994 Dec;**124**(Suppl. 12):2712S–5S.

62. Graham PA, Maskell E, Rawlings JM, Nash AS, Markwell PJ. Influence of a high fibre diet on glycaemic control and quality of life in dogs with diabetes mellitus. *J Small Anim Pract* 2002 Feb;**43**(2):67–73.

63. Mazzaferro EM, Greco DS, Turner AS, Fettman MJ. Treatment of feline diabetes mellitus using an alpha-glucosidase inhibitor and a low-carbohydrate diet. *J Feline Med Surg* 2003 Jun;**5**(3):183–9.

64. Hall TD, Mahony O, Rozanski EA, Freeman LM. Effects of diet on glucose control in cats with diabetes mellitus treated with twice daily insulin glargine. *J Feline Med Surg* 2009 Feb;**11**(2):125–30.

65. Peikes H, Morris DO, Hess RS. Dermatologic disorders in dogs with diabetes mellitus: 45 cases (1986–2000). *J Am Vet Med Assoc* 2001 Jul 15;**219**(2): 203–8.

66. Nelson RW, Griffey SM, Feldman EC, Ford SL. Transient clinical diabetes mellitus in cats: 10 cases (1989–1991). *J Vet Intern Med* 1999 Jan-Feb;**13**(1): 28–35.

67. Alt N, Kley S, Tschuor F, Zapf J, Reusch CE. Evaluation of IGF-1 levels in cats with transient and permanent diabetes mellitus. *Res Vet Sci* 2007 Dec;**83**(3):331–5.

68. Zini E, Hafner M, Osto M, Franchini M, Ackermann M, Lutz TA, et al. Predictors of clinical remission in cats with diabetes mellitus. *J Vet Intern Med* 2010 Nov-Dec;**24**(6):1314–21.

69. Sieber-Ruckstuhl NS, Kley S, Tschuor F, Zini E, Ohlerth S, Boretti FS, et al. Remission of diabetes mellitus in cats with diabetic ketoacidosis. *J Vet Intern Med* 2008 Nov-Dec;**22**(6):1326–32.

70. Norman EJ, Wolsky KJ, MacKay GA. Pregnancy-related diabetes mellitus in two dogs. *N Z Vet J* 2006 Dec;**54**(6):360–4.

71. Moretti S, Zini E, Tschuor F, Reusch CE. First experiences with the continuous real-time glucose monitoring system (Guardian REAL-time CGMS) in a cat with diabetes mellitus. *Schweiz Arch Tierheilkd* 2009 Jan;**151**(1):27–30.

72. Moretti S, Tschuor F, Osto M, Franchini M, Wichert B, Ackermann M, et al. Evaluation of a novel real-time continuous glucose-monitoring system for use in cats. *J Vet Intern Med* 2010 Jan-Feb;**24**(1):120–6.

73. Reineke EL, Fletcher DJ, King LG, Drobatz KJ. Accuracy of a continuous glucose monitoring system in dogs and cats with diabetic ketoacidosis. *J Vet Emerg Crit Care (San Antonio)* 2010 Jun;**20**(3): 303–12.

74. Ristic JM, Herrtage ME, Walti-Lauger SM, Slater LA, Church DB, Davison LJ, et al. Evaluation of a continuous glucose monitoring system in cats with diabetes mellitus. *J Feline Med Surg* 2005 Jun;**7**(3):153–62.

75. Wiedmeyer CE, Johnson PJ, Cohn LA, Meadows RL. Evaluation of a continuous glucose monitoring system for use in dogs, cats, and horses. *J Am Vet Med Assoc* 2003 Oct 1;**223**(7):987–92.

76. Goossens MM, Nelson RW, Feldman EC, Griffey SM. Response to insulin treatment and survival in 104 cats with diabetes mellitus (1985–1995). *J Vet Intern Med* 1998 Jan-Feb;**12**(1):1–6.

77. Bulgin M.S., Anderson B.C. Verminous arteritis and pancreatic necrosis with diabetes mellitus in a pony. *Comp Cont Edu Pract Vet* **5**:S482–5.

78. Jeffrey JR. Diabetes mellitus secondary to chronic pancreatitis in a pony. *J Am Vet Med Assoc* 1968 Nov 1;**153**(9):1168–75.

79. Baker JR, Ritchie HE. Diabetes mellitus in the horse: a case report and review of the literature. *Equine Vet J* 1974 Jan;**6**(1):7–11.

80. Holscher MA, Linnabary RL, Netsky MG, Owen HD. Adenoma of the pars intermedia and hirsutism in a pony. *Vet Med Small Anim Clin* 1978 Sep;**73**(9):1197–200.

81. King JM, Kavanaugh JF, Bentinck-Smith J. Diabetes mellitus with pituitary neoplasms in a horse and a dog. *Cornell Vet* 1962 Jan;**52**:133–45.

82. Loeb WF, Capen CC, Johnson LE. Adenomas of the pars intermedia associated with hyperglycemia and glycosuria in two horses. *Cornell Vet* 1966 Oct;**56**(4):623–39.

83. McCoy DJ. Diabetes mellitus associated with bilateral granulosa cell tumors in a mare. *J Am Vet Med Assoc* 1986 Apr 1;**188**(7):733–5.

84. Muylle E, van den Hende C, Deprez P, Nuytten J, Oyaert W. Non-insulin dependent diabetes mellitus in a horse. *Equine Vet J* 1986 Mar;**18**(2):145–6.

85. Munoz MC, Doreste F, Ferrer O, Gonzalez J, Montoya JA. Pergolide treatment for Cushing's syndrome in a horse. *Vet Rec* 1996 Jul 13;**139**(2):41–3.

86. Firshman AM, Valberg SJ. Factors affecting clinical assessment of insulin sensitivity in horses. *Equine Vet J* 2007 Nov;**39**(6):567–75.

87. Johnson PJ, Scotty NC, Wiedmeyer C, Messer NT, Kreeger JM. Diabetes mellitus in a domesticated Spanish mustang. *J Am Vet Med Assoc* 2005 Feb 15;**226**(4):584–8, 542.

88. van der Kolk JH, Rijnen KE, Rey F, de Graaf-Roelfsema E, Grinwis GC, Wijnberg ID. Evaluation of glucose metabolism in three horses with lower motor neuron degeneration. *Am J Vet Res* 2005 Feb;**66**(2):271–6.

89. Tasker JB, Whiteman CE, Martin BR. Diabetes mellitus in the horse. *J Am Vet Med Assoc* 1966;**149**:393–9.

90. Ruoff WW, Baker DC, Morgan SJ, Abbitt B. Type II diabetes mellitus in a horse. *Equine Vet J* 1986 Mar;**18**(2):143–4.

91. Menzies-Gow N. Diabetes in the horse: a condition of increasing clinical awareness for differential diagnosis and interpretation of tests. *Equine Vet J* 2009 Dec;**41**(9): 841–3.

Living with Diabetes: A Running Commentary

Debasis Bagchi [1], *Nair Sreejayan* [2]

[1] University of Houston College of Pharmacy, Houston, TX [2] University of Wyoming, School of Pharmacy, Laramie, WY, USA

Diabetes is a chronic disease.[1] The body's main fuel is a form of sugar called glucose, which is derived from the food we consume. To appropriately utilize glucose, the body produces a hormone called insulin, which is produced by the pancreas. Insulin facilitates glucose transport from the bloodstream to the cells where it produces energy. Diabetes is a compromised condition of elevated levels of blood sugar as a consequence of inadequate insulin and/or the body's resistance to insulin. Basically, diabetes is associated with an impaired glucose cycle, altering metabolism.[1-3]

As discussed extensively in this book, there are mainly two types of diabetes (1) type 1 and (2) type 2 diabetes. Furthermore, it is important to note that *Gestational Diabetes Mellitus* (GDM) occurs in 2−5% of pregnant women as a result of relatively insufficient insulin production and responsiveness and is similar to type 2 diabetes. GDM will either disappear or improve after delivery.[4]

Type 1 diabetes is an autoimmune disorder characterized by the loss of pancreatic beta cells. Consequently the body either stops producing insulin or produces very little insulin. Under this circumstance, glucose cannot get into the cells and remain in the blood causing hyperglycemia or high blood sugar. Most people develop type 1 diabetes before the age of 30 and it occurs equally among men and women.[4]

Type 2 diabetes is a metabolic disorder that is characterized by high blood glucose from the perspective of insulin resistance and relative insulin deficiency. Elevated blood glucose increases the risk of heart attacks including several cardiovascular complications and stroke, impairs wound healing, causes hearing and vision loss including blindness, and can lead to cognitive dysfunction, kidney failure and non-traumatic lower limb amputations.[4] Obesity is associated with 55% of type 2 diabetes cases.[4] It is worthwhile to mention that increased prevalence in childhood obesity has led to the increase in type 2 diabetes in children and adolescents. Environmental pollutants and toxins including bisphenol A, a constituent in plastics, have also been reported to increase the incidence of type 2 diabetes.

Approximately 10% of total cases of diabetes in the US comprise of type 1 diabetes, while 90% of the diabetic cases are type 2.[4]

The ideal blood glucose level [4] in humans should be

- 70–100 mg/dl before meals
- less than 140 mg/dl, 90 min after a meal
- around 140 mg/dl at bedtime.

Under normal conditions, the blood glucose level fluctuates throughout the day and is the lowest in the morning. A higher range indicates diabetes.

However, if properly managed with healthy lifestyle changes such as regular physical activity, non-smoking, low or no alcohol consumption and a healthy diet, type 2 diabetes can be managed in 82% of the cases. Decreasing consumption of saturated fats and trans-fat while replacing them with unsaturated fats may reduce the risk of diabetes.

A significant number of medicinal plants including *Allium cepa, Allium sativum, Aloe vera, Brassica juncea, Cajanus cajan, Coccinia indica, Caesalpinia bonducella, Eugenia jambolana, Ficus bengalenesis, Gymnema sylvestre, Momordica charantia L., Mucuna pruriens, Murraya koeingii, Ocimum sanctum, Pterocarpus marsupium Roxb., Swertia chirayita, Syzigium cumini, Tinospora cordifolia and Trigonella foenum graecum L.* have demonstrated varying degrees of hypoglycemic and antihyperglycemic activity in experimental and clinical antidiabetic models.[5-7] A number of phytochemicals including alkaloids, flavonoids, phenolics, and terpenoids have shown significant antidiabetic potential. Particularly, schulzeines A, B, and C, radicamines A and B, 2,5-imino-1,2,5-trideoxy-L-glucitol, beta-homofuconojirimycin, myrciacitrin IV, dehydrotrametenolic acid, corosolic acid, 4-(alpha-rhamnopyranosyl)ellagic acid, and 1,2,3,4,6-pentagalloylglucose have shown significant antidiabetic activities.[6] A database for antidiabetic plants with clinical/experimental trials has already been established.[7]

Proper nutrition, consumption of fresh fruits and green leafy vegetables and requisite antioxidants, in conjunction with regular physical exercise can modulate the incidence of type 2 diabetes. A number of treatment regimens have been discussed in this book with mechanistic insights which may help the diabetic patients.

References

1. http://www.endocrineweb.com/news/type-1-diabetes/6222-type-1-diabetes-type-2-diabetes-grow-prevalence Type 1 diabetes and type 2 diabetes grow in prevalence. [accessed 28.06.11].
2. National diabetes statistics, http://diabetes.niddk.nih.gov/dm/pubs/statistics/2011 [accessed 27.06.11].
3. One in three diabetes patients don't adhere to treatment. World News, http://www.pharmatimes.com/Article/11-06-28/One_in_three_diabetes_patients_don_t_adhere_to_treatment.aspx [accessed 28.06.11].
4. Diabetes treatment, diabetes diet, symptoms of diabetes, http://diabetesdirectory.org/ [accessed 2.05.11].
5. Grover JK, Yadav S, Vats V. Medicinal plants of India with anti-diabetic potential. *J Ethnopharmacol* 2002;**81**:81–100.
6. Jung M, Park M, Lee HC, Kang YH, Kang ES, Kim SK. Antidiabetic agents from medicinal plants. *Curr Med Chem* 2006;**13**:1203–18.
7. Singh S, Gupta SK, Sabir G, Gupta MK, Seth PK. A database for anti-diabetic plants with clinical/experimental trials. *Bioinformation* 2009;**4**:263–8.

Index

Note: Page numbers followed by f indicate figures and t indicate tables.

Color Plates

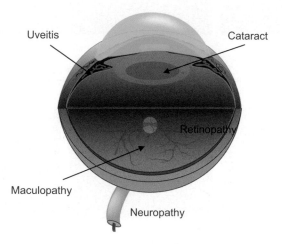

FIGURE 13.1 Ocular complications of diabetes. Ocular diabetic complications include keratitis, cataract, uveitis, retinopathy, maculopathy and ocular neuropathy. Diabetic retinopathy and maculopathy are the most important ocular complications because they lead to vision loss.

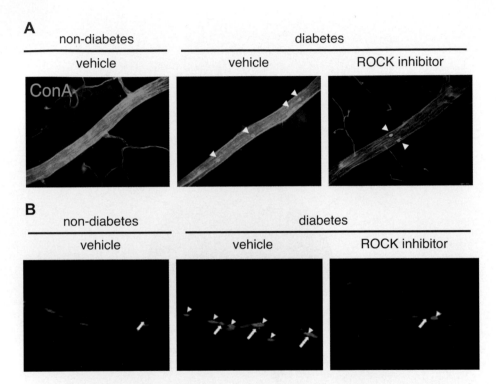

FIGURE 13.3 ROCK as a target for diabetic retinopathy. A: More leukocyte adhesion is observed in diabetic retina compared with normal retina. ROCK inhibitor fasudil blocks the leukocyte adhesion on retinal vessels. White arrowheads indicate firmly adhering leukocytes. B: Dead or injured endothelial cells [red, propidium iodide (PI)] and endothelial nuclei (blue, DAPI). Injured retinal endothelium (white arrowhead) with adherent leukocytes (white arrow) is increased in diabetic retina which is blocked by ROCK inhibitor.

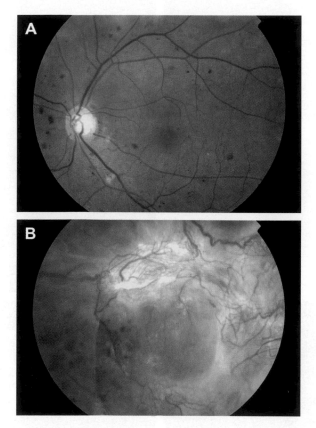

FIGURE 13.5 Clinical features of diabetic retinopathy. A: Non-proliferative diabetic retinopathy. Cardinal signs are retinal microaneurysms, hemorrhages and hard exudates. B: Proliferative diabetic retinopathy is characterized by angiogenesis and fibrovascular membranes.

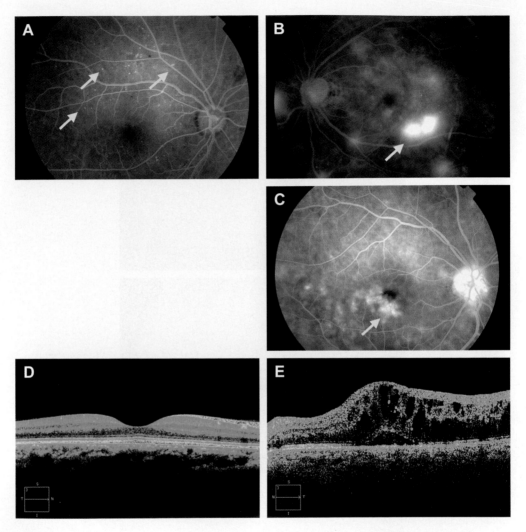

FIGURE 13.6 Imaging of diabetic retinopathy. A–C: Fluorescein retinal angiography (FA). A: FA images of non-proliferative diabetic retinopathy which is characterized by microaneurysms (arrows). B: FA images of non-proliferative diabetic retinopathy. Fluorescein leakage is angiogenesis (arrows). C: Pooling of fluorescein dye by macular edema (arrows). D, E: Optical coherence tomography (OCT). OCT images of normal retina (D) and diabetic macular edema (E).

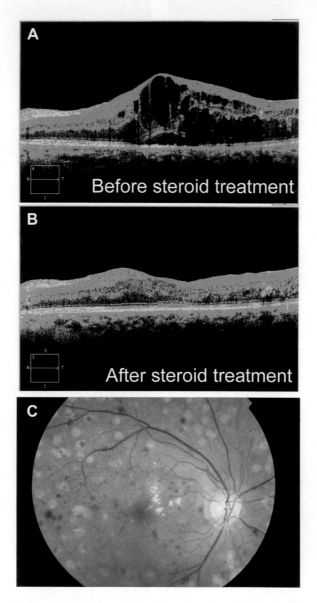

FIGURE 13.7   Therapy for diabetic retinopathy. A: Steroid therapy for diabetic macular edema. B: OCT images before and after steroid (triamcinolone acetonide) treatment. Steroid treatment resolves diabetic macular edema. OCT is a useful tool to estimate the efficiency of steroid for diabetic macular edema. B: Laser photocoagulation. Laser photocoagulation reduces retinal oxygen demand. This treatment causes regression of retinal neovascularization and reduces central macular thickening.

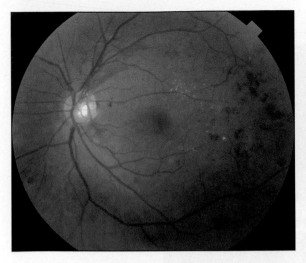

FIGURE 14.1 Proliferative diabetic retinopathy. Fundus photograph, left eye, demonstrating proliferative diabetic retinopathy with prominent neovascularization of the disc.

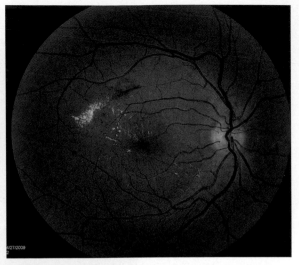

FIGURE 14.3 Diabetic macular edema. Fundus photograph, right eye, demonstrating diabetic macular edema with retinal thickening and hard exudates.

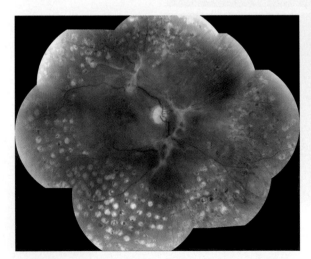

FIGURE 14.2 Panretinal photocoagulation. Montage fundus photograph, right eye, demonstrating regressed proliferative diabetic retinopathy following treatment with panretinal photocoagulation.

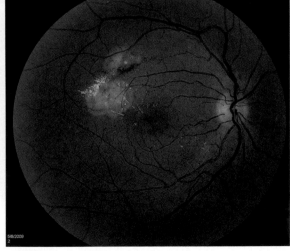

FIGURE 14.4 Focal photocoagulation. Fundus photograph, right eye, demonstrating the same patient as in Figure 14.3, immediately following focal photocoagulation of diabetic macular edema.

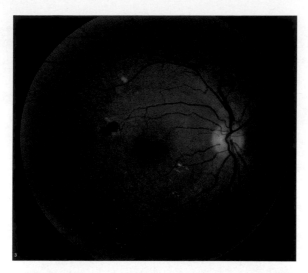

FIGURE 14.5 Focal photocoagulation. Fundus photograph, right eye, demonstrating the same patient as in Figures 14.3 and 14.4, approximately one year following focal photocoagulation of diabetic macular edema.

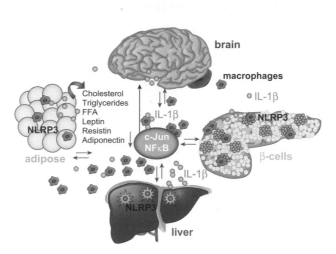

FIGURE 19.1 The inflammatory axis in metabolic diseases and interplay between macrophage-derived IL-1β and its action in adipose, brain, pancreas, and liver (from[9, 54]). Macrophages migrate into insulin-sensitive organs and produce pro-inflammatory signals, which change the cell fate. In adipose, this leads to increased production of cholesterol, triglycerides, adipokines, and cytokines. Insulin sensitivity is impaired and glucose uptake disturbed. Mediated through intracellular signaling cascades, NFκB and c-Jun and the NALP3 inflammasome are activated and insulin resistance in the liver, fat, and brain and impaired insulin secretion in the β-cells develop. Reproduced with kind permission of Springer Science & Business Media.

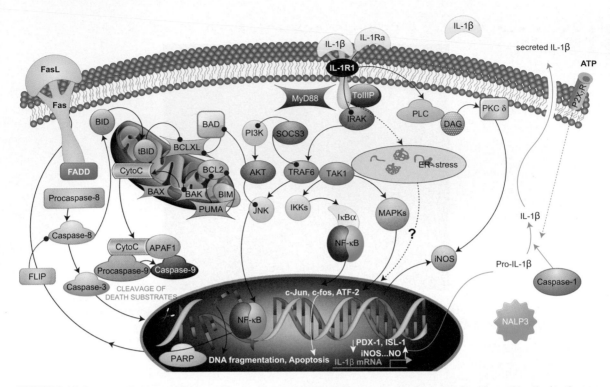

FIGURE 19.2 **Cross-linking extrinsic and intrinsic pathways by IL-1β signaling in the β-cell.** Details are described in the text.

FIGURE 19.3 **Genes and environment: IL-1β affects the transcription factors TCF7L2 and PDX1 and induces β-cell apoptosis and impaired function.** IL-1β signals in the β-cell induce JNK and inhibit AKT activation, this enhances FoxO1 translocation after phosphorylation by JNK (c-Jun N-terminal kinase). TCF7L2 levels are reduced and inhibit GLP signaling. Decreases in the pool of free *β*-catenin (and inhibition of nuclear translocation)leads to reduced TCF7L2-mediated transcription. Decreased phosphorylation and activation of GSK-3β promotes proteosomal degradation, and degradation of TCF7L2 itself. Loss of TCF7L2 leads to a decrease in GLP-1R, AKT phosphorylation is reduced and increases the activity of FoxO1 and its translocation to the nucleus, while PDX-1 is oppositely regulated and glucose-mediated insulin transcription is disturbed. Together, these effects all result in impaired insulin secretion and β-cell survival.

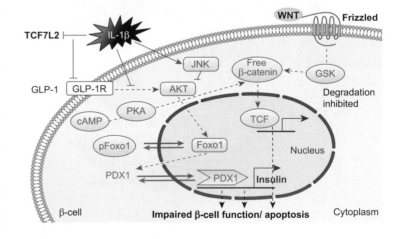

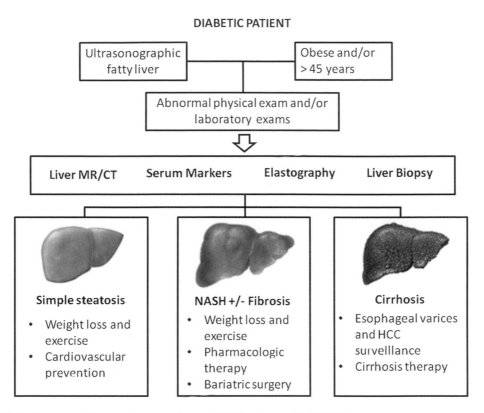

FIGURE 23.1   Suggested diagnostic approach to a T2DM patient with NAFLD.

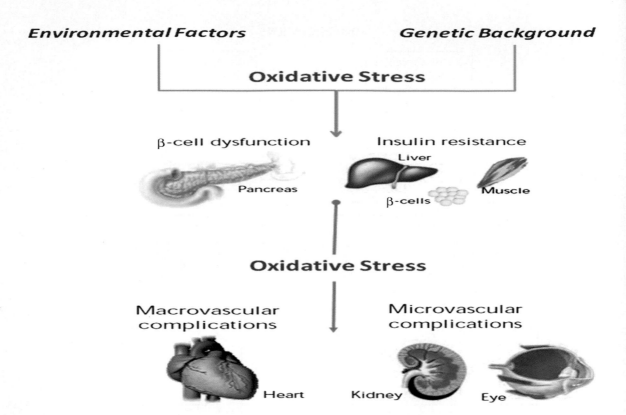

FIGURE 24.1   Oxidative stress and diabetes.

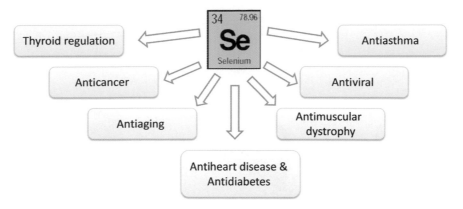

FIGURE 26.1 **Some examples of the health benefits of selenium in mammalian body.** Selenium basically detoxifies cancer-causing agents, stabilizes DNA and preserves DNA integrity, reduces cellular as well as motochondrial oxidative stress, and has antioxidant effects as selenoenzymes which have vital roles in the body.

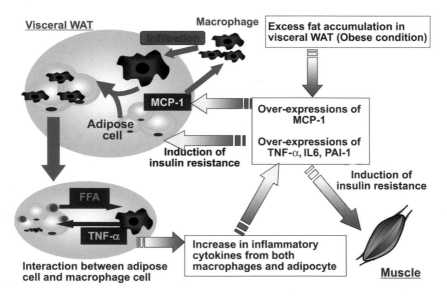

FIGURE 29.3 Involvement of inflammatory cytokines from both macrophages and adipocytes in insulin resistance.

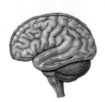
Brain
Increase satiety
GLP-1 agonists

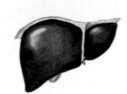
Liver
↓ *Glucose production*
Metformin
Thiazolidiones
GLP-1 agonists
DPP-4 inhibitors

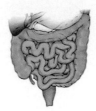
Intestin
↓ *Glucose absorption*
Alpha-glucosidase inhibitors

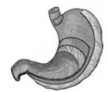
Stomach
Slow gastric emptying
GLP-1 agonists

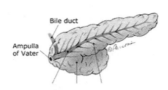
Bile duct
Ampulla of Vater
Pancreas
↑ *Insulin secretion*
Sulfonylureas
Non-sulfonylureas secretagogues
GLP-1 agonists
DPP-4 inhibitors

Adipose tissue, Muscle
↑ *Peripheral glucose uptake*
Metformin
Thiazolidiones

FIGURE 37.1 Mechanism of action of the currently available oral agents for type 2 diabetes.

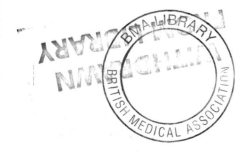